Queen Elizabeth Hospital

UH00000677

WK 270

64.50
9.10.06

D1336740

UHB TRUST LIBRARY
WITHDRAWN FROM STOCK

This book is _ _ _ _ _ on or before the last date show'

UHB TRUST LIBRARY
QUEEN ELIZABETH HOSPITAL
NUFFIELD HOUSE
EDGBASTON
BIRMINGHAM B15 2TH

Practical Management of Thyroid Cancer

Ernest L. Mazzaferri, Clive Harmer, Ujjal K. Mallick
and Pat Kendall-Taylor (Eds)

Practical Management of Thyroid Cancer

A Multidisciplinary Approach

With 121 Figures

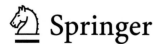 Springer

Ernest L. Mazzaferri, MD, MACP
Emeritus Professor and Chairman of Internal
Medicine, The Ohio State University,
Columbus, OH, USA
and
Professor of Medicine, University of Florida,
Gainsville, FL, USA

Ujjal K. Mallick, MS, FRCR
Northern Centre for Cancer Treatment,
Newcastle upon Tyne,UK; Vice-Chair, Thyroid
Cancer Subgroup, National Cancer Research
Institute, UK
and
Chairman, Northern Cancer Network Thyroid
Cancer Group, UK

Clive Harmer, FRCR, FRCP
Head of Thyroid Unit, Department of
Radiotherapy, Royal Marsden Hospital,
London, UK

Pat Kendall-Taylor, MD, FRCP
Emeritus Professor, Department of Medicine,
University of Newcastle upon Tyne, UK

A catalogue record for this book is available from the British Library.

Library of Congress Control Number: 2005924409

ISBN-10: 1-85233-910-1   e-ISBN: 1-84628-013-3
ISBN-13: 978-1-85233-910-4

Printed on acid-free paper

© Springer-Verlag London Limited 2006

Apart from any fair dealing for the purposes of research or private study, or criticism or review, as permitted
under the Copyright, Designs and Patents Act 1988, this publication may only be reproduced, stored or transmitted, in any form or by any means, with the prior permission in writing of the publishers, or in the case of
reprographic reproduction in accordance with the terms of licences issued by the Copyright Licensing Agency.
Enquiries concerning reproduction outside those terms should be sent to the publishers.

The use of registered names, trademarks, etc. in this publication does not imply, even in the absence of a specific
statement, that such names are exempt from the relevant laws and regulations and therefore free for general
use.

Product liability: The publisher can give no guarantee for information about drug dosage and application
thereof contained in this book. In every individual case the respective user must check its accuracy by consulting other pharmaceutical literature.

Printed in the United States of America.   (BS/EB)

9 8 7 6 5 4 3 2 1

Springer Science+Business Media
springeronline.com

Foreword

Cancer of the thyroid gland may be a less common condition than carcinoma of the breast, lung, or colon, but it occurs with sufficient frequency to constitute a major problem that is of concern to general practitioners, physicians, and particularly surgeons. Some idea of the frequency of thyroid carcinoma is given by its incidence in the United States. Every year some 26,000 patients are diagnosed there as suffering from thyroid cancer. Comparable figures apply to most countries in Europe although the incidence does vary somewhat from country to country, perhaps depending on the endogenous iodine intake. Of the 21,000 patients diagnosed annually in the United States, two thirds will be women, and some 800 will die of the disease during the year.

This book should do much to improve the outcome in the treatment of thyroid cancer. First because it is written by a small team of experts of international repute. Secondly their wide experience of the condition allows them to write with authority and thirdly they express their views in clear and commendable English.

There is no evasion of the difficulties that confront those who have to treat thyroid cancer. The condition usually declares itself by the appearance of a lump, often very small, in the patient's neck. The general practitioner who is usually the first port of call for the patient seldom has the facilities to investigate the matter further, but it is essential that he or she is familiar with the further diagnostic steps that must be taken. This knowledge brings increased interest to the general practitioner's professional life and allows him or her to support the patient on the long path the patient will have to follow in the weeks or months to come.

At last we have in this book a really authoritative, comprehensive and very readable book on a condition that all members of the medical profession are likely to encounter at some time in their professional lives. Recent advances in the availability of different radioisotopes of iodine, new techniques for the imagining of these isotopes and for the rapid measurement of thyroid hormones and thyroid autoantibodies have revolutionized the diagnosis and management of cancer of the thyroid gland. With our enhanced understanding and knowledge, the prognosis for patients with thyroid cancer has much improved and will improve even further when the knowledge contained in this book has been widely absorbed by members of the medical and nursing professions at large. To these professionals this book will be a delight because there is nowadays very little disagreement as to what is the best and most effective way to treat thyroid cancers and these ways are clearly set out in this highly commendable book.

Sir Richard Bayliss

Preface

This book is intended for practitioners who manage patients with thyroid cancer and students who are learning about the disease. It aims to provide practical information about this diverse group of tumors to physicians, surgeons, and other healthcare providers involved in the day-to-day management of patients, while supplying a sufficient depth of intellectual material to spark the interest of serious students of the disease. An admittedly audacious goal, we believe this series of concise reviews by experts in the field, laced with more than two thousand figures, tables, and references, forms a robust basis for our overall approach to thyroid cancer. A broad variety of practitioners was necessary to write this book, reflecting the multidisciplinary team required to manage our patients. The careful reader will see some diverse views among authors, reflecting the usual differences of opinion in medicine, disagreements that we should embrace because they spark the fire of debate that generates new ideas.

We thank Sir Richard Bayliss for his kind words in the foreword of this book and my fellow editors for their thoughtful ideas and contributions. We all owe a great debt of gratitude to our multinational authors who focused their cumulative expertise and vast experience to bear on the ideas expressed in this book, while showing their passion for medicine on virtually every page – and they did this by generously contributing hundreds of hours of their time.

Chapter 5 is written by Jenny Pitman, a thyroid cancer patient who shares her emotional journey with our readers, one that grips virtually every patient with this disease. This is the story of a brave lady who reached deep into her soul to find the personal strength that was necessary to deal with the news that she had cancer . . . and then she shared this strength with other patients at the Royal Marsden and with our readers. We thank her for her contributions not only to the book, but to her fellow patients. She inspires all of us.

Ernest L. Mazzaferri, MD, MACP

Contents

Section X. Aggressive Thyroid Cancers

Section XI. Future Developments and Directions for Research in Thyroid Cancer

List of Contributors

Sir Richard Bayliss, KCVO, MD, FRCP, FRCPath, FMed Sci
Lister Hospital, London, UK

Nadine R. Caron, MD, MPH, FRCS
Department of Surgery, University of British Columbia, Prince George, BC, Canada

Orlo H. Clark, MD, FACS
Department of Surgery, University of California, San Francisco, UCSF Comprehensive Cancer Center at Mt Zion Hospital, San Francisco, CA, USA

Susan E. M. Clarke, MSc, FRCP, FRCR
Department of Nuclear Medicine, Guy's and St Thomas' Hospital NHS Foundation Trust, London, UK

Mary Comiskey, MB BCh, FRCP
Northern Centre for Cancer Treatment and Marie Curie Hospice Newcastle, Newcastle upon Tyne Hospitals NHS Trust and Marie Curie Cancer Care, Newcastle upon Tyne, UK

William D. Drucker, MD
Endocrine Service, Department of Medicine, Memorial Sloan-Kettering Cancer Center, New York, NY, USA

Rossella Elisei, MD
Department of Endocrinology and Metabolism, University of Pisa, University Hospital, Pisa, Italy

James A. Fagin, MD
Division of Endocrinology and Metabolism, University of Cincinnati, Cincinnati, OH, USA

Shireen Fatemi, MD
Department of Endocrinology, Southern California Permanente Medical Group, Panorama City, CA, USA

Masud S. Haq, BSc, MBBS, MRCP
Thyroid Unit, Royal Marsden Hospital, London, UK

Clive Harmer, FRCR FRCP
Thyroid Unit, Royal Marsden Hospital, London, UK

Richard S. Houlston, MD, PhD, FRCP, FRCPath
Section of Cancer Genetics, Institute of Cancer Research, Sutton, UK

Wellington Hung, MD, PhD, FACE, FAAP, FACP
Developmental Endocrinology Branch, National Institute of Child Health and Human, Development, National Institutes of Health, Bethesda, MD, USA

Julian E. Kabala, MB ChB, MRCP, FRCR
Department of Clinical Radiology, Bristol Royal Infirmary, Bristol, UK

Pat Kendall-Taylor, MD, FRCP
Department of Medicine, University of Newcastle upon Tyne, UK

Katherine Kendell, BA, MSc
Northern Centre for Cancer Treatment, Newcastle General Hospital, Newcastle upon Tyne, UK

Sophie M. Leboulleux, MD
Department of Nuclear Medicine and
Endocrine Tumours, Institut Gustave Roussy,
Villejuif, France

Duncan Leith, MBBS
Cramlington Medical Group, Cramlington, UK

Thomas W. J. Lennard, MD, FRCS
School of Surgical and Reproductive Sciences,
The Medical School, University of Newcastle
upon Tyne, Newcastle upon Tyne, UK

Göran Lundell, MD, PhD
Department of Oncology, Karolinska
University Hospital, Stockholm, Sweden

Ujjal K. Mallick, MS, FRCR
Northern Centre for Cancer Treatment,
Newcastle General Hospital, Newcastle upon
Tyne and Northern Cancer Network Thyroid
Cancer Group, UK

Ernest L. Mazzaferri, MD, MACP
Department of Internal Medicine, The Ohio
State University, Columbus, OH and
Department of Medicine, University of
Florida, Gainesville, FL, USA

Anne Marie McNicol, BSc, MB ChB, MD,
MRCP, FRCP, FRCPath
Divison of Cancer Sciences and Molecular
Pathology, University of Glasgow, and
Department of Pathology, Royal Infirmary,
Glasgow

Geoffrey Mitchell, MBBS, FRACGP, FAChPM
School of Medicine, University of Queensland,
Brisbane, Queensland, Australia

Yuri E. Nikiforov, MD, PhD
Department of Pathology and Laboratory
Medicine, University of Cincinnati Medical
Center, Cincinnati, OH, USA

Caroline Owen-Hafiz, RGN, MSc
Department of ENT/Head and Neck Surgery,
The Regional Cancer Unit, Queen Elizabeth
Hospital, University of Birmingham NHS
Trust, Birmingham, UK

Furio Pacini, MD
Department of Internal Medicine,
Endocrinology and Metabolism, and
Biochemistry, University of Siena, Siena, Italy

Petros Perros, BSc, MBBS, MD, FRCP
Department of Endocrinology, Freeman
Hospital, Newcastle upon Tyne, UK

Aldo Pinchera, MD, FRCP
Department of Endocrinology and
Metabolism, University of Pisa, University
Hospital, Pisa, Italy

Jennifer S. Pitman
Novelist and Former Racehorse Trainer
Hungerford, UK

Sanjay Popat, BSc, MB BS, MRCP, PhD
Section of Cancer Genetics, Institute of
Cancer Research, Sutton, UK

Christoph Reiners, MD
Clinic and Policlinic for Nuclear Medicine,
University of Würzburg, Würzburg, Germany

David L. Richardson, MB BS, FRCR
Department of Radiology, Royal Victoria
Infirmary, Newcastle upon Tyne, UK

Matthew D. Ringel, MD
Divisions of Endocrinology, Oncology, and
Human Cancer Genetics, The Ohio State
University, College of Medicine, Columbus,
OH, USA

Richard J. Robbins, MD
Endocrine Service, Department of Medicine,
Memorial Sloan-Kettering Cancer Center, New
York, NY, USA

Nicholas J. Sarlis, MD, PhD, FACE, FACP
Department of Endocrine Neoplasia and
Hormonal Disorders, The University of Texas
M. D. Anderson Cancer Center, Houston, TX,
USA

Martin J. Schlumberger, MD
Department of Nuclear Medicine and
Endocrine Tumours, Institut Gustave Roussy,
Villejuif, France

Steven I. Sherman, MD
Department of Endocrine Neoplasia and
Hormonal Disorders, University of Texas
M. D. Anderson Cancer Center, Houston, TX,
USA

Carole A. Spencer, PhD, MT, FACB
Department of Medicine, University of
Southern California, Los Angeles, CA, USA

Cord Sturgeon, MD
Department of Surgery, Division of
Gastrointestinal and Endocrine Surgery,
Northwestern University Feinberg School of
Medicine, Chicago, IL, USA

Jan Tennvall, MD, PhD
Department of Oncology, Lund University
Hospital, Lund, Sweden

Douglas B. Villaret, MD, FACS
Department of Otolaryngology-Head and
Neck Surgery, University of Florida,
Gainesville, FL, USA

Louiza Vini, MD, FRCR
Department of Radiotherapy, Athens Medical
Center, Athens, Greece

Göran Wallin, MD, PhD
Department of Surgery, Karolinska University
Hospital, Stockholm, Sweden

John C. Watkinson, MSc, MS, FRCS, DLO
Department of ENT/Head and Neck and
Thyroid Surgery, Queen Elizabeth Hospital,
University Hospital Birmingham NHS Trust,
Birmingham, UK

Wilmar M. Wiersinga, MD, PhD
Department of Endocrinology and
Metabolism, Academic Medical Center,
University of Amsterdam, Amsterdam, The
Netherlands

1

An Overview of the Management of Thyroid Cancer

Ernest L. Mazzaferri

Abbreviations

ATC	Anaplastic thyroid carcinoma
DTC	Differentiated thyroid cancer
DxWBS	Diagnostic whole-body ^{131}I scan
^{18}FDG-PET	^{18}Fluorodeoxyglucose positron emission tomography
FNA	Fine-needle aspiration
FNMTC	Familial nonmedullary thyroid cancer
FTC	Follicular thyroid cancer
HAB	Heterophile antibody
HTC	Hürthle cell cancer
IMA	Immunometric assay
MTC	Medullary thyroid cancer
PTC	Papillary thyroid cancer
RET	Rearranged during transfection proto-oncogene
rhTSH	Recombinant human TSH
RIA	Radioimmunoassay
RxWBS	Posttherapy whole-body ^{131}I scan
Tg	Thyroglobulin
TgAb	Antithyroglobulin antibody
THST	Thyroid hormone suppression of TSH
THW	Thyroid hormone withdrawal
TSH	Thyrotropin

Introduction

The management of thyroid cancer has changed substantially over the past several decades, largely as a result of our expanding knowledge of this unique group of tumors and the availability of newer diagnostic and therapeutic modalities. Patients with thyroid cancer require the assistance of a diversified group of health-care providers during literally every phase of their care, from the time of diagnosis to the extended period of follow-up. This book is a statement of the breadth of the collective knowledge and skills that are required to properly assist patients with these tumors. Our goal is to summarize, in a practical way, how patients with thyroid cancer are optimally managed and how the fabric of their care is carefully woven by a group of providers with specialized skills, each of whom adds a unique part to the patient's overall care. Without this broad multidisciplinary approach, gaps may occur at every turn in management, which may pose serious obstacles to achieving the best long-term results for our patients.

While it is true that the more differentiated forms of thyroid cancer are generally characterized by an indolent course with low morbidity and mortality and are among the most curable of cancers, patients are sometimes advised that this is not a serious problem, which could not be more wrong. As a result of such advice, patients sometimes forgo long-term follow-up that is essential to their management. Moreover, this attitude trivializes the importance of the disease and certainly is not the view of any patient that I have ever seen. Chapter 4 is written by a patient who gives her poignant account of thyroid cancer from the perspective of someone who is living with it. She underscores the emotional impact that it has on a person and how she managed to cope with our medical system and the problems associated with her disease. Her chapter is near the front of the book to remind us all why we practice medicine.

Thyroid cancer comprises a group of tumors with strikingly different features. Papillary thyroid carcinoma (PTC), follicular thyroid carcinoma (FTC), and Hürthle cell carcinoma (HTC), tumors of the thyroid follicular cell often collectively referred to as differentiated thyroid cancer (DTC), have unique characteristics that become blurred when classified together as DTC. While their management is similar, important diagnostic, therapeutic, and prognostic differences exist among the three tumor types. Two other forms of thyroid cancer also pose unique problems. They are medullary thyroid carci-

noma (MTC), a tumor of the thyroid C cell that secretes calcitonin, and anaplastic thyroid carcinoma (ATC), which often arises from benign thyroid tumors or DTC. This chapter will provide a broad overview of the management of thyroid cancer, which is discussed in considerably more detail in the following chapters.

Incidence and Mortality Rates

Incidence Rates

Contemporary Rates

An estimated 122803 cases of thyroid cancer occurred around the world in the year 2000, causing an estimated 8570 deaths [1]. Yet thyroid cancer is relatively uncommon, striking only about 1.18 people per 100000 persons worldwide, with a somewhat higher incidence in Europe and North America [1]. Thyroid cancer accounted for only about 1.6% of all new cancer cases in the USA during 2003 [2], but it strikes at all ages. Its incidence rate in women is about threefold that in men, peaking in midlife in women and more than two decades later in men (Figure 1.1). In the first decade of life its incidence is the same in boys and girls.

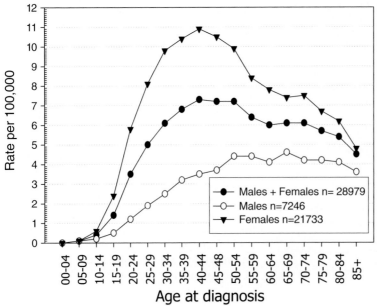

The Incidence of Thyroid Cancer According to Patient Age

Legend:
- ●— Males + Females n= 28979
- ○— Males n=7246
- ▼— Females n=21733

Figure 1.1 Age at which thyroid cancer was identified in 28979 persons in the United States between 1973 and 2001. The peak age at the time of diagnosis in women is between ages 40 and 44 years and in men between 65 and 69 years. (Figures 1.1, 1.2, and 1.4 are drawn from data in the Surveillance, Epidemiology, and End Results (SEER) Public Use Program [3], patients with thyroid cancer, single primary, and histologically confirmed.)

Figure 1.2 Annual incidence rate of thyroid cancer in 28 979 patients according to the year of diagnosis from 1973 to 2001. (From SEER Public Use Program [3].)

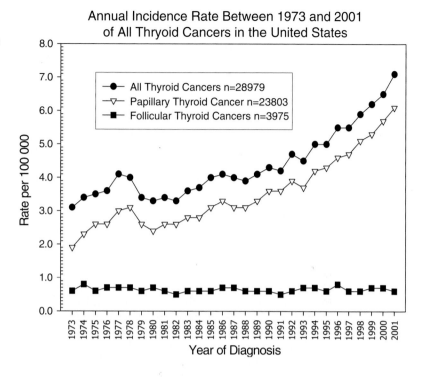

Historical Changes in Incidence Rates

The incidence rates of thyroid cancer in many places around the world have increased significantly over the past three decades [1]. Between 1973 and 2001, the rates more than doubled in the USA, going from about 3.0 to 7.0 cases per 100 000 persons ($P < 0.05$), due almost exclusively to a rise in the incidence of PTC without a concurrent change in that of FTC [3] (Figure 1.2). A study from France found a similar change in the incidence of thyroid cancer between 1978 and 1997 that was also mainly due to PTC [4]. Similar observations are reported from England [5], Canada [6], and other areas [7–10], but not in every part of the world [1]. This increased incidence of PTC has been attributed to exposure to ionizing radiation [11–13], iodine prophylaxis [10], alterations in histological diagnostic criteria of clinically unimportant thyroid neoplasia [8], and the increasingly more common discovery of asymptomatic small cancers on imaging studies, so-called "incidentalomas" because they usually have an indolent behavior [14]. Yet if incidentalomas were the only cause of the rising incidence of thyroid cancer, tumor stage should have concurrently decreased during all three decades, which did not happen in the USA [3]. Some of the increase in incidence may have been due to external beam irradiation and ^{131}I from a variety of sources [5,15,16], but this is a complex issue that requires more study.

Mortality Rates

Contemporary Mortality Rates

Ten-year thyroid cancer mortality rates in 53 856 patients treated between 1985 and 1995 in the USA were lowest for PTC and highest for ATC (Table 1.1) [17]. Yet the majority of deaths were due to PTC, simply because it comprises the vast majority of thyroid cancers (Table 1.1) [17]. Thyroid cancer death rates are higher in patients older than about 45 years at the time of diagnosis (Figure 1.3) [18,19]. Still, when categorized into low and high risk groups by the AMES (age, metastases, extension, and size) criteria, most (~60%) of the deaths due to thyroid cancer occurred in the low risk group [17].

Table 1.1 Distribution of histologic tumor types and deaths due to thyroid cancer among 53 856 patients treated between 1985 and 1995 in the USA[a]

Type of tumor	Patients (n)	Percent of all thyroid cancers	10-year relative survival	Cancer deaths (n)	Deaths due to tumor type[b] (%)
Papillary	42 686	80%	93%	2988	53%
Follicular	6 764	11%	85%	1015	18%
Hürthle	1 585	3%	76%	380	7%
Medullary	1 928	4%	75%	482	9%
Anaplastic	893	2%	14%	768	14%
Total	53 856			5633	

[a] Data from Hundahl et al.[17] Percentages rounded to nearest integer.
[b] The total number of deaths attributable to each type of thyroid cancer between 1985 and 1995.

Historical Changes in Mortality Rates

Despite the significant rise in the incidence of thyroid cancer, its mortality rates have declined almost 50% in the past three decades, mainly as the result of a fall in mortality rates for PTC that is most apparent in patients 40 years of age or older at the time of diagnosis, the group most likely to die of cancer (Figure 1.4A) [3]. Why this occurred is unknown, but may in part be due to earlier treatment of less advanced tumors in recent decades or other as yet unidentified factors. Declining mortality rates are mainly due to improvement in survival with PTC (Figure 1.4B).

There are striking differences in the incidence and mortality rates of thyroid cancer in men and women. While thyroid cancer is the most rapidly rising cause of cancer in women living in the USA [3], its mortality rates have declined over 30% in women (Figure 1.5), more than that of almost any cancer except those of the stomach and uterine cervix, and Hodgkin's disease [3]. In sharp contrast, mortality rates of

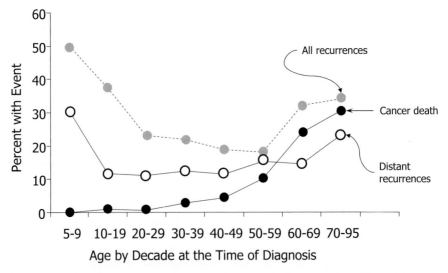

Figure 1.3 Thyroid cancer death rates and recurrence rates according to decade of age at the time of diagnosis in 1556 patients with PTC or FTC. (Drawn from the data of Mazzaferri and Jhiang [18,19].)

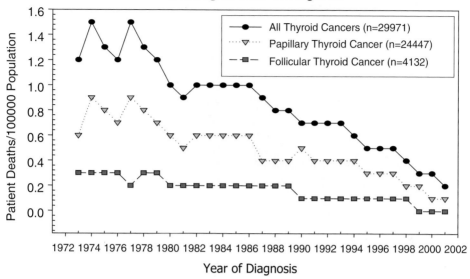

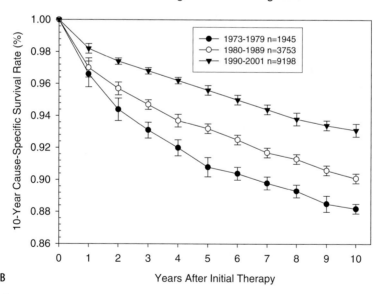

Figure 1.4 **A** Thyroid cancer death rates per 100 000 persons in the USA according to the year of diagnosis. **B** Ten-year cause-specific survival rates in patients aged 40 years and older with PTC or FTC diagnosed in years 1973 to 2001 (From SEER Public Use Program [3].)

thyroid cancer in men have risen 3.9% in the past three decades (Figure 1.5) and, over time, are twice those in women (Figure 1.6), largely because men present at an older age (Figure 1.1) with more advanced tumors than those in women (Figure 1.7), making it the most rapidly rising cause of cancer death in men in the USA [3]. This is due to late diagnosis and delayed therapy, which reflects how men utilize the healthcare system. Indeed, Leenhardt et al.

Gender Differences in Incidence and Mortality 1973 to 1996

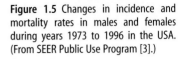

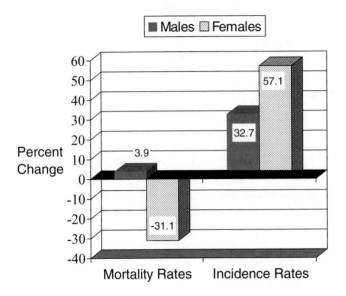

Figure 1.5 Changes in incidence and mortality rates in males and females during years 1973 to 1996 in the USA. (From SEER Public Use Program [3].)

Cause Specific Survival of Females and Males Age 40 and Older with Papillary and Follicular Thyroid Cancer

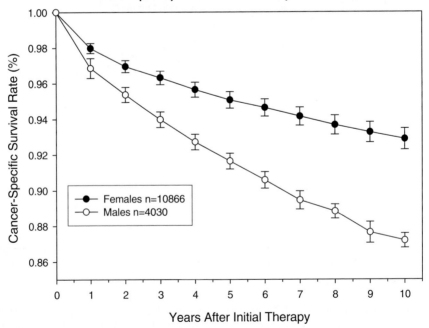

Figure 1.6 Ten-year cause-specific survival rates in men and women aged 40 years and older with PTC or FTC. (From SEER Public Use Program [3].)

Figure 1.7 Changes in tumor stage of PTC and FTC in males (dark bars) and females (light bars) diagnosed in years 1973 to 1996. (From SEER Public Use Program [3].)

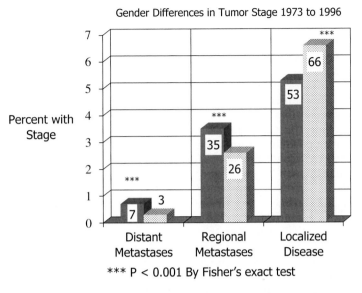

Gender Differences in Tumor Stage 1973 to 1996

Percent with Stage

*** P < 0.001 By Fisher's exact test

[14] found that the proportion of women referred for evaluation of a thyroid nodule in France has increased over the past two decades, which did not happen in men, a finding which they attributed to two factors: first, thyroid disorders are more common in women, and second, women are the main consumers of healthcare [20]. Thus there is robust evidence that the mortality rate of thyroid cancer is twice as high in men as in women because the diagnosis is delayed in men and treatment often is initiated after the tumor has spread beyond the thyroid gland.

Causes of Death from Thyroid Cancer

Because the mortality rates from thyroid cancer are low, there are few clinical descriptions of how patients die from their tumors. One study of 161 fatal cases found that respiratory insufficiency accounted for the most deaths (43%), followed by circulatory failure (15%), hemorrhage (15%), and airway obstruction (13%) [21]. Respiratory insufficiency is due to bulky pulmonary metastases that replace normal lung tissue, while massive hemorrhage and airway obstruction are due to unbridled tumor growth in the neck and mediastinum [21]. Circulatory failure is caused by compression of the vena cava by mediastinal or sternal metastases [21]. These observations provide guidance for improving survival and

the quality of life for patients with advanced tumor.

Features That Shape Prognosis

Tumor Recurrence

Depending upon the initial therapy and tumor stage, 20–30% of patients have tumor recurrences over several decades [18]. Indeed in the past when follow-up tests were less sensitive than those used today, 5% of regional recurrences and 25% of distant recurrences were found 20 years or more after initial therapy (see Chapter 20) [19]. Among our patients who had local recurrences, 74% were in cervical lymph nodes, 20% had them in thyroid remnants and 6% were in trachea or muscle, and 7% died of cancer [19]. Twenty-one percent of our patients had recurrences in distant sites, usually in the lungs, and half died of cancer. Recurrent tumor caused over half the cancer deaths in our patients. The others were due to persistent tumor that was readily apparent from the initial operative and clinical notes.

Histology and Other Tumor Features

It is important to know the key features of the tumors that collectively comprise malignant tumors of the thyroid gland. Each is unique and has its own features that may portend either a difficult and nagging problem of persistent disease, or a relatively easy and swift course that ends happily for the patient. Knowing the characteristics of the tumor and its probable clinical behavior is the first place to begin anticipating a patient's needs and long term prognosis. In Chapter 9, Dr McNicol reviews the salient pathology features that play a role in the long-term outcome of patients with thyroid cancer.

Papillary (PTC)

Tumors that arise from thyroid follicular cells secrete thyroglobulin (Tg) and tend to grow slowly and have a good prognosis [19]. However, tumor recurrences are common with PTC, ranging as high as 30% if the initial therapy is incomplete [18]. Classic PTC, the most common form of thyroid cancer, is often a mixed papillary-follicular tumor but a few have a purely papillary pattern, features that have no bearing on prognosis but may cause confusion about its pathological classification [22]. PTC is generally unencapsulated and about 2 to 3 cm in diameter and tends to infiltrate the thyroid and may extend through the capsule of the gland [23]. It invades lymphatics and blood vessels and is commonly found in multiple sites within the thyroid and in regional lymph nodes. Late in its course, lung metastases from PTC appear as diffuse bilateral pulmonary nodules on chest X-ray, whereas they are visible only by ^{131}I scans in the earliest stages. Hematogenous spread to bone, central nervous system, and other sites can also occur. The distinctive cellular features of PTC can be recognized by fine-needle aspiration (FNA) biopsy or frozen-section in over 95% of cases [24,25] and it is thus easy to identify early in its course, making it amenable to prompt therapy.

PTC Variants

Certain tumor variants digress from the classic features of PTC. The most common is follicular variant PTC, which is characterized by architectural features of FTC (malignant microfollicles) and cellular features of PTC. It may be difficult to identify by FNA or intraoperative frozen tumor sections [26] but usually has a prognosis similar to classic PTC [27–29]. Classic PTC often has a large follicular component that may be mistaken for its follicular variant, a diagnosis that requires complete involvement of the tumor with malignant follicles that have cytological features of PTC [22]. Diffuse sclerosing variant of PTC, which may be mistaken for Hashimoto's thyroiditis because it often presents as a diffuse goiter with fibrosis and positive antithyroid antibodies, is associated with some unfavorable features at presentation (large tumor and extensive lymph node metastasis) but also has a prognosis that is usually similar to that of classic PTC [30,31]. Oxyphilic (Hürthle cell) PTC may have a more aggressive course than classic PTC [32]. Tall cell [33] and columnar cell [34] PTC variants, which typically occur in older patients, usually are large tumors that are often metastatic and fail to concentrate [131]I. This tumor has a poor prognosis as does insular thyroid cancer, another subtype of thyroid cancer that may be mistaken for ATC and often fails to concentrate [131]I [31].

Follicular (FTC)

This is usually a solitary encapsulated tumor with a microfollicular pattern that is more aggressive than PTC. Patients tend to be older with tumor of more advanced stage at the time of diagnosis than those with PTC. Widely invasive FTC has a poor prognosis and is easily recognized by its aggressive extension into surrounding tissues. Up to 80% of those with such tumors develop metastases and more than 15% die of their disease within 10 years [17,18]. However, nowadays most are minimally invasive encapsulated tumors that closely resemble follicular adenomas, a diagnostic problem that also plagues Hürthle cell tumors. The distinction between low grade FTC and follicular adenoma can be only be made by review of the permanent histological sections and not by FNA or frozen section study [26], which poses a serious management predicament at the time of surgery. The main criteria that differentiate follicular adenoma from FTC are malignant cells penetrating the tumor capsule or invading blood vessels within or beyond its capsule, which has a worse prognosis than capsular penetration alone [35,36]. Still, a few patients with minimally invasive FTC die of their disease [37].

Hürthle (Oncocytic) Cell Cancer (HTC)

When most (>75%) or all of a tumor contains Hürthle cells, it is classified as HTC unless it has papillary architecture. In the past there has been some controversy about the diagnosis and management of HTC but more recent series have clarified the main issues. A large study found that the 10-year cancer mortality rate was 25% for HTC, compared with 15% for FTC [17]. Pulmonary metastases occur in 20–35% of patients with HTC, about twice the rate that occurs with FTC [38]. Diagnosis of low grade HTC requires histological study of multiple permanent surgical histopathology sections.

Anaplastic Thyroid Cancer (ATC)

Arguably the worst cancer to affect humans, ATC usually causes death within 3 to 5 months of diagnosis [39]. Survival is better with tumors that contain an admixture of anaplastic and differentiated thyroid cancer [40,41], supporting the notion that ATC often arises from benign or differentiated malignant thyroid tumors. This underscores why long delays in the recognition of more differentiated thyroid cancers is dangerous [42,43]. Treatment strategies are often ineffective and few specialists have extensive expertise in the management of this tumor. Chapter 30 by Drs Haq and Harmer and Chapter 31 by Professor Tennvall and colleagues, all experts in its management, summarize current therapy.

Medullary Thyroid Cancer (MTC)

This tumor arises from thyroid C cells that secrete calcitonin. First described in 1959 as a distinct tumor type with amyloid struma [44], its cell of origin was not recognized until 1967 when E. D. Williams in a landmark study [45] identified the parafollicular cell as the progenitor of MTC. Other investigators [46,47] shortly demonstrated that high calcitonin levels were present in both the blood and tumors of patients with MTC, which quickly led to the identification of a large number of affected kindreds [48–50]. In 1988 two groups found that a susceptibility locus for inherited MTC resides on chromosome 10 [51,52], where the responsible genes map to the pericentromeric region [53]. In 1993 several groups [54–57] proved that

mutations of a single gene on chromosome 10, the rearranged during transfection (*RET*) proto-oncogene, were responsible for the inherited forms of MTC. Up to 40% are heritable tumors transmitted as an autosomal dominant trait. Genetic testing now identifies affected kindreds and, along with analysis of tumor behavior within the kindred, allows for propitious timing of prophylactic thyroidectomy. Chapter 21 by Professor Pinchera and Dr Elisei provides explicit advice on the diagnosis and management of this difficult tumor.

Tumor Features That Influence Prognosis

Tumor Size

PTC smaller than 1 cm, termed microcarcinoma, is often found unexpectedly during surgery for benign thyroid conditions. While most pose no threat to survival and require no further surgery [58], about 20% are multifocal and as many as 60% have cervical lymph node metastases, some of which are palpable [59]. Lung metastases occur rarely, especially with multifocal tumors with cervical metastases, which are the only microcarcinomas with significant morbidity and mortality [59,60]. With these exceptions, the recurrence and cancer mortality rates are near zero [58,59]. In our series, 30-year recurrence rates with DTC smaller than 1.5 cm were less than one-third those associated with larger tumors [19]. There is a linear relationship between tumor size and cancer recurrence and mortality for both papillary and follicular carcinomas [19]. Still, management decisions for patients with these tumors are exceedingly complex, and are extensively reviewed by Drs Drucker and Robbins in Chapter 29.

Multiple Microscopic Intrathyroidal Tumors

About 20% of PTCs are found to be multicentric when the thyroid is examined routinely and up to 80% have more than one tumor if the thyroid is examined with extreme care [18]. Regarded only as intrathyroidal metastases in the past, multiple variants of the PTC/ret oncogenes in PTCs within the same thyroid are proof that many are individual tumors arising in a background of genetic or environmental susceptibility [61].

The presence of multicentric tumor cannot be predicted on the basis of clinical risk stratification [62]. They are not apparent until the final histological sections of the entire thyroid gland have been clinically studied, which has a direct bearing upon the need to surgically excise the contralateral lobe and to ablate the thyroid remnant with ^{131}I in most cases. Among patients undergoing routine completion thyroidectomy for presumed unilateral DTC, about half have tumor in the contralateral lobe [18,62,63]. Moreover, when multifocal tumor is present in the thyroid lobe first excised, or when the tumor has recurred, bilateral multifocal tumor is almost always found [64].

Patients with multiple intrathyroidal tumors have almost twice the incidence of nodal metastases [65] and three times the rate of lung and other distant metastases, and are threefold more likely to develop persistent disease than those with single tumors [66]. Thirty-year cancer mortality rates in our patients with multiple tumors were two times those of patients with a single tumor [19].

Local Tumor Invasion

About 5–10% of tumors grow directly into surrounding tissues, increasing both morbidity and mortality. Microscopic or gross tumor invasion, which can occur with both PTC and FTC [19], may involve neck muscles, blood vessels, recurrent laryngeal nerves, larynx, pharynx, and esophagus, or tumor can extend into the spinal cord and brachial plexus. The symptoms are usually hoarseness, cough, dysphagia, hemoptysis, and airway insufficiency or neurological dysfunction. Extrathyroidal tumor extension usually leads to lymph node and distant metastasis [67]. The tumor was locally invasive in 115 of our patients (8% of those with papillary and 12% of those with follicular carcinoma); 10-year recurrence rates were 1.5 times and cancer-specific death rates were five times those of patients without local tumor invasion, and nearly all with tumor invasion died within the first decade [19].

Regional Metastases

Lymph node PTC metastases occur at a higher rate than is often appreciated and are often in unpredictable sites. In one study, for example,

60% of patients with PTC had cervical lymph node metastases: one third were bilateral and almost 25% were in the contralateral paratracheal area [68]. Cervical lymph node micrometastases are often found at sites that bear little relation to the site of the thyroid tumor [69], especially in patients with microcarcinoma [70]. Lymph node metastases can be identified by detecting sentinel lymph nodes with isosulfan blue dye or other markers at the time of surgery [71]. Performing a careful neck ultrasonography before surgery also helps. In one study, for example, preoperative ultrasonography detected lymph node or soft tissue metastases in neck compartments believed to be uninvolved by physical examination in nearly 40% of the patients, thus altering the surgical procedure [72]. While some believe that regional lymph node metastases have little bearing on prognosis, most find they have an important effect on outcome. For instance, one study found that the presence of lymph node metastases increased the rate of distant metastases more than 11-fold [60]. In our long-term studies, cervical lymph node metastases, especially when they were bilateral and mediastinal, were an independent risk factor for recurrence, distant metastases, and survival [18].

Distant Metastases

About 10% of patients with PTC and up to 25% of those with FTC develop distant metastases, half of which are apparent at the time of diagnosis [73]. They occur more often (35%) with HTC than with PTC or FTC and after the age of 40 years [38]. Among 1231 patients reported in 13 studies, 49% of the metastases were to lung, 25% to bone, 15% to both lung and bone, and 10% to the central nervous system or other soft tissues [73]. The eventual outcome is influenced mainly by the patient's age, the tumor's metastatic site(s) and their ability to concentrate ^{131}I, and mere tumor bulk [74,75]. Although some patients with distant metastases survive for decades, especially younger patients, about half die within 5 years regardless of tumor histology [73]. In a study from France, survival rates with distant metastases were 53% at 5 years, 38% at 10 years, and 30% at 15 years [76]. Survival is longest with diffuse microscopic lung metastases seen only on posttreatment ^{131}I imaging and not by X-ray [76–78]. The prognosis is much worse when the metastases do not concentrate ^{131}I or appear as large lung nodules and is intermediate when the tumors are small nodules on X-ray that concentrate [131]I [74,78].

Patient Features Affecting Prognosis

Patient Age

Nearly every study shows that the patient's age at the time of diagnosis is an important prognostic variable and that thyroid carcinoma is more lethal after about age 40 years. The risk of death from cancer increases with each subsequent decade of life, dramatically rising after age 60 years (Figure 1.3). The pattern of tumor recurrence is quite different. Recurrence rates are highest (40%) at the extremes of life, before age 20 and after age 60 years (Figure 1.3) [19,73,79]. Yet despite the clear effect of age upon survival, there is disagreement about how it should be factored into the treatment plan, especially in children and young adults. Children commonly present with more advanced disease than adults and have more tumor recurrences after therapy, but their prognosis for survival is good [79]. Some believe that young age has such a favorable influence upon survival that it overshadows the prognosis predicted by the tumor characteristics [80]. The majority, however, believe that the tumor stage and histological differentiation are as important as the patient's age in determining prognosis and management [19,79,81]. In Chapter 23, Drs Sarlis and Hung provide an extensive discussion and review current management recommendations for children with thyroid cancer.

Gender

Death rates from thyroid cancer are twice as high in men as in women (Figure 1.6) [19,80]. Men with thyroid cancer thus should be regarded with special concern, especially those over age 50 years, when many present with advanced stage tumors.

Graves' Disease

Thyrotropin receptor antibodies may promote tumor growth in patients with Graves' disease. Some find thyroid carcinoma in almost half of the palpable nodules in patients with Graves' disease [82]. The tumors are larger and display aggressive behavior [82]. Some find that thyroid carcinoma occurring in patients with Graves' disease is more often invasive and metastatic to regional lymph nodes, even when the primary tumor is small [82,83].

Familial Nonmedullary Thyroid Cancer (FNMTC)

This syndrome can be clinically divided into two groups. In one, NMTC is a relatively infrequent component of a familial tumor syndrome (familial adenomatous polyposis [84] and Cowden syndrome with multiple hamartomas and breast cancer). The PTC is found in younger patients but not in infants, and is characterized by multicentric and often microscopic tumor that usually has an excellent prognosis [84].

In the other group, which comprises about 5% of all PTCs, a familial susceptibility occurs without a familial tumor syndrome. Although unequivocal evidence of FNMTC as a distinct entity awaits the identification of the susceptibility genes [85], the clinical and genetic evidence is sufficiently compelling that insight can be derived from current studies [86,87]. It has been suggested that there are three familial PTC syndromes in which PTC is the predominant clinical feature of a familial syndrome that has an autosomal dominant inheritance with partial penetrance [87]. In this instance, patients tend to have multicentric tumors that are often microcarcinomas that generally tend to be more aggressive than usual [88–90] and should be treated accordingly. First degree family members should be carefully examined for the disease. These syndromes are thoroughly discussed in Chapter 22 by Drs Popat and Houlston.

Clinical Staging Systems and Prognostic Indexes

Although the patient's age and tumor stage at the time of diagnosis are the most important variables predicting outcome, their relative importance is debated. Several clinical staging and prognostic scoring systems have been proposed that use age over 40 years as a major feature to identify risk. When more emphasis is assigned to the patient's age, the relative importance of tumor stage tends to be diminished. This concept, however, does not appear to be widely accepted among practicing physicians because young patients with low prognostic scores often have tumor recurrence. At an international consensus conference in 1987, only 5 of 160 participants treated younger patients more conservatively [91]. Similarly, in a 1988 international survey of thyroid specialists [92] and a 1996 survey of clinical members of the American Thyroid Association [93], age was not used by the majority of respondents in their therapeutic decisions. Current recommendations for the treatment of children now suggest the same therapy as is given to adults with similarly staged tumors [79]. (See Chapter 23.)

Current Diagnostic Approach

The diagnostic approach to thyroid nodules differs somewhat according to the type of physician who first sees the patient in consultation and the availability of specialist teams. This is apparent in Section II, which reviews the diagnosis of thyroid cancer in four separate chapters by Drs Perros, Mitchell and Leith, McNicol, and Wiersinga (Chapters 7–10). Each has the same general approach but with a somewhat different slant, according to the circumstances of their practice and specialty. Still, the overall approach is the same in most urban areas.

History and Physical Examination

Although most patients with thyroid nodules have no serious symptoms, a few have such a distinctive presentation that the diagnosis of thyroid cancer is obvious (Table 1.2). Patients who present with rapidly growing tumors, vocal cord paralysis, tumor that is fixed to surrounding tissues, or large multiple cervical lymph nodes are so likely to have thyroid cancer that even with a negative biopsy, the patient should undergo surgery. This is also true for familial medullary thyroid carcinoma (FMTC) syndrome, MEN2A or MEN2B syndromes or familial nonmedullary thyroid cancer [94,95], or one of the syndromes associated with nonmedullary thyroid cancer (familial adenomatous polyposis (FAP) or Gardner syndrome [96], Cowden syndrome [97]) (Table 1.2, Figure 1.8) [98]. (See Chapters 21 and 22.)

Table 1.2 Clinical findings suggesting the diagnosis of thyroid cancer in a patient with a thyroid nodule

Highly suspicious
Family history of thyroid cancer (medullary thyroid[a] cancer or nonmedullary thyroid cancer[b])
Rapid tumor growth
A nodule that is very firm or hard
Fixation of the nodule to adjacent structures
Paralysis of vocal cords
Stridor
Large regional lymph nodes
Distant metastases

Moderately suspicious
Age <20 years or >70 years
Male sex (adults)
History of head and neck irradiation
Symptoms of compression, including dysphagia, hoarseness, dyspnea, and cough

[a] Familial medullary thyroid carcinoma (FMTC) syndrome, MEN 2A or MEN2B syndromes.
[b] More than one first degree relative with nonmedullary thyroid cancer [94,95], or one of the syndromes associated with nonmedullary thyroid cancer (familial adenomatous polyposis (FAP) or Gardner syndrome [96], Cowden syndrome [97]). See Chapter 22.

Thyroid Ultrasonography

Now a mainstay in the diagnosis of thyroid nodules, ultrasonography provides a high pretest probability of cancer when certain characteristics exist in a nodule, namely a solid or partly cystic nodule with irregular and blurred margins, mixed hypoechoic isoechoic areas and microcalcifications, and intranodular vascular pattern [99]. Malignant cervical lymph nodes have a characteristic pattern, appearing round, without a hilar area and containing intranodular vascular flow. A Solbiati index (SI = ratio of largest to smallest diameter) of about one and a complex echoic pattern or irregular hyperechoic small intranodular structures and irregular diffuse intranodular blood flow are the best indicators of malignancy in a lymph node [100], which often provides information that alters the surgical approach [72]. These features are reviewed in detail in Chapter 26 by Dr Richardson.

Fine-Needle Aspiration Biopsy (FNA)

Patients with either an isolated thyroid nodule or a multinodular goiter should be considered for FNA because the incidence of thyroid cancer

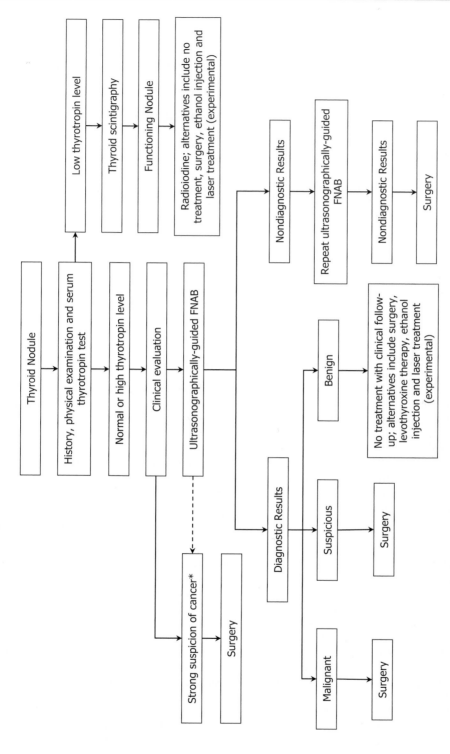

Figure 1.8 Algorithm for the cost-effective evaluation and treatment of a patient with a thyroid nodule. (From Hegedus L. Clinical practice. The thyroid nodule. N Engl J Med 2004;351(17):1764–1771. Copyright © 2004 Massachusetts Medical Society. All rights reserved.) * In the original algorithm, FNA is not suggested for patients with strong suspicion of cancer; however, in our clinic we perform this procedure even in patients we are certain have thyroid cancer.

in thyroid nodules is the same, usually between 5% and 10% in both solitary nodules and in multinodular goiters [101,102]. However, the exact rate varies, and averaged about 9% among 7724 patients in one review, which varied according to FNA technique and the selection of patients for FNA, ranging from 5% to 17% in patients with solitary thyroid nodules and from 5% to 14% in those with multiple nodules [102]. Although nodule size of 1 cm or more has been the cutoff used to identify those that require FNA, studies show that smaller nodules with suspicious features should undergo biopsy [99]. Many now perform FNA on nodules as small as 8 mm if they appear highly suspicious on ultrasonography [99].

The cytology from FNA shows one of four general characteristics: (1) insufficient material for diagnosis, (2) PTC, or (3) indeterminate cytology (follicular tumor) representing either follicular adenoma or low grade FTC, or (4) benign cytology from either a colloid nodule or thyroiditis [103]. When the cytology is insufficient for diagnosis, repeat aspiration will yield adequate material for diagnosis in about half the cases; those that do not should be surgically removed because about 5% are malignant [104,105]. In Europe, serum calcitonin measurements are often done in the course of evaluating patients with multinodular goiter [106], a practice that has not yet been fully embraced by American endocrinologists [107]. The current algorithm used for the diagnosis of thyroid nodules is shown in Figure 1.8.

Initial Therapy

In addition to the factors mentioned above, timely and appropriate treatment has an important bearing on prognosis. In this section, treatment will be considered only for differentiated tumors of follicular epithelium, PTC, FTC, and HTC. Therapy of MTC is quite different and is the subject of unique guidelines and is discussed in full in Chapter 21 [108,109]. Likewise, therapy of ATC is discussed in Chapter 30 by Drs Haq and Harmer, and in Chapter 31 by Professor Tennvall and colleagues. Current guidelines on the treatment of DTC from the United States [110] and Europe [111] advise total or near-total thyroidectomy followed by ^{131}I ablation of the

thyroid remnant for most patients. Although the treatment of children has been more controversial, many now recommend that they be treated the same as adults [79]. This is disussed in detail in Chaper 23 by Sarlis and Hung.

Delay in Therapy

The median time from the detection of the tumor to initial therapy in our patients was 4 months, but ranged from less than one month to 20 years [19]. Delay in diagnosis correlated with cancer mortality. The median delay was 18 months in patients who died of carcinoma compared with 4 months in those still living ($P < 0.001$). Cancer mortality was 4% when patients underwent initial therapy within a year and 10% in the others; 30-year cancer mortality rates in these two groups, respectively, were 6% and 13% ($P < 0.001$).

Surgery

Thyroid Surgery

Most believe that optimal initial surgery is total or near total thyroidectomy when thyroid cancer is identified preoperatively [18] and this is performed by the majority of surgeons in the USA [112]. Although some surgeons propose hemithyroidectomy for patients considered to be at low risk for cancer death [113], the recurrence rates are high in this group, including lung metastases, and there is no sensitive test to detect tumor in the follow-up evaluations of such patients [18,114]. For MTC, total thyroidectomy with removal of the posterior thyroid capsule is usually advised, especially for familial cases [108].

When hemithyroidectomy has been performed, removal of the contralateral lobe (completion thyroidectomy) is usually advised when the ipsilateral tumor is larger than 1 cm, or when it is metastatic or invades the thyroid capsule, or the patient has been exposed to radiation, or has familial or multicentric tumor [18]. About half the time cancer is found in the contralateral lobe [18]. Patients who undergo completion thyroidectomy within 6 months of the primary operation have significantly fewer recurrences, fewer lymph node and hematogenous metastases and survive significantly longer than those in whom the second operation is delayed [63].

We thus advise completion thyroidectomy as soon as possible after hemithyroidectomy. At 30 years, the recurrence rate among 436 patients who had undergone subtotal thyroidectomy was significantly higher than that among 698 patients who had undergone total or near-total thyroidectomy (40% versus 26%, $P < 0.002$); cancer-specific mortality rates were also higher in the subtotal thyroidectomy group (9% and 6%, $P = 0.02$) [19]. This is discussed in detail by Dr Villaret and Professor Mazzaferri in Chapter 12. Choice of a surgeons specializing in thyroid cancer surgery is particularly important in the outcome of patients with these tumors, and is reviewed in Chapter 11 by Professor Clark and his associates. Initial thyroid surgery is discussed in detail in Chapters 11, 12, 13, and 14.

Lymph Node Surgery

When cervical lymph node metastases are found, modified neck dissection sparing the sternocleidomastoid muscle is usually advised [114]. This should not be done prophylactically when lymph node metastases are not present. Patients with cervical lymph nodes metastases, those with primary tumor invading beyond the thyroid capsule, and women older than 60 years appear to benefit most from modified radical neck dissection [115]. Lymph node surgery is discussed in detail in Chapter 13 by Mr John Watkinson.

Radioactive Iodine (^{131}I) Therapy

Thyroid Remnant Ablation

This is defined as ^{131}I therapy administered to destroy presumably normal residual thyroid tissue. Routine ^{131}I remnant ablation, although questioned by some [116], is widely used and has appeal for several reasons. First, it may destroy occult microscopic cancer [18,62]. Second, it enables earlier detection of persistent tumor by post ^{131}I treatment whole-body scans (RxWBS) [81]. Third, it greatly facilitates the use of serum Tg measurements during follow-up. Few metastases can be visualized by ^{131}I scanning when appreciable amounts of normal thyroid tissue remain after surgery. Lastly, serum Tg concentration, which is the most sensitive marker of persistent disease, is unreliable

when a large thyroid remnant is present [117]. Thus ^{131}I is given postoperatively even to patients without known residual disease who have a good prognosis [38,118,119]. Still, this approach continues to engender debate and calls for randomized clinical trials [120], but they are so difficult to design that they are likely not to be done in the near future [121,122].

Remnant ablation was initially done with 2775 and 5550 MBq ^{131}I (75 to 150 mCi), but later clinicians began using 925 to 1110 mg (25 to 30 mCi) to avoid hospitalization, which is no longer necessary in the USA because of a change in federal regulations that permits much larger activities of ^{131}I in ambulatory patients. Smaller amounts of ^{131}I <1110 MBq (30 mCi), which can ablate thyroid remnants if the mass of residual thyroid tissue is small, has appeal because of the lower cost and lower whole-body radiation dose. One randomized prospective study of this question found that the first dose ablated thyroid bed uptake in 81% of patients given 225 MBq (30 mCi) and in 84% treated with 3700 MBq (100 mCi) [123]. Another randomized study [124] found that any activity of ^{131}I between 925 and 1850 MBq (25 to 50 mCi) appears to be adequate for remnant ablation [124]. Both studies were performed with a thyroid hormone withdrawal (THW) protocol in which the patient receives triiodothyronine (liothyronine, Cytomel) for 4 weeks and no thyroid hormone and a low iodine diet during the last 2 weeks before ^{131}I therapy.

More recently, ^{131}I remnant ablation has been done after intramuscular administration of recombinant human thyrotropin-α (rhTSH, Thyrogen), which stimulates thyroidal ^{131}I uptake and Tg release while the patient continues thyroid hormone (T_4) therapy, thus avoiding symptomatic hypothyroidism [125]. Although now approved only for diagnostic use, rhTSH, 0.9 mg, has been given intramuscularly every day for 2 days followed by 1110 to 3700 MBq (30 to 100 mCi) ^{131}I on the third day and RxWBS about 5 days later. This protocol has been shown to successfully prepare patients for ^{131}I remnant ablation. At the present time, the drug is approved in Europe and is likely to be approved in late 2005 for this purpose in the USA. Complete ablation, defined as an absence of uptake on an 85 MBq (5 mCi) ^{131}I diagnostic whole-body scan (DxWBS) image about one year later, was achieved in over 84% of patients prepared with T_4 withdrawal and in over 86% of those given rhTSH, who were treated, respectively, with an average of 4662 and 4403 MBq (126 and 119 mCi) of ^{131}I [119]. Another study found that 1110 MBq (30 mCi) ^{131}I given 48 hours instead of 24 hours after the last rhTSH injection failed to ablate the thyroid remnant when rhTSH was given [126]. Still another study showed that 1110 MBq (30 mCi) of ^{131}I was successful when T_4 was stopped the day before the first injection of rhTSH and started again the day after the ^{131}I was administered, which was associated with a fall in urine iodine levels attributed to the ~50 μg iodine content in a daily dose of T_4 compared with the 5 μg content of ^{131}I [127]. Patients tolerate rhTSH well, with only occasional transient mild headache and nausea. This is extensively reviewed in Chapter 17 by Professors Pacini and Schlumberger.

Long-Term Effects of Remnant Ablation and Treatment of Persistent Tumor with ^{131}I

Although some studies find that total thyroidectomy and ^{131}I therapy does not have a better effect upon outcome than does postoperative treatment with thyroxine alone [128], long-term studies generally find a beneficial effect of ^{131}I therapy. A study of 1599 patients treated between 1948 and 1989 found that ^{131}I therapy was the single most powerful prognostic indicator for increased disease-free survival [129]. Multivariate analyses show that ^{131}I has an independent prognostic effect when administered either to ablate the thyroid remnant or to treat metastases [18,38,130]. We found tumor recurrences in 7% of patients treated with 1073 to 3750 MBq (29 to 50 mCi) and in 9% treated with 1887 to 7400 MBq (51 to 200 mCi) of ^{131}I given to ablate thyroid remnants. In our study, ^{131}I given either to ablate the thyroid bed or to treat metastases each independently lowered the rates of all recurrences, distant recurrence, and cancer deaths. In studies with shorter follow-up than ours, multivariate analyses show that ^{131}I therapy lowers death rates in patients with bone [75,131] and lung [132] metastases providing they concentrate ^{131}I, and reduces locoregional recurrences, whether given to treat metastases or to ablate the thyroid remnant [130,133,134].

Therapeutic ^{131}I Dosimetry

Of the three dosimetry methods available, the simplest and most widely used is to administer an empiric fixed amount of ^{131}I. From 1110 to 3700 MBq (30 to 100 mCi) ^{131}I is given to ablate a thyroid remnant [135]. Patients with lymph node metastases removed by surgery are treated with 3700 to 6475 MBq (100 to 175 mCi), and microscopic tumor extending through the thyroid capsule is treated with 5550 to 7400 MBq (150 to 200 mCi). Diffuse pulmonary metastases that concentrate 50% or more of the test dose of ^{131}I, which is very uncommon [136], are treated with 150 mCi ^{131}I (5550 MBq) or less to avoid lung injury that may occur when more than 80 mCi (2960 MBq) are retained in the whole body 48 hours after the dose. Distant metastases are usually treated with 200 mCi (7400 MBq) ^{131}I.

A second approach is to use quantitative dosimetry to predict radiation doses to the target tissues, namely thyroid remnant or metastases, and to radiosensitive tissues to which the radiation dose must be limited, including the bone marrow and lungs in those with diffuse pulmonary metastases, and the whole-body radiation dose. This is favored by some because radiation exposure from arbitrarily fixed doses of ^{131}I can vary considerably [137]. If the lesional dose is less than 35 Gy (3500 rads), it is unlikely that the tumor will respond to ^{131}I therapy [137;138]. Conversely, ^{131}I activities that deliver 80 to 120 Gy (8000 to 12 000 rads) to the thyroid remnant or deliver 300 Gy (30 000 rads) to metastatic foci are likely to be effective. To make these calculations it is necessary to estimate tumor size, which in some situations is not possible.

A third approach is to calculate an upper ^{131}I activity limit that delivers a maximum of 2 Gy (200 rad) to the whole blood while keeping the whole-body ^{131}I retention less than 4440 MBq (120 mCi) at 48 hours or less than 2960 MBq (80 mCi) when there is diffuse lung uptake. Dosimetry is complicated and is performed in a limited number of large medical centers. Moreover, comparison of outcomes between empiric fixed dose methods and dosimetric approaches is difficult and unreliable, and prospective trials to address the optimal therapeutic approach have not been done [139]. The complications of ^{131}I therapy are reviewed in detail in Chapter 15

Figure 1.9 The therapeutic response to ^{131}I is due to three things: the effective T$_{1/2}$ (biological retention of the isotope in a tumor), the half-life of the isotope (~8 days for ^{131}I) and the activity (amount) of ^{131}I administered. The most common reason for failure of ^{131}I treatment is a short biological half-life (T$_{1/2}$) of ^{131}I in a tumor. The most common way that the therapeutic response is enhanced is by increasing the ^{131}I activity (dose). However, lithium increases the biological T$_{1/2}$ by as much as threefold, permitting the use of the smallest effective amount of ^{131}I, thus reducing the complications of ^{131}I therapy.

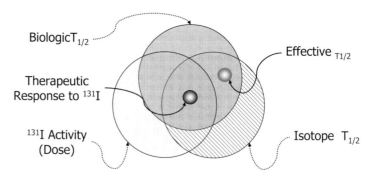

Factors Affecting the Therapeutic Response To ^{131}I Administration

by Drs Haq and Harmer and in Chapter 16 by Dr Vini.

Lithium Pretreatment

The therapeutic response to ^{131}I is related to the amount of radiation that is delivered to the follicular cell, which is a function of: (1) the amount of ^{131}I administered, (2) the biological half-time (T$_{1/2}$), which is the retention time of ^{131}I within the cell, and (3) the isotope physical half-life (Figure 1.9). The *effective T$_{1/2}$* is the combination of the biological T$_{1/2}$ and the physical T$_{1/2}$ of ^{131}I. Maxon et al. found that the main reason for failure of ^{131}I therapy was a short *effective T$_{1/2}$* of ^{131}I [140]. The biological retention T$_{1/2}$ of iodine in the thyroid is 60 days, but is only about 10 h in tumors [140].

Studies by Robbins and associates [141] from the USA National Institutes of Health show that lithium given at a dosage of 300–900 mg daily (10 mg/kg) for 7 days prolongs the biological T$_{1/2}$ and thus the effective T$_{1/2}$ in PTC and FTC [141]. The mean increase in the biological T$_{1/2}$, which was 50% in tumors and 90% in remnants, was proportionately greater in lesions with poor ^{131}I retention [141]. When the control T$_{1/2}$ was less than 3 days, lithium prolonged the effective T$_{1/2}$ by more than 50%. More ^{131}I accumulated during lithium therapy, probably as a consequence of its effect on iodine release without increasing radiation to other organs. Serum lithium levels should be measured daily and maintained in the usual therapeutic range between 0.8 and 1.2 nmol/L.

Potential Adverse Effects of ^{131}I Therapy

Acute Complications

Radiation Thyroiditis

Up to 20% of patients, usually those with a large thyroid remnant, given sufficient ^{131}I to deliver about 500 Gy (50 000 rads) develop thyroiditis [142], which occurs less often when 1110 MBq (30 mCi) of ^{131}I is administered [143]. Within a week, painful swallowing, neck and ear pain, thyroid tenderness and swelling, and transient mild thyrotoxicosis may occur, which is usually transient, requiring no therapy.

Radiation Sialadenitis

Up to one-third of patients develop acute and/or chronic parotid or submandibular gland sialadenitis after ^{131}I therapy [144]. Symptoms may occur within 24 hours and are more likely when large amounts of ^{131}I have been given to a patient with a small thyroid remnant [144]. Chewing gum, sucking on lemon candies, 24 hours after ^{131}I administration, and hydration may prevent the sialadenitis and xerostomia. Still, most patients experience intermittent painless salivary gland swelling that is caused by an epithelial plug in the salivary duct, beginning several months after ^{131}I therapy and lasting a few hours, reminiscent of a salivary duct stone. There is a salty taste when the salivary pressure is reduced spontaneously or by manual pressure on the parotid. Often misdiagnosed as infectious parotitis, it requires no therapy and usually improves spontaneously within about a year; however, it may be associated with a chronic xerostomia [144]. Most patients have reduced taste for several weeks, sometimes with transient tongue pain [144].

Ocular Dryness and Nasolacrimal Obstruction

A recent study found that conjunctivitis and nasolacrimal drainage system obstruction occurred 3 to 16 months after administering larger amounts of [131]I (6660 ± 555 MBq, 180 ± 15 mCi) [145]. This occurred in 3.4% of 563 patients in one study [146] but its incidence may be higher since these patients were not systematically evaluated nor questioned about tearing. The reported patients, who were likely to be the worst cases, often required surgical therapy [146].

Radiation Sickness

About two-thirds of patients given 7400 MBq (200 mCi) or more develop mild radiation sickness with headache, nausea and occasional vomiting that begins about 4 hours after ^{131}I administration and resolves in about 24 hours. It rarely occurs with less [131]I [138].

Acute Tumor Edema or Hemorrhage

This is the most serious acute complication, which may result from ^{131}I therapy or TSH stimulation, induced either by thyroid hormone withdrawal or rhTSH stimulation [147]. Serious symptoms can occur rapidly when the tumor is in a critical location such as the brain, spinal cord, or airway [147,148]. Likewise, pain may occur in bone metastases. Pretreatment with corticosteroids may minimize these problems, but surgery for spinal lesions and isolated brain metastases should be considered before TSH stimulation or ^{131}I therapy [149]. Vocal cord paralysis is reported in patients with a large amount of functioning thyroid tissue in close proximity to the vocal cords [138]. Transient peripheral facial nerve palsy also occurs rarely after high dose ^{131}I therapy [150].

Hematological Changes

A slight reduction in platelets and white blood cell counts may follow ^{131}I therapy but is typically transient and asymptomatic [151]. Pancytopenia can follow very large doses of ^{131}I, which may require transfusions, but this is usually reversible [151,152].

Late Complications

The main long-term complications of ^{131}I are damage to the gonads, bone marrow, and lungs, and the induction of other carcinomas.

Ovarian Damage

The risk of permanent damage to the ovaries after ablative radioiodine treatment appears to be low and most patients can be reassured they can have normal pregnancies after ^{131}I treatment. During the first year after ^{131}I therapy, middle-aged women may developed temporary amenorrhea and elevated serum gonadotropin concentrations [153] and women of all ages have a higher than expected rate of spontaneous miscarriage [154], yet there are no measurable effects of ^{131}I on fertility, birth defect, birthweight and prematurity rates [155]. Still, ^{131}I therapy may be associated with early menopause [156]. In a study by Vini et al. [157] of 496 women under the age of 40 at the time of diagnosis, 65% of whom had received 3 GBq (81 mCi) of ^{131}I while the remainder had received subsequent treatment with a cumulative activity of 8.5–59 GBq (230–1595 mCi) for persistent disease, transient amenorrhea or menstrual irregularities lasting up to 10 months occurred in 83 patients (17%). No cases of permanent ovarian failure were recorded. There were 427 children born to 276 women; only one patient was unable to achieve a successful pregnancy. Four premature births and 14 miscarriages occurred but no congenital abnormalities were reported. In a study of 33 children treated at an average age of 14.6 years with a mean dose of 7252 MBq (196 mCi) of ^{131}I, the frequency of infertility (12%), miscarriage (1.4%), prematurity (8%), and major congenital anomalies (1.4%) after an average follow-up of almost 19 years was not significantly different from that in the general population [158]. See Chapter 16 for an excellent review of this by Dr Vini.

Testicular Damage

In men, gonadal damage may be more severe [159], with permanent testicular damage or transiently reduced sperm counts roughly proportional to the ^{131}I dose administered [160]. Serum follicle-stimulating hormone (FSH) levels usually do not change or rise transiently, although they may remain high [161]. Serum testosterone concentrations and fertility are usually not affected [162]. In a longitudinal analysis of 21 men, six had no change or only a slight increase in serum FSH after ^{131}I therapy while 11 others had a transient rise above normal 6 to 12 months after treatment. Four men treated with several doses of ^{131}I had a progressive increase in serum FSH, which eventually became permanent. Semen analysis performed in a small subgroup of men showed a consistent reduction in sperm motility, but the serum testosterone concentrations in the treated and normal men were similar. A survey of 59 men treated with ^{131}I found they had fathered 106 children, none of whom was reported to have had major congenital malformations [162]. In another study, fertility was normal in 30 patients who were aged 30 years or less when treated; they had 44 live births [163]. Two men who had received a total of 35.9 and 52.98 GBq (972 and 1432 mCi) between ages 10 and 19 years had fathered two and three children, respectively, up to 13 and 24 years later. Another treated at age 24 with 25.2 GBq (680 mCi) had oligospermia with an elevated serum FSH. Thus, ^{131}I therapy occasionally impairs testicular germinal cell function, posing a significant risk of infertility. Young men should consider banking sperm specimens before therapy, particularly if larger cumulative doses of ^{131}I are to be given [159].

Bone Marrow Damage

This and the induction of other tumors are the most serious late hazards of ^{131}I therapy. Large amounts of [131]I (>37 000 MBq, 1000 mCi) can cause a small but significant excess of deaths, especially from bladder cancer and leukemia [163]. Bladder cancer occurs more often in those with relatively little ^{131}I uptake in the neck or metastases [163]. In one report, 80% of 35 patients treated with ^{131}I had bone marrow abnormalities, including three with acute

myeloid leukemia [164]. Those with pancytopenia had received cumulative ^{131}I activities over 37.0 GBq (1000 mCi) [164]. In 13 large series comprising a total of 2753 patients with thyroid carcinoma, 14 cases of leukemia were detected [165], resulting in a prevalence of about five cases per 1000 patients (0.5%), which is higher than expected in the general population. Acute myeloid leukemia tends to occur within 10 years of treatment and is less likely when ^{131}I is given annually rather than every few months, and when total blood doses per administration are less than 2 Gy (200 rad) [165]. The lifetime risk of leukemia is so small (0.33%) that it does not outweigh the benefit of ^{131}I therapy [166]. The risk of life lost because of recurrent thyroid cancer exceeds that from leukemia by fourfold to 40-fold, and is greatest in younger patients [166]. Few cases of leukemia occur when ^{131}I is given at 12-month intervals and cumulative amounts are less than 22.0 to 29.6 GBq (600 to 800 mCi) [151]. Still, ^{131}I therapy is not stopped for patients with serious metastatic tumor who have reached these limits.

Pulmonary Fibrosis

This rarely occurs in patients with diffuse pulmonary metastases treated with [131]I [167]. It can be avoided by using ^{131}I in amounts that result in a whole-body retention of less than 2.96 GBq (80 mCi) 48 hours after its administration when there is diffuse ^{131}I uptake in the lungs seen on the DxWBS. However, retention of >50% at 48 hours is uncommon [136].

Thyroid Hormone Therapy

TSH Suppression

The idea that TSH stimulates both the iodine transport and growth of thyroid carcinoma (only DTC) is the basis for the wide use of T_4 in treating this disease. Like normal thyroid tissue, most PTCs and FTCs have functional TSH receptors, but whether postoperative T_4 alone improves survival is less certain. Although there have been no prospective randomized trials of this question, there is evidence that TSH stimulates tumor growth [168]. PTC in patients with Graves' disease may be more aggressive, presumably as a result of stimulatory effects of circulating TSH receptor antibodies [82]. Rapid tumor growth sometimes follows T_4 withdrawal [169] or the use of rhTSH in preparation for ^{131}I therapy [168]. Moreover, T_4 given as an adjuvant to surgical and ^{131}I therapy is effective [122,170]. After 30 years' follow-up, we found that there were significantly fewer recurrences in patients treated with T_4 as compared with no adjunctive therapy ($P < 0.01$) and there were fewer cancer deaths in the T_4 group (6% versus 12%, $P < 0.001$) [19].

Potential Adverse Effects of T_4 Therapy

Patients with thyroid cancer are usually treated with T_4 to lower TSH secretion below normal, thereby deliberately causing subclinical if not overt thyrotoxicosis. One potential consequence of this is bone mineral loss, even in children [79], but especially in postmenopausal women with thyroid carcinoma [171–173]. This may be prevented by estrogen or bisphosphonate therapy. More importantly, using the smallest T_4 dose necessary to suppress TSH has no significant effects on bone metabolism and bone mass in men or women with thyroid cancer [174].

Cardiovascular abnormalities occur in patients taking suppressive doses of T_4 and may be ameliorated by beta-adrenergic blockade. Subclinical thyrotoxicosis causes an increased risk of atrial fibrillation [175], a higher 24-hour heart rate, more atrial premature contractions, increased cardiac contractility and ventricular hypertrophy, systolic and diastolic dysfunction, and increased cardiovascular mortality [176–179], especially when the TSH is <0.1 mIU/L.

Thyroxine (T_4) Dosage

Patients with thyroid cancer who have undergone total thyroid ablation require more T_4 than those with spontaneously occurring primary hypothyroidism. In one study, for example, the average dose of T_4 that resulted in an undetectable basal serum TSH concentration and no increase in serum TSH after thyrotropin-releasing hormone (TRH) was 2.7 ± 0.4 (SD) µg/kg/day [180]. Younger patients needed larger T_4 doses than older patients did and TSH suppression was more likely when the therapy had been prolonged. In a study of patients with thyroid cancer and other forms of hypothyroidism, the dose of T_4 needed to bring serum

TSH concentrations to normal was 2.11 and 1.62 µg/Kg/day, respectively [181].

One study found that a constantly suppressed TSH (≤0.05 mIU/L) was associated with a longer relapse-free survival than when serum TSH levels were always 1 mIU/L or higher, and that the degree of TSH suppression was an independent predictor of recurrence [182]. Another large study found that disease stage, patient age, and ^{131}I therapy independently predicted disease progression, but that the degree of TSH suppression did not [183].

The most appropriate amount of T_4 for most patients with thyroid cancer reduces the serum TSH concentration to just below the lower limit of normal or the low normal range (e.g. 0.3 or 0.4 mIU/L) if careful follow-up examinations show the patient is free of tumor. Some prefer greater suppression, lowering TSH levels to between 0.05 and 0.1 mIU/L in low risk patients and to less than 0.01 mIU/L in high risk patients [171]. However, there is no published evidence that maintaining serum TSH levels lower than 0.01 mIU/L has benefits and it does have some risks.

Follow-up Studies

Prevalence of Thyroid Cancer in the Population

There are about 300 000 patients in the USA [3] and 200 000 in Europe [184] living with thyroid cancer. Virtually all require lifelong follow-up, which until recently, was done mainly with serum Tg determinations obtained during T_4 suppression of TSH and [131]I DxWBS performed after thyroid hormone withdrawal. More recently, follow-up has become more complex, and is substantially more accurate. Older antithyroglobulin antibody assays did not detect low levels of anti-Tg antibody [184], which factitiously lower serum Tg results from immunometric assays. Also, 3 to 5 mCi [131]I DxWBS, computed tomography (CT), and magnetic resonance imaging (MRI) were the mainstays of imaging, but are now known to be far less capable of locating tumor than are newer more sensitive ultrasound and Doppler techniques, and [131]I RxWBS and [18]FDG-PET imaging studies. Identifying persistent DTC late in its course was the consequence of using insensitive tests that often identified tumor relapse decades after initial treatment [185]. Many were probably persistent tumors that had fallen below the detection limits of older tests. Newer follow-up paradigms identify persistent tumor 6 to 18 months after total thyroid ablation, permitting the application of earlier therapy with the hope of improving outcome (Professor Schlumberger and associates review this in considerable depth in Chapter 19).

Serum Thyroglobulin (Tg)

Paradigms for the follow-up of patients who appear to be free of tumor after total thyroidectomy and thyroid remnant ablation have shifted to performing neck ultrasonography and measuring Tg during TSH suppression and after rhTSH stimulation, or T_4 withdrawal (which produces symptomatic hypothyroidism that many patients choose to avoid) [184,186]. These paradigms are used by many US physicians (Figures 1.10, 1.11, and 1.12). Accurate serum Tg measurement is the cornerstone of this follow-up paradigm (Professor Spencer and Dr Fatemi

review this in Chapter 18). Serum Tg and ultrasonography identifies almost all patients with residual tumor, thus preventing unnecessary additional testing in those without residual tumor. For those who are cured, as confirmed by a serum Tg that fails to rise in response to rhTSH and a negative thyroid ultrasound examination, the T_4 dose can be reduced to maintain the TSH level in the low normal range, thus avoiding the potential harmful effects of subclinical thyrotoxicosis.

High Serum Tg Levels and Negative Whole-Body [131]I Imaging

The main consequence of applying sensitive diagnostic tests during follow-up is identifying patients with elevated serum Tg levels and negative ^{131}I imaging studies. This is a complex problem that requires careful evaluation but sometimes identifies patients with early metastatic tumor that is often highly amenable to ^{131}I therapy. This problem is reviewed in depth in Chapter 20. The new management and

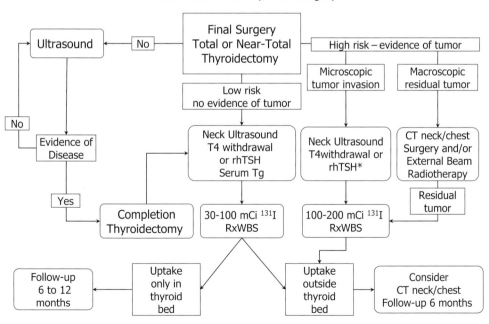

Figure 1.10 The first phase of follow-up of DTC occurs about 1–2 months after surgery. * This indication for rhTSH is not approved by the US FDA, but the drug can be used in selected patients (see text).

UHB TRUST LIBRARY
QEH

Phase 2 Followup after ^{131}I Remnant Ablation

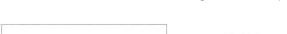

Figure 1.11 The second phase of follow-up of DTC occurs about 6–12 months after surgery.

Phase 3 Long-term Followup

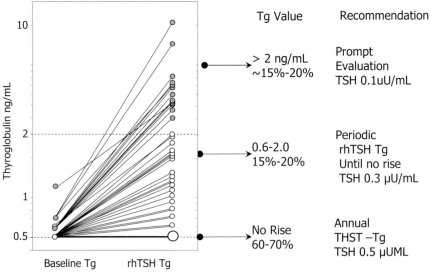

Figure 1.12 The third phase of follow-up of DTC occurs after the patient has no evidence of tumor.

follow-up paradigms described in this book offer substantial improvement over those used in the past.

References

1. Ferlay J, Bray F, Pisani P, Parkin DM. GLOBCAN 2000: Cancer Incidence, Mortality and Prevalence Worldwide Ver.1.0 JARC Cancer Base No. 5 Lyon, IARC Press, 2001. Last updated on 03/02/2001. http://www-dep.iarc.fr/globocan/globocan.html [1.0]. 2001.
2. Ries LAG, Eisner MP, Kosary CL, et al. SEER Cancer Statistics Review, 1975–2001, National Cancer Institute. Bethesda, MD. http://seer.cancer.gov/csr/1975_2001/. 2004.
3. Surveillance, Epidemiology, and End Results (SEER) Program (www.seer.cancer.gov) SEER*Stat Database: Incidence – SEER 9 Regs Public-Use, Nov 2003 Sub (1973–2001), National Cancer Institute, DCCPS, Surveillance Research Program, Cancer Statistics Branch, released April 2004, based on the November 2003 submission. National Cancer Institute, 2004.
4. Colonna M, Grosclaude P, Remontet L, et al. Incidence of thyroid cancer in adults recorded by French cancer registries (1978–1997). Eur J Cancer 2002; 38(13):1762–1768.
5. Cotterill SJ, Pearce MS, Parker L. Thyroid cancer in children and young adults in the North of England. Is increasing incidence related to the Chernobyl accident? Eur J Cancer 2001; 37(8):1020–1026.
6. Liu S, Semenciw R, Ugnat AM, Mao Y. Increasing thyroid cancer incidence in Canada, 1970–1996: time trends and age-period-cohort effects. Br J Cancer 2001; 85(9):1335–1339.
7. Lundgren CI, Hall P, Ekbom A, Frisell J, Zedenius J, Dickman PW. Incidence and survival of Swedish patients with differentiated thyroid cancer. Int J Cancer 2003; 106(4):569–573.
8. Verkooijen HM, Fioretta G, Pache JC, et al. Diagnostic changes as a reason for the increase in papillary thyroid cancer incidence in Geneva, Switzerland. Cancer Causes Control 2003; 14(1):13–17.
9. Merhy J, Driscoll HK, Leidy JW, Chertow BS. Increasing incidence and characteristics of differentiated thyroid cancer in Huntington, West Virginia. Thyroid 2001; 11(11):1063–1069.
10. Huszno B, Szybinski Z, Przybylik-Mazurek E, et al. Influence of iodine deficiency and iodine prophylaxis on thyroid cancer histotypes and incidence in endemic goiter area. J Endocrinol Invest 2003; 26(2 Suppl): 71–76.
11. Heidenreich WF, Kenigsberg J, Jacob P, et al. Time trends of thyroid cancer incidence in Belarus after the Chernobyl accident. Radiat Res 1999; 151:617–625.
12. Zheng TZ, Holford TR, Chen YT, et al. Time trend and age-period-cohort effect on incidence of thyroid cancer in Connecticut, 1935–1992. Int J Cancer 1996; 67:504–509.
13. Estimated exposures and thyroid doses received by the American people from iodine-131 in fallout following Nevada atmospheric nuclear bomb tests. A report from the National Cancer Institute. Washington, DC: US Department of Health and Human Services. National Institutes of Health. National Cancer Institute, 1997.
14. Leenhardt L, Bernier MO, Boin-Pineau MH, et al. Advances in diagnostic practices affect thyroid cancer incidence in France. Eur J Endocrinol 2004; 150(2): 133–139.
15. Institute of Medicine, Committee on Thyroid Screening Related to, National Research Council (US), Committee on Exposure of the American People to Iodine-131 from Nevada nuclear-bomb tests review of the National Cancer Institute report and public health implications. Washington, DC: National Academy Press, 1999.
16. Rahu M. Health effects of the Chernobyl accident: fears, rumours and the truth. Eur J Cancer 2003; 39(3):295–299.
17. Hundahl SA, Fleming ID, Fremgen AM, Menck HR. A National Cancer Data Base report on 53 856 cases of thyroid carcinoma treated in the US, 1985–1995. Cancer 1998; 83:2638–2648.
18. Mazzaferri EL, Kloos RT. Current approaches to primary therapy for papillary and follicular thyroid cancer. J Clin Endocrinol Metab 2001; 86(4):1447–1463.
19. Mazzaferri EL, Jhiang SM. Long-term impact of initial surgical and medical therapy on papillary and follicular thyroid cancer. Am J Med 1994; 97:418–428.
20. Pinn VW. Sex and gender factors in medical studies: implications for health and clinical practice. JAMA 2003; 289(4):397–400.
21. Kitamura Y, Shimizu K, Nagahama M, et al. Immediate causes of death in thyroid carcinoma: Clinicopathological analysis of 161 fatal cases. J Clin Endocrinol Metab 1999; 84:4043–4049.
22. LiVolsi VA. Pure versus follicular variant of papillary thyroid carcinoma: clinical features, prognostic factors, treatment, and survival. Cancer 2003; 98(9): 1997–1998.
23. Burman KD, Ringel MD, Wartofsky L. Unusual types of thyroid neoplasms. Endocrinol Metabol Clin North Am 1996; 25:49–68.
24. LiVolsi VA. Unusual variants of papillary thyroid carcinoma. In: Mazzaferri EL, Kreisberg RA, Bar RS (eds) Advances in endocrinology and metabolism. St Louis: Mosby-Year Book, Inc., 1995: 39–54.
25. Yang GC, Liebeskind D, Messina AV. Ultrasound-guided fine-needle aspiration of the thyroid assessed by ultrafast Papanicolaou stain: data from 1135 biopsies with a two- to six-year follow-up. Thyroid 2001; 11(6):581–589.
26. Kesmodel SB, Terhune KP, Canter RJ, et al. The diagnostic dilemma of follicular variant of papillary thyroid carcinoma. Surgery 2003; 134(6):1005–1012.
27. Sobrinho-Simoes M, Soares J, Carneiro F. Diffuse follicular variant of papillary carcinoma of the thyroid: report of eight cases of a distinct aggressive type of tumor. Surg Pathol 1990; 3:189–203.
28. Zidan J, Karen D, Stein M, Rosenblatt E, Basher W, Kuten A. Pure versus follicular variant of papillary thyroid carcinoma. Cancer 2003; 97(5):1181–1185.
29. Passler C, Prager G, Scheuba C, et al. Follicular variant of papillary thyroid carcinoma: a long-term follow-up. Arch Surg 2003; 138(12):1362–1366.

30. Chow SM, Chan JK, Law SC, et al. Diffuse sclerosing variant of papillary thyroid carcinoma – clinical features and outcome. Eur J Surg Oncol 2003; 29(5): 446–449.

31. Albareda M, Puig-Domingo M, Wengrowicz S, et al. Clinical forms of presentation and evolution of diffuse sclerosing variant of papillary carcinoma and insular variant of follicular carcinoma of the thyroid. Thyroid 1998; 8(5):385–391.

32. Herrera MF, Hay ID, Wu PS, et al. Hurthle cell (oxyphilic) papillary thyroid carcinoma: a variant with more aggressive biologic behavior. World J Surg 1994; 16:669–674.

33. Prendiville S, Burman KD, Ringel MD, et al. Tall cell variant: An aggressive form of papillary thyroid carcinoma. Otolaryngol Head Neck Surg 2000; 122(3): 352–357.

34. Ferreiro JA, Hay ID, Lloyd RV. Columnar cell carcinoma of the thyroid: Report of three additional cases. Hum Pathol 1996; 27:1156–1160.

35. van Heerden JA, Hay ID, Goellner JR, et al. Follicular thyroid carcinoma with capsular invasion alone: A nonthreatening malignancy. Surgery 1992; 112:1130–1138.

36. D'Avanzo A, Treseler P, Ituarte PH, et al. Follicular thyroid carcinoma: histology and prognosis. Cancer 2004; 100(6):1123–1129.

37. Thompson LD, Wieneke JA, Paal E, Frommelt RA, Adair CF, Heffess CS. A clinicopathologic study of minimally invasive follicular carcinoma of the thyroid gland with a review of the English literature 2. Cancer 2001; 91(3):505–524.

38. Lopez-Penabad L, Chiu AC, Hoff AO, et al. Prognostic factors in patients with Hurthle cell neoplasms of the thyroid. Cancer 2003; 97(5):1186–1194.

39. McIver B, Hay ID, Giuffrida DF, et al. Anaplastic thyroid carcinoma: A 50-year experience at a single institution. Surgery 2001; 130(6):1028–1034.

40. Rodriguez JM, Pinero A, Ortiz S, et al. Clinical and histological differences in anaplastic thyroid carcinoma. Eur J Surg 2000; 166(1):34–38.

41. Voutilainen PE, Multanen M, Haapiainen RK, Leppäniemi AK, Sivula AH. Anaplastic thyroid carcinoma survival. World J Surg 1999; 23:975–979.

42. Miura D, Wada N, Chin K, et al. Anaplastic thyroid cancer: cytogenetic patterns by comparative genomic hybridization. Thyroid 2003; 13(3):283–290.

43. Camargo R, Limbert E, Gillam M, et al. Aggressive metastatic follicular thyroid carcinoma with anaplastic transformation arising from a long-standing goiter in a patient with Pendred's syndrome. Thyroid 2001; 11(10):981–988.

44. Hazard JB, Hawk WA, Crile G Jr. Medullary (solid) carcinoma of the thyroid: A clinicopathologic entity. J Clin Endocrinol Metab 1959; 19:152–161.

45. Williams ED. Medullary thyroid carcinoma of the thyroid gland. J Clin Pathol 1967; 20:395–398.

46. Melvin KE, Tashjian AH Jr. The syndrome of excessive thyrocalcitonin produced by medullary carcinoma of the thyroid. Proc Natl Acad Sci USA 1968; 59:1216–1222.

47. Tashjian AH Jr, Melvin EW. Medullary carcinoma of the thyroid gland. Studies of thyrocalcitonin in plasma and tumor extracts. N Engl J Med 1968; 279:279–283.

48. Jackson CE, Tashjian AH Jr, Block MA. Diagnostic dependability of calcitonin assay in family studies for medullary thyroid carcinoma. J Lab Clin Med 1971; 78:817–818.

49. Melvin KE, Miller HH, Tashjian AH Jr. Early diagnosis of medullary carcinoma of the thyroid gland by means of calcitonin assay. N Engl J Med 1971; 285:1115–1120.

50. Melvin KE, Tashjian AH Jr, Miller HA. Studies in familial thyroid cancer. Trans Assoc Am Physicians 1971; 84:144–151.

51. Simpson NE, Kidd KK, Goodfellow PJ, et al. Assignment of multiple endocrine neoplasia type 2A to chromosome 10 by linkage. Nature 1987; 328:528–530.

52. Mathew CGP, Chin KE, Easton DF, et al. A linked genetic marker form multiple endocrine neoplasia type 2A on chromosome 10. Nature 1987; 328:527–528.

53. Lairmore TC, Howe JR, Korte JA, et al. Familial medullary thyroid carcinoma and multiple endocrine neoplasia type 2B map to the same region of chromosome 10 as multiple endocrine neoplasia type 2A. Genomics 1991; 9:181–192.

54. Mulligan LM, Kwok JBJ, Healey CS, et al. Germ-line mutations of the RET proto-oncogene in multiple endocrine neoplasia type 2A. Nature 1993; 363:458–460.

55. Hofstra RMW, Landsvater RM, Ceccherini I, et al. A mutation in the RET proto-oncogene associated with multiple endocrine neoplasia type 2B and sporadic medullary thyroid carcinoma. Nature 1994; 367:375–376.

56. Wells SA Jr, Donis-Keller H. Current perspectives on the diagnosis and management of patients with multiple endocrine neoplasia type 2 syndromes. Endocrinol Metabol Clin North Am 1994; 23:215–228.

57. Carlson KM, Dou S, Chi D, et al. Single missense mutation in the tyrosine kinase catalytic domain of the RET protooncogene is associated with multiple endocrine neoplasia type 2B. Proc Natl Acad Sci USA 1994; 91: 1579–1583.

58. Moosa M, Mazzaferri EL. Occult thyroid carcinoma. Cancer J 1997; 10:180–188.

59. Baudin E, Travagli JP, Ropers J, et al. Microcarcinoma of the thyroid gland – The Gustave-Roussy Institute Experience. Cancer 1998; 83:553–559.

60. Chow SM, Law SC, Chan JK, et al. Papillary microcarcinoma of the thyroid – prognostic significance of lymph node metastasis and multifocality. Cancer 2003; 98(1):31–40.

61. Sugg SL, Ezzat S, Rosen IB, Freeman JL, Asa SL. Distinct multiple RET/PTC gene rearrangements in multifocal papillary thyroid neoplasia. J Clin Endocrinol Metab 1998; 83:4116–4122.

62. Pacini F, Elisei R, Capezzone M, et al. Contralateral papillary thyroid cancer is frequent at completion thyroidectomy with no difference in low- and high-risk patients. Thyroid 2001; 11(9):877–881.

63. Scheumann GFW, Seeliger H, Musholt TJ, et al. Completion thyroidectomy in 131 patients with differentiated thyroid carcinoma. Eur J Surg 1996; 162:677–684.

64. Pasieka JL, Thompson NW, McLeod MK, Burney RE, Macha M. The incidence of bilateral well-differentiated thyroid cancer found at completion thyroidectomy. World J Surg 1992; 16:711–716.

65. Loh KC, Greenspan FS, Gee L, Miller TR, Yeo PPB. Pathological tumor-node-metastasis (pTNM) staging

for papillary and follicular thyroid carcinomas: A retrospective analysis of 700 patients. J Clin Endocrinol Metab 1997; 82:3553–3562.

66. Massin JP, Savoie JC, Garnier H, et al. Pulmonary metastases in differentiated thyroid carcinoma. Study of 58 cases with implications for the primary tumor treatment. Cancer 1984; 53:982–992.

67. Machens A, Holzhausen HJ, Lautenschlager C, Thanh PN, Dralle H. Enhancement of lymph node metastasis and distant metastasis of thyroid carcinoma. Cancer 2003; 98(4):712–719.

68. Mirallie E, Visset J, Sagan C, Hamy A, Le Bodic MF, Paineau J. Localization of cervical node metastasis of papillary thyroid carcinoma. World J Surg 1999; 23(9): 970–973.

69. Qubain SW, Nakano S, Baba M, Takao S, Aikou T. Distribution of lymph node micrometastasis in pN0 well-differentiated thyroid carcinoma. Surgery 2002; 131(3):249–256.

70. Wada N, Duh QY, Sugino K, et al. Lymph node metastasis from 259 papillary thyroid microcarcinomas: frequency, pattern of occurrence and recurrence, and optimal strategy for neck dissection. Ann Surg 2003; 237(3):399–407.

71. Arch-Ferrer J, Velazquez D, Fajardo R, et al. Accuracy of sentinel lymph node in papillary thyroid carcinoma. Surgery 2001; 130(6):907–913.

72. Kouvaraki MA, Shapiro SE, Fornage BD, et al. Role of preoperative ultrasonography in the surgical management of patients with thyroid cancer. Surgery 2003; 134(6):946–954.

73. Mazzaferri EL. Thyroid carcinoma: Papillary and follicular. In: Mazzaferri EL, Samaan N (eds) Endocrine tumors. Cambridge, MA: Blackwell Scientific Publications Inc., 1993: 278–333.

74. Schlumberger M, Challeton C, De Vathaire F, Parmentier C. Treatment of distant metastases of differentiated thyroid carcinoma. J Endocrinol Invest 1995; 18:170–172.

75. Pittas AG, Adler M, Fazzari M, et al. Bone metastases from thyroid carcinoma: clinical characteristics and prognostic variables in one hundred forty-six patients. Thyroid 2000; 10(3):261–268.

76. Schlumberger M, Tubiana M, De Vathaire F, et al. Long-term results of treatment of 283 patients with lung and bone metastases from differentiated thyroid carcinoma. J Clin Endocrinol Metab 1986; 63:960–967.

77. Sisson JC, Giordano TJ, Jamadar DA, et al. 131-I treatment of micronodular pulmonary metastases from papillary thyroid carcinoma. Cancer 1996; 78:2184–2192.

78. Schlumberger MJ. Diagnostic follow-up of well-differentiated thyroid carcinoma: Historical perspective and current status. J Endocrinol Invest 1999; 22(suppl to no. 11):3–7.

79. Hung W, Sarlis NJ. Current controversies in the management of pediatric patients with well-differentiated non-medullary thyroid cancer: A review. Thyroid 2002; 12:683–702.

80. Cady B. Staging in thyroid carcinoma. Cancer 1998; 83:844–847.

81. Miccoli P, Antonelli A, Spinelli C, Ferdeghini M, Fallahi P, Baschieri L. Completion total thyroidectomy in children with thyroid cancer secondary to the Chernobyl accident. Arch Surg 1998; 133:89–93.

82. Belfiore A, Russo D, Vigneri R, Filetti S. Graves' disease, thyroid nodules and thyroid cancer. Clin Endocrinol (Oxf) 2001; 55(6):711–718.

83. Ohta K, Pang XP, Berg L, Hershman JM. Growth inhibition of new human thyroid carcinoma cell lines by activation of adenylate cyclase through the β-adrenergic receptor. J Clin Endocrinol Metab 1997; 82:2633–2638.

84. Bell B, Mazzaferri EL. Familial adenomatous polyposis (Gardner's syndrome) and thyroid carcinoma: A case report and review of the literature. Dig Dis Sci 1993; 38:185–190.

85. Fagin JA. Editorial familial nonmedullary thyroid carcinoma – the case for genetic susceptibility. J Clin Endocrinol Metab 1997; 82:342–344.

86. Loh KC. Familial nonmedullary thyroid carcinoma: a meta-review of case series. Thyroid 1997; 7(1):107–113.

87. Malchoff CD, Malchoff DM. The genetics of hereditary nonmedullary thyroid carcinoma. J Clin Endocrinol Metab 2002; 87(6):2455–2459.

88. Lupoli G, Vitale G, Caraglia M, et al. Familial papillary thyroid microcarcinoma: a new clinical entity. Lancet 1999; 353:637–639.

89. Alsanea O, Wada N, Ain K, et al. Is familial nonmedullary thyroid carcinoma more aggressive than sporadic thyroid cancer? A multicenter series. Surgery 2000; 128(6):1043–1050.

90. Uchino S, Noguchi S, Kawamoto H, et al. Familial nonmedullary thyroid carcinoma characterized by multifocality and a high recurrence rate in a large study population. World J Surg 2002; 26(8):897–902.

91. Van De Velde CJH, Hamming JF, Goslings BM, et al. Report of the consensus development conference on the management of differentiated thyroid cancer in the Netherlands. Eur J Cancer Clin Oncol 1988; 24:287–292.

92. Baldet L, Manderscheid JC, Glinoer D, Jaffiol C, Coste Seignovert B, Percheron C. The management of differentiated thyroid cancer in Europe in 1988. Results of an international survey. Acta Endocrinol (Copenh) 1989; 120:547–558.

93. Solomon BL, Wartofsky L, Burman KD. Current trends in the management of well differentiated papillary thyroid carcinoma. J Clin Endocrinol Metab 1996; 81: 333–339.

94. Frankenthaler RA, Sellin RV, Cangir A, Goepfert H. Lymph node metastasis from papillary-follicular thyroid carcinoma in young patients. Am J Surg 1990; 160:341–343.

95. Agostini L, Mazzi P, Cavaliere A. Multiple primary malignant tumours: gemistocytic astrocytoma with leptomeningeal spreading and papillary thyroid carcinoma. A case report. Acta Neurol (Napoli) 1990; 12:305–310.

96. Soravia C, Sugg SL, Berk T, et al. Familial adenomatous polyposis-associated thyroid cancer – A clinical, pathological, and molecular genetics study. Am J Pathol 1999; 154:127–135.

97. Marsh DJ, Dahia PLM, Caron S, et al. Germline PTEN mutations in Cowden syndrome-like families. J Med Genet 1998; 35:881–885.

98. Hegedus L. Clinical practice. The thyroid nodule. N Engl J Med 2004; 351(17):1764–1771.

99. Papini E, Guglielmi R, Bianchini A, et al. Risk of malignancy in nonpalpable thyroid nodules: predictive value of ultrasound and color-Doppler features. J Clin Endocrinol Metab 2002; 87(5):1941–1946.

100. Gorges R, Eising EG, Fotescu D, et al. Diagnostic value of high-resolution B-mode and power-mode sonography in the follow-up of thyroid cancer. Eur J Ultrasound 2003; 16(3):191–206.

101. Belfiore A, La Rosa GL, LaPorta GA, et al. Cancer risk in patients with cold thyroid nodules: Relevance of iodine intake, sex, age and multinodularity. Am J Med 1992; 93:363–369.

102. Mandel SJ. A 64-year-old woman with a thyroid nodule. JAMA 2004; 292(21):2632–2642.

103. Mazzaferri EL. Management of a solitary thyroid nodule. N Engl J Med 1993; 328:553–559.

104. Alexander EK, Heering JP, Benson CB, et al. Assessment of nondiagnostic ultrasound-guided fine needle aspirations of thyroid nodules. J Clin Endocrinol Metab 2002; 87(11):4924–4927.

105. Massoll N, Nizam MS, Mazzaferri EL. Cystic thyroid nodules: diagnostic and therapeutic dilemmas. Endocrinologist 2002; 12(3):185–198.

106. Elisei R, Bottici V, Luchetti F, et al. Impact of routine measurement of serum calcitonin on the diagnosis and outcome of medullary thyroid cancer: experience in 10 864 patients with nodular thyroid disorders. J Clin Endocrinol Metab 2004; 89(1):163–168.

107. Bonnema SJ, Bennedbaek FN, Ladenson PW, Hegedus L. Management of the nontoxic multinodular goiter: a North American survey. J Clin Endocrinol Metab 2002; 87(1):112–117.

108. Brandi ML, Gagel RF, Angeli A, et al. CONSENSUS: Guidelines for Diagnosis and Therapy of MEN Type 1 and Type 2. J Clin Endocrinol Metab 2001; 86(12):5658–5671.

109. Machens A, Niccoli-Sire P, Hoegel J, et al. Early malignant progression of hereditary medullary thyroid cancer. N Engl J Med 2003; 349(16):1517–1525.

110. NCCN Thyroid Cancer Practice Guidelines. Oncology 13 Supplement 11A, NCCN Proceedings http://www.nccn.org/physician_gls/f_guidelines.html. 1999.

111. British Thyroid Association. Guidelines for the Management of Differentiated Thyroid Cancer in adults. http://www.british-thyroid-association.org/guidelines.htm. 2002.

112. Hundahl SA, Cady B, Cunningham MP, et al. Initial results from a prospective cohort study of 5583 cases of thyroid carcinoma treated in the united states during 1996. US and German Thyroid Cancer Study Group. An American College of Surgeons Commission on Cancer Patient Care Evaluation study. Cancer 2000; 89(1):202–217.

113. Shah JP, Loree TR, Dharker D, et al. Prognostic factors in differentiated carcinoma of the thyroid gland. Am J Surg 1993; 164:658–661.

114. Mazzaferri EL. NCCN thyroid carcinoma practice guidelines. Oncology 1999; 13 Supplement 11A, NCCN Proceedings http://www.nccn.org/physician_gls/f_guidelines.html:391–442.

115. Noguchi S, Murakami N, Yamashita H, Toda M, Kawamoto H. Papillary thyroid carcinoma – modified radical neck dissection improves prognosis. Arch Surg 1998; 133:276–280.

116. Hay ID. Papillary thyroid carcinoma. Endocrinol Metab Clin North Am 1990; 19(3):545–576.

117. Baloch Z, Carayon P, Conte-Devolx B, et al. Laboratory medicine practice guidelines. Laboratory support for the diagnosis and monitoring of thyroid disease. Thyroid 2003; 13(1):3–126.

118. Koh JM, Kim ES, Ryu JS, Hong SJ, Kim WB, Shong YK. Effects of therapeutic doses of 131I in thyroid papillary carcinoma patients with elevated thyroglobulin level and negative 131I whole-body scan: comparative study. Clin Endocrinol (Oxf) 2003; 58(4):421–427.

119. Robbins RJ, Larson SM, Sinha N, et al. A retrospective review of the effectiveness of recombinant human TSH as a preparation for radioiodine thyroid remnant ablation. J Nucl Med 2002; 43(11):1482–1488.

120. Dragoiescu C, Hoekstra OS, Kuik DJ, et al. Feasibility of a randomized trial on adjuvant radio-iodine therapy in differentiated thyroid cancer. Clin Endocrinol (Oxf) 2003; 58(4):451–455.

121. Mazzaferri E. A randomized trial of remnant ablation–in search of an impossible dream? J Clin Endocrinol Metab 2004; 89(8):3662–3664.

122. Sawka AM, Thephamongkhol K, Brouwers M, Thabane L, Browman G, Gerstein HC. Clinical review 170: A systematic review and metaanalysis of the effectiveness of radioactive iodine remnant ablation for well-differentiated thyroid cancer. J Clin Endocrinol Metab 2004; 89(8):3668–3676.

123. Johansen K, Woodhouse NJ, Odugbesan O. Comparison of 1073 MBq and 3700 MBq iodine-131 in postoperative ablation of residual thyroid tissue in patients with differentiated thyroid cancer. J Nucl Med 1991; 32:252–254.

124. Bal CS, Kumar A, Pant GS. Radioiodine dose for remnant ablation in differentiated thyroid carcinoma: a randomized clinical trial in 509 patients. J Clin Endocrinol Metab 2004; 89(4):1666–1673.

125. Ladenson PW, Braverman LE, Mazzaferri EL, et al. Comparison of administration of recombinant human thyrotropin with withdrawal of thyroid hormone for radioactive iodine scanning in patients with thyroid carcinoma. N Engl J Med 1997; 337:888–896.

126. Pacini F, Molinaro E, Castagna MG, et al. Ablation of thyroid residues with 30 mCi (131)I: a comparison in thyroid cancer patients prepared with recombinant human TSH or thyroid hormone withdrawal. J Clin Endocrinol Metab 2002; 87(9):4063–4068.

127. Barbaro D, Boni G, Meucci G, et al. Radioiodine treatment with 30 mCi after recombinant human thyrotropin stimulation in thyroid cancer: effectiveness for postsurgical remnants ablation and possible role of iodine content in L-thyroxine in the outcome of ablation. J Clin Endocrinol Metab 2003; 88(9):4110–4115.

128. Hay ID, Thompson GB, Grant CS, et al. Papillary thyroid carcinoma managed at the Mayo Clinic during six decades (1940–1999): temporal trends in initial therapy and long-term outcome in 2444 consecutively treated patients. World J Surg 2002; 26(8):879–885.

129. Samaan NA, Schultz PN, Hickey RC, Haynie TP, Johnston DA, Ordonez NG. Well-differentiated thyroid carcinoma and the results of various modalities of treatment. A retrospective review of 1599 patients. J Clin Endocrinol Metab 1992; 75:714–720.

130. Chow SM, Law SC, Mendenhall WM, et al. Papillary thyroid carcinoma: prognostic factors and the role of radioiodine and external radiotherapy. Int J Radiat Oncol Biol Phys 2002; 52(3):784–795.

131. Bernier MO, Leenhardt L, Hoang C, et al. Survival and therapeutic modalities in patients with bone metastases of differentiated thyroid carcinomas. J Clin Endocrinol Metab 2001; 86(4):1568–1573.

132. Schlumberger M, Challeton C, De Vathaire F, et al. Radioactive iodine treatment and external radiotherapy for lung and bone metastases from thyroid carcinoma. J Nucl Med 1996; 37:598–605.

133. Taylor T, Specker B, Robbins J, et al. Outcome after treatment of high-risk papillary and non-Hurthle-cell follicular thyroid carcinoma. Ann Intern Med 1998; 129:622–627.

134. Tsang TW, Brierley JD, Simpson WJ, Panzarella T, Gospodarowicz MK, Sutcliffe SB. The effects of surgery, radioiodine, and external radiation therapy on the clinical outcome of patients with differentiated thyroid carcinoma. Cancer 1998; 82:375–388.

135. Hodgson DC, Brierley JD, Tsang RW, Panzarella T. Prescribing [131]iodine based on neck uptake produces effective thyroid ablation and reduced hospital stay. Radiother Oncol 1998; 47:325–330.

136. Sisson JC. Practical dosimetry of 131I in patients with thyroid carcinoma. Cancer Biother Radiopharm 2002; 17(1):101–105.

137. Maxon HR, Englaro EE, Thomas SR, et al. Radioiodine-131 therapy for well-differentiated thyroid cancer – a quantitative radiation dosimetric approach: outcome and validation in 85 patients. J Nucl Med 1992; 33: 1132–1136.

138. Brierley J, Maxon HR. Radioiodine and external radiation therapy. In: Fagin JA (ed.) Thyroid cancer. Boston/Dordrecht, London: Kluwer Academic Publishers, 1998: 285–317.

139. Van Nostrand D, Atkins F, Yeganeh F, Acio E, Bursaw R, Wartofsky L. Dosimetrically determined doses of radioiodine for the treatment of metastatic thyroid carcinoma. Thyroid 2002; 12(2):121–134.

140. Maxon HR, Thomas SR, Hertzberg VS, et al. Relation between effective radiation dose and outcome of radioiodine therapy for thyroid cancer. N Engl J Med 1983; 309:937–941.

141. Koong SS, Reynolds JC, Movius EG, et al. Lithium as a potential adjuvant to ^{131}I therapy of metastatic, well differentiated thyroid carcinoma. J Clin Endocrinol Metab 1999; 84:912–916.

142. Randolph GW, Daniels GH. Radioactive iodine lobe ablation as an alternative to completion thyroidectomy for follicular carcinoma of the thyroid. Thyroid 2002; 12(11):989–996.

143. Burmeister LA, duCret RP, Mariash CN. Local reactions to radioiodine in the treatment of thyroid cancer. Am J Med 1991; 90:217–222.

144. Alexander C, Bader JB, Schaefer A, Finke C, Kirsch CM. Intermediate and long-term side effects of high-dose radioiodine therapy for thyroid carcinoma. J Nucl Med 1998; 39:1551–1554.

145. Kloos RT, Duvuuri V, Jhiang SM, Cahill KV, Foster JA, Burns JA. Nasolacrimal drainage system obstruction from radioactive iodine therapy for thyroid carcinoma. J Clin Endocrinol Metab 2002; 87(12):5817–5820.

146. Burns JA, Morgenstern KE, Cahill KV, Foster JA, Jhiang SM, Kloos RT. Nasolacrimal obstruction secondary to I(131) therapy. Ophthal Plast Reconstr Surg 2004; 20(2):126–129.

147. Vargas GE, Uy H, Bazan C, Guise TA, Bruder JM. Hemiplegia after thyrotropin alfa in a hypothyroid patient with thyroid carcinoma metastatic to the brain. J Clin Endocrinol Metab 1999; 84:3867–3871.

148. Datz FL. Cerebral edema following iodine-131 therapy for thyroid carcinoma metastatic to the brain. J Nucl Med 1986; 27:637–640.

149. Chiu AC, Delpassand ES, Sherman SI. Prognosis and treatment of brain metastases in thyroid carcinoma. J Clin Endocrinol Metab 1997; 82:3637–3642.

150. Levenson D, Gulec S, Sonenberg M, Lai E, Goldsmith SJ, Larson SM. Peripheral facial nerve palsy after high-dose radioiodine therapy in patients with papillary thyroid carcinoma. Ann Intern Med 1994; 120:576–578.

151. Van Nostrand D, Neutze J, Atkins F. Side effects of "rational dose" iodine-131 therapy for metastatic well-differentiated thyroid carcinoma. J Nucl Med 1986; 27: 1519–1527.

152. Dorn R, Kopp J, Vogt H, Heidenreich P, Carroll RG, Gulec SA. Dosimetry-guided radioactive iodine treatment in patients with metastatic differentiated thyroid cancer: largest safe dose using a risk-adapted approach. J Nucl Med 2003; 44(3):451–456.

153. Raymond JP, Izembart M, Marliac V, et al. Temporary ovarian failure in thyroid cancer patients after thyroid remnant ablation with radioactive iodine. J Clin Endocrinol Metab 1989; 69:186–190.

154. Schlumberger M, De Vathaire F, Ceccarelli C, et al. Exposure to radioactive iodine-131 for scintigraphy or therapy does not preclude pregnancy in thyroid cancer patients. J Nucl Med 1996; 37:606–612.

155. Dottorini ME, Lomuscio G, Mazzucchelli L, Vignati A, Colombo L. Assessment of female fertility and carcinogenesis after iodine-131 therapy for differentiated thyroid carcinoma. J Nucl Med 1995; 36:21–27.

156. Ceccarelli C, Bencivelli W, Morciano D, Pinchera A, Pacini F. 131I therapy for differentiated thyroid cancer leads to an earlier onset of menopause: results of a retrospective study. J Clin Endocrinol Metab 2001; 86(8): 3512–3515.

157. Vini L, Hyer S, Al Saadi A, Pratt B, Harmer C. Prognosis for fertility and ovarian function after treatment with radioiodine for thyroid cancer. Postgrad Med J 2002; 78(916):92–93.

158. Sarkar SD, Beierwaltes WH, Gill SP, Cowley BJ. Subsequent fertility and birth histories of children and adolescents treated with 131I for thyroid cancer. J Nucl Med 1976; 17:460–464.

159. Mazzaferri EL. Gonadal damage from 131I therapy for thyroid cancer. Clin Endocrinol (Oxf) 2002; 57(3):313–314.

160. Handelsman DJ, Turtle JR. Testicular damage after radioactive iodine (I-131) therapy for thyroid cancer. Clin Endocrinol 1983; 18:465–472.

161. Pacini F, Gasperi M, Fugazzola L, et al. Testicular function in patients with differentiated thyroid carcinoma treated with radioiodine. J Nucl Med 1994; 35:1418–1422.

162. Hyer S, Vini L, O'Connell M, Pratt B, Harmer C. Testicular dose and fertility in men following I(131) therapy for thyroid cancer. Clin Endocrinol (Oxf) 2002; 56(6): 755–758.

163. Edmonds CJ, Smith T. The long-term hazards of the treatment of thyroid cancer with radioiodine. Br J Radiol 1986; 59:45–51.

164. Gunter HH, Schober O, Schwarzrock R, Hundeshagen H. Hematologic long-term modifications after radio-iodine therapy in carcinoma of the thyroid gland. II. Modifications of the bone marrow including leukemia. Strahlentherapie und Onkologie 1986; 163:475–485.

165. Maxon H, III, Smith HS. Radioiodine-131 in the diagnosis and treatment of metastatic well differentiated thyroid cancer. Endocrinol Metabol Clin North Am 1990; 19:685–718.

166. Wong JB, Kaplan MM, Meyer KB, Pauker SG. Ablative radioactive iodine therapy for apparently localized thyroid carcinoma. A decision analytic perspective. Endocrinol Metabol Clin North Am 1990; 19:741–760.

167. Brown AP, Greening WP, McCready VR, Shaw HJ, Harmer CL. Radioiodine treatment of metastatic thyroid carcinoma: the Royal Marsden Hospital experience. Br J Radiol 1984; 57:323–327.

168. Cooper DS, Specker B, Ho M, et al. Thyrotropin suppression and disease progression in patients with differentiated thyroid cancer: results from the National Thyroid Cancer Treatment Cooperative Registry. Thyroid 1998; 8(9):737–744.

169. Maloof F, Vickery AL, Rapp B. An evaluation of various factors influencing the treatment of metastatic thyroid carcinoma with I 131. J Clin Endocrinol Metab 1956; 16(1):1–27.

170. Mazzaferri EL. Thyroid cancer in thyroglossal duct remnants: a diagnostic and therapeutic dilemma. Thyroid 2004; 14(5):335–336.

171. Dulgeroff AJ, Hershman JM. Medical therapy for differentiated thyroid carcinoma. Endocrinol Rev 1994; 15:500–515.

172. Faber J, Galloe AM. Changes in bone mass during prolonged subclinical hyperthyroidism due to L-thyroxine treatment: A meta-analysis. Acta Endocrinol (Copenh) 1994; 130:350–356.

173. Uzzan B, Campos J, Cucherat M, Nony P, Boissel JP, Perret GY. Effects on bone mass of long term treatment with thyroid hormones: A meta-analysis. J Clin Endocrinol Metab 1996; 81:4278–4289.

174. Marcocci C, Golia F, Vignali E, Pinchera A. Skeletal integrity in men chronically treated with suppressive doses of L-thyroxine. J Bone Miner Res 1997; 12:72–77.

175. Sawin CT, Geller A, Wolf PA, et al. Low serum thyrotropin concentrations as a risk factor for atrial fibrillation in older persons. N Engl J Med 1994; 331: 1249–1252.

176. Parle JV, Maisonneuve P, Sheppard MC, Boyle P, Franklyn JA. Prediction of all-cause and cardiovascular mortality in elderly people from one low serum thyrotropin result: a 10-year cohort study. Lancet 2001; 358(9285):861–865.

177. Biondi B, Fazio S, Carella C, et al. Cardiac effects of long term thyrotropin-suppressive therapy with levothyroxine. J Clin Endocrinol Metab 1993; 77:334–338.

178. Fazio S, Biondi B, Carella C, et al. Diastolic dysfunction in patients on thyroid-stimulating hormone suppressive therapy with levothyroxine: Beneficial effect of β-blockade. J Clin Endocrinol Metab 1995; 80:2222–2226.

179. Shapiro LE, Sievert R, Ong L, et al. Minimal cardiac effects in asymptomatic athyreotic patients chronically treated with thyrotropin-suppressive doses of L-thyroxine. J Clin Endocrinol Metab 1997; 82:2592–2595.

180. Bartalena L, Martino E, Pacchiarotti A, et al. Factors affecting suppression of endogenous thyrotropin secretion by thyroxine treatment: retrospective analysis in athyreotic and goitrous patients. J Clin Endocrinol Metab 1987; 64:849–855.

181. Burmeister LA, Goumaz MO, Mariash CN, Oppenheimer JH. Levothyroxine dose requirements for thyrotropin suppression in the treatment of differentiated thyroid cancer. J Clin Endocrinol Metab 1992; 75:344–350.

182. Pujol P, Daures JP, Nsakala N, Baldet L, Bringer J, Jaffiol C. Degree of thyrotropin suppression as a prognostic determinant in differentiated thyroid cancer. J Clin Endocrinol Metab 1996; 81:4318–4323.

183. Cooper DS, Specker B, Ho M, et al. Thyrotropin suppression and disease progression in patients with differentiated thyroid cancer: Results from the National Thyroid Cancer Treatment Cooperative Registry. Thyroid 1999; 8:737–744.

184. Schlumberger M, Berg G, Cohen O, et al. Follow-up of low-risk patients with differentiated thyroid carcinoma: a European perspective. Eur J Endocrinol 2004; 150(2):105–112.

185. Mazzaferri EL, Kloos RT. Using recombinant human TSH in the management of well-differentiated thyroid cancer: current strategies and future directions. Thyroid 2000; 10(9):767–778.

186. Haugen BR, Pacini F, Reiners C, et al. A comparison of recombinant human thyrotropin and thyroid hormone withdrawal for the detection of thyroid remnant or cancer. J Clin Endocrinol Metab 1999; 84:3877–3885.

Section I

The UK Multidisciplinary Approach to Management of Thyroid Cancer

2

The UK Evidence-Based Guidelines for the Management of Thyroid Cancer: Key Recommendations

Pat Kendall-Taylor

Introduction

National UK evidence-based guidelines for the management of thyroid cancer were completed in 2001 and published in March 2002 [1]. The guidelines cover management of differentiated (papillary and follicular) thyroid cancer (DTC) and medullary thyroid cancer (MTC); they are intended for the use of all disciplines involved in any way in the care of patients with thyroid cancer. In addition to the detailed guidelines, the document includes key recommendations, guidelines for the primary care physician, and detailed information (in the form of three booklets) for patients. The guidelines have been welcomed by cancer networks in the UK, by individuals responsible for treating such patients and in addition have been adopted in several other countries.

In the United States the management of thyroid cancer follows guidelines published by the American Thyroid Association in 1996 [2], by the National Comprehensive Cancer Network (NCCN) in 1999 [3], and the American Association of Clinical Endocrinologists (AACE) in 2001 [4]. In the UK, the National Institute for Clinical Excellence (NICE) is in the process of developing guidelines for "Head and Neck Cancers" which include thyroid cancer (see www.nice.org.uk); these are expected in late 2004 and deal in detail with matters relating to referral and the organization of the multidisciplinary team (MDT).

In this chapter I shall review briefly the background to the development of the UK guidelines and outline the key recommendations.

Development of the Guidelines

The guidelines were compiled under the auspices of the British Thyroid Association by a panel of national experts representing all relevant disciplines, colleges, and societies in the UK. Patient representatives were fully involved in the process of guideline development, as well as the preparation of patient information literature.

The development followed the process recommended in the literature available at the time for the development and use of guidelines, such as the series in the *British Medical Journal* (1999 volume 318, edited by M. Eccles and J. Grimshaw). A systematic review of the literature was undertaken. The definition of Types of Evidence and the Grading of Recommendations follows that of the Agency for Health Care Policy and Research (AHCPR, 1994). Randomized trials are generally not available for thyroid cancer, and evidence is therefore based on large retrospective studies such that the level of evidence according to AHCPR is generally II or III; as a result there is still controversy regarding some aspects of treatment. After completion the guidelines and the accompanying patient information booklets were subjected to extensive external peer review. The comments and recommendations were reviewed and appropriate revisions made. The document is formatted so that the reader may obtain an overview of treatment, backed by the Level of Recommendation (AHCPR), and obtain extensive references to more detailed publications.

The recommendations are in accord with the UK requirements for cancer management as detailed in the NHS Manual of Cancer Services Standards [5].

Case of Need for Guidelines

Although differentiated thyroid cancers are not common they are of similar frequency to cervical cancer and multiple myeloma and are the commonest malignant endocrine tumors. Furthermore they are among the few curable cancers. When managed according to best practice, the vast majority of patients can expect cure, and thus good management is mandatory. The annual reported incidence in the UK for 1971–1995 was 2.3 per 100 000 women and 0.9 per 100 000 men, with approximately 900 new cases and 220 deaths recorded every year in England and Wales [6]. More recent data give the incidence in England for year 2000 as 3.3 women and 1.3 men per 100 000, suggesting a possible increase (see NICE Guidelines at www.nice.org.uk). In the USA an estimated 17 000 new cases are diagnosed and 1300 deaths from thyroid cancer occur annually [7]. From large American series the 10-year survival rates for papillary and follicular thyroid cancer were 93–94% and 84–85% respectively [8,9]; local or regional recurrences develop in up to 30% of patients and distant metastases in up to 20% [10,11]; recurrence rate increases with time and 40-year recurrence rates are about 35% [11]. Overall 8–10% of patients with a diagnosis of thyroid cancer die of their disease [9,10]. Figures for European countries showed that 5-year survival for adults with thyroid cancer in England prior to 1998 (64% men, 75% women) was below the European average (72% for men, 80% for women) [12].

Patients at high risk of recurrence and death from thyroid cancer can be identified at the time of diagnosis by considering well-established prognostic factors, the principal indicators for poor prognosis being extremes of age, male gender, poorly differentiated histological features of the tumor, and tumor stage [10]. Treatment also clearly influences prognosis [11]; in particular the adequacy of surgical treatment and the use of ^{131}I ablation therapy have been shown to result in reduced recurrence rate and lower disease-specific mortality [9,13]. Large retrospective studies [13] have suggested a tendency for improved outcome over the last few years, which again is thought to be a consequence of the increasing use of total thyroidectomy and ^{131}I ablation, as well as other significant factors such as use of serum thyroglobulin (Tg) to monitor for recurrence, and more effective suppression of thyroid-stimulating hormone (TSH) by thyroxine (T_4). Not only has detailed analysis of the data powerfully demonstrated the important effect of meticulous initial therapy on prognosis [11,13], but it also documents the effects of delays in diagnosis and treatment on the mortality rate [9].

The reasons for the relatively poor outcome of DTC in the UK may be multifactorial, but there is evidence that thyroid cancer management in the UK has not been optimal. Audits from several groups have identified severe deficiencies in practice [14–16], which include inadequate surgery, failure to administer radioiodine in cases where it is indicated, inadequate suppression of TSH by T_4, and deficient use of Tg for follow-up; poor communication between specialists and the lack of identified specialist clinics have been highlighted as major contributory factors. In one specialist center deficiencies could be demonstrated in up to 20% of cases, whereas outside the specialist center between 21% and 60% of cases were inadequately managed [16]. Another audit, done prior to the introduction of local guidelines, found that in more than 50% of cases surgery was not done by a member of the multidisciplinary team (MDT), tumor size was not recorded in the case notes, and the extent of tumor removed was inadequate; these figures improved markedly and significantly after guidelines were introduced [17]. In addition, it became apparent from patients' feedback that their quality of life could be improved, particularly with respect to better communication and information.

These various factors – the outcome, the management process, and level of patient satisfaction – indicated the need for guidelines to be developed, for locally agreed protocols to be implemented, and for centralization of expertise and patient management. In developing the guidelines the chief aims were: to improve the long-term overall and disease-free survival of patients with thyroid cancer; to enhance the health-related quality of life of patients with thyroid cancer; to improve the referral pattern and management of patients with thyroid cancer. The guidelines were also intended to provide a basis for local and national audit, and each section offers recommendations that are suitable for the audit process.

In addition to the key recommendations and overview of management, the areas covered by the guidelines include: an introduction which discusses the epidemiology and prognostic factors; presentation, diagnosis, and referral; fine-needle biopsy as the keystone for diagnosis; surgery; radioiodine therapy; posttreatment follow-up; recurrent disease; pathology reporting, grading, and staging of thyroid cancers. Appendices give details of staging, assay methodology and the use of rhTSH. A separate guide for primary care physicians includes advice about diagnosis and referral, together with a summary of treatment and follow-up.

Key Recommendations

The Multidisciplinary Team (MDT)

The most important of the key recommendations is that patients with thyroid cancer should be referred to and managed by a designated MDT (see Chapter 3). The point is made that all clinicians should now accept that management of patients with thyroid cancer outside the framework of the designated MDT is inappropriate. Patients with newly diagnosed or suspected thyroid cancer should be referred to a member of the MDT. Decisions about treatment should be made by the MDT, preferably in the setting of a combined clinic, and follow-up should be done by members of the team. Membership of the MDT will normally be appointed in the UK by the Regional Cancer Network. More details about the functioning of the MDT can be found in Chapter 3 and also in the NICE guidelines for head and neck cancers.

The core team comprises: endocrinologist, surgeon, and oncologist or radiotherapist (or in some instances nuclear medicine physician), all of whom should have received training in, and have expertise and interest in, the management of thyroid cancer, and should maintain continuing professional development. These specialists are supported by: pathologist, medical physicist, biochemist, radiologist, and specialist nurse, all of whom should likewise have special training and experience in the management of patients with thyroid cancer.

Patient Focus

Good communication with the patient is regarded as mandatory, and patients should be included in the decision-making process. Careful thought must be given to the prompt and sensitive communication of the diagnosis to the patient and also to the primary care physician.

Patients should be offered full verbal and written information about their condition and given the opportunity to discuss any aspect of their treatment; also information about support groups and websites. Patients should have continuing access to a member of the team for guidance and support.

To accompany the guidelines three information booklets for patients were produced, in which the information given is staged, to avoid overburdening of the patient at the time of diagnosis. Thus the first booklet is introductory and deals mainly with tests and diagnosis, the second relates to thyroid surgery, and the third to the use of radioiodine. The intention was that every clinic seeing patients with thyroid cancer would have a supply to be used in conjunction with the guidelines.

Diagnosis and Referral

Patients with suspected or newly diagnosed thyroid cancer should be referred to a member of the MDT. Guidelines for the investigation and management of thyroid swellings can be found in Chapter 7. Clinical features which should give rise to suspicion, and which indicate the need for urgent referral (within 2 weeks), are any of the following in association with a thyroid lump: newly presenting lump or increasing in size, a family history of thyroid cancer, a history of previous neck irradiation, young patients (<10 years) or old patients (usually >65 years) especially men, and unexplained hoarseness or voice change. Cervical lymphadenopathy is another indication for prompt referral. Stridor is a late presenting sign and any patient with stridor should be seen immediately.

Diagnostic assessment will include clinical examination, thyroid function tests, thyroid autoantibodies, and fine-needle aspiration cytology (FNAC) with or without ultrasound scan guidance.

Fine-Needle Aspiration Cytology (FNAC) and Pathology

FNAC is an essential diagnostic procedure that is used in the planning of surgery. The cytology should be reported by a cytopathologist who has a special interest in thyroid disease and is a member of the MDT. An adequate sample is required and reports should be based on descriptive text, but should include a numerical coding as a guide towards specific further investigation or therapeutic action.

Surgical samples must be fully documented both macroscopically and microscopically and tumors classified according to the TNM status; the disease can then be staged I to IV.

Initial Treatment

After the initial FNAC for diagnosis and treatment planning, most patients with DTC, especially those with tumors greater than 1 cm, multifocal disease, extrathyroidal spread, familial disease, and those with clinically involved nodes, will undergo total thyroidectomy followed by ^{131}I ablation and TSH suppression.

Surgery

The mainstay of treatment for differentiated thyroid cancer is surgery. The adequacy of the surgical procedure is an important factor determining the outcome: Mazzaferri and Jhiang [9] found a significant difference in mortality rate in patients who received less than near-total thyroidectomy (Figure 2.1), and Hay et al. [13] found a highly significant difference in recurrence rate between unilateral lobectomy and bilateral lobar resection (Figure 2.2).

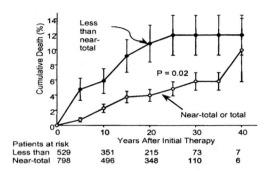

Figure 2.1 Disease-specific mortality in patients treated with total or near-total thyroidectomy compared with patients who underwent less extensive surgery. (Reproduced from Mazzaferri EL, Thyroid cancer: impact of therapeutic modalities on prognosis, Chapter 10 in *Thyroid Cancer* (ed. Fagin JA), Kluwer Academic Publishers, Boston/Dordrecht London, 1998, pages 255–284.)

Patients with a small cancer of 1 cm diameter or less and node negative can be adequately treated by lobectomy followed by TSH suppression (T_4 therapy). Lobectomy alone may also be appropriate treatment for certain other cases known to be at low risk, but this decision should be endorsed by the MDT.

[131]I Therapy

The majority of patients with a tumor size of more than 1 cm diameter should have ^{131}I ablation therapy. Pregnancy or breast-feeding must be excluded before radioactive iodine is administered.

Reassessment with a whole-body radioiodine scan (after stopping T_4 for 4 weeks) is indicated 4–6 months after ^{131}I ablation, although in low risk patients measurement of Tg alone may be adequate. If significant uptake of the tracer is detectable, a further ^{131}I therapy dose should be given and a posttreatment scan obtained. Following this the patient should restart T_4. If there is suspicion of residual disease, further scans should be carried out.

Radioiodine therapy should only be carried out in centers with appropriate facilities and will be administered by an oncologist (or nuclear medicine physician) who is a member of the MDT and holds an appropriate ARSAC (Administration of Radioactive Substances Advisory Committee) certificate.

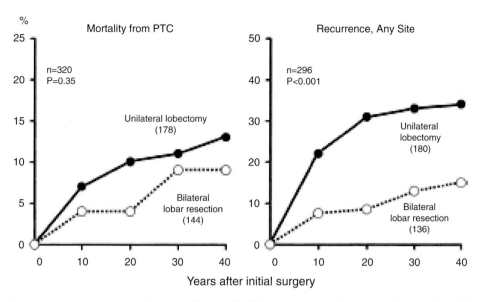

Figure 2.2 Comparison of cumulative disease-specific mortality (left-hand panel) and recurrence (right-hand panel) between patients treated for papillary thyroid cancer by either unilateral lobectomy or bilobar resection. (From Hay ID, McConahey WM, Goellner JR Managing patients with papillary thyroid carcinoma: insights gained from the Mayo Clinic's experience of treating 2512 consecutive patients during 1940 through 2000. *Transactions of the American Clinical and Climatological Association* 2002; 113:241–260.)

TSH Suppression

Life-long suppression of the trophic effect of TSH on tumor cells is one of the main components of treatment. This point was well demonstrated by Mazzaferri [18], who found the cumulative recurrence rate to be significantly less when thyroxine had been given compared with those in whom it was not given (Figure 2.3). Patients should be started on T_4 3 days after ^{131}I therapy and maintained at a dose sufficient to suppress TSH to <0.1 mu/L. T_4 is better than T_3 for long-term treatment and the dose must be sufficient to suppress TSH to <0.1 mu/L (usually 175 μg or 200 μg per day). Thyroxine must be discontinued for 4 weeks before ^{131}I scan or therapy.

Subsequent Management

Follow-up

Surveillance for recurrence of disease is essential and is based on: annual clinical examination, annual measurement of serum Tg and

TSH, and diagnostic scanning when indicated (isotopic imaging and/or ultrasound or CT scan). Follow-up should be life-long because thyroid cancer has a long natural history: late recurrences do occur, which can be successfully treated. Support and counseling are necessary, particularly in relation to pregnancy.

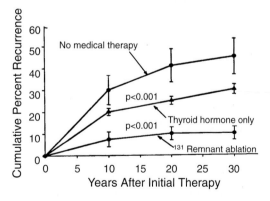

Figure 2.3 Cumulative recurrence rate for DTC related to treatment given after initial surgery. (Reproduced from Mazzaferri EL, Thyroid cancer: impact of therapeutic modalities on prognosis, Chapter 10 in *Thyroid Cancer* (ed. Fagin JA), Kluwer Academic Publishers, Boston/Dordrecht London, 1998, pages 255–284.)

Serum thyroglobulin (Tg) is a very useful tumor marker that is used to monitor for recurrence, in patients who have been treated with thyroidectomy and ^{131}I ablation.

Tg should be checked in all postoperative patients with differentiated thyroid cancer. It is best measured after TSH stimulation, but for routine follow-up of patients in remission it is acceptable to measure it while TSH is suppressed. If the Tg becomes elevated then steps must be taken to identify any focus of recurrent tumor.

Recombinant human TSH is now available and has an evolving role in the management of selected cases [19]. Recombinant human TSH (rhTSH) is used instead of stopping T_3 or T_4 prior to ^{131}I scan or measurement of thyroglobulin, thus avoiding hypothyroidism with its debilitating symptoms. It is clearly indicated in patients who are unable to mount a TSH response to thyroid hormone withdrawal, and also those for whom an episode of hypothyroidism is particularly undesirable, but may be used for any low risk patient for diagnostic purpose, provided serum Tg is undetectable on suppressive thyroxine therapy and anti-Tg antibodies are absent. Its potential therapeutic role has not yet been fully evaluated.

Progressive Disease

External beam radiotherapy is only occasionally used, for patients with T4 (TNM staging) tumors, or distant metastases. There are a number of potential new therapies for the treatment of progressive disease, based on developing knowledge of thyroid cancer biology [for review see 20] and many of these are currently undergoing clinical trial.

Medullary Thyroid Cancer (MTC)

A section of the guidelines is devoted to medullary thyroid cancer (MTC), a rare disease that requires a dedicated, multidisciplinary regional service, dovetailing with that for MEN1 and MEN2. Developments in the molecular genetics of MTC have facilitated a rational framework for management, but the use and interpretation of molecular diagnostics requires careful application in individual patients and their families. Access to a Clinical Genetics Service and *RET* gene testing is therefore essential.

The initial evaluation of suspected MTC includes FNAC and measurement of plasma calcitonin [21,22]. A comprehensive family history is required, to search for features of endocrinopathies of the MEN2 spectrum [23,24]. Endocrinopathies associated with MEN should be sought and all new patients should be screened biochemically for pheochromocytoma. All new patients with MTC should be referred for *RET* mutation testing whether or not there is an evident family history, and this should include exons 10, 11, 13, 14, and 15; screening of exons 10 and 11 alone is an incomplete test.

The mainstay of treatment for MTC is total thyroidectomy and central node dissection; the adequacy of the initial operation largely determines the long-term outcome of the disease. Prophylactic surgery is recommended for disease-free carriers of germline *RET* mutations; the precise mutation found will guide the timing of the surgery [25]. Life-long follow-up is essential and includes monitoring of the tumor marker calcitonin. More detailed consensus guidelines for the diagnosis and management of the MEN2 syndromes are available [25].

The Guidelines Now

Implementation

The intention was that the guidelines be adopted by the individual Regional Cancer Networks in the UK, and that they should be an essential reference for all who are involved in any way with the treatment of patients with thyroid cancer, whether managers, hospital specialists, specialist nurses, primary care physicians, or professional organizations. The onus is on clinicians and managers and other members of the MDTs, to ensure that the necessary recommendations and changes to organization and practice are put into effect. It is much to be hoped that implementation of the guidelines through local protocols is resulting in the fulfillment of the stated objectives and the delivery of high quality care across the UK, with subsequent improvement in survival and quality of life for patients with thyroid cancer.

Audit

Regular audit of outcomes and processes should be carried out. All patients with thyroid cancer should be registered, and an appropriate national dataset for this purpose is in the process of development in the UK by the NHS Information Authority. Prospective data collection will allow audit of national outcomes and will provide the potential for assessment of different treatment modalities.

Revision and Update

It was the expectation that a full review of the guidelines would take place 3 years after their publication. This will need to take particular note of new developments and recent publications. In this context the sections that will clearly require modification are those relating to use of rhTSH, the measurement of thyroglobulin, the use of ^{18}fluorodeoxyglucose positron emission tomography (^{18}F-FDG-PET) scanning in recurrent or metastatic disease, and the treatment of progressive disease.

Summary

This chapter has reviewed the UK guidelines for the management of thyroid cancer and made reference to other available guidelines. The objective for clinicians involved in treating thyroid cancer must be to achieve lower recurrence rate and lower mortality rate. This will require early diagnosis and treatment, specialist management of patients by an MDT, adherence to guidelines, better detection of recurrence, and more effective treatment for progressive disease. In addition, clinicians should aim for improved wellbeing of the patient, and to that end consideration must be given to improving communication as well as the avoidance of hypothyroidism.

References

1. British Thyroid Association. Guidelines for the management of thyroid cancer in adults. London: Royal College of Physicians, 2002.
2. Singer PA, Cooper DS, Daniels GH, et al. Treatment guidelines for patients with thyroid nodules and well-differentiated thyroid cancer. Arch Intern Med 1996; 156:2165–2172.
3. Mazzaferri EL. NCCN thyroid carcinoma practice guidelines. Oncology 1999; 13:391–442.
4. Cobin RH, Gharib H. AACE/AAES Medical/surgical guidelines for clinical practice: management of thyroid carcinoma. Endocr Pract 2001; 7:202–220.
5. NHS Manual of Cancer Services Standards 2000: http://www.doh.gov.uk/cancer/mcss.htm.
6. Coleman PM, Babb P, Damiecki P, et al. Cancer survival trends in England and Wales 1971–1995: Deprivation and NHS region. (Series SMPS No. 61.) London: Stationery Office, 1999: 471–478.
7. Landis SH, Murray T, Bolden S, Wingo PA. Cancer statistics. CA Cancer J Clin 1998; 48:6–29.
8. Hundahl SA, Fleming ID, Fremgen AM, Menck HR. A National Cancer Data Base report on 53 856 cases of thyroid carcinoma treated in the US, 1985–1995. Cancer 1998; 83:2638–2648.
9. Mazzaferri EL, Jhiang SM. Long-term impact of initial surgical and medical therapy on papillary and follicular thyroid cancer. Am J Med 1994; 97:418–428.
10. Schlumberger MJ. Papillary and follicular thyroid carcinoma. N Engl J Med 1998; 338:297–306.
11. Mazzaferri EL, Kloos RT. Clinical review. Current approaches to primary therapy for papillary and follicular thyroid cancer. J Clin Endocrinol Metab 2001; 86: 1447–1463.
12. Teppo L, Hakulinen and Eurocare Working Group. Variation in survival of adult patients with thyroid cancer in Europe. Eur J Cancer 1998; 34:2238–2252.
13. Hay ID, McConahey WM, Goellner JR. Managing patients with papillary thyroid carcinoma: insights gained from the Mayo Clinic's experience of treating 2512 consecutive patients during 1940 through 2000. Trans Am Clin Climatol Assoc 2002; 113:241–260.
14. Hardy KJ, Walker BR, Lindsay RS, Kennedy RL, Seckl JR, Padfield PL. Thyroid cancer Management. Clin Endocrinol 1995; 42:651–655.
15. Vanderpump MPJ, Alexander L, Scarpello JHB, Clayton RN. An audit of management of thyroid cancer in a district general hospital. Clin Endocrinol 1998; 48:419–424.
16. Kumar H, Daykin J, Holder R, Watkinson JC, Sheppard MC, Franklyn JA. An audit of the management of differentiated thyroid cancer in specialist and non-specialist clinic settings. Clin Endocrinol 2001; 54:719–723.
17. Phillips AW, Fenwick JD, Mallick UK, Perros P. The impact of clinical guidelines on surgical management in patients with thyroid cancer. Clin Oncol 2003; 15:485–489.
18. Mazzaferri EL. Thyroid cancer: impact of therapeutic modalities on prognosis. In: Fagin JA (ed.) Thyroid cancer. Boston/Dordrecht, London: Kluwer Academic Publishers, 1998: 255–284.
19. Robbins RJ, Robbins AK. Recombinant human thyrotropin and thyroid cancer management. J Clin Endocrinol Metab 2003; 88:1933–1938.
20. Braga-Basaria M, Ringel MD. Beyond radioiodine: a review of potential new therapeutic approaches for thyroid cancer. J Clin Endocrinol Metab 2003; 88(5): 1947–1960.

21. Wells SA, Dilley WG, Farndon JR, et al. Early diagnosis and treatment of medullary thyroid carcinoma. Arch Intern Med 1985; 145:1248–1252.
22. Marsh DJ, McDowall D, Hyland VJ, et al. The identification of false positive responses to the penta-gastrin stimulation test in RET mutation negative members of MEN 2A families. Clin Endocrinol 1996; 44:213–220.
23. Gagel RF, Cote GJ, Martin Bughalo MJG, et al. Clinical use of molecular information in the management of multiple endocrine neoplasia type. Am J Intern Med 1995; 238:333–341.
24. Carlson KM, Bracamontes J, Jackson CE, et al. Parent of origin effects in multiple endocrine neoplasia type 2B. Am J Hum Genet 1994; 55:1076–1078.
25. Brandi ML, Gagel RF, Angeli A, et al Guidelines for diag-nosis and therapy of MEN type 1 and type 2. J Clin Endocrinol Metab 2001; 86:5658–5671.

Obtaining Information

"Guidelines for the management of thyroid cancer in adults" can be obtained from the Publications Department, Royal College of Physicians, 11 St Andrews Place, London NW1 4LE, UK.

The Patient Information booklets can be obtained from the British Thyroid Founda-tion, PO Box 97, Clifford, Wetherby, West Yorkshire LS23 6XD, UK.

Guidelines and patient information booklets can also be viewed at: www.British-Thyroid-Association.org.

3

Thyroid Cancer Multidisciplinary Team and the Organizational Paradigm

Ujjal K. Mallick

"Once a paradigm through which to view nature has been found there is no such thing as research in the absence of any paradigm. To reject one paradigm without simultaneously substituting another is to reject science itself." (Thomas S. Kuhn [1])

Abbreviations and Definitions

AACE	American Association of Clinical Endocrinologists
ARSAC	Administration of Radioactive Substances Advisory Committee
BAES	British Association of Endocrine Surgeons
BAHNO	British Association of Head and Neck Oncologists
BTA	British Thyroid Association
Calman –Hine	In 1995 an expert advisory group on cancer (EAGC) was set up with the chief medical officers of health for England and for Wales Sir Kenneth Calman and Dame Deidre Hine, respectively. It made major recommendations about how to improve the organization and delivery of cancer services across the country emphasizing the three major elements of cancer care – primary care, cancer unit, and cancer centers
Cancer center	Larger hospitals dealing with common as well as rarer cancers referred from cancer units. They also provide special diagnostic and therapeutic techniques, like radiotherapy
Cancer network	An organization modeled for cancer services to implement the cancer plan bringing together health service commissioners (health authorities, primary care groups and hospital trusts) and providers (primary and community care and hospitals), the voluntary sector and local authorities. Each network typically serve a population of around 1–2 million people. Cancer networks work together to develop strategic service delivery plans to develop all aspects of cancer services, prevention, screening, diagnosis, treatment, supportive care, and specialist palliative care

Cancer unit	These are established in those district general hospitals that are large enough to have clinical teams with the expertise and facilities to deal with the more common cancers, such as breast, lung, and colorectal (bowel) cancers
DTC	Differentiated thyroid cancer
FNAC	Fine-needle aspiration cytology
IMA	Immunometric assay
IMRT	Intensity modulated radiotherapy – special technique of external beam radiotherapy where high doses can be given to tumors close to vital structures like spinal cord twithout exceeding the tolerance dosage of the vital organ by controlling the energy deposited in real time in different parts of the radiation field by complex computer based treatment planning
IOG	Improving Outcomes Guidance
IR(ME)R	The Ionising Radiation (Medical Exposures) Regulations 2000
IRR	Ionising Radiations Regulations
MCS	Manual of Cancer Services Standards
MDT	Multidisciplinary team
NCCN	National Comprehensive Cancer Network, USA
NICE	National Institute of Clinical Excellence. Gives health professionals advice on providing their NHS patients with the highest clinical standards of care. It gives guidance on health technologies, management of specific conditions and safety, cost effectiveness, and efficacy of interventional diagnostic and therapeutic procedures
NSSG	Network (Tumour) Site specific Group
NYCRIS	Northern and Yorkshire Cancer Registry and Information Service
PET	Positron emission tomography
rhTSH	Recombinant human TSH
RIA	Radioimmunoassay

Introduction

The story of management of differentiated thyroid carcinoma in recent years has been a story of shifting paradigms. In many areas new ones have been developed or are being developed, indicating significant advances in the approach to the management of thyroid cancer. These are covered in several chapters in this book and a short list is given below:

1. Preoperative molecular diagnosis on fine-needle aspiration (FNA) cytology.
2. Genome-wide expression profiling (genomics), transcriptomics, proteomics, and metabolomics for molecular risk categorization.
3. Development of consensus guidelines in several countries for optimal management of thyroid cancer.
4. Extent of initial surgery.
5. The role of high dose versus low dose radioiodine treatment for differentiated thyroid cancer.
6. Consensus in strategies of follow-up for differentiated thyroid cancer.
7. Role of recombinant human TSH (rhTSH) in diagnosis and management.
8. The role of sodium iodide symporter gene and molecular targeting in thyroid cancer.
9. Development of service standards and organizational framework for the multidisciplinary team management of thyroid cancer.
10. Patient and carer involvement in management decisions.

The development of service standards and the multidisciplinary team management of thyroid cancer has been another major conceptual shift in the overall management of thyroid cancer, certainly in the UK.

Thyroid Cancer Management – Patterns of Care Studies

Until recently we had a kind of Panglossian view about the outcome of thyroid cancer [2]. It was thought that thyroid cancer was rare and highly curable and that the management process was very satisfactory with the best possible outcome. However, there is evidence that the incidence of papillary thyroid cancer is rising worldwide [3] and the survival figures for thyroid cancer in the UK are worse than the European average [4]. While factors such as registration and case mix might partly explain this difference it is also likely that differences in management strategies have a significant effect on overall survival.

The thyroid cancer service in the UK in the past has been rather patchy, inconsistent, and fragmented and did not follow any specific guidelines. Recent publications have suggested that there is considerable room for improvement. Reports from other countries also suggested the need for more organization of multidisciplinary management and treatment according to consensus guidelines [5–11].

The author was involved with a recent study in the north of England which looked at all thyroid cancer patients diagnosed between 1998 and 1999 (234 patients) and examined responses from 48 consultants and 10 other healthcare professionals involved in treating thyroid cancer patients in 2001 and 2002. The conclusion was that prior to the publication of local and national guidelines, practice in this region was not very satisfactory. It was found that 18% of pathology results were incorrect. After review of histology, 18% of patients had a different prognosis and 8% had a different treatment plan as a result. FNA cytology was not widely used and experienced cytologists were not available; 33% of patients were operated on by a surgeon who performed fewer than five surgical procedures for thyroid cancer a year. However, in 2001 half the surgeons questioned were operating on more than 20 cases of nonmalignant thyroid disease. Fewer than half the patients had satisfactory discussion that was documented in the notes or had adequate written information provided about their illness [7].

Volume–Outcome Relationships, Centralization (Regionalization) of Service

A group called "The Leapfrog Group" (www.leapfroggroup.org) has been set up in the USA recommending that patients are referred to high volume hospitals for major surgical interventions such as esophagectomy, pancreatectomy, and coronary arterial bypass graft on the basis that outcomes of high risk procedures in high volume hospitals are better than in low volume hospitals.

While much discussion is taking place about the implications of this approach it is also becoming clear from many publications that outcomes of major and specialized cancer surgery and treatment of rare cancers like thyroid cancer have a positive volume–outcome relationship in that outcomes might be better in high volume hospitals than in hospitals that see only a few patients a year [12–16].

On the basis of these and other publications it may be that in the future thyroid cancer surgery and management will be centralized or concentrated in higher volume settings, which in other countries is a concept known as "regionalization" [17,18].

Multidisciplinary Team (MDT) – Advantages and Disadvantages

In the Introduction to "NHS Cancer Plan, Three Year Progress Report – Maintaining the Momentum" the National Cancer Director, Professor Mike Richards, said that the establishment of specialist cancer teams across the country has been one of the most important developments in recent years. "These multidisciplinary teams bringing together surgeons, radiologists, pathologists, oncologists, palliative care specialists and other professionals are now helping to ensure that patients receive appropriate investigations and treatment and they are helping to deliver co-ordinated care within the hospitals." He also said "The primary secondary and tertiary level services need to work closely together and that is what has been achieved by the Cancer Networks, which facilitate service planning and co-ordination across the institutional boundaries" [19].

The advantages of a multidisciplinary team looking after thyroid cancer are well known and have been detailed in the recent Improving Outcomes Guidance (IOG) by NICE [20]. The most important benefit of multidisciplinary working is that each individual patient gets the most appropriate treatment decision made by a team of experts. It is possible to consider each single patient from a range of view points from people with different areas of expertise. This ensures that each patient is offered the best possible treatment currently available. Structured organization of MDT meetings is crucial so that different professionals can make their contribution without being present for the whole of the meeting if this is not necessary, thereby saving staff time. The key requirement is that each discipline is able to contribute independently to the decisions so that individual patients get the most appropriate treatment decision.

It can also improve communication and coordination of communication between professionals and patients and carers and coordination throughout the service. It is an effective framework for maintaining uniformity of treatment delivery across the country. Auditable standards will lead to improving the service continually. Continuing professional development of members and adherence to published guidelines can be supported and monitored.

It also speeds up and streamlines the referral process and thereby reduces undesirable delay in starting treatment.

The disadvantage of course is that this is quite time intensive and is resource dependent. Proper resourcing of manpower and facilities are required for the professionals to provide the time necessary for regular multidisciplinary meetings.

Each thyroid MDT should be typically covering a population base of 1 million in the UK and it may not be possible to institute all the recommendations at once. Therefore prioritization is going to have to be made and desirable MDT functioning can only be achieved gradually over a period of time. It is estimated that the cost of setting up MDT functioning in the UK might be more than two to three million pounds for head and neck cancer only. For thyroid cancer MDT the expenses would be mainly the appointment of adequate staff including specialist nurses, MDT coordinators and support staff to allow them to have their MDT meetings and to participate in regular audit and studies [20]. The cost of provision of services, such as the provision of neck lump clinics, recombinant human TSH, and access to PET scans etc., would also be significant.

Importance of the MDT in Thyroid Cancer Management

The importance of MDT working for thyroid cancer is well recognized and is recommended by most thyroid clinicians across the world. In the UK the British Thyroid Association Guidelines have recommended that MDT working should be a mandatory requirement for any center involved in the management of thyroid cancer [21–30].

The recent executive report published by the Northern and Yorkshire Cancer Registry and Information Service (NYCRIS) in June 2004 revealed that fewer than half the clinicians who responded did belong to an MDT in 2001–2002. It also concluded that the value of MDTs cannot be overstated and the suboptimal service that existed in the past can only be improved by the institution of MDT management as recommended by the national guidelines [7].

Multidisciplinary Team Organization in Different Countries

The MDT in the USA mostly comprises of endocrinologists, nuclear medicine specialists who do the nuclear medicine components, pathologists who are familiar with these tumors, radiologists who perform the other imaging studies such as positron emission tomography (PET), endocrine and head and neck surgeons, and radiotherapy specialists who get involved with external beam radiotherapy. The primary care practitioners do not get very involved in management, but are key players in the identification of thyroid nodules. Oncology nurses are not usually involved in the care of patients with thyroid cancer. Most medical centers have a tumor board comprising these specialists and that group tends to help formulate the overall plan of management for thyroid cancer. In most cases, endocrinologists take the lead and arrange long-term follow-up. Many of the endocrinologists also do office ultrasonography (E. Mazzaferri, personal communication).

In Italy the thyroid cancer service is provided mainly by five or six major centers and all of them have well-established MDTs. The endocrinologists take a lead role and nuclear medicine physicians deal with the radioiodine treatments. The composition of teams is more or less the same as in the UK and USA. Meetings take place according to caseload, for example once a month or more frequently. The catchment population varies as some centers act as national and international centers of excellence. In smaller centers not all cases are necessarily discussed in the MDT but patients with complex management problems are discussed. As elsewhere specialist nurses and primary care physicians are not regularly involved in all centers (F. Pacini, personal communication).

In Germany several Regional Tumour Registries were set up many years ago but they were not directly involved with day-to-day treatment. Over the last 2–3 years MDTs for thyroid cancer have been operational in university hospitals. Currently about a third of the university hospitals have established MDTs. They tend to follow national consensus guidelines for management, which were developed about 5 years ago. Smaller centers tend to refer thyroid cancer patients to these university hospitals for management. The group composition is the same as elsewhere, with nuclear medicine specialists taking the lead role. They arrange radioiodine treatments and subsequent follow-up after surgery (C. Reiners, personal communication).

In France all the ten large cancer networks have MDTs for thyroid cancer. The team consists of a nuclear medicine physician, endocrinologist, pathologist, surgeon, and a radiotherapist and oncologist. Endocrinologists, largely, and sometimes nuclear medicine physicians, take a lead role in follow-up. The radioiodine is administered by the nuclear medicine physicians. Large centers have a weekly MDT meeting and some see up to 300 new patients a year. Specialist nurses and general practitioners are not always involved (E. Baudin, personal communication).

In the UK most big centers and some big cancer units now have MDTs as a mandatory requirement within the National Cancer Plan. Compliance with the standards is currently very variable. Large centers achieve most of the priority 1* standards while the smaller units still find it difficult. The main problem is time constraints for staff in hard-pressed specialties who have to attend several cancer MDTs, for example

oncologists radiologists, pathologists, and lack of specialist nurses and support for the MDT. However, commitment and support is being provided by networks and hospital trusts and publication of the NICE IOG will certainly improve the situation. Mostly clinical oncologists and in some centers nuclear medicine specialists conduct the radioiodine treatment. Clinical oncologists, surgeons, and endocrinologists arrange shared or joint clinic follow-up. Further details are provided later in the chapter and especially in the summary table (see Table 3.1).

In India thyroid cancer is generally managed by a team consisting of nuclear medicine physicians, surgeons, radiotherapist, endocrinologist, and very rarely, a medical oncologist. The nuclear medicine physician generally is the lead and arranges long-term follow-up. These teams are restricted only to very few major specialist centers in big cities. Some big centers treat up to 400–500 patients with radioiodine each year. Generally the team meets weekly, depending on caseload (C. S. Bal, personal communication).

In Australia the multidisciplinary teams and clinics are confined to capital cities and major regional centers. They usually consist of an endocrinologist, radiation oncologist, a surgeon, and generally a pathologist. They usually meet weekly, depending on the caseload. In some centers about five to six new cases are seen a week from a population of about 3.75 million. In situations like this, where there is such a center covering 1.6 million square kilometers in area and such a big population, the local general practitioners often have to arrange additional diagnostic tests locally before appropriate referral to the center (G. Mitchell, personal communication).

The Structure and Function of the Thyroid Cancer MDT in the UK – the NICE Guidance

The National Institute of Clinical Excellence published an "improvement in outcomes" guidance for head and neck cancer in November 2004. This is a most comprehensive assessment of the service and will provide detailed and definitive advice about service configuration and commissioning of cancer services for thyroid cancer as well. The following is a summary. For the details the reader is advised to consult the manual [20] or the website – www.nice.org.uk.

The responsibility of the thyroid MDT would be to provide a service usually for a population base of over 1 million and generally should be established in a cancer center or involve several cancer units.

Thyroid cancer MDT can either be part of a currently existing head and neck cancer team or operate as a separate endocrine oncology team who discuss predominantly malignant but also benign thyroid conditions.

The MDT should be responsible for the diagnosis, assessment, decisions about treatment and overall management of patients throughout the course of the disease and also provide support.

The MDT should decide what would be the most appropriate treatment for individual patients and where and by whom it should be carried out.

Teams should be responsible for providing the highest quality of care promptly and efficiently and provide information to patients, their primary care physicians, and all professionals concerned.

The MDT should also support, advise, and educate professionals who provide services for these patients outside of the cancer center and therefore may have to provide an outreach service.

The MDT should make arrangements for referral at each stage of the patient's treatment, which should be streamlined.

A named member of the core team should be the principal clinician to whom the patient should relate at one particular time.

MDT coordinators should organize a meeting at a specific time and on a regular basis.

Audit would be a central feature regarding clinical outcomes, and patient and carer surveys should also be carried out.

The MDT should also take responsibility for making sure that comprehensive data collection takes place regarding the patient's stage, treatment decision, and outcomes, and that regular audits are undertaken.

There have been a lot of publications about a positive volume and outcome relationship, particularly in oncology, and it would appear that outcome is likely to be better in centers with a larger volume of work in thyroid cancer surgery and management than in centers that see only a few patients a year, as already indicated earlier in this chapter. In the long term, it is likely that surgery will be centralized so that it is done by specialized surgeons.

Also more reliable and meaningful audits or studies can be carried out and skills can be maintained and improved in rare cancers like thyroid cancer if large numbers are concentrated in a center and treated by a small number of experts [20].

These measures will lead to the provision of uniform and high quality care across the country.

MDT Standards and Manual of Cancer Services Standards (MCS) UK, 2004

The MCS 2004 [31] details MDT measures which review many aspects of the MDT including structure and function recommended by the NICE IOG and some key points are mentioned below. It currently covers the generic MDT and MDT for common cancers such as breast or lung for which the IOG have been published for some time. The thyroid and head and neck cancer MDT measures will be published soon.

Definition of MDT

The most practical definition suggested by the Manual of Cancer Services Standards UK, published in July 2004, is given below.

This is best answered from the patient's point of view. If you were a patient, who would you consider to be your MDT?

Primarily it is that group of people of different health care disciplines, which meets together at a given time (whether physically in one place, or by video or tele-conferencing) to discuss a given patient and who are each able to contribute independently to the diagnostic and treatment decisions about the patient. They constitute that patient's MDT [31].

The actual composition of the MDT of course will vary, depending on which tumor site the team is supposed to manage, and for the thyroid cancer specific MDT is detailed in Table 3.1.

The Objectives of MDT

The key objective is to provide each individual patient with the best possible management decisions currently available. Again the definition of this as mentioned in the MCS is as follows:

- To ensure that designated specialists work effectively together in teams such that decisions regarding all aspects of diagnosis, treatment, and care of individual patients and decisions regarding the team's operational policies are multidisciplinary decisions.
- To ensure that care is given according to recognized guidelines (including guidelines for onward referrals) with appropriate information being collected to inform clinical decision-making and to support clinical governance/audit.
- To ensure that mechanisms are in place to support entry of eligible patients into clinical trials, subject to patients giving fully informed consent [31].

The Proposed Structure and MDT Standards for Thyroid Cancer

The details of the standards and the measures to achieve the required compliance are obviously not relevant to clinicians in other countries but there is similarity in many aspects and it may provide a basis for further developments.

A proposed thyroid MDT standards list is given in Table 3.1. This has been modified from the Breast Cancer Standards 2004 and therefore is not the definitive document. Thyroid cancer MDT measures based on the NICE IOG will be published by the Department of Health in due course. However, Table 3.1 will give some idea about the comprehensive nature of the standards that an MDT will have to follow and can act as a discussion paper for development of multidisciplinary practice for any center wanting to develop a reliable service framework.

The unique feature is that these standards are auditable and can be monitored.

For further details the reader is advised to go to the website – www.dh.gov.uk.

Peer Review

The functions of the MDT are supported by cancer centers and cancer units, and audit of the standards is facilitated by external peer review visits to assess compliance and to provide support and suggestions for improvement. If there are any areas of noncompliance with suboptimal service provision the trust and the networks are provided with support with resources to correct this before the peer review visit, which will take place every 3 years.

The National Manual of Quality Measures for Cancer Peer Review 2004 (www.dh.gov.uk/ policy and guidance) has also been published following the positive evaluation of the first round of cancer peer review in 2001.

Cancer peer review visits "aim to improve care for people with cancer and their families by ensuring that services are as safe as possible, improving the quality and effectiveness and care, improving the patient and carer experience, undertaking independent fair reviews of services, providing development and learning for all involved and encouraging the dissemination of good practice." The process of peer review will encompass not only quality measures but also the whole system of patient care and the patient and carer experience.

It is expected that a peer review will mandatorily review all MTDs for cancer types that have so far been covered by the Improving Outcomes Guidance processes detailed by NICE. Therefore it will eventually cover functioning of thyroid cancer MDTs in due course. It will assess compliance with the MDT standards as indicated in Table 3.1 in addition to other aspects of the service as indicated above [31,32].

The Future and Development of International Best Practice Models

In the absence of randomized controlled trials the treatment of thyroid cancer across the world is largely based on national guidelines and consensus statements. Although different centers in different countries have their own framework for commissioning and service delivery for thyroid cancer, there are some common

Table 3.1 The multidisciplinary team (MDT) for local thyroid cancer

Measure number	Measure	Level
	MDT leadership	
1	Single named lead clinician	1*
2	Agreed responsibilities with host hospital trust lead clinician	1*
	Team criteria	
3	MDT listed as part of the named services within the network locality	1*
	MDT structure	
4	Named core members of the MDT specialist surgeon, endocrinologist, oncologists, or nuclear medicine physician, pathologist, medical physicist, radiologist, specialist nurse.	1*
5	Team attendance at NSSG meetings	1*
6	Named lead histopathologist	1*
7	Named lead imaging consultant	1*
8	All consultants core members of at least one MDT	1*
9	Two named core team members from each professional group	1
	MDT meeting	
10	If separate prediagnostic MDT membership named	1*
11	*Thyroid-specific standard*	1*
	Meet regularly (weekly, fortnightly, or monthly depending on caseload) and record core attendance and protocols for referral before next scheduled meeting	
12	Core member (or cover) present for half of meetings	1*
13	Core members (or cover) present for two-thirds of meetings	1
14	MDT agreed cover arrangements for core member	1*
	Operational policies	
15	Annual meeting to discuss operational policy	1*
16	Policy for all new patients to be reviewed by MDT	1*
17	Policy for communication of diagnosis to GP	1
18	Completed audit of timeliness of diagnosis notification	1
19	Written policy to provide general practitioners or primary care trusts with data on timeliness of urgent referrals	1
20	Operational policy for named key worker	1*
21	Implementation of key worker policy	1
22	*Thyroid-specific standard*	
	Core MDT clinical consultants spend at least one to two direct clinical care session for thyroid cancer every week (for discussion depending on caseload and local variables)	1
23	*Thyroid-specific standard*	
	Core MDT nurse spends at least 50% of time on thyroid cancer (for discussion)	1
24	*Thyroid-specific standard*	
	Thyroid cancer clinicians would be trained to appropriate guidelines, for example BAHNO (British Association of Head and Neck Oncologists, Otolaryngologists), British Association of Endocrine Surgeons, British Thyroid Association, ARSAC, IRR, IR(ME)R etc.	1*
25	Written agreement between MDT and other clinicians who are not regular core members of the MDT	1
26	*Thyroid-specific standard*	
	Core MDT nuclear medicine specialist has reported a minimum number of I^{131} scans and delivered a minimum number of high dose I^{131} therapy. The number to be discussed by professional organizations according to region and workload	1*
27	*Thyroid-specific standard*	
	Lead clinician ensures with relevant core members that sensitive and reliable thyroglobulin assay (IMA or RIA) and thyroglobulin antibody assessments are available	1*
28	*Thyroid-specific standard*	
	Lead clinician ensures that facilities for recombinant human TSH, PET scanning are available (depending on local variables)	1
29	*Thyroid-specific standard*	
	Lead clinician ensures that a written protocol for radio iodine administration agreed by the MDT is available	1*
	Lead clinician ensures optimum facilities are available for delivering high dose radioiodine ablation and treatment by trained clinicians following the Ionising	1*
	Radiation Regulations, which are carried out in the referral hospital which acts as a catchment area for this MDT and maintains their caseload	1*
	MDT nurse specialist	

Table 3.1 *Continued*

Measure number	Measure	Level
30	Core nurse member undertaking or enrolled for specialist study	1*
31	Core nurse member completed specialist study	1
32	Core nurse member undertaking or enrolled for communication skills study	1*
33	Core nurse member completed communication skills study	1
34	Agreed responsibility for core nurse members	1*
35	Agreed list of additional responsibilities for management and research for the core nurse member	1*
36	*Thyroid-specific standard*	
	Extended membership of MDT: Specialist palliative care, consultant clinical psychologist, biochemist, medical oncologist, geneticist	1*
	Team function	
37	Agreement for communication to patients and policy for access to MDT by patients/carers	1*
38	Patient permanent consultation record	1*
39	Patient experience survey	1*
40	Presentation and discussion of patient experience survey	1
41	Implementation of action point arising from survey	1
42	Provision of written patient information	1*
43	Patient notes checklist	1
44	Agree and record individual patient treatment planning decision	1*
	Clinical guidelines	
45	Network site-specific group agreed clinical guidelines	1*
46	Network site-specific group agreed referral guidelines	1*
	Imaging guidelines	
47	Network site-specific group agreed diagnosis, assessment imaging guidelines	1*
	Pathology guidelines	
48	Network site-specific group agreed diagnosis, assessment pathology guidelines	1*
	Follow-up guidelines	
49	*Thyroid-specific standard*	1*
	MDT/Network agreed guidelines for thyroid cancer follow-up	
	Data collection	
50	MDT/Network agreed collection of minimum data set	1*
51	MDT/Network site-specific group agreed policy for the electronic collection of specific portions of minimum data set (MDS)	1*
52	One year's cancer registry % return	1*
53	Registry return compared to patient numbers discussed at MDT	1*
	Network audit	
54	MDT/Network site-specific group agreed participation in network audit	1*
55	MDT present results from participation in audit to NSSG	1
	Trial	
56	MDT/Network-site specific group agreed list of approved studies and trials (although rare for thyroid cancer)	1
	Service improvement	
57	MDT agreed core member responsible for integration of service improvement	1*
58	Patient cancer journey process mapping and action plan	1*
59	One resulting service improvement action point with supporting data	1*
60	Network service improvement lead capacity/demand study	1
61	Patient choice to pre-book 2-week wait referral appointment	1*
62	Patient choice to pre-book first diagnostic test appointment	2
63	Patient choice to choose and pre-book elective admission date	1*
64	Patient choice to choose and pre-book first treatment date	2
65	*Thyroid-specific standard – for discussion*	1*
	Workload of at least 25 new patients per year (benign and malignant) for surgeons. Possibly the same number of new thyroid cancer patients for the other core members of the MDT. It would of course vary from area to area and geographic location and the size of the catchment population	

Key to table: Level of standards have been classified such that the level 1 and level 2 indicate relative priority that cancer networks should give to the achievement. Some level 1 standards, which are asterisked, are standards the network should as a priority ensure are in place.

Crown copyright material is reproduced with the permission of the Controller of HMSO and the Queen's Printer for Scotland.

themes. It is therefore also possible that a synthesis from these existing frameworks may in the future lead to a consensus and development of international best practice models for service delivery, service redesign, and modernization. This of course needs to take into consideration geographical and societal factors, healthcare systems and healthcare priorities of the local population and financial constraints.

MDT Management Pathway for Differentiated Thyroid Cancer at a Glance – an Example

Introduction

- Management decisions for thyroid cancer are based largely on retrospective studies with level of evidence at III/IV and grades of recommendation at level B/C.
- Appropriate national guidelines, for example BTA, AACE, NCCN, or other consensus guidelines should be followed.
- Setting up a regular MDT meeting with a core group of specialists as indicated in Table 3.1 is the first step. Members of the extended team should be contacted as and when necessary.
- Clinicians who are not members of the MDT should refer patients onwards to a core member of the MDT.
- Cytology and pathology, surgery, radioiodine therapy, and endocrine and genetic aspects of management in particular should be restricted to specialists.
- Structured organization of MDT meetings is crucial to prevent wastage of staff time.
- All new and old patients with management problems should be discussed in the MDT for truly multidisciplinary decisions which are properly recorded and disseminated promptly to appropriate members.
- The patient should be provided with adequate written information or other sources, such as video or CD–ROM, approved by the team. The patient should be offered the opportunity to pre-visit the

radioiodine suite and meet another patient who has had treatment if the patient so wishes.

- The treatment plan, the supporting evidence, outcome, and side effects should be fully and openly discussed with each patient before being asked to give informed consent.
- The importance of Involving the informed patient in the decision-making process is paramount.
- Patients should have easy access to the key MDT member at each stage of treatment and have support and counseling.
- Continuing professional development of members is essential.
- Many of the above suggestions are part of professional self-regulation and largely resource-neutral and achievable even in developing countries where other clinical priorities may make the following suggestions unrealistic and impossible at present.
- Complying with the thyroid-specific standards and priority 1* standards as far as practicable commensurate with local variables, caseload, financial and staffing resources is the next step.
- At least two audit projects and patient surveys a year and taking action on the basis of these are recommended.
- This exists in many developed countries in different formats and many parts of the UK but achieving all standards will need time, resources, and support from the cancer networks.
- It is helpful to have the views of patient support groups or patient panels for policy decisions regarding service development issues.

These are summary points. Please consult relevant chapters for the evidentiary scientific basis, detailed discussion, and references about the options mentioned below, which represent one viewpoint but not how an individual patient should be treated.

Primary Care

- Referral guidelines and guidelines for primary care should be followed.

- Primary care has an important role in multidisciplinary management of thyroid cancer in the UK.
- Easy and quick access to key MDT members is vital.
- Suspicious thyroid nodules or lumps (especially with the following features) should be referred to a surgeon or endocrinologist of the MDT.
  (a) New nodule or old nodule increasing in size.
  (b) Nodule in a patient with a family history of thyroid cancer.
  (c) Nodule in a patient with a history of neck irradiation.
  (d) Nodule in the extremes of age, <10, >65.
  (e) Nodule with unexplained hoarseness and voice changes.
  (f) Nodule with cervical lymph node.
  (g) Rarely stridor with a large thyroid swelling (urgent referral needed) [21].
- Only thyroid function tests required before referral (in some places ultrasound may be appropriate).
- Help from primary care may be required with optimal TSH suppression (TSH <0.1) in most cases (or low normal if appropriate).
- Support required from primary care during pregnancy, recurrent disease, for hypocalcemia, and regarding long-term effects of high dose thyroxine on bone and cardiovascular system etc.

Initial Treatment

- Clinical assessment and FNA cytology (with/without ultrasound, sometimes core biopsy) by the surgeon or endocrinologist is the gold standard investigation.
- Other preoperative investigations as appropriate according to approved guidelines.
- Discussion of cytology/biopsy in diagnostic MDT if available or MDT.
- Decision about extent of surgery according to the agreed guidelines of the MDT.
  Near-total or total thyroidectomy + level VI node dissection (preferred by majority).

Mazzaferri, [40] British Thyroid Association (BTA) guidelines, Clark, [41] Hay [42] (low + high risk), Cady [43] (high risk only).

Hemithyroidectomy.

Cady (low risk) [43].

- Decision on the need for completion thyroidectomy if follicular carcinoma after hemithyroidectomy for indeterminate cytology.
- Discussion of histology in the MDT following surgery.
- Risk categorization by pTNM (more widely used) or AMES or MACIS.
- Decision on ablation versus no ablation as per MDT guideline.
  (Chapters 1, 17); Sawka et al. [34], Mazzaferri [35].

Mazzaferri, [40] BTA guidelines – routine for >1.5 cm tumors.

Hay [44] – only for MACIS >6 (high risk).

Cady – only for high risk AMES.

- Discussion of diagnosis and treatment plan fully with patient in the presence of a specialist nurse or counselor for support.
- Serious diagnosis of cancer or its complications should be notified to the primary care team within 24 hours in the UK.
- Agreed nuclear medicine departmental protocol for radioiodine administration should be available.
- Decision on low dose(1.1 GBq) or high dose(3 GBq) ablation according to agreed MDT guideline.

Bal (1996 and 2004), Creutzig, [47] Johansen [48] – Low dose (preferred in many countries but not widely practiced yet in the UK).

Doi (meta-analysis) [49] – low dose equally effective mainly after optimal thyroidectomy with a small remnant.

Sirisalipoch (multicenter trial) – low dose not as effective (Chapters 1, 17, 20]) [33].

Follow-up

- Joint clinic or shared follow-up.
- To ensure availability of reliable assay of thyroglobulin (IMA or RIA) and thyroglobulin antibodies [Chapter 18] [36].

- Assessment of ablation at 6–12 months by thyroglobulin (rhTSH or off TSH) with or without diagnostic scan (the latter is becoming routine) (Chapters 1, 17) [37,38].
- rhTSH stimulated thyroglobulin assessment gives reliable information about disease control certainly in low risk cases. The level of thyroglobulin rise may be about half of that after thyroxine withdrawal.
- During subsequent follow-up for low risk cancers if stimulated thyroglobulin (Tg) is >2 (when Tg on T_4 is undetectable, happens in about 20% of cases) further investigation should be considered [37].
- Routine diagnostic scans do not necessarily provide additional information regarding management (except when thyroglobulin antibodies are present).
- Follow up strategies should be based on American or European consensus guidance [37,38].
- Ensuring availability of recombinant human TSH (rhTSH) for follow-up and treatment in appropriate cases.
- Neck ultrasound by an experienced radiologist is very valuable for follow-up and is highly sensitive in detecting residual or recurrent disease along with thyroglobulin assessment after recombinant human TSH [Chapter 17].
- To consider whether full TSH suppression (<0.1) is necessary long term for low risk cases after rhTSH stimulated thyroglobulin becomes undetectable after initial treatment in view of long-term effects of high thyroxine on bone and heart [38].
- Support and advice required regarding childbearing in appropriate cases.
- Support and advice required regarding long-term side effects, especially ^{131}I-related late effects, surgery-related voice changes and long-term hypocalcemia; osteoporosis, and cardiac effects of long-term TSH suppression.
- Strategy for long-term follow-up in conjunction with primary care needs to be agreed.

Recurrent Disease

- Discussion of all recurrent and metastatic disease in the MDT which may need multidisciplinary management of complex problems.
- PET scan should be available, especially for patients with raised thyroglobulin and negative scan.
- Surgery, radioiodine, external beam radiotherapy, and combinations are the main treatment options for recurrent disease; in a small proportion of patients embolization, redifferentiation therapy, and therapeutic radiolabeled octreotide may be of use.
- Radioactive iodine – it is preferable to keep the cumulative radioiodine doses to <20 GBq (Schlumberger, [50] especially if the patient has also had external beam radiotherapy) or at least below 40 GBq if clinical situation allows. The time interval between repeated radioiodine treatment doses should be kept to about 12 months and not less than 6 months if possible unless there is rapidly progressive disease. This probably minimizes long-term side effects of radioiodine. Fixed dose (5–7 GBq) is common or dosimetry-based doses can be used (Chapters 1, 15).
- External beam radiotherapy – three-dimensional conformal radiotherapy should be used in appropriate cases as an adjuvant (if gross macroscopic and microscopic residual disease and further surgery is not suitable) or for recurrent cancer in the neck if further surgery or radioactive iodine is not appropriate. Dose: 50–60 Gy over 5–6 weeks or its radio-biological equivalent. Up to 66 Gy to large volume disease if necessary. Maximum spinal cord dose 46 Gy in 2 Gy fractions or equivalent. Field size – (depending on cases):

  Superior – tip of the mastoid or hyoid.

  Inferior – carina or suprasternal notch.

  Lateral – whole width of the neck or tumor with margin.

  Intensity modulated radiotherapy (IMRT) may be used in the future to improve dose distribution (Chapters 1, 15).
- Raised thyroglobulin and negative iodine scan (Chapter 18).

Check strict preparation for the scanning procedure and exclude false-negative scan and false-positive thyroglobulin (presence of heterophil antibodies and residual normal thyroid remnant). Thyroglobulin assessment quite soon after high dose radioiodine treatment might also give high levels which gradually disappear over months, sometimes a year or two.

Routine empirical high dose iodine treatment – Schlumberger, [51] Pineda and others – effective in some cases (Chapter 20).

Selective high dose iodine therapy if necessary after further investigation with neck ultrasound, CT scan, PET etc.– Mazzaferri, Pacini, Wartofsky (see Chapter 1).

- Chemotherapy – Adriamycin or Adriamycin and platinum are active agents. Raised TSH can be used (see Chapter 30). This is for iodine-negative advanced disease when no other options are available. Others are under investigation, for example liposomal anthracycline etc. [33].
- Molecular targeted therapy – small molecule tyrosine kinase inhibitors (gefitinib or Iressa) are under investigation for end-stage radioiodine refractory disease [33].
- Although trials and studies are rare, efforts should be made to design and take part in collaborative clinical and translational studies [39].
- Specialist palliative care and symptom control for end-stage disease and support from clinical psychologists.

Summary

Thyroid cancer should be managed by a multidisciplinary team of experts. This can only provide the best possible care for individual patients for this rare and highly curable cancer.

This does take place in many countries and in recent years this has been made more formalized in the UK as a part of the NHS National Cancer Plan.

Recommendations have been made by NICE (IOG) about the detailed structure and function of a multidisciplinary team specializing in thyroid cancer management in the UK, which should treat a population base of approximately 1 million.

Every MDT in the UK has to comply with the highest possible standards and one of the most comprehensive list (MCS) of these has also been published for most cancers (thyroid awaited). The unique feature is that compliance with these standards is auditable and will be monitored while support will be provided to achieve these objectives.

Treatment should be based on evidence-based guidelines, which should be regularly reviewed, and outcomes should be regularly monitored.

The members of the team should have continuing professional development and should be engaged in regular audit and participation in clinical studies and trials.

The patients must always be given proper information and support and should take part in the decision-making process.

The essential theme is that the treatment should be patient focused and that the service provided should be high quality, fast track, caring and cost-effective to achieve the highest cure rate and the best possible quality of life for our patients.

This particular detailed framework is clearly not relevant for all countries but there may be common themes and it can initiate some helpful discussions, providing a basis for sharing good practice, and indeed can lead to the development of a model for international best practice.

Postscript – Tableau No IV; Lozenge Composition with Red, Gray, Blue, Yellow, and Black by Piet Mondrian

Finally MDT management of thyroid cancer and other cancers is evidenced-based science but it is also an art. Individual team members' contributions develop and compose the most effective and comprehensive treatment plan for each patient (delivering it with utmost care, humanity, and compassion which in itself is an art), as is portrayed in the following famous painting by Piet Mondrian (Figure 3.1).

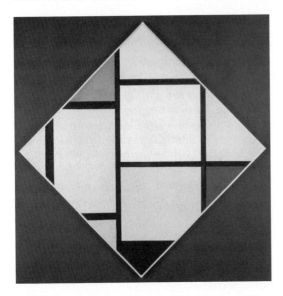

Figure 3.1 Piet Mondrian. Tableau No. IV; Lozenge Composition with Red, Gray, Blue, Yellow, and Black, Gift of Herbert and Nannette Rothschild, Image © 2005 Board of Trustees, National Gallery of Art, Washington, c. 1924/1925, oil on canvas on hardboard.

Acknowledgments. The author gratefully acknowledges relying on and quoting from Department of Health publications and NICE IOG on the subject and especially using the summary table (Table 3.1), which has been modified to design thyroid MDT standards.

The author is very grateful to Professor Mazzaferri, Professor Pacini, Dr Baudin, Professor Reiners, Professor Bal, and Professor Mitchell for helpful information and to the members of the Northern Cancer Network thyroid cancer team for helpful discussions.

Grateful thanks to Mrs Paula Simpson and Mrs Gina Brailey for the preparation of this manuscript.

References

1. Kuhn TS. The Structure of Scientific Revolutions, 2nd edn, Enlarged, Vol 2, No 2 National Encyclopaedia of Unified Science. Chicago: The University of Chicago Press, 1970: 79.
2. Voltaire FMA. Candide, translated by John Butt. London: Penguin Books, 1947.
3. Rossi RL, Majlis S, Rossi RM. Thyroid cancer. Surg Clin North Am 2000; 80:571–580.
4. Teppo L, Hakulinen E and Eurocare Working Group. Variation in survival of adult patients with thyroid cancer in Europe. Eur J Cancer 1998; 34(14):2238–2252.
5. Vanderpump MPJ, Alexander L, Scarpellow JHB, Clayton RM. An audit of management of thyroid cancer in a district general hospital. Clin Endocrinol 1998; 48:419–424.
6. Kumar H, Daykin J, Holder R, Watkinson JC, Sheppard MC, Franklyn JA. An audit of the management of differentiated thyroid cancer in specialist and non-specialist clinical settings. Clin Endocrinol 2001; 54:719–723.
7. Management of Thyroid Cancer in the Northern and Yorkshire Region, 1998–1999. Executive Report June 2004. Northern and Yorkshire Cancer Registry and Information Service. www.nycris.org.uk.
8. Hundahl SA, Fleming ID, Fremgen AM, Menck HR. A National Cancer Data Base report on 53 856 cases of thyroid carcinoma treated in the US, 1985–1995. Cancer 1998; 83(12):2638–2648.
9. Hundahl SA, Cady B, Cunningham MP, et al. Initial results from a prospective cohort study of 5583 cases of thyroid carcinoma treated in the United States during 1996. US and German Thyroid Cancer Study Group. An American College of Surgeons Commission on Cancer Patient Care Evaluation Study. Cancer 2000; 89(1):202–217.
10. Holzer S, Reiners C, Mann K, et al. Patterns of care for patients with primary differentiated carcinoma of the thyroid gland treated in Germany during 1996. US and German Thyroid Cancer Group. Cancer 2000; 89(1):192–201.
11. Hoelzer S, Steiners D, Bauer R, et al. Current practice of radioiodine treatment in the management of differentiated thyroid cancer in Germany. Eur J Nucl Med 2000; 27(10):1465–1472.
12. Birkmeyer JD. Understanding surgeon performance and improving patient outcomes. J Clin Oncol 2004; 22(14):2765–2766.
13. Sosa JA, Bowman HM, Tielach JM, Powe NR, Gordon TA, Udelsman R. The importance of surgeon experience for clinical and economic outcomes from thyroidectomy. Ann Surg 1998; 228:320–328.
14. Lamade W, Renz K, Willeke F, Klar E, Herfarth C. Effect of training on the incidence of nerve damage in thyroid surgery. Br J Surg 86:388–391.
15. Smith TJ, Hillner BE, Bear HD. Taking action on the volume–quality relationship: How long can we hide our heads in the colostomy bag? J Natl Cancer Inst 2003; 95(10):695–697.
16. Zarnegar R, Brunaud L, Clark OH. Prevention, evaluation and management of complications following thyroidectomy for thyroid carcinoma. Endocrinol Metab Clin North Am 2003; 32(2):483–502.
17. Wang L. The volume–outcome relationship: Busier hospitals are indeed better, but why? J Natl Cancer Inst 2003; 95(10):700–702.
18. Kuijpens JL, Hansen B, Hamming JF, Ribot JG, Haak HR, Coebergh J-WW. Trends in treatment and long-term survival of thyroid cancer in Southeastern Netherlands, 1960–1992. Eur J Cancer 1998; 34(8):1235–1241.
19. The NHS Cancer Plan, Three year progress report. Maintaining the momentum. Department of Health, October 2003; The NHS Cancer Plan 2000. www.dh.gov.uk/cancer.

20. Improving Outcomes in Head and Neck Cancer. The Manual, November 2004. National Institute of Clinical Excellence: www.nice.org.uk.
21. British Thyroid Association. Guidelines for the management of thyroid cancer in adults. London: Royal College of Physicians, 2002.
22. Vini L, Harmer C. Management of thyroid cancer. Lancet Oncol 2002; 3(7):407–414.
23. Mallick UK, Lucraft HH, Proud G, et al. Optimising the management of differentiated thyroid cancer. Clin Oncol 2000; 12:363–364.
24. Sherman SI. Thyroid carcinoma. Lancet 2003; 361(9356): 501–511.
25. Tuttle M, Robbins R, Larsen SM. Challenging cases in thyroid cancer: A multidisciplinary approach. Eur J Nucl Med Mol Imaging 2004, 31(4):605–612.
26. Northern Cancer Network Site Specific Thyroid Cancer Group. Management guidelines for thyroid cancer. Newcastle upon Tyne: NCN. Clin Oncol 2000; 12:373–391.
27. Delisle MJ, Schvartz C, Theobald S, Maes B, Vaudrey C, Pochart JM. Cancers of the thyroid. Value of a regional registry on 627 patients diagnosed, treated and followed by a multidisciplinary team. Ann Endocrinol 1996; 57(1):41–49.
28. Kondo T, Tomita K. Thyroid tumour clinical path. Nippon Jibiinkoka Gakkai Kaiho 2001; 104(10):1017–1024.
29. AACE/AAES Medical/Surgical Guidelines for Clinical Practice: Management of Thyroid Carcinoma, Endocr Pract 2001; 7(3):200–220.
30. National Comprehensive Cancer Network. 2003. www.NCCN.org.
31. The Manual of Cancer Services Standards – July 2004: www.dh.gov.uk/cancer.
32. National Manual of Quality Measures for Cancer Peer Review 2004. www.dh.gov.uk/policyandguidance.
33. Mallick UK, Charalambous H. Current issues in the management of differentiated thyroid cancer Nucl Med Commun 2004; 25(9):873–881.
34. Sawka AM, Thephamongkhol K, Brouwers M, Thabane L, Browman G, Gerstein H. A systematic review and metaanalysis of the effectiveness of radioactive iodine remnant ablation for well differentiated thyroid cancer. J Clin Endocrinol Metab 2004; 89(8):3668–3678.
35. Mazzaferri E. A randomised trial of remnant ablation – in search of an impossible dream. J Clin Endocrinol Metab 2004; 89(8):3662–3664.
36. Spencer CA. Challenges of serum thyroglobulin (Tg) measurement in the presence of Tg autoantibodies. J Clin Endocrinol Metab 2004; 89(8):3702–3704.
37. Mazzaferri EL, Robbins RJ, Spencer CA, et al. A consensus report of the role of serum thyroglobulin as a monitoring method for low risk patients with papillary thyroid carcinoma. J Clin Endocrinol Metab 2003; 88(4): 1433–1441.
38. Schlumberger M, Berg G, Cohen O, et al. Follow-up of low risk patients with differentiated thyroid carcinoma: a European perspective. Eur J Endocrinol 2004; 150: 105–112.
39. International Cancer Research Portfolio – www.cancerportfolio.org.
40. Mazzaferri EL, Kloos RT. Current approaches to primary therapy for papillary and follicular thyroid cancer. J Clin Endocrinol Metab 2001; 86:1447–1463.
41. Clark OH, Levin K, Zeng QH, et al. Thyroid cancer: the case for total thyroidectomy. Eur J Cancer Clin Oncol 1988; 24:305–313.
42. Hay ID, Grant CS, Bergstralh EJ, et al. Unilateral total lobectomy: is it sufficient surgical treatment for patients with AMES low-risk papillary thyroid carcinoma? Surgery 1998; 124:958–966.
43. Cady B. Our AMES is true: How an old concept still hits the mark: or, risk group assignment points the arrow to rational therapy selection in differentiated thyroid cancer. Am J Surg 1997; 174:462–468.
44. Hay ID. Papillary thyroid carcinoma. Endocrinol Metab Clin North Am 1990; 19:545–576.
45. Bal C, Padhy AK, Jana S, et al. Prospective randomized clinical trial to evaluate the optimal dose of ^{131}I for remnant ablation in patients with differentiated thyroid carcinoma. Cancer 1996; 77:2574–2580.
46. Bal CS, Kumar A, Pant GS. Radioiodine dose for remnant ablation in differentiated thyroid carcinoma: a randomized clinical trial in 509 patients. J Clin Endocrinol Metab 2004; 89:1666–1673.
47. Creutzig H. High or low dose radioiodine ablation of thyroid remnants? Eur J Nucl Med 1987; 12:500–502.
48. Johansen K, Woodhouse NJ, Odugbesan O. Comparison of 1073 MBq and 3700 MBq iodine-131 in postoperative ablation of residual thyroid tissue in patients with differentiated thyroid cancer. J Nucl Med 1991; 32:252–254.
49. Doi SA, Woodhouse NJ. Ablation of the thyroid remnant and 131I dose in differentiated thyroid cancer. Clin Endocrinol (Oxf) 2000; 52:765–773.
50. Schlumberger MJ. Medical progress – Papillary and follicular thyroid carcinoma. N Engl J Med 1998; 338:297–306.
51. Schlumberger M, Mancusi F, Baudin E, et al. 131-I Therapy for elevated thyroglobulin levels. Thyroid 1997; 7:273–276.

4

Thyroid Cancer from the Perspective of a Patient

Jennifer S. Pitman

In October 1997, following a bit of a cold, I noticed a tiny lump, about the size of a pea, in the middle of my throat. That night I rang Professor Newman-Taylor, who had been such a help in the past, and told him about my discovery. He asked me some questions "did it move up and down when I swallowed?" He then said he thought it was my thyroid and asked me to keep him informed when I had seen my GP.

The next morning our "vet" Charlie Schreiber was at our racing yard blood testing some horses, so I asked him if he could pop into the house when he had finished, where I told him about the lump. He had a good look and also advised me to see my doctor, who arranged an appointment for me with a specialist in Swindon.

When I eventually saw the ENT specialist, he suggested that I was suffering from a virus and advised me to rest; he thought the lump would eventually go away. When Charlie Schreiber called in a few days later he asked how I got on. I told him the advice I had been given by the specialist was to "rest" and casually added "I don't know if that comes in tablet form or it's a liquid!" I remember Charlie was very quiet at first, and kept looking at the floor. Then he said, "I don't like to say this kind of thing Mrs P, but I feel you should seek a second opinion." It so happened I already had an appointment with Professor Newman-Taylor in London at the Royal Brompton Hospital in December to discuss a long-standing allergy problem. He said he

thought I looked really well but when I mentioned the lump in my throat he asked if he could take a look. I said I had already seen a specialist and told him the advice I had been given. Following a gentle and detailed examination the Professor looked skywards and said "That will not go away" and would I mind if he made an appointment for me to visit the Royal Marsden Hospital across the road the same day.

At this point I knew that my husband David and I were struggling, trying not to panic. When someone mentions the Royal Marsden you are bound to be a bit scared. Further examination by Dr Harmer suggested that the lump was a small cyst, some fluid was taken from it, and I was asked to return in 3 months time.

By the time I returned in March, it seemed to me that the cyst had grown a "baby." Once more fluid was removed and I was asked to come back in a further 3 months. The constant worry of this problem hanging over us was becoming unbearable and I was also being nagged by my vets to get the lump removed, which didn't help! Eventually, in May I rang the surgeon, Mr Peter Rhys Evans, and explained that I couldn't cope any longer with the strain that the uncertainty was causing David. I added that in my experience the best way to deal with the problems I had in my life was to remove them, so could he please remove the cyst.

The operation was carried out on 1 June 1998 and at first Mr Rhys Evans seemed happy with the outcome of the surgery. But on 17 June he rang to say he needed to see me again. The cyst on my thyroid, he explained, had been benign, but I was horrified to hear him add that the attached tissue was abnormal – and you don't need a degree in medicine to know what that means. They had found traces of cancer. If Frank Bruno had punched me I would not have been more winded. I had been feeling light-hearted that morning because I had been working hard at my fitness – and with a great deal of success – but now I sat at the desk in my office in a state of shock as Mr Rhys Evans quietly confirmed that a second operation would be necessary. I gently replaced the phone. I was so angry, I felt my whole body was letting me down. Through the office window I could see David washing the car, singing away with the music. I was in tears, and began kicking the bottom of the desk and swearing at my body. How on earth could I tell him or my sons Mark and Paul, I knew they would be devastated. It was all developing into a terrible nightmare and my body felt like it was about to explode.

I rang Mark, who fortunately was in his office only a mile away, and asked him if he would come round to see me. He came immediately having sensed my despair. When Mark and David rushed into the house the look on David's face was heart wrenching, truly dreadful. He kept asking, "What's happened? What's happened?" I told him about the phone call as clearly as I could, before he decided to ring Mr Rhys Evans himself.

Despite our fears we decided to continue with our arrangements to go on the mini cruise which had been planned for some weeks, before attending the Derby sale at Fairyhouse, where I bought most of my young horses. I returned to hospital for my second operation on 30 June, and this time they removed the entire thyroid gland and some lymph nodes. On reflection I've always felt the very mention of the word cancer was far more terrifying than the treatment I received to cure it, and in the darkest days, my family and friends were there to support me when I needed them most.

At first I didn't want anyone to know about my cancer. At the time I felt I wasn't coping very well. I was tired and every time I closed my eyes the "Grim Reaper" was staring me in the face, but I guess you wouldn't be human if you were not full of doubts and fears. At one point I really thought I would end up in a straitjacket if I didn't pull myself together. But now, looking back, I appreciate that all the strange thoughts and obscure fears that troubled me will have happened to lots of others in the same position. The problem is you don't want to talk about your feelings to your closest family so an invisible barrier appears. I now know that is a big mistake.

I had to go back to the Royal Marsden Hospital at the end of July for the radiotherapy treatment to deal with any lingering traces of the cancer. I was given leaflets which explained the procedure for the treatment in the Nuclear Medicine Department and discovered that whatever I took into the room, I would not be allowed to bring out because it could be contaminated. The room was quite comfortable, but no-one was allowed to enter, so it was a bit like being in solitary confinement for 4 days.

A barrier was placed across the doorway, so when David came to visit he was only able to stand or sit on the far side while we talked. There was no question of his reaching out and touching my hand. All my food and drink was placed on a tray at the barrier and I felt a bit like Oliver in *Oliver Twist*.

My treatment came in the form of a large capsule, which I was required to swallow. I have to confess that by the time it was produced, I was ready to bolt. Frankly, having read the leaflet, I was absolutely terrified and would have disappeared given half a chance.

When Dr Glenn Flux, the senior physicist, arrived with the capsule, I put it in my mouth with some serious misgivings and swallowed it. I now knew that my opportunity to bolt had gone. Once the 3000 units of radioactive iodine were in my system I was not going to be leaving for 4 days no matter how scared I felt because I would be radioactive.

My stay at the Marsden proved to be the longest 4 days and 4 nights of my life. It was a time when I desperately needed someone, preferably David, to put his arms around me, hug me and say that I would be all right. But that was not possible. Coping physically with the treatment was not a problem. I did, in fact, sail through it, but emotionally, I was a wreck.

It didn't help that I had bought some magazines from our local newsagents to help me while away the seemingly endless hours on my own. The first one I picked up contained an article by a woman who had beaten cancer, but who had drifted apart from her husband in the process and, ultimately, she lost him. Of course, having read the headlines, I had to read the entire article, even though it was hardly designed to cheer me up.

When I had the energy, I worked like mad on the exercise bicycle in my room in a determined attempt to force the iodine through my system at the earliest rate of knots possible. I knew the sooner it finished its work, the sooner I'd be allowed to leave. Frankly, I could not bear the thought of staying there a second longer than was strictly necessary.

I don't mind admitting that I felt a bit of a "Jesse" during my stay at the Sutton hospital. Outside at lunchtime, I could hear children who I thought were patients laughing and joking. But I was feeling that sorry for myself, I didn't want to depress myself any further by seeing them from my window. Yet, curiously, for a place where there were so many sick people, there was an air of brightness in the hospital that I found difficult to understand. I deduced it came from the staff, who were most professional and supportive in their approach.

Nevertheless it was a huge relief when Dave came to take me home on Friday 31 July. At that stage I was still not allowed to come into contact with old people or young children. The next morning was a lovely bright sunny day so I decided to mow the lawns. Dave was horrified at the very suggestion and refused to get the mower out for me. I persisted despite his protests, and after I'd been mowing for a while, with the warmth of the sun and a slight breeze on my face, I began to feel I was the luckiest person in the whole world, as I suddenly realized that health is the greatest gift of all.

I had to go back into hospital for a crucial scan on 27 November. I had gone down to the Royal Marsden Hospital earlier in the week to be given what I hoped would be one final, small capsule of radioiodine. I then returned on the Friday for the scan which would determine the success or failure of the previous treatment.

Lying there while the scan takes place you begin to dread more bad news. What if I needed another operation or more treatment? People say you are brave in this type of situation, but quite honestly, you don't have a choice if you want to survive. You have to be brave.

The last few weeks of the year are really hectic for National Hunt trainers; with so many race meetings taking place, it was difficult to make

an appointment with Dr Harmer, who was in charge of my treatment, and who would be able to give me the results of my final scan. As he was also away for a week or two, we pencilled in a date close to Christmas. In the end I felt I couldn't wait that long to hear the result, so I rang the hospital after about ten days, explaining that I needed to know if I would require more treatment as contingency plans would need to be in place regarding my work if that was the case. I couldn't just abandon my horses. That is *not* how life works when you are dealing with animals, whether they have two legs or four.

Officially, the medical staff were not allowed to tell me, but unofficially they gave me the wonderful news that I would not need to go back for more treatment. When I eventually saw Dr Harmer on 23 December he confirmed the news. It was to be the best possible Christmas present ever and I can remember his words as if it was yesterday.

"What I can write here, Jenny, is that you are CURED," he said. Despite my earlier contact with the hospital I was still a bit apprehensive until he said those few words. When I came out of the consulting room I felt as if I was walking on air. But this sense of elation was shortlived, for as I was leaving I met someone I knew who was arriving for treatment. I was immediately overwhelmed by an enormous sense of guilt.

It was a feeling that returned time and again over the next few weeks. Eventually one Sunday evening I broke down crying. When Dave asked what was wrong, I couldn't answer him. He persisted as usual, so in the end I had to explain that I felt so guilty at recovering while others were still suffering.

"Well if you think I am going to apologize because you are better, then you are very wrong. You cannot keep carrying everyone else's burden as well as your own," he said with a quiet anger and much feeling.

When I was first told that I had cancer I felt ashamed. I had a great desire to stand in the shower and wash it all away. Following my return home after the second operation, my voice was so poor that my grand-daughter, Darcy Rose, backed away from me when I invited her to help me feed the fish in our garden. She was so unsure of me. But a few weeks later, as I sat on the lawn watching the children play, she ran up behind me, put her head on my back and wrapped her arms around my neck. I could have thrown myself on the ground and wept in relief.

I'm sure the worst ordeal was not mine. David was the one who really suffered, yet for a long time we didn't talk about my illness and its implications, until the situation had reached the point where there seemed to be a barrier between us. I felt I couldn't tell him what I was thinking because I didn't want to upset him. The tension between us became quite unbearable until one night, when we were lying in bed, I felt that we had to break down the barrier and talk it through.

The biggest part of the problem was that David's father had died from cancer, yet he had never discussed this with me. Now, although we were both worried about upsetting one another, I realized it had to be dealt with. That night it all came tumbling out and we sat in bed talking for several hours. It was an enormous relief to be able to hear his fears and to share our problems. Three and a half hours later when I popped downstairs to make us both a cup of tea it was well into the early hours of the morning but I had the best and most restful sleep for months.

A few months later Dr Harmer asked me if I would join the Thyroid and Isotope Therapy Tumour Working Group to represent the patients at the Royal Marsden. My husband and I duly agreed, but I didn't relish the first meeting. Did I really want to know about the success and failure of the treatment for thyroid cancer? Yes, sadly there is failure. My view was that I had cancer but after the operation to remove my thyroid I was someone who no longer had cancer. A view I hold to this day.

One important topic that arose during one of Dr Harmer's meetings was students – how they beg consultants for a particular topic to write a thesis but, it appears, in many cases these are not completed and the research is not handed over if a student moves on. So a lot of time and effort is spent backtracking. I would like to emphasize how important to me and future cancer sufferers this information is. One small piece of research can produce the missing link in the puzzle that can literally save lives.

What have I learnt from all this? Values. The importance of your family and friends – and my wonderful horses that have been my medication and meditation; they didn't judge me and they never told tales! You can surround yourself with material things which in the end amount to nothing. Labels on clothes, the latest car, TV or gadgets have no real value. I feel I have a greater understanding of other people. I have met great people from all walks of life and I have a huge debt to the medical and veterinary professions, who almost certainly saved my life. Which has enabled me to treasure my family and grandchildren for a few more years to come.

5

The Role of the Specialist Nurse

Caroline Owen-Hafiz

The Development of the Specialist Nurse Role

Most patients with thyroid cancer, particularly differentiated thyroid cancer (DTC), have a good prognosis [1,2]. The standard combined treatments are considered to be well tolerated, with low health-related quality of life (HRQOL) morbidity. Some patients have been told that DTC is "the best cancer to have" [3].

In patients with such a good prognosis and low symptom morbidity, what is the role of a specialist nurse (SN)? To date the role of the SN in thyroid cancer care has developed into three main branches:

- the enhancement of the provision of patient/carer information;
- psychological support;
- help with symptom control/rehabilitation.

These three aspects have evolved from the patient and health professional's directive and more recently from evidenced-based research as discussed below.

A recently expressed criticism of modern thyroid cancer care is the perceived failure to focus on "the human being who bears the burden of the cancer" [3–5]. As one patient put it "doctors and others seem to treat thyroid cancer lightly (in an emotional sense) because it is usually quite curable. That's not at all how it felt to me" [6]. There is a growing body of research to suggest that patients and carers do suffer a significant amount of psychological distress with HRQOL morbidity following thyroid cancer diagnosis and treatment [3,7–11] (Table 5.1). Dow describes thyroid cancer survivors as the "forgotten segment of the cancer survivor population" [12]. Compared with other oncology patients, they have less access to cancer support services, which probably reflects their better prognosis and gentler treatment [4,6]. Therefore an increased effort is now being made to provide this group with information, psychological support, and symptom control/rehabilitation.

The Role of the SN in Patient/Carer Psychological Support and Information

It is suggested by the British Thyroid Association that in order to best meet a patient's psychological/information needs, a patient should be encouraged to attend consultations with a family member, friend, or carer, who should also have full access to support from the multidisciplinary team (MDT). It is also recommended that an SN should be made available for support [13]. It is hoped that the SN can engage in open and honest discussion to create a forum where each patient/carer's psychological/information needs can be best identified. It is anticipated

Table 5.1 Reported psychological reactions by patients following thyroid cancer diagnosis and treatment planning [3–4,6,9]

Shock
Anxiety or panic or development/worsening of anxiety disorders
Frustration
Anger
Denial
Low mood or clinical diagnosed depression (moderate to severe)
Isolation
Overwhelming dread of dying
Inability to retain information (short-term memory loss)
Confusion, misconceptions, or information gaps
Afraid or too embarrassed to ask physician to repeat (or better communicate) information
Emotional pain
Loss of control over personal destiny
Fear of the disease and/or the treatments (surgery or radioactive iodine)
Stigma of disease/treatment
Adjustment process
Focusing and planning process
Multiple expectations
Coping with diagnosis
Coping with processing multiple complex information (needed for informed consent)
Sadness and fear for the end of cherished relationships
Living with fear of recurrence
Rarely (but at times) palliative living adjustment
Hope

that the formal acknowledgment of patients' needs and the provision of information will help the patient/carer feel more supported, informed, in control, and that their needs and concerns are being addressed. The psychological/information support provided by the SN needs to respect patient/carer autonomy and guard against dependency. Therefore the role of the SN is to provide psychological/information support that works alongside/towards the enhancement of patient/carer information, coping skills, adjustment, self-development, and independence.

The SN can also promote patient choice and availability of useful resources: patient support groups, patient information websites, and useful contacts [14]. The SN needs a good clinical insight into all types of thyroid cancer such as papillary, follicular, medullary, and the different

treatment pathways in order to give appropriate support. An experienced and knowledgeable SN can help the patient cope with multiple and complex information that is needed for patient informed consent. The SN can also make available to the patient written information in an appropriate, manageable, and sequential way. Such written information can be obtained from the MDT producing agreed patient information fact sheets or by the use of the British Thyroid Association set of three patient information booklets [15]:

1. The thyroid gland and thyroid cancer;
2. Thyroid surgery;
3. Radioactive iodine ablation treatment.

An example of how the role of the SN can complement the existing support provided by the MDT can be seen in Table 5.2, based on the British Thyroid Association's guidelines on informing the patient [13]. The suggested role of the SN is given in the right-hand column.

The Role of the SN in Symptom Control and Rehabilitation

Resent research suggests that patient support should be in the form of early rehabilitation programs and should be provided by the MDT. This should be delivered in a holistic way, ideally during the first year after diagnosis. It should include counseling with a psychotherapeutic approach to improve mental health, emotional functioning, and social competence [8]. Growing research also suggests that psychotherapy, especially group psychotherapy, can reduce psychological distress and in some cases improve survival [5–7]. An SN can work with the MDT to review/help with the provision of such services.

Some patients have experienced neck or shoulder stiffness/restricted movement and/or pain that may be prolonged or lasting. Therefore it is recommended that rehabilitation should also include early physical exercise (endurance and strength training performed in groups) to improve physical performance and help patients fulfill their social roles (family, household, work) [8,15]. In order to be most effective in symptom control/rehabilitation the SN needs to

Table 5.2 The role of the SN working alongside the British Thyroid Association guidelines informing the patient

Guideline	Suggested role of the SN
The patient will be informed of the diagnosis by a member of the MDT; facilities should be available for this to be done during a private, uninterrupted consultation.	At the time of the diagnosis and treatment planning an SN can be present for support and to take notes. Subsequently at the patient's request the SN can be available to repeat this information exactly, if the patient has not been able to fully retain all the information at one sitting or needs a safe supportive environment to compose themselves before going home. This helps free the specialist to answer more specific and complicated questions for others. The presence of the SN at the initial diagnosis and treatment planning is also thought to promote the development of a good working relationship between SN and patient/carer. The SN can subsequently act as a useful advocate/support as requested throughout the patient/carer treatment journey.
A trained nurse specialist will be available to provide additional counseling if required.	The SN can provide patients/carers with a confidential, objective, and advanced form of psychological support. An SN needs to have a good clinical insight into a patient's investigations, diagnosis, and treatment pathway to enable the support to be appropriate. Most thyroid cancers are very amenable to treatment and curable but there is a possibility of recurrence, especially in the very young and in the elderly. This can occur at any stage, but recurrence can be treated successfully, so lifelong clinical follow-up and availability of support is important.
Whenever possible a relative or friend should attend the consultation and accompany the patient home.	An SN can provide support for carers while maintaining the consent and confidentiality of the patient. It must be remembered that carers may have a great deal of stress and play a key role in the patient's support/recovery. In the rare cases of medullary cell carcinoma it is sometimes, but not always, hereditary and the SN can help support the family while awaiting genetic counseling.
Written information concerning thyroid cancer and its treatment and possible complications will be available to the patient.	An SN can help coordinate the updating, accessibility, and replenishment of such specialist written information/resources. An SN can ensure patient/carer access to full resources such as: patient information booklets, patient support groups, patient information web sites, and useful contacts [14]. An SN needs to be aware of the treatment stages and that patients may feel at times vulnerable and overwhelmed with information that is needed for full consent. The SN is in a key position to gain experience in helping the MDT best judge the sequential timing of the delivery of such information balanced with each individual patient's wishes, coping/adjustment ability, and treatment schedule.
A prognosis should not be offered before adequate staging information is available.	An SN needs to acquire advanced skills in helping support patients/carers through the stress of waiting for a diagnosis by not giving false information and helping the client cope with the unknown. The SN needs to develop skills in helping patients prepare realistically for variable outcomes.
Patients may have difficulty understanding all this information at a single consultation and an opportunity for further exploration/discussion should be offered.	It must be remembered that patients/carers are individuals and have a myriad of positive and negative reactions to a diagnosis and treatment planning: some may be in shock. An SN can aid the MDT in clinic and subsequently by making herself available to patient/carers when they feel they are ready for more information. The SN can introduce herself to the patient/carer and leave contact details to facilitate this.

Source: Royal College of Physicians, British Thyroid Association. Guidelines for the management of thyroid cancer in adults. London: RCP, 2001.

separate psychological from physical symptoms in order to best assess and re-refer the patient to the most appropriate MDT resources. This can be particularly challenging in a patient following DTC treatment as many common psychological symptoms of stress, low mood or clinical depression can also be found in thyroid hormonal imbalance or directly following surgery, as demonstrated in Tables 5.1 and 5.3.

There are many reported psychological and physical symptoms that patients may experience following thyroid cancer and its treatment apart from those reported in Tables 5.1 and 5.3. Therefore an SN needs a good clinical insight into psychological and physical symptoms in order to give appropriate support, aid the MDT to pick up any worrying clinical signs early, and to seek advice or refer to the most appropriate

Table 5.3 Reported physical and psychological symptoms of hormone replacement or calcium imbalance [4,6,12,13]

Dry skin
Fatigue
Decreased concentration
Sleep disturbance
Reduced social, work, and family activity
Poor appetite
Constipation
Reduced motor skills
Fluid retention
Low mood or depression
Hair loss
Palpitations/shaky
Feeling anxious
Undesired weight change
Overactive
Heat and cold intolerance
Migraine/headaches
Pins and needles in hands/face/feet (low calcium?)
Generally feeling unwell (low calcium?)

Table 5.4 Reported patient key concerns regarding radioactive iodine therapy [9,17]

Isolation
Separation
Feeling weak/tired
Anxiety/panic
Low mood
Tightness in the throat and/or feel flushed – usually no more than 24 hours (may be relieved by an anti-inflammatory drug)
Temporary slight loss in taste
Low iodine intake concerns
Discharge precaution information
Fear of radiation danger to self, family members, fertility, and future children

member of the MDT. This may be particularly beneficial in newly treated patients with symptoms of thyroxine or calcium imbalance or postoperative complications in order to maximize symptom control and rehabilitation. Occasionally the SN may need to help with palliative care/support. The SN may be a useful support until the appropriate formal hospital and or community palliative care team are fully in place in order to guard against the patient/carer feeling abandoned.

The Role of the SN Following Thyroid Ablation with Radioactive Iodine Therapy

Some patients will require thyroid ablation with radioactive iodine therapy. This understandably has been reported as psychologically and physically very stressful for patients and their carers on top of the hormonal physical changes due to the reduction, change, or temporary cessation of hormone replacement therapy [16]. The role of the SN again is to offer psychological support and information alongside the MDT to deal with patient/carer concerns about treatment. The SN's role is to reduce the psychological and physical impact of the therapy by providing

support/information that enables the patient/carer to prepare mentally and physically for such treatment. Commonly reported patient concerns regarding radioactive iodine therapy are listed in Table 5.4.

The Role of the SN During Thyroid Hormone Withdrawal (in Preparation for Treatment or Scanning Procedures)

During thyroid hormone withdrawal patients may experience symptoms that are physical and psychological which can also affect their social wellbeing [9,15]. The role of the SN is to help prepare and educate patients/carers about hormone withdrawal side effects, the fostering of realistic expectations during scanning procedures or treatment and help with balancing or temporarily rearranging family and work activities during and around this period [17,18].

In Summary

The role of the SN in thyroid cancer care has developed into three main branches: the provision of information, the provision of psychological support, and help with/coordination of symptom control/rehabilitation. The SN needs to have advanced interpersonal, communication, and psychological support skills plus a sound knowledge of thyroid cancer, its treatment and symptom control. The SN should also be aware of all the available formal and voluntary support group resources. The SN can complement the existing MDT in order to minimize the HRQOL impact of thyroid cancer and its treatment.

References

1. Mazzaferri EL, Kloos RT. Long-term outcome of patients with differentiated thyroid carcinoma: effect of therapy. Endocr Pract 2000; 6:469–476.
2. Vassilopoulou-Sellin R. Management of papillary thyroid cancer. Oncology 1995; 9:45–151.
3. Schultz PN, Stava C, Vassilopoulou-Sellin R. Health profiles and quality of life of 518 survivors of thyroid cancer. Head Neck 2003; 25(5):349–356.
4. Shey J. Why I started the Thyroid Cancer Foundation. [Editorial]. Cancer 2001; 91(4):623–624.
5. Meyer TJ, Mark MM. Effects of psychosocial interventions with adult cancer patients: a meta-analysis of randomized experiments. Health Psychol 1995; 14:101–108.
6. Hassey Dow K, Ferrell BR, Anello C. Balancing demands of cancer surveillance among survivors of thyroid cancer. Cancer Pract 1997; 5(5):289–295.
7. Hammerlid E, Persson LO, Sullivan M. Quality of life effects of psychosocial intervention in patients with head and neck cancer. Otolaryngol Head Neck Surg 1999; 120:507–516.
8. Schultz PN, Beck ML, Vassilopoulou-Sellin R. Cancer survivors: work related issues. AAOHN J 2002; 50(5): 220–226.
9. Fitch MI, McGrath PN. The needs of family members of patients receiving radioactive iodine. Can Oncol Nurs J 2003; 13(4):220–231.
10. Wood LC. Support groups for patients with Graves' disease and other thyroid conditions. Endocrinol Metab Clin North Am 1998; 27(1):101–107.
11. Owen C, Watkinson JC, Pracy P, Glaholm J. The psychosocial impact of head and neck cancer. Clin Otolaryngol 2001; 26:351–356.
12. Dow KH, Ferrell BR, Anello C. Balancing demands of cancer surveillance among survivors of thyroid cancer. Cancer Pract 1997; 5(5):289–295.
13. British Thyroid Association. Guidelines for the management of thyroid cancer in adults. Informing the patient. March 2002: 6.
14. Patient support groups: BACUP 3 Bath Place, Rivington Street, London EC2A 3JR; British Thyroid Foundation, PO Box 97, Clifford, Wetherby, West Yorkshire LS23 6XD. Useful contacts: Macmillan information line 0845 601 6161; Cancerlink Freephone Information Helpline 0800 132905; Asian language line 0171 713 786; Cancer Bacup 0800 800 1234, www.cancerbacup.org.uk; CancerHelp UK http://medweb.bham.ac.uk/cancerhelp; Thyroid Cancer Survivors' Association www.thyca.org. Useful sites can be found on the BTA links page www.british-thyroid-association.org.
15. British Thyroid Association. Guidelines for the management of Thyroid Cancer in Adults. Patient information booklets: The thyroid gland and thyroid cancer; Thyroid surgery; Radioactive iodine ablation treatment. March 2002; Appendix 7. www.british-thyroid-association.org.
16. Crevenna R, Zettinig G, Keilani M, et al. Quality of life in patients with non-metastatic differentiated thyroid cancer under thyroxin supplementation therapy. Support Care Cancer 2003; 11:597–603.
17. Stajduhar KI, Neithercut J, Pham P, Rohde J, Sicotte A, Young K. Thyroid cancer: Patients' experience of receiving iodine-131 therapy. Oncol Nurs Forum 2000; 27(8):1213–1218.
18. Dow KH, Ferrell BR, Anello C. Quality of life changes in patients with thyroid cancer after withdrawal of thyroid hormone therapy. Thyroid 1997; 7(4):613–619.

6

The Role of the Clinical Psychologist

Katherine Kendell

Prevalence of Psychological Distress

For most people a diagnosis of cancer is a distressing life event. For many, the initial reaction is that they have been given a death sentence. In fact the majority of patients diagnosed with cancer will adjust psychologically, cope with subsequent treatment, and adapt their lives appropriately. Nevertheless, a substantial minority of patients will experience clinical levels of psychological distress that merit some level of professional intervention.

Estimates of the prevalence of psychological/psychiatric disorder in a population with cancer vary widely, due to differences in the subgroups studied and use of different criteria for defining disorders. Derogatis et al. [1] found that 47% of adult inpatients with cancer had formal psychiatric disorders. Zabora et al. [2] screened a large ($n = 4496$), heterogeneous population of cancer patients with the Brief Symptom Inventory [3] (a psychometrically sound self-report measure) and found that 35.1% were suffering clinical levels of psychological distress. Greer et al. [4] studied 1260 patients with various cancers, within 12 weeks of diagnosis, and found 23% to have clinically significant anxiety or depression. Hence it can be assumed that between a quarter and a third

of cancer patients will experience clinically relevant levels of psychological distress at some point in their cancer experience. The great majority of that distress will be directly related to disease or treatment.

Risk factors for developing psychological disorder, in the face of cancer, include: previous history of psychological problems; inadequate social support; serious negative life events in addition to cancer; maladaptive coping style [5] as well as younger age at diagnosis; pre-existing marital problems; low expectations regarding the effectiveness of treatment; a prior adverse experience of cancer in the family; lack of involvement in satisfying activities; and inability to accept the physical changes associated with the disease or its treatment [6]. Adjustment disorders, depression, and anxiety are the most common psychological disorders within a cancer population. Other problems encountered include: post-traumatic stress disorder; phobic avoidance of treatment; relational problems; sexual dysfunction; and delirium. Patients are more likely to be psychologically vulnerable at certain key points in their cancer journey, for example at diagnosis, at discharge from treatment, and if recurrence of disease occurs. Unfortunately studies indicate that the majority of psychological distress in cancer patients goes undetected and therefore untreated [7,8].

A Psychological Model of Adjustment to Cancer

When someone first receives the news that they have cancer, the greatest concern is usually survival. Patients often ask "am I going to die?" In younger people particularly, there is likely to be a period of shock and disbelief as implicit assumptions about invincibility are shattered. The individual then goes through a process of appraisal which will greatly influence their adjustment to the disease. As individuals make sense of their diagnosis they address three key questions: How great is the threat? What can be done about it? What is the prognosis? Moorey and Greer [9] have identified four different conclusions that people may come to about their diagnosis. These are outlined in Figure 6.1.

A person perceiving cancer as a challenge is likely to feel relatively optimistic and be more likely to engage in treatment. A perception of threat is likely to lead to anxiety. A perception that harm has already occurred may lead to hopelessness and lack of engagement in treatment. Denial of any threat may enable an individual to feel better but, if too great, could prevent engagement in treatment.

At some point after the initial threat to survival has been appraised, the wider implications of cancer and its treatment are likely to be considered and may become significant sources of

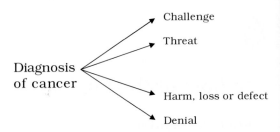

Figure 6.1 The appraisal of the diagnosis of cancer. (From *Cognitive Behaviour Therapy for People with Cancer* (2002) by Stirling Moorey and Steven Greer, p. 12. By permission of Oxford University Press.)

distress. Moorey and Greer have labeled the morbidity associated with disease and treatment "the threat to the self," in which they include: debilitating physical symptoms; inability to carry out former work, leisure or family roles; and disfigurement (Figure 6.2).

According to Moorey and Greer's cognitive model of adjustment, the "personal meaning of cancer," based on an idiosyncratic appraisal of the threat to survival and the threat to the self, is an important determinant of an individual's adaptation to their disease. Moorey and Greer's model helps to explain why any two individuals with the same disease may react very differently to a diagnosis of cancer. For someone who has relied heavily on their appearance for self-esteem, treatment associated with hair loss or scarring may be devastating. Someone else who

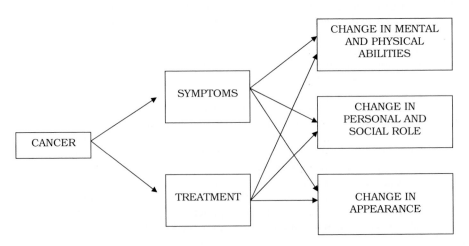

Figure 6.2 Negative consequences of the diagnosis of cancer. (From *Cognitive Behaviour Therapy for People with Cancer* (2002) by Stirling Moorey and Steven Greer, p. 15. By permission of Oxford University Press.)

has always perceived themselves to be in control of their life, may be unfazed by disfiguring surgery but find it extremely hard to live with uncertainty about potential relapse.

Psychological adjustment, based on an individual's appraisal of cancer, is associated with emotional response. Greer and Watson [10] have described five distinct styles of adjustment: fighting spirit; avoidance or denial; fatalism; helplessness and hopelessness; and anxious preoccupation. Fighting spirit is characterized by a perception that cancer is a threat to be actively challenged. It is associated with less risk of developing anxiety and depression. The helpless and hopeless adjustment style, characterized by a perception of major loss and a lack of active coping behaviors, is associated with clinical depression. An anxiously preoccupied adjustment style characterized by excessive worrying and compulsively seeking reassurance is associated with clinical anxiety [9].

Psychological Aspects of Thyroid Cancer

Thyroid cancer is a relatively rare disease, with an incidence of 3.1 per 100 000 per year [11]. Differentiated thyroid cancer, accounting for the majority of cases, is curable in 90% of patients given appropriate treatment [12]. On this basis many patients are told that thyroid cancer is a "good cancer" to have. However, medullary carcinoma, accounting for 4% of cases, has a 10-year survival rate of 75%. Undifferentiated, or anaplastic, carcinomas account for only 2% of cases, but carry a very poor prognosis, with a 3-year survival rate of only 3% [11].

There is limited published information related to the long-term physical health of survivors of thyroid cancer, and very little published material describing psychological and social outcomes [13]. However, there are a number of descriptive studies offering accounts of patients' perspectives and nursing care needs.

As part of a wider survey of adult survivors of cancer, Shultz and colleagues [13] described medical and psychosocial outcomes of 518 survivors of thyroid cancer. Interestingly, these authors found that survivors of thyroid cancer reported that their disease had affected their overall health, more frequently than did any other diagnostic group. Thyroid cancer patients who had been treated with radiation were almost twice as likely to report an overall effect on their health as those who had not received radiation. Almost a quarter of the sample described symptoms that could be associated with thyroid dysregulation, for example: dry skin; hair loss; poor concentration; sleep disturbance; fatigue; weight change; palpitations; heat/cold intolerance; diarrhea/constipation; depression; anxiety. Thyroid cancer survivors reported psychological problems, memory loss, and migraine headaches more frequently than survivors of other types of cancer. The authors conclude that the morbidity associated with a diagnosis of thyroid cancer is significantly more pronounced than generally understood [13].

An Italian study used a standardized instrument (structured clinical interview for Diagnostic and Statistical Manual of Mental Disorders – III – Revised) to evaluate the lifetime prevalence of psychiatric disorders in 93 inpatients with different thyroid diseases. They found higher rates of several psychiatric disorders in thyroid patients than in the general population. These authors suggest that underlying biochemical abnormalities may explain the co-occurrence of psychiatric disorder and thyroid diseases [14].

A number of descriptive studies have explored patients' perspectives of undergoing treatment with radioactive iodine [15,16]. For the purpose of this treatment, patients are placed in isolation and their contact with staff and visitors is strictly limited, in order to minimize the spread of contamination from bodily fluids. Thus patients are socially as well as physically isolated, at a time when they may be in particular need of support due to distressing physical symptoms and fear of their disease. The special precautions taken with these patients, and the isolation itself, often result in increasing anxiety and fear in patients, about the nature of their disease.

Stajduhar et al. [15] elicited feedback from a small number of patients ($n = 27$) who had undergone treatment with radioactive iodine. Profound physical and social isolation was the greatest concern for these patients. They reported not having had adequate information or preparation prior to treatment, in order to enable them to cope effectively. They were aware of inconsistencies in staff members' understanding of the risks of radioactive iodine and the treatment process. Patients sensed a reluctance of some staff to be in contact with them. These patients also described how physical aspects of the treatment room served to compound their distress. The authors make three general recommendations on the basis of their study: (1) a program of education for patients and families prior to admission for treatment; (2) a comprehensive staff education program developed by a multidisciplinary healthcare team, in collaboration with patients; (3) modifications to the treatment room to make it more comfortable and less clinical.

Another descriptive study, using a somewhat larger population of patients ($n = 190$) who each completed a standardized survey, was conducted by McGrath and Fitch [16]. This study also highlighted the distressing effects of isolation and the need for careful preparation of patients prior to treatment. Patients called for written as well as verbal information. Again, they were aware that nursing staff were sometimes inexperienced and held inconsistent views about the dangers of treatment.

Both patient groups and nurses have highlighted the need for education and preparation of nursing staff who deal with thyroid cancer patients. Due to the rare nature of the disease, staff may not work with thyroid cancer patients on a regular basis [17]. Nurses who lack understanding of the relative risks of exposure to patients during treatment may avoid patients unnecessarily and therefore cause unnecessary patient distress. McGrath and Fitch sensibly suggest standard guidelines for staff and visitor contact, which are based on evidence and reflect realistic risk, as well as patients' needs, rights, and responsibilities [16].

Patients have suggested modifications to the treatment room that may improve morale, including: having a window; enough room to exercise; shower facilities; television and video player; telephone; an intercom to enable conversations with staff [15,16]. Patients have also identified a need for support groups set up specifically for people with thyroid cancer, rather than for cancer patients in general. These groups can address the particular needs and concerns of this group and provide "buddy systems" to help support patients undergoing treatment [15,18].

Following treatment for thyroid cancer, patients are required to undergo regular monitoring of their disease status for the rest of their lives. The morbidity associated with lifetime surveillance is highlighted in a number of studies [13,19,20]. Surveillance generally involves thyroid hormone withdrawal followed by body scanning. The induced hypothyroid state results in symptoms of: fatigue; sleep disturbance; impaired psychomotor skills; reduced ability to concentrate; anorexia; pain and fluid retention [19]. As is true for survivors of other types of cancer, the process of monitoring generally raises patients' concerns about the threat of recurrence.

The combination of debilitating physical symptoms and fear of recurrence can profoundly affect psychological and social wellbeing. In a qualitative study of a small number ($n = 34$) of thyroid cancer survivors, feelings of loss, anxiety, depression, and impaired concentration were reported [20]. The process of surveillance is socially very disruptive. As thyroid cancer typically affects a relatively young population, the majority of whom are of working and child-rearing age, the resulting social disruption is particularly pertinent. Thyroid cancer patients are more likely to be gainfully employed (63%) than a general population of cancer survivors (35%) [13]. However, surveillance results in time taken off work or decreased performance at work. In addition, patients' ability to carry out household tasks and engage in childcare, family and social relationships is impaired.

A disease-specific measure of quality of life (QOL – thyroid scale) was used with 34 thyroid cancer patients undergoing surveillance. Negative changes to patients' self-reported quality of life were found to be greatest between peak hormone withdrawal and thyroxine therapy. Common patient concerns included: symptoms associated with thyroid hormone withdrawal; fertility issues; distress associated with treatment; fear of cancer recurrence. However, these authors elicited some positive changes too, such as hopefulness and renewed sense of purpose in life [19]. Shultz and colleagues also reported patient perceptions that in the longer term their experiences were associated with improved family relationships [13].

It has been argued that the long-term monitoring indicated for people treated for thyroid cancer may be more difficult to endure than treatment itself [20]. A combination of physical, psychological, and social factors may give rise to emotional disturbance, for example symptoms of anxiety and depression.

Clinical Psychology in Oncology

Clinical psychologists are applied scientists specializing in cognitive, emotional, behavioral, and social aspects of human behavior. They are trained to work with individuals, couples, families, and groups and to provide a consultative service to other healthcare professions. Direct clinical work includes detailed psychological assessments and design and provision of therapeutic interventions. Other roles include: teaching other healthcare staff about psychological issues; training non-psychology staff in direct clinical skills; providing support and supervision to other healthcare professionals who offer psychological support; providing consultation and advice to clinicians and managers; collaboration with multidisciplinary colleagues on research.

The aim of clinical psychology in oncology is to promote psychological wellbeing and reduce the distress associated with diagnosis, treatment, and living with disease. Encouraging the recognition and detection of psychological distress is a high priority. Enabling other healthcare staff to provide psychological support to patients and their families is a key role. Due to the high prevalence of psychological distress and the scarcity of clinical psychology resources, direct clinical interventions need to be targeted towards patients and carers with the most complex psychological needs and those most likely to benefit from a formal psychological intervention.

Role of the Clinical Psychologist in Thyroid Cancer

It is apparent that patients undergoing treatment and surveillance for thyroid cancer may be experiencing much greater levels of psychological distress than healthcare staff have generally anticipated, based on a relatively good prognosis. A significant minority of people with any type of cancer experience clinical levels of distress at some point in their cancer journey and it may well be that those with thyroid cancer experience higher levels of distress than some other subgroups.

Therefore a key role of the clinical psychologist is to educate other staff about psychological responses to diagnosis, treatment, and surveillance. This may start with advice to managers in order to influence the provision of resources and facilities; for example, understanding of patients' need for careful preparation for treatment may support the case for having specialist nurses allocated to thyroid cancer. Considering the impact of the immediate environment on psychological wellbeing may strengthen the case for modifying treatment rooms.

A clinical psychologist should be involved in the design and implementation of a program of education for healthcare staff involved with thyroid cancer patients. The education program should include psychological needs of patients, communication skills, and evidence-based information on risks of radiation exposure and relevant precautions. Nuclear medicine technicians as well as doctors and nurses should be included in the educational program. The clinical psychologist could also offer consultation and advice on preparation of patients for treatment and the provision of both oral and written information.

Provision of supervision and support for specialist nurses who would themselves be offering frontline psychological support to patients is an important role of the clinical psychologist. This may involve training nurses in specific clinical skills, for example counseling skills or cognitive behavioral techniques.

A clinical psychologist may offer advice and consultation to specialist nurses and/or former patients who wish to establish a patient support group. The clinical psychologist could usefully provide a regular presentation on psychological aspects of thyroid cancer and coping skills to the support group. If the support group operates a "buddy system" for new patients undergoing treatment, the clinical psychologist may offer support and supervision to the buddies.

Psychological assessment and direct clinical interventions should be provided by the clinical psychologist for more complex psychological problems, for example clinical depression or anxiety, post-traumatic stress disorder, phobic avoidance of treatment. Enabling other clinical staff to recognize and detect such distress and make appropriate referrals is part of this role.

Following referral, the clinical psychologist would offer the patient a comprehensive assessment. On the basis of assessment the patient may be offered a course of therapy (e.g. cognitive therapy, interpersonal therapy, brief psychotherapy). If therapy is not deemed appropriate, advice on management may be offered to the referrer. Psychological therapy would be based on the patient's idiosyncratic needs, but may focus on: preparing for and coping with treatment; re-establishing roles following treatment; overcoming depression; addressing marital and sexual difficulties; living with ongoing surveillance and threat of recurrence.

For patients complaining of memory problems, a neuropsychological assessment, using formal psychometric tools, such as the Wechsler Memory Scale III [21], may be useful. This would be followed by careful feedback to both the patient and the referrer, and appropriate advice on management of memory problems.

As cancer is understood to have psychological and social ramifications for partners and families, as well as for patients themselves, it is sometimes advantageous to involve significant others in assessment and therapy. (This would only occur with the patient's consent.) Other family members often offer valuable perspectives on problems and potential solutions. Addressing marital and sexual difficulties is usually more successful when both partners are engaged in therapy. Occasionally a whole family group may be involved in a systemic intervention, aimed at improving communication and renegotiating roles and boundaries. Systemic psychological interventions may be particularly appropriate for families affected by medullary thyroid carcinoma associated with the inherited disease multiple endocrine neoplasia type 2a.

For some patients and their families, particularly in cases of medullary or anaplastic carcinomas, psychological support through terminal care and bereavement may be indicated. Psychological support for terminally ill patients and their families focuses on enabling people to maximize their quality of life and address unresolved psychosocial issues. Following a patient's death, the clinical psychologist could be asked to intervene where other family members experience complicated or prolonged grief.

It is clear from the existing literature that there is much scope for further research into psychosocial aspects of thyroid cancer. Given the relatively rare nature of this disease and the need for larger population studies, cross center studies would be more useful than single center studies. Clinical psychologists should collaborate with colleagues in medicine, nursing and academia to implement carefully designed studies. Clinical psychologists can also usefully contribute to audit of services. For example, monitoring the prevalence of depression and anxiety in patients being treated for thyroid cancer or comparing different methods that non-psychology staff may use to detect psychological distress are examples of useful audit projects to be undertaken at a local service level.

The expectation is that the clinical psychologist would be a valuable resource to colleagues in other professions treating the patient with thyroid cancer. The aim is to promote psychological wellbeing, detect and alleviate psychological distress, enhance staff morale, and promote holistic patient care.

References

1. Derogatis LR, Morrow GR, Fetting J, et al. The prevalence of psychiatric disorders among cancer patients. JAMA 1983; 249:751–757.
2. Zabora J, Brintzenhofeszoc K, Curbow B, Hooker C, Piatadosi S. The prevalence of psychological distress by cancer site. Psycho-oncology 2001; 10:19–28.
3. Derogatis LR. The Brief Symptom Inventory (BSI): Administration, scoring and procedures manual, 3rd edn. Minneapolis, MN: National Computer Systems, 1993.
4. Greer S, Moorey S, Baruch JDR, et al. Adjuvant psychological therapy for patients with cancer: a prospective randomised trial. BMJ 1992; 304:675–680.
5. DCP Briefing Paper no 13. Clinical Psychology Services in Oncology: A guide for Purchasers of Clinical Psychology Services. The British Psychological Society Division of Clinical Psychology, 1997.
6. Burton M, Watson M. Counselling people with cancer. Chichester: John Wiley, 1998.
7. Burton MV, Parker RW. A randomised controlled trial of preoperative psychological preparation for mastectomy. Psycho-oncology 1995; 4:1–19.

8. Maguire P. Improving the detection of psychiatric problems in cancer patients. Soc Sci Med 1985; 20:819–823.
9. Moorey S, Greer S. Cognitive behaviour therapy for people with cancer. Oxford: Oxford University Press, 2002.
10. Greer S, Watson M. Mental adjustment to cancer: its measurement and prognostic importance. Cancer Surv 1987; 6:439–453.
11. Mokbel K Concise notes in oncology, 2nd edn. Petroc Press, 2001.
12. Mazzaferri EL. Long term outcome of patients with differentiated thyroid carcinoma: effect of therapy. Endocr Pract 2000; 6:469–476.
13. Shultz PN, Stava C, Vassilopoulou-Sellin R. Health Profiles and quality of life of 518 survivors of thyroid cancer. Head Neck 2003; May:349–356.
14. Placidi GPA, Boldrini M, Patronelli A, et al. Prevalence of psychiatric disorders in thyroid diseased patients. Neuropsychobiology 1998; 38:222–255.
15. Stajduhar KI, Neithercut J, Chu E, et al. Thyroid cancer: patients' experiences of receiving iodine-131 therapy. Oncol Nurs Forum 2000; 27(8):1213–1218.
16. McGrath PN, Fitch MI. Patient perspectives on the impact of receiving radioactive iodine: Implications for practice. Can Oncol Nurs J 2003; 13(3):152–163.
17. Baker KH, Feldman JE. Thyroid cancer: a review. Oncol Nurs Forum 1993; 20(1):95–104.
18. Shey J. Why I started the Thyroid Cancer Foundation. Cancer 2001; 91(4):623–624.
19. Hassey Dow K, Ferrell BR, Anello C. Quality of life changes in patients with thyroid cancer after withdrawal of thyroid hormone therapy. Thyroid 1997; 7(4):613–619.
20. Hassey Dow K, Ferrell BR, Anello C. Balancing demands of cancer surveillance among survivors of thyroid cancer. Cancer Pract 1997; 5(5):289–295.
21. Wechsler D. Wechsler Memory Scale, 3rd edn. London: The Psychological Corporation, 1998.

Section II

The Diagnosis of Thyroid Cancer

7

Thyroid Nodules

Petros Perros

Thyroid nodules are common in the general adult population. In contrast, thyroid cancer is relatively rare and disease-specific mortality is low [1,2]. The challenge that faces clinicians who manage patients with thyroid nodules is to identify the minority of patients who harbor thyroid cancers, while causing minimum harm to those who have benign disease [3,4].

Epidemiology

The prevalence of thyroid nodules increases with age. They are commoner in women than men and very common in areas of iodine deficiency. The prevalence of palpable thyroid nodules in most series is 3–7% [5–8] and the annual incidence 0.1% [7]. Using sensitive imaging techniques such as high resolution ultrasound, it has been shown that over 50% of all adults have thyroid nodules [9–11]. Similarly high prevalence of nodules has been noted in postmortem studies [12]. The malignancy rate of palpable solitary nodules is 5% with a range of 3.4–29% [13]. Nearly half of all patients thought to have a solitary nodule by clinical examination are found to have multiple nodules on ultrasonography [14]. The incidence of malignancy in multinodular goiters is similar to that of solitary nodules [15,16]. Different pathologies presenting as thyroid nodules are shown in Table 7.1.

Natural History

Most thyroid lumps are benign colloid nodules. The natural history of colloid nodules has been reported in several studies. In iodine replete areas the majority remain unchanged after 10 years of follow-up. Some decrease in size and may disappear. On average 22% of patients with thyroid nodules regress spontaneously over a 6-month to 3-year follow-up period [17,18] and in one series 46% of benign nodules disappeared after 30 months following fine-needle aspiration biopsy [19]. Some nodules (less than 20%) grow bigger and the prevalence of malignancy in nodules that continue to grow was reported to be 26% [20]. A more recent series from an iodine replete area found a much higher incidence of increase in thyroid nodule size (69%) judged ultrasonographically [21]. Thyroid function may alter very slowly over several years in patients with multinodular colloid nodules and some patients develop thyroid autonomy [22]. Initially the serum thyrotropin (TSH) falls to the lower end of the reference range, while serum thyroid hormone concentrations remain normal. The serum TSH may continue to fall and become undetectable, while normal thyroid hormone levels persist ("subclinical hyperthyroidism"). Eventually serum thyroid hormone concentrations rise and the patient may develop hyperthyroid symptoms.

Thyroid nodules due to autoimmune (Hashimoto's) thyroiditis have a variable course;

Table 7.1 Different pathologies presenting as a thyroid nodule

Colloid nodule
Colloid cyst
Follicular adenoma
Multinodular goiter
Malignancy
Papillary
Follicular
Medullary
Anaplastic
Lymphoma
Metastasis
Hashimoto's thyroiditis
Subacute thyroiditis
Effect of prior operation or ^{131}I therapy
Thyroid hemiagenesis
Parathyroid cyst or adenoma

over several years the thyroid tends to atrophy and the goiter decreases in size [23]. Occasionally Hashimoto goiters enlarge with the passage of time, and in such cases an underlying lymphoma needs to be excluded, particularly in older patients [17].

Thyroid nodules due to differentiated thyroid cancer, if left untreated, usually continue to grow, or may remain unchanged for several years. More aggressive types of thyroid cancer (medullary thyroid cancer, thyroid lymphoma, anaplastic thyroid cancer) grow rapidly. Thyroid nodules due to thyroid cancer do not regress spontaneously. Sudden enlargement of a nodule associated with localized pain and sometimes systemic symptoms is usually due to hemorrhage into a benign nodule or cyst [24].

Pathogenesis

Colloid Nodules

Histologically colloid nodules are composed of large areas of colloid-filled spaces lined by flattened, inactive looking follicular epithelial cells and lacking a fibrous capsule. Both clonal and polyclonal proliferation is thought to take place [22,25]. Defects in the reabsorption of thyroglobulin from the lumen of the follicle or abnormal storage of thyroglobulin have been suggested as possible mechanisms [25]. Genetic and environmental influences are also thought to be involved [25,26].

Other Types of Nodule

Functioning thyroid adenomas ("toxic nodules") often have somatic constitutively activating mutations of the TSH receptor [27]. Molecular rearrangements or mutations in the pathogenesis of differentiated thyroid cancer (RET/PTC, BRAF) have been implicated [26,28]. Medullary thyroid cancer is frequently associated with activating somatic or germline mutations of the RET gene. Mutations in tumor suppressor genes (p53) have been reported in anaplastic thyroid cancer [29]. External beam irradiation to the thyroid in childhood increases the incidence of both benign and malignant thyroid nodules [30].

Initial Assessment

Patients with thyroid nodules should be referred to a specialist (endocrinologist or thyroid surgeon) for further assessment. Such a strategy speeds the process of reaching a diagnosis and is cost-effective [31]. Clinical assessment by history-taking and examination usually does not lead to a precise diagnosis. Patients are often asymptomatic except for being aware of the nodule. Clinical features that warrant urgent referral are shown in Table 7.2. Rarely thyroid cancer can be inferred with confidence on clinical grounds alone; in such cases the nodule is hard [32], irregular, and associated with palpable cervical lymphadenopathy, but this is an extremely uncommon presentation. The initial clinical assessment is important in selecting which patients require additional investigations for exclusion of cancer. The only essential inves-

Table 7.2 Clinical features in patients with thyroid nodules warranting urgent referral

History of increase in size (rapid growth)
Family history of thyroid cancer
History of previous neck irradiation
Very young (<20) or very old (>70) patients
Unexplained hoarseness or voice change
Cervical lymphadenopathy
Compression symptoms including dysphagia, dysphonia, hoarseness, dyspnea, and cough
Stridor
A nodule that is very firm or hard
Nodule fixation to adjacent structures

tigation by the primary care physician is bio-chemical assessment of thyroid function. Other tests, including imaging, at this stage are unnecessary and may delay reaching a diagnosis.

Biochemistry and Immunology

Patients with a toxic adenoma, toxic multinodular goiter, Hashimoto's thyroiditis, or relapsed Graves' disease after subtotal thyroidectomy need not be investigated further with regard to the nature of the nodule, unless there are worrying features on palpation or there is a clear history of recent increase in size. Patients with abnormal thyroid function should be referred routinely to an endocrinologist.

Thyroid function tests are therefore an important useful early screening test for selecting patients who require further assessment in order to exclude cancer, and should be performed by the primary care physician in all patients presenting with a thyroid nodule.

Serum calcitonin may be elevated in patients with nodules due to medullary thyroid cancer, a rare cause of thyroid nodule with a prevalence of about 0.5–0.7% [33]. Routine measurement of serum calcitonin in all patients with thyroid nodules has been advocated by some and retrospective evidence suggests a better outcome in cases that are thus detected than in those diagnosed by conventional means [34]. This strategy, however, remains controversial and cannot yet be recommended.

Thyroid antibodies (antithyroid peroxidase and antithyroglobulin antibodies) are useful to identify patients with autoimmune thyroid disease, but the results of these tests are not necessary in making a decision about referral.

Fine-Needle Aspiration Biopsy

Surgical removal of nodules was used extensively several years ago as a means of excluding thyroid cancer. This, however, was an unnecessary procedure in 95% of cases where the histology turned out to be benign [35]. The introduction of fine-needle aspiration biopsy (FNAB) has been shown to reduce the rate of thyroidectomies, increase the incidence of thyroid cancer in resected thyroid lobes, and to be cost-effective [36]. The sensitivity, specificity, and accuracy of FNAB vary between 70% and 100% in different series [37,38]. The experience

of the person performing the biopsy and of the cytologist, as well as the threshold for accepting a specimen as adequate, determine the diagnostic utility of this test [37,39]. False-positive FNABs are generally rare [38], although the false-negative rate can be as high as 6%, but in most series it is approximately 1% [19,39,40]. FNABs are usually classified into one of six categories: no follicular thyroid cells present (Thy0); follicular thyroid cells present, but inadequate in number for an accurate diagnosis (Thy1); benign (Thy2); follicular neoplasm or hyperplastic nodule (Thy3); suspicious of malignancy (Thy4); malignant (Thy5) [41]. Two common problems limit the usefulness of FNAB: inadequate specimens (i.e. smears containing insufficient numbers of follicular thyroid cells, Thy0 and Thy1) and the inability of FNAB to distinguish between a benign hyperplastic nodule and a follicular carcinoma, which together constitute a significant minority of all FNABs (Thy3).

Inadequate specimens require repeating the FNAB either by palpation (42% chance of repeat biopsy being inadequate, [42]) or with ultrasound guidance (95% chance of an adequate sample [43]).

Ultrasonography

Ultrasound-guided FNAB increases the diagnostic yield to more than 95% and this approach has been adopted by many centers [44,45]. It is, however, costly and the results are operator dependent [42]. Ultrasonography often reveals additional useful features which may help in the clinical management. Irregular margins, increased vascularity, and the presence of calcification increase the likelihood of cancer [46]. However, none of these features are pathognomonic of thyroid cancer and FNAB remains the first investigation of choice in secondary care.

Thyroid Scintigraphy

Thyroid scintiscans may in specific circumstances help to distinguish a benign hyperplastic nodule from a potential follicular neoplasm. Hyperplastic nodules are characteristically "hot" on scintiscans, whereas thyroid cancers are typically "cold." Hot nodules have a very low incidence of malignancy [39]. However, technetium-99 thyroid scanning may be misleading and ^{123}I scanning is preferable for classifying thyroid nodules as hot or cold. [123]I is expensive, and the classification of a nodule into the hot or cold category may subjective [47]. For these reasons most centers do not perform thyroid scintiscans as part of the initial assessment of thyroid nodules.

Management of Thyroid Nodules

Malignant Nodules

If the nodule is shown to be due to differentiated thyroid cancer (papillary or follicular) or medullary thyroid cancer (Thy5), definitive surgery should be performed, which in all but exceptional cases should be total or near-total thyroidectomy. Thyroid lymphomas usually require further staging and conventional treatment with chemotherapy and/or radiotherapy. Surgery is seldom necessary for thyroid lymphomas or anaplastic thyroid carcinomas. The latter have an extremely bleak prognosis and usually require palliative treatments.

Benign Nodules

Hot nodules causing hyperthyroidism may be treated with radioidine, which usually restores euthyroidism and causes reduction of the size of the nodule over several months [48]. Good results are also reported with percutaneous ethanol injection in centers with experience in this [49].

Benign thyroid nodules in euthyroid patients do not require treatment unless they are symptomatic. Treatment may be considered if patients are concerned about the cosmetic effect of the nodule or if the nodule is sufficiently large to cause obstructive symptoms. Suppressive thyroxine therapy has been used to reduce the size of benign thyroid nodules in euthyroid subjects, but a meta-analysis has failed to show a consistent beneficial effect and this treatment cannot be recommended [3]. Percutaneous ethanol injection can be helpful in both cystic and solid benign nodules in centers with experience in this technique [46,50]. Radioiodine can be effective in reducing the size of nontoxic

goiters and is particularly valuable in elderly and unfit patients where surgery may be risky [51]. Surgery is indicated in patients with large nodules or multinodular goiters causing obstructive symptoms or cosmetic problems.

Management of Patients with Nondiagnostic Cytology

Patients with adequate cytology which is intermediate (Thy3 and Thy4), require surgery in order to obtain an accurate diagnosis. The risk of malignancy is approximately 20–25% in Thy3 nodules [52,53] and 40–50% in Thy4 lesions [41]. Lobectomy is the operation of choice for nodules with indeterminate cytology (Thy3 or Thy4). If the histology is benign, the contralateral thyroid lobe will be adequate in most cases for maintaining euthyroidism without a need for thyroxine therapy. If, however, the lesion is malignant, the surgeon can proceed to a completion thyroidectomy without having to re-explore the same lobe, thus minimizing the risks of hypoparathyroidism and recurrent laryngeal nerve injury.

In a very small proportion of patients the FNA may not yield adequate numbers of cells for diagnosis even after multiple attempts, or the patient may refuse to have an FNA. The management and follow-up of these patients depends on the index of suspicion of an underlying cancer and their own individual circumstances and comorbidity. The case for surgery (usually hemithyroidectomy) is strengthened in patients who give a history of rapid growth, if the nodule is large (>3 cm), hard or fixed, in recurrent cystic nodules and nodules that are considered to be high risk (Table 7.2). In all other cases of deferred surgery, follow-up is mandatory with regular clinical and ultrasonographic assessments.

Management of Thyroid "Incidentalomas"

Small nonpalpable thyroid nodules are common in the general population and with increasing use of imaging techniques such lesions are frequently detected in asymptomatic subjects. The prevalence of thyroid cancer in such lesions is thought to be low (about 1–2%) [54]. However, recent data suggest that in some series the incidence of cancer may be as high as 12% and often associated with cervical lymph node metastases or multifocal tumors [55,56]. These findings are contradictory to the experience in other centers and until wider evidence to the contrary is available, observation of small (<1 cm), impalpable nodules in patients who are not otherwise in a high risk category (Table 7.2) is recommended [57]. The incidence of thyroid cancer in non-palpable thyroid nodules >10 mm diameter appears to be similar to palpable nodules [58] and such nodules ought to be investigated.

Follow-up of Benign Thyroid Nodules

Some authors recommend that a benign FNAB should be confirmed by a second FNAB 6–12 months later, because of a false-negative rate of up to 6% of the initial FNAB [59]. The decision to subject patients to a second FNA has to be balanced against the probability of nondiagnostic aspirate, false-positive results (e.g. Thy3 in up to 7% of cases) necessitating surgery, reduction in cost-effectiveness, and heightened patient anxiety [35]. A small proportion of patients will develop new nodules or enlargement of their existing nodule, and some will develop thyroid dysfunction; therefore some form of follow-up seems appropriate, although the optimal means of achieving this is unknown.

Organizational Aspects of a Thyroid Nodule Service

Ideally a "one stop" clinic with access to biochemical testing of thyroid function (if not already available), cytology, and diagnostic ultrasound can provide rapid diagnosis and planning for those cases that require treatment. Patients can be assessed clinically, FNAB performed, cytology reported and if necessary repeated until an adequate sample can be obtained. Those patients who require surgery either for diagnosis or for treatment can have a consultation with the surgeon and the operation planned. Only a few centers are able to provide such a facility because of limited resources. The crucial aspect of a thyroid nodule service,

however, is that it is staffed by clinicians and cytologists who are appropriately trained and experienced in dealing with thyroid nodules.

Performing a biopsy implies suspicion of cancer and most patients experience anxiety about the procedure and the outcome. Before the biopsy the reason for performing this test should be discussed openly with the patient and informed consent obtained. Patients should understand that the result of the biopsy may not provide a definitive answer and that further tests (including surgery) may be required. It is good practice to give patients the opportunity to discuss these issues, and to arrange prospectively a time and place for the communication of the result of the biopsy. This may include breaking bad news, in which case a relative and a nurse should be present. It is preferable therefore for the discussion of the results of the biopsy to take place in person. Informing patients of a diagnosis of cancer by letter or by telephone is an unsatisfactory approach, in the author's opinion, except in specific circumstances and only if that is the patient's own preference.

The Future

Several molecular markers of thyroid cancer are known and the list is continuously growing. Detection of molecular markers of thyroid cancer in FNAB specimens can potentially improve the diagnostic yield and reduce the incidence of indeterminate biopsies. Early experience, particularly with respect to galectin-3 and thyroid peroxidase, is encouraging [60,61]. However, with the exception of calcitonin immunostaining for medullary carcinoma, there are no reliable immunohistological or molecular tests at this time for distinguishing between benign and malignant nodules using FNAB material [62].

References

1. Gharib H. Changing concepts in the diagnosis and management of thyroid nodules. Endocrinol Metab Clin North Am 1997; 26:777–800.
2. Weiss RE, Lado-Abeal J. Thyroid nodules: diagnosis and therapy. Cur Opin Oncol 2002; 14:46–52.
3. Castro MR, Caraballo PJ, Morris JC. Effectiveness of thyroid hormone suppressive therapy in benign solitary

thyroid nodules: a meta-analysis. J Clin Endocrinol Metab 2002; 87:4154–4159.

4. Lawrence W Jr, Kaplan BJ. Diagnosis and management of patients with thyroid nodules. J Surg Oncol 2002; 80(Suppl):157–170.

5. Vander JB, Gaston EA, Dawber TR. The significance of nontoxic thyroid nodules: Final report of a 15-year study of the incidence of thyroid malignancy. Ann Intern Med 1968; 69:537–540.

6. Mazzaferri EL. Management of a solitary thyroid nodule. N Engl J Med 1993; 328:553–559.

7. Tunbridge WM, Evered DC, Hall R, et al. The spectrum of thyroid disease in a community: the Whickham survey. Clin Endocrinol 1977; 7:481–493.

8. Aghini-Lombardi F, Antonangeli L, Martino E, et al. The spectrum of thyroid disorders in an iodine-deficient community: the Pescopanano Survey. J Clin Endocrinol Metab 1999; 84:561–566.

9. Horlocker TT, Hay JE, James EM, Reading CC, Charboneau JW. Prevalence of incidental nodular thyroid disease detected during high resolution parathyroid ultrasonography. In: Medeiros-Neto G, Gaitan E (eds) Frontiers in thyroidology, Vol 2. New York: Plenum Medical, 1985:1309–1312.

10. Stark DD, Clark OH, Gooding GA, Moss AA. High resolution ultrasonography and computed tomography of thyroid lesions in patients with hyperparathyroidism. Surgery 1983; 94:863–868.

11. Ezzat S, Sarti DA, Cain DR, Braunstein GD. Thyroid incidentalomas. Prevalence by palpation and ultrasonography. Arch Intern Med 1994; 154:1834–1840.

12. Mortensen JD, Woolner LB, Bennett WA. Gross and microscopic findings in clinically normal thyroid glands. J Clin Endocrinol Metab 1955; 15:1270–1280.

13. Walsh RM, Watkinson JC, Franklyn J. The management of the solitary thyroid nodule: a review. Clin Otolaryngol 1999; 24:388–397.

14. Rojeski MT, Gharib H. Nodular thyroid disease. Evaluation and management. N Engl J Med 1985; 313:428–436.

15. Franklyn JA, Daykin J, Young J, Oates GD, Sheppard MC. Fine needle aspiration cytology in diffuse or multinodular goitre compared to solitary thyroid nodules. BMJ 1993; 307:240.

16. Tollin SR, Mery GM, Jelveh N, et al. The use of fine-needle aspiration biopsy under ultrasound guidance to assess the risk of malignancy in patients with a multinodular goiter. Thyroid 2000; 10:235–241.

17. Burch HB. Evaluation and management of the solid thyroid nodule. Endocrinol Metab Clin North Am 1995; 24:663–710.

18. Gharib H, Mazzaferri EL. Thyroxine suppressive therapy in patients with nodular thyroid disease. Ann Intern Med 1998; 128:386–394.

19. Boey J, Hsu C, Collins RJ. False-negative errors in fine-needle aspiration biopsy of dominant nodules: a prospective follow-up study. World J Surg 1986; 10:623–630.

20. Kuma K, Matsuzuka F, Kobayashi A, et al. Outcome of long standing solitary thyroid nodules. World J Surg 1992; 16:583–587.

21. Alexander EK, Hurwitz S, Heering JP, et al. Natural history of benign solid and cystic thyroid nodules. Ann Intern Med 2003; 138:315–318.

22. Derwahl M, Studer H. Nodular goiter and goiter nodules: Where iodine deficiency falls short of explaining the facts. Exp Clin Endocrinol Diabetes 2001; 109:250–260.

23. Weetman AP, McGregor AM. Autoimmune thyroid disease: further developments in our understanding. Endocr Rev 1994; 15:788–830.

24. Paleri V, Maroju RS, Ali MS, Ruckley RW. Spontaneous retro- and parapharyngeal haematoma caused by intrathyroid bleed. J Laryngol Otol 2002; 116:854–858.

25. Salabe GB. Pathogenesis of thyroid nodules: histological classification? Biomed Pharmacother 2001; 55:39–53.

26. Moretti F, Nanni S, Pontecorvi A. Molecular pathogenesis of thyroid nodules and cancer. Baillière's Clin Endocrinol Metab 2000; 14:517–539.

27. Dremier S, Coppee F, Delange F, Vassart G, Dumont JE, Van Sande J. Thyroid autonomy. Mechanism and clinical effects. J Clin Endocrinol Metab 1996; 81:4187–4193.

28. Kimura ET, Nikiforova MN, Zhu Z, Knauf JA, Nikiforov YE, Fagin JA. High prevalence of BRAF mutations in thyroid cancer: genetic evidence for constitutive activation of the RET/PTC-RAS-BRAF signalling pathway in papillary thyroid carcinoma. Cancer Res 2003; 63:1454–1457.

29. Fagin JA. Branded from the start – distinct oncogenic initiating events may determine tumor fate in the thyroid. Mol Endocrinol 2002; 16:903–911.

30. Schneider AB. Radiation-induced thyroid tumors. Endocrinol Metab Clin North Am 1990; 19:495–508.

31. Ortiz R, Hupart KH, DeFesi CR, Surks MI. Effect of early referral to an endocrinologist on efficiency and cost of evaluation and development of treatment plan in patients with thyroid nodules. J Clin Endocrinol Metab 1998; 83:3803–3807.

32. Raber W, Kaserer K, Niederle B, Vierhapper H. Risk factors for malignancy of thyroid nodules initially identified as follicular neoplasia by fine-needle aspiration: results of a prospective study of one hundred and twenty patients. Thyroid 2000; 10:709–712.

33. Hahm JR, Lee MS, Min YK, et al. Routine measurement of serum calcitonin is useful for early detection of medullary thyroid carcinoma in patients with nodular thyroid diseases. Thyroid 2001; 11:73–80.

34. Elisei R, Bottici V, Luchetti F, et al. Impact of routine measurement of serum calcitonin on the diagnosis and outcome of medullary thyroid cancer: experience in 10,864 patients with nodular thyroid disorders. J Clin Endocrinol Metab 2004; 89:163–168.

35. Belfiore A, La Rosa GL. Fine-needle aspiration biopsy of the thyroid. Endocrinol Metab Clin North Am 2001; 30:361–400.

36. Caplan RH, Wester SM, Lambert PJ, Rooney BL. Efficient evaluation of thyroid nodules by primary care providers and thyroid specialists. Am J Managed Care 2000; 6:1134–1140.

37. Burch HB, Burman KD, Reed HL, Buckner L, Raber T, Ownbey JL. Fine needle aspiration of thyroid nodules. Determinants of insufficiency rate and malignancy yield at thyroidectomy. Acta Cytol 1996; 40:1176–1183.

38. Morgan JL, Serpell JW, Cheng MSP. Fine-needle aspiration cytology of thyroid nodules: how useful is it? Aust N Z J Surg 2003; 73:480–483.

39. Tabaqchali MA, Hanson JM, Johnson SJ, Wadehra V, Lennard TW, Proud G. Thyroid aspiration cytology in

Newcastle: a six year cytology/histology correlation study. Ann R Coll Surg Eng 2000; 82:149–155.

40. Sclabas GM, Staerkel GA, Shapiro SE, et al. Fine-needle aspiration of the thyroid and correlation with histopathology in a contemporary series of 240 patients. Am J Surg 2003; 186:702–709.

41. Poller DN, Ibrahim AK, Cummings MH, Mikel JJ, Boote D, Perry M. Fine-needle aspiration of the thyroid. Cancer 2000; 90:239–244.

42. Chow LS, Gharib H, Goellner JR, van Heerden JA. Nondiagnostic thyroid fine-needle aspiration cytology: management dilemmas. Thyroid 2001; 11:1147.

43. Karstrup S, Balslev E, Juul N, Eskildsen PC, Baumbach L. US-guided fine needle aspiration versus coarse needle biopsy of thyroid nodules. Eur J Ultrasound 2001; 13:1–5.

44. Hatada T, Okada K, Ishii H, Ichii S, Utsunomiya J. Evaluation of ultrasound-guided fine-needle aspiration biopsy for thyroid nodules. Am J Surg 1998; 175:133–136.

45. Danese D, Sciacchitano S, Farsetti A, Andreoli M, Pontecorvi A. Diagnostic accuracy of conventional versus sonography-guided fine-needle aspiration biopsy of thyroid nodules. Thyroid 1998; 8:15–21.

46. Kim EK, Park CS, Chung WY, et al. New sonographic criteria for recommending fine-needle aspiration biopsy of nonpalpable solid nodules of the thyroid. Am J Roentgenol 2002; 178:687–691.

47. Hedayati N, McHenry CR. The clinical significance of an isofunctioning thyroid nodule. Am Surg 2003; 69:311–315.

48. Burch HB, Shakir F, Fitzsimmons TR, Jaques DP, Shriver CD. Diagnosis and management of the autonomously functioning thyroid nodule: the Walter Reed Army Medical Center experience, 1975–1996. Thyroid 1998; 8:871–880.

49. Monzani F, Caraccio N, Goletti O, et al. Five-year follow-up of percutaneous ethanol injection for the treatment of hyperfunctioning thyroid nodules: a study of 117 patients. Clin Endocrinol 1997; 46:9–15.

50. Del Prete S, Caraglia M, Russo D, et al. Percutaneous ethanol injection efficacy in the treatment of large symptomatic thyroid cystic nodules: ten-year follow-up of a large series. Thyroid 2002; 12:815–821.

51. Manders JM, Corstens FH. Radioiodine therapy of euthyroid multinodular goitres. Eur J Nucl Med Mol Imaging 2002; 29(Suppl 2):S466–470.

52. Bahar G, Braslavsky D, Shpitzer T, et al. The cytological and clinical value of the thyroid "follicular lesion". Am J Otolaryngol 2003; 24:217–220.

53. Monzani F, Caraccio N, Iacconi P, et al. Prevalence of cancer in follicular thyroid nodules: is there still a role for intraoperative frozen section analysis? Thyroid 2003; 13:389–394.

54. Nabriski D, Ness-Abramof R, Brosh TO, Konen O, Shapiro MS, Shenkman L. Clinical relevance of nonpalpable thyroid nodules as assessed by ultrasound-guided fine needle aspiration biopsy. J Endocrinol Invest 2003; 26:61–64.

55. Papini E, Guglielmi R, Bianchini A, et al. Risk of malignancy in nonpalpable thyroid nodules: predictive value of ultrasound and color-Doppler features. J Clin Endocrinol Metab 2002; 87:1941–1946.

56. Nam-Goong IS, Kim H, Gong G, et al. Ultrasonography-guided fine-needle aspiration of thyroid incidentaloma: correlation with pathological findings. Clinical endocrinology. Clin Endocrinol 2004; 60:21–28.

57. AACE clinical practice guidelines for the diagnosis and management of thyroid nodules. http://www.aace.com/clin/guidelines/thyroid_nodules.pdf.

58. Hagag P, Strauss S, Weiss M. Role of ultrasound-guided fine-needle aspiration biopsy in evaluation of nonpalpable thyroid nodules. Thyroid 1998; 8:989–995.

59. Blum M. Why do clinicians continue to debate the use of levothyroxine in the diagnosis and management of thyroid nodules? Ann Intern Med 1995; 122:63–64.

60. Bartolazzi A, Gasbarri A, Papotti M, et al. Application of an immunodiagnostic method for improving preoperative diagnosis of nodular thyroid lesions. Lancet 2001; 357:1644–1650.

61. Haugen BR, Woodmansee WW, McDermott MT. Towards improving the utility of fine-needle aspiration biopsy for the diagnosis of thyroid tumours. Clin Endocrinol 2002; 56:281–290.

62. Hegedus L. Clinical practice. The thyroid nodule. N Engl J Med 2004; 351:1764–1771.

8

Thyroid Cancer and the General Practitioner

Geoffrey Mitchell and Duncan Leith

The different ways general practice operates across the world causes some difficulties in attempting to describe a primary care approach to thyroid cancer. The approach of practitioners in areas where the specialist team may be immature or nonexistent will differ to that where the specialist team is highly developed and close at hand. We have identified the highest diagnostic and management level that a general practitioner (GP) might be expected to exercise in a remote context. GPs in better served areas may not need to exercise these skills, but should be aware of the tasks required for comprehensive care of these patients.

For example, in Australia, there are specialist teams in the capital cities, and GPs can refer to them with little need for workup. However, a quarter of the population of 20 million does not live in capital cities but is scattered across vast rural areas. The patient may be days away from a specialist. (As an idea of Australia's size, Perth to Brisbane is the same distance as Dublin to Moscow!) These patients need a workup at a local level which ensures that any trip undertaken is not wasted. Australian GPs frequently do a lot more diagnostic work before specialist referral than would happen in Britain, and have more extensive follow-up responsibilities. The GP *is* the health service in many Australian locations!

The Diagnostic Context of General Practice

To appreciate the issues GPs face in dealing with rare conditions, it is important to look at the context in which primary care is practiced. Definitions of primary care all emphasize the comprehensive nature of primary care. The American Academy of Family Physicians, for example, states that family (general) practice is:

- The medical specialty that provides continuing and comprehensive health care for the individual and the family.
- The specialty in breadth that integrates the biological, clinical, and behavioral sciences and in scope that encompasses all ages, both sexes, each organ system and disease entity [1].

Primary practitioners serve all comers, with all their complaints – both medical and nonmedical. They deal with the condition in the context of the person and their social milieu.

Hence for thyroid cancer, the challenges are to identify the condition, arrange appropriate investigation and referral for definitive treatment, have a role in follow-up, and participate in palliative care. The GP interprets the disease and the processes for the patient, and acts as advocate for the patient in a confusing and intimidating health system at a time when the patient and their loved ones are extremely vulnerable.

Diagnostic Frameworks for General Practice

Because GPs must be able to distinguish rare, life (or lifestyle) threatening conditions from more common conditions, it is essential to have a diagnostic framework that accomplishes this efficiently. This framework must be sensitive enough not to miss these major conditions, but specific enough to ensure that patients and the community are not subjected to unnecessary, expensive investigations and inconvenience. It needs to identify the patient's concerns and possible psychosocial basis for presentation of physical symptoms. Such a framework has been developed by Murtagh [2]. It directs the practitioner to ask five questions when confronted with a clinical problem.

1. What is the probability diagnosis?
2. What serious disorders must not be missed?
3. What disorders are commonly missed?
4. Is this one of the masqueraders[1] in medical practice?
5. Is this patient trying to tell me something?

The *probability diagnosis* is that condition most likely to explain the presenting complaint. It highlights the relationship between the prevalence of a condition and the likelihood that the condition is truly present. A symptom or sign reflective of a high prevalence condition will most likely be due to that complaint. A symptom reflective of a rare condition is much more likely to be a false-positive finding. Since

---

[1]The masqueraders can be grouped into primary and secondary groups. The primary (most common) masqueraders are: depression, diabetes mellitus, drugs, anemia, thyroid disease, spinal dysfunction, and urinary tract infection. A secondary (less common) list includes: chronic renal failure, HIV/AIDS, rare bacterial infections (e.g. subacute bacterial endocarditis, tuberculosis), systemic viral infections (e.g. infectious mononucleosis, hepatitis A, B, C, D, E), neurological dilemmas (e.g. Parkinson's disease, multiple sclerosis), connective tissue disorders (e.g. systemic lupus erythematosus, polymyalgia rheumatica).

GPs work in the community, they are familiar with what is common in that community. By expecting the common, they will rarely be mistaken.

However, they must not miss the rare but *serious causes* of a symptom. This may mean testing a little more intensely to rule out the condition, or having a strategy that identifies the rare and important as its true identity declares itself over time (see below).

Some causes of a condition are *commonly misdiagnosed*, and should be considered. An example is constipation as a cause of a child's abdominal pain. There are also symptom complexes that present in a variety of nonspecific ways that can be missed if not considered. These are the *masqueraders*. An example is hypothyroidism, which can present as depression, dementia, weight gain, tiredness, hoarse voice, or even cardiac failure.

Finally, it is a common occurrence that physical symptoms can be the presenting symptoms of psychosocial or spiritual distress. If the pattern of illness does not ring true, or if there is dissonance between the described severity and objective signs and symptoms, the GP is alerted to the presence of potential personal distress.

A great strength of general practice is the longitudinal care of patients, which allows both the opportunity to develop a comprehensive picture of the patient's social context, and opportunities to observe the natural history of disease. This creates opportunities to add a "safety net" to the diagnostic process. Many of the conditions that GPs see have differing time disease trajectories, but present with markedly similar conditions in the early stages. Because primary practice allows for repeated visits, the "return visit" becomes a powerful diagnostic tool. The clinical picture becomes clearer as time progresses. Conditions with a steady progression of symptoms with time can be distinguished from ones that are self-limiting, simply by a review in a week or a month. It is much more difficult to put in place such a means of review in secondary or tertiary care facilities, due to organizational, manpower, and funding constraints.

It is in this context that problems in identifying and managing cancer of the thyroid in general practice become obvious.

Making the Diagnosis of Thyroid Cancer in General Practice

Thyroid cancer is rare. It presents as an isolated thyroid nodule, and has an annual incidence of between 0.5 and 10 per 100 000 population [3]. In Australia in 1998, the average GP in a major city had a practice of 1028 patients (up to 1960 in remote areas) [4]. Therefore, a full-time GP will see one thyroid cancer every 10 years at most. If the lower figure is taken there will be some GPs who will never see a case in a 40-year working life.

By contrast, the prevalence of clinically detectable (i.e. detectable by clinical examination) benign thyroid nodules is much higher in the general population than is thyroid cancer, the main differential diagnosis. A population-based study in Finland found thyroid nodules by ultrasound in 27.3% of subjects tested. Of these, only 5% were clinically detectable. This equates to a prevalence of 1.4% in the general population [5]. The average Australian GP practice will thus have 14 patients with a clinically detectable nodule. A Spanish study of the incidence of thyroid disorders in five general practices with 5834 people identified 19 cases of thyroid nodule in the period January 1985 to June 1993. Three of these were thyroid cancers (two papillary and one follicular cancer) [6]. It is thus clear that this is an uncommon GP problem, with thyroid cancer being an exceedingly rare occurrence.

Following Murtagh's diagnostic method, the GP must therefore be aware of the probability diagnosis of a lump in the thyroid (and surrounding structures).

High Probability

Single nodule:

Simple colloid nodule
Follicular adenoma
Regional lymph node

Multiple nodules:

Hashimoto's thyroiditis
Multinodular goiter (nontoxic or toxic)

Colloid nodule (dominant nodule in a multinodular goiter)

Other neck structures:

Regional lymph nodes

Low Probability

Thyroid nodules:

Parathyroid adenoma
Thyroid cancer
Secondary cancer in thyroid

Other neck structures:

Thyroglossal cyst
Secondary cancer in lymph nodes

At the same time GPs must have a strategy that will identify important causes not to be missed, including thyroid cancer.

History

Most thyroid nodules will be asymptomatic, and present after being noticed by the patient. Alternatively the nodule may be discovered by the doctor while examining the neck for unrelated conditions.

The key elements of history helping to distinguish thyroid cancer from other causes of a thyroid nodule relate to the known risk factors. These include age <20 or >70, external irradiation to the neck during childhood or adolescence, family history of thyroid cancer (seen in medullary cancer of the thyroid or multiple endocrine neoplasia type 2). The presence of an accompanying hoarse voice, dysphagia or neck pain, rapid nodule enlargement, symptoms of compression, including stridor and dyspnea, or enlarged lymph nodes are signs of potential invasion of the cancer to local structures [7].

Historical features that reduce the chance of a cancer include: family history of Hashimoto's thyroiditis or autoimmune thyroid disease; family history of benign thyroid nodule or goiter; symptoms of hypothyroidism or hyperthyroidism [7]. Living in an area of iodine deficiency increases the chance of multinodular goiter [8].

Examination [9,10]

Thyroid cancer usually presents with a lump in the neck. Some features make the diagnosis of cancer more likely, while others tend to negate this possibility.

General inspection of the patient should seek features of hyperthyroidism (typically a constellation of anxious demeanor, weight loss, tachycardia, sweating, eye signs including lid lag, lid retraction, and exophthalmos), or hypothyroidism (slowed mentation, weight gain, coarse skin and hair, bradycardia).The presence of either syndrome makes thyroid cancer unlikely. However, weight loss or a hoarse voice may point to the diagnosis of thyroid cancer.

After general inspection, the first challenge for the GP is to determine whether the lump is within the thyroid gland or not. Inspection and palpation should be both used to determine this. Good light and plenty of access to observe the patient from "in front" as well as "behind" is required. A normal thyroid gland is usually not visible. Sometimes, however, the gland can be seen in a thin patient, whilst obesity makes the detection of a lump within the gland even harder. In inspecting the thyroid gland it is useful to ask the patient to swallow. A thyroid swelling will move up and down during this act. Asking the patient to "stick out their tongue" will also cause a lump within the gland to rise unless it is fixed to surrounding tissues by tumor.

Palpation is best performed by standing behind the patient. The patient should lower the chin slightly as this will aid relaxation of the neck muscles. Both hands, each with its thumb in the nape of the neck, should be used simultaneously to palpate the gland. The patient can be asked to repeat the swallowing exercise at intervals as described above. However, for the patient's comfort it may be necessary to give the patient a drink of water to make swallowing easier.

Careful examination of the nodule ought to distinguish the isolated single nodule from a dominant nodule in a multinodular goiter. The risk of malignancy in an isolated thyroid nodule and multinodular thyroid gland is the same. The nodule should be examined to distinguish between softness (versus hard for cancer), smooth borders (versus irregular), mobility of the nodule (versus fixed to other structures). Tenderness of the nodule and surrounding structures may be present. It is not as reliable a sign, as both an acutely active thyroiditis and an invasive cancer may be tender.

There are often no other symptoms or signs in thyroid cancer. The presence of associated symptoms may indicate that the tumor is more aggressive or has spread to a distant site.

Patients more at risk of cancer are males, and whose ages are less than 20 or greater than 70 years old. While males have a higher proportion of malignant to benign nodules; the gender ratio for all thyroid cancers is 3:1 [11].

Nodules less than 1 cm in diameter may be missed clinically. Larger nodules may also be difficult to palpate when they are situated deep in the gland.

The next dilemma for the general practitioner is to identify those lumps that need investigation or referral from those that do not – and of those that need referral which need urgent referral.

Investigations

History and examination will rarely do more than raise the possibility of a thyroid cancer diagnosis. They will also occasionally point to the likely diagnosis of nonmalignant thyroid nodules. Investigations will be required to clinch the diagnosis. The algorithm in Figure 8.1 will assist in distinguishing alternate diagnoses. This algorithm assumes the GP has ready access to basic thyroid function tests, and the ability to refer to specialists if required for further evaluation. A diagram outlining specialist diagnosis and management procedures (Figure 1.8) is given in Chapter 1.

The sensitive thyroid-stimulating hormone assay (TSH) is an important initial test. It will distinguish between potentially overactive thyroid nodules and others.

Whether further tests over and above TSH should be performed depends on context. Further tests are inappropriate where: (1) a multidisciplinary team exists, (2) other tests are not readily available to the GP, and (3) the patient can be seen by specialists in a reasonable time frame. Initiation of other investigations by the GP should be performed (1) in the absence of specialist services, (2) where the tests are available to the GP, and (3) where they can be performed ahead of the referral and taken to the specialist. This may actually save time.

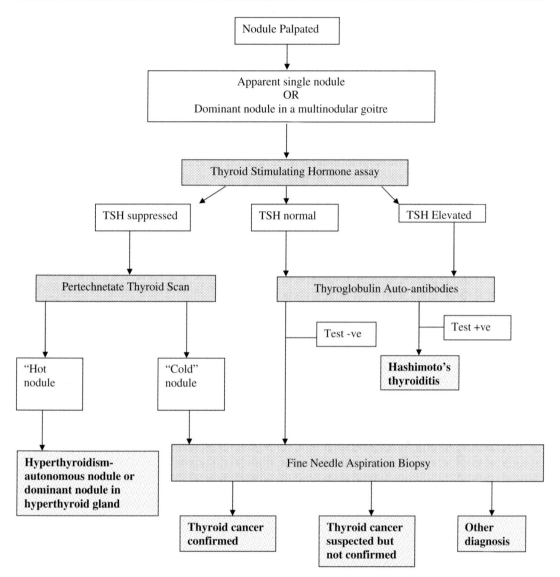

Figure 8.1 General practitioner diagnosis of potential malignant thyroid nodule. Heavily shaded boxes = diagnostic tests, light shaded boxes = potential diagnosis.

If the TSH is suppressed, a pertechnetate (^{99m}Tc) or ^{123}I scan should be ordered. An active nodule will demonstrate increased uptake of the radioactive material, which confirms the diagnosis of a hyperfunctioning isolated nodule, or dominant nodule in a hyperfunctioning gland. However, most nodules will not demonstrate increased uptake (so-called "cold" nodules). These will require fine-needle aspiration biopsy to determine their composition.

If the TSH is normal or elevated, the diagnosis then is between an autoimmune thyroiditis and other forms of nodule including cancer. Thyroid autoantibody assays (antithyroid peroxidase and antithyroglobulin) will determine the presence of immune activity. Although cancers and Hashimoto's thyroiditis can coexist, this is rare [7]. Serum calcitonin would be added to the investigations performed if there is a family history of medullary thyroid carcinoma.

Fine-needle aspiration biopsy is the only test that can confirm the presence of thyroid cancer. The test has a false-negative rate of 1–11%, a false-positive rate of 1–8%, a sensitivity of 65–98%, and a specificity of 72–100%. Limitations of fine-needle aspiration are related to the skill of the aspirator, the expertise of the cytologist, and the difficulty in distinguishing some benign cellular adenomas from their malignant counterparts [12]. Ultrasound guided biopsy is useful in aspiration of impalpable lesions.

When to Refer – and How Urgently

In the UK the presence of any of the following is an indication for urgent referral [13]. The clinical information should be faxed to secondary care within 24 hours of the decision to refer so that the patient can be seen within 2 weeks:

1. Thyroid lump – newly presenting or increasing in size.
2. Thyroid lump in a patient with a family history of thyroid cancer.
3. Thyroid lump in a patient with a history of previous neck irradiation.
4. Thyroid lump in very young (usually <10 years) or very old patients (usually >65 years) [13] especially men.
5. Unexplained hoarseness or voice changes associated with a goiter.
6. Cervical lymphadenopathy (usually deep cervical or supraclavicular region).
7. Stridor (this is a late presenting sign and patients should be seen immediately).

Where to Refer Patients with Possible Thyroid Cancer

Euthyroid patients with a thyroid nodule may have thyroid cancer and should be referred to a member of a multidisciplinary thyroid cancer team if it is available. Patients with hyper- or hypothyroidism and a nodule or nodular goiter should be referred routinely to an endocrinologist.

Patients should be referred to a surgeon or endocrinologist who has a specialist interest in thyroid cancer and preferably is a member of a multidisciplinary team (MDT) if one is available. A clinical oncologist or nuclear medicine physician, preferably a member of an MDT, may also be appropriate.

Patients with unexplained hoarse voice may have a thyroid cancer, and should be considered for referral as above. However, smokers with a hoarse voice (and no goiter) are more likely to have laryngeal pathology, and should be referred to an ear, nose, and throat surgeon in the first instance for examination of the vocal cords and laryngeal structures.

"Incidentalomas"

GPs may order ultrasounds of the neck in order to identify the nature of a goiter or other neck mass. Scans are also ordered to exclude retrosternal goiter as a cause of dysphagia, or unexplained dyspnea. Such scans may reveal impalpable thyroid nodules as incidental findings.

These are termed "incidentalomas." They present a management dilemma, as occult thyroid cancers are found in autopsy specimens at a rate of 36 per 1000 patients (compared with a clinical rate of 0.5–10 per 100 000 per annum) [14]. It may be, therefore, that the doctor is forced to investigate these lesions. If the nodule is one of many in a multinodular thyroid, the likelihood of cancer is very small. Moreover, as clinical cancer of the thyroid accounts for <1% of cancer deaths [3], there must be a large number of cancers that are present but clinically insignificant.

Thus there is a similarity between the clinical decisions required to be made in thyroid cancer and prostate cancer. Up to 75% of all prostate cancers may never be diagnosed [15]. The dilemma faced by medical practitioners, especially GPs who find such a lesion is: what will be the cost-benefit of investigating an incidentaloma? In a younger person, there will be little argument. However, in older people, what is going to be the benefit of investigation, treatment, and ongoing surveillance of a condition that may have caused no extra morbidity?

Role of the GP in Initial Diagnosis

GPs will often be the first port of call for a patient who has found a thyroid nodule, and may be the one who identifies the nodule incidentally either on physical examination or on ultrasound.

Much of the patient's workup can be conducted in general practice, depending on local access to biochemical and pathological testing, specialist teams, and local protocols. This work can reduce the time required for specialists to perform their diagnostic procedures.

Should a diagnosis of thyroid cancer be possible, it is essential that the possibility is canvassed with the patient before referral to the specialist. Responses to the diagnosis in other cancers when patients are not forewarned can range from disbelief to anger, and specialist colleagues are put in an invidious position when there is no preparation [16].

Informing the Patient

The patient should be informed of the diagnosis by a member of the specialist team. Written information concerning thyroid cancer and its treatment should be available to the patient in the specialist clinic. Patients may have difficulty understanding all this information at a single consultation and an opportunity for further explanation/discussion should be offered by the specialist team. However given the easier access and often longstanding relationship with their GP, patients may approach primary care for further information, interpretation of the specialist consultation, and help. It is therefore essential that the GP and his nursing colleagues have access to and understand the information being given to the patient by secondary care.

In the UK, patients may receive information from secondary care in the form of leaflets explaining (1) tests and treatment, (2) thyroidectomy, and (3) radioactive iodine ablation therapy. These have been formulated into three patient information booklets which are available on the British Thyroid Association website – www.british-thyroid-association.org.

How to Break Bad News

While providing patients with the facts about an adverse diagnosis such as thyroid cancer is important, the manner in which the news is conveyed is vital. Poorly conveyed bad news can leave long-lasting adverse psychological consequences [17].

Meticulous attention to detail will minimize the impact of the news. If the patient is coming as an outpatient to receive the diagnosis, they should be advised to have their spouse or a trusted adult come with them to the consultation.

Adequate time should be set aside. The GP should be prepared for shows of emotion, both from the patient as the news is conveyed, as well as some internal discomfort of his own. The news should be delivered in private. Information similar to that discussed above should be given to the patient. The GP should sit at the same level as the patient, and speak slowly and clearly. Be prepared to repeat information. Patients recall only a fraction of what is said when bad news is broken, so giving the information in written form is vital. Always arrange a repeat visit to reinforce the message and allow unanswered questions to be answered.

What to say:

1. Start by summarizing what the patient knows. For example, "As you know, we found a lump in your thyroid gland. We needed to do a series of tests to work out what the problem might be."

2. Ask what they think the problem is. "Have you got any thoughts about what the problem might be?"

3. Name the problem: "I'm afraid your fears that it might be cancer might be correct. We need to arrange for tests to make sure you don't have a form of thyroid cancer."

4. Discuss where we go from here. Be honest with the answers. In particular with prognosis, state that the prognosis cannot be determined until the nature of the cancer (if it is cancer) has been determined. Highlight the generally good prognosis most forms of thyroid cancer have.

5. Be prepared to repeat information – arrange for a follow-up appointment and suggest the patient writes down questions he or she might have.

The Need for Specialists to Inform the Primary Care Team

Secondary care providers have a responsibility to inform the primary care team at regular intervals during diagnosis and treatment. Good practice and present guidelines encourage the following:

1. The GP should be informed within 24 hours (by telephone or fax) of the diagnosis being communicated to the patient. The GP should also be made aware of the

information which has been given to the patient and of the planned treatment.

2. Subsequent alterations in prognosis, management, or drug treatment should be communicated promptly to the GP as patients/carers will often approach their GP for confirmation or extra information.

Support of Patients During Treatment and Follow-up

GPs should be familiar with the treatment procedure during and after the initial phase of diagnosis. Ablation of all thyroid tissue with ^{131}I is usually performed at the time that TSH production is maximal – usually around 4 weeks post surgery. Thereafter, the patient will require replacement therapy with thyroxine (T_4). This will only be ceased in the weeks prior to periodic reassessment with radioactive iodine scans. GPs will need to monitor thyroxine levels. Serum thyroglobulin levels can also be monitored as this hormone is a sensitive marker of well-differentiated thyroid tumors [3].

Serum calcium and parathyroid hormone surveillance should be considered until it is established that the parathyroid gland preserved at the time of surgery is functioning adequately. If a total thyroidectomy is required, autologous transfer of a parathyroid gland into a muscle mass will be performed.

The most common forms of thyroid cancer – follicular and papillary – have excellent survival rates, even when there has been spread beyond the thyroid [14]. GPs can therefore be very optimistic when talking to most patients about prognosis. While patients will accept this outlook, the emotional response to suffering cancer needs to be considered. Anxiety will rise with every follow-up check and will not abate until news that "no recurrence has been found" is delivered. Moreover, the physical symptoms related to thyroid hormone withdrawal required prior to reassessment are profound, severe, and debilitating. Dow and colleagues found that patients with thyroid cancer had to learn through their own personal experiences what physical limitations were imposed during the period of surveillance testing. As well, the physical changes and anticipation of body scanning

exerted a profound effect on their psychological and social wellbeing. Feelings of loss, anxiety, depression, and loss of concentration were very difficult to endure [18,19].

One challenge for all practitioners dealing with cancer patients is that of offering shared decision-making capacity. With thyroid cancer, the treatment protocols for most will be relatively inflexible, and patient choice will be limited to whether to agree to treatment or not. However, studies in breast cancer patients indicate some women want an active role in decision-making. Degner et al. showed that women with higher levels of education and who were younger wanted to be more actively involved in decision-making. However only 30–40% of patients achieved the role they preferred for themselves [20]. These findings may not be transferable to other cancer patients: it has been shown that patients with colorectal cancer had a lower proportion of patients wanting to have an active decision-making role than was the case with breast cancer patients [21].

Long-Term Follow-up

Regular follow-up is necessary, particularly for detection of early recurrence, initiation of appropriate treatment, TSH suppression, and management of hypocalcemia. This is usually undertaken by either a member of the MDT, working in a multidisciplinary setting and according to the established local guidelines, or by the GP where that facility does not exist. Once the thyroid remnant has been ablated, the frequency of attendance will be decided in each case individually: usually 3-monthly for the first 2 years, decreasing to 6-monthly for 3 years, and annually thereafter. Support and counseling may be necessary, particularly for younger patients, and in relation to pregnancy.

Follow-up should be life-long because:

- The disease has a long natural history.
- Late recurrences can occur, which can be successfully treated with a view to cure or long-term survival.
- The consequences of supraphysiological T_4 replacement (such as atrial fibrillation and osteoporosis) need monitoring, especially as the patient ages.

- Late side-effects of ^{131}I treatment may develop, such as leukemia or second tumors.

At each visit the following tasks should be completed:

- Patient history should be taken.
- A clinical examination should be performed.
- Assessment of the adequacy of TSH suppression and of possible effects of thyroxine excess.
- Measurement of thyroglobulin (Tg) as a marker of tumor recurrence. (Undetectable Tg without TSH stimulation does not, however, exclude the possibility of recurrent tumor. Serum calcium should be measured if indicated.)

Recurrent Disease

Local recurrence of thyroid cancer is common, occurring in up to 30% of patients thought to be disease-free after treatment [22]. Distant metastases develop in 5–20% of patients with differentiated thyroid carcinoma, mainly in the lungs and bones. Early detection of recurrent or metastatic disease can lead to cure or certainly long-term survival – particularly if it is operable or takes up radioactive iodine.

Palliative Care

Palliative care is not necessary in the vast majority of patients with differentiated thyroid cancer because they are cured. However, in a very small proportion of patients with recurrent end-stage disease (and in patients with anaplastic thyroid cancer) palliative care will be necessary. The GP should work with a palliative care consultant, in conjunction with the MDT.

Symptoms of stridor and fear of choking are very distressing and can be alleviated by pharmacological means, palliative surgery, and counseling. These patients should be referred early to the local palliative care team. There are excellent guides for primary palliative care. Local practice guidelines are available in many Western settings [23–25].

Special Situations

Pregnancy

A minimum of 4 months is recommended before conception post treatment. However a risk of spontaneous abortion may persist for up to one year post treatment. TSH should be monitored to ensure TSH remains suppressed as T_4 requirements may increase in pregnancy [13].

The diagnosis of thyroid nodules in pregnant women can usually be managed in the same way as in nonpregnant patients [26], except that radionuclide scanning is contraindicated [7]. A thyroid nodule presenting in pregnancy should be investigated by FNA biopsy. Surgical removal of thyroid nodules is relatively safe during the second trimester, which is the safest time for surgery during pregnancy. (Surgery during the first trimester carries a high risk of abortion.) ^{131}I studies can follow in the postpartum period. Surgery also can usually be deferred until after the pregnancy. Only very rarely is termination of pregnancy followed by thyroidectomy, ^{131}I studies, and treatment needed [13].

Childhood

While the prevalence of thyroid nodules is less common in children, the risk of malignancy appears to be much higher (14–40% in children as opposed to 5% in adults) [26]. Recent reports suggest FNA biopsy has an important role in the diagnosis and management of thyroid nodules in children. However, studies involving children have been limited, and false-negative results have raised concerns about the accuracy of this test in children [26]. Therefore surgical excision may be appropriate even if FNA suggests benign disease [13].

Family History

Medullary thyroid cancer is a rare disease accounting for 5–10% of all thyroid cancers. Twenty-five percent of these cancers are familial, inherited in an autosomal dominant manner, necessitating a comprehensive and integrated approach to patient and family.

The Advantage of a Strong Primary Care Sector

Starfield has shown conclusively that the stronger the country's primary care sector, and the more money per capita is spent on the sector, the better health outcomes are achieved [27]. In complex conditions such as thyroid cancer, the gatekeeper role and the role of the patient advocate are critical.

Gatekeeper Role

This is the role whereby a well-trained GP has the responsibility of determining which resources are the most appropriate for the patient's needs. This role gives the GP the responsibility of allocating scarce health resources most appropriately, by directing the patient to the tests and specialists most suited to the patient's needs. Ideally the GP has the ability to diagnose the problems accurately, know the resources available in a community, and match the need to the resources. It is not always obvious which tests and resources are most appropriate for the patient. In systems where the patient has the capacity to make these decisions autonomously, at best a lot of money can be wasted, and at worst, serious treatment errors can be made and life can be put at risk [28].

Patient Advocate

Thyroid cancer is a serious and frightening condition, where the management is complex and ongoing. Navigating the complexities of treatment in an ever more complex health system can be confusing and frightening. The GP has a pivotal role in ensuring the patient gets the right attention by the right service in the right time frame. He or she therefore can assume the role of a "health advocate" or "case manager." This role also involves interpreting the disease, the treatments, and the prognosis for the patient. It is an enabling role which is critical for the empowerment of the patient, and for assisting the patient understand the condition and what is being proposed. Understanding the disease process allows the patient to "live with" the illness better. Empowerment of the patient in

this way will lead to better health outcomes [25,29,30].

Conclusion

Thyroid cancer is rare, and many GPs will not see it in a professional lifetime. However it is life-threatening, and GPs must have diagnostic strategies that enable it to be identified promptly, efficiently, and cost-effectively. How this is done, and to what extent the GP is involved in workup and follow-up, varies enormously throughout the world and the various health systems. Some GPs will have ready access to multidisciplinary teams, while others will have to conduct much of the diagnostic and follow-up work on their own in rural and remote settings.

The core skills of accurate history-taking and diagnosis are common in all locations. The central roles of the GP as a gatekeeper and patient advocate should be common to all settings.

References

1. American Academy of Family Physicians. American Academy of Family Physicians: Policy and Advocacy. www.aafp.org, 2003.
2. Murtagh J. A safe diagnostic strategy. In: Murtagh J (ed.) General practice. Sydney: McGraw Hill, 1998: 101–105.
3. Cobin RH, Gharib H for Thyroid Carcinoma Task Force. AACE/AAES Medical/surgical guidelines for clinical practice: Management of thyroid carcinoma. Endocr Pract 2001; 7:203–220.
4. Harding J. The supply and distribution of general practitioners. In: General practice in Australia: 2000. Canberra: Commonwealth Department of Health and Aged Care, 2000: 41–74.
5. Brander A, Viikinkoski P, Nickels J, Kivisaari L. Thyroid gland: US screening in a random adult population. Radiology 1991; 181(3):683–687.
6. Serra M, Méndez MA, Davins J, et al. [Thyroid pathology in a health center]. Aten Primaria 1995; 15(7):457–460.
7. Feld S for Thyroid Nodule Task Force. AACE clinical practice guidelines for the diagnosis and management of thyroid nodules. Endocr Pract 1996; 2:80–84.
8. Mackenzie EJ, Mortimer RH. 6: Thyroid nodules and thyroid cancer. Med J Aust 2004; 180(5):242–247.
9. MacLeod J. The general examination and the external features of disease. In: MacLeod J (ed.) Clinical examination. Edinburgh: Churchill Livingstone, 1977: 83–86.
10. Bailey H. The thyroid gland. In: Clain A (ed.) Demonstrations of physical signs in clinical surgery. Bristol: Wright & Sons, 1980: 156–156.
11. Australian Institute of Health and Welfare. Thyroid cancer. In: Cancer survival in Australia 2001. Part 1 –

National Summary Statistics. Canberra: NIHW, 2002: 84–87.

12. Gharib H, Goellner JR, Johnson DA. Fine-needle aspiration cytology of the thyroid. A 12-year experience with 11 000 biopsies. Clin Lab Med 1993; 13(3):699–709.

13. Working Party: Royal College of Physicians. Key recommendations and overview of management of thyroid cancer (differentiated and medullary). www.rcplondon.ac.uk, 2002.

14. Schlumberger MJ, Torlantano M. Papillary and follicular thyroid carcinoma. Baillieres Best Pract Res Clin Endocrinol Metab 2000; 14(4):601–613.

15. Etzioni R, Cha R, Feuer EJ, Davidov O. Asymptomatic incidence and duration of prostate cancer. Am J Epidemiol 1998; 148:775–784.

16. Mitchell G, Mitchell C. Lung cancer. Aust Fam Physician 2004; 33:321–325.

17. Del Mar CB, Henderson M. Communicating bad news to patients and relatives. In: Mitchell C, Sanders M, Byrne G (eds) Medical consultation skills. Melbourne: Addison-Wesley, 1996: 103–117.

18. Dow KH, Ferrell BR, Anello C. Balancing demands of cancer surveillance among survivors of thyroid cancer. Cancer Pract 1997; 5(5):289–295.

19. Dow KH, Ferrell BR, Anello C. Quality-of-life changes in patients with thyroid cancer after withdrawal of thyroid hormone therapy. Thyroid 1997; 7(4):613–619.

20. Degner LF, Kristjanson LJ, Bowman D, et al. Information needs and decisional preferences in women with breast cancer. JAMA 1997; 277(18):1485–1492.

21. Beaver K, Bogg J, Luker KA. Decision-making role preferences and information needs: a comparison of colorectal and breast cancer. Health Expect 1999; 2:266–276.

22. Treatment statement for health professionals – thyroid cancer. 2004, National Cancer Institute. www.cancer.org.

23. Mitchell G, Bowman J, McEniery J, Eastwood H. The blue book of palliative care: evidence based clinical guidelines for primary practitioners. Ipswich: Ipswich and West Moreton Division of General Practice, 1999.

24. Writing Group, Therapeutic Guidelines: Palliative care. Therapeutic Guidelines. Melbourne: Therapeutic Guidelines, 2001.

25. Regnard C, Tempest S. A guide to symptom relief in advanced disease, 4th edn. Hale, England: Hochland and Hochland, 1998.

26. Welker MJ, Orlov D. Thyroid nodules. Am Fam Physician 2003; 67(3):559–566.

27. Starfield B. Continuous confusion? Am J Public Health 1980; 70:117–119.

28. Mitchell G, Pachmajer U. Critical Event Analysis as a means of defining the value of General Practice to a health system: a proposal. Eur J Gen Pract 2001; 7:115–117.

29. McWhinney I. Illness, suffering and healing. In: A textbook of family medicine. New York: Oxford University Press, 1989: 72–87.

30. McWhinney I. Core values in a changing world. BMJ 1998; 316:1807–1809.

9

The Role of the Pathologist

Anne Marie McNicol

Introduction

The multidisciplinary team dealing with patients with thyroid nodules must include a pathologist. The aim is to make the correct diagnosis as soon as possible after presentation, to prevent surgery where it is not required, and to allow treatment to be planned when malignancy is diagnosed. The first investigation should now be fine-needle aspiration (FNA) cytology. With adequate specimens, the pathologist can give a relatively clear indication of the nature of the lesion. A diagnosis of benign disease indicates that the nodule need not be removed other than for local pressure effects or cosmetic reasons. This has reduced surgical intervention for thyroid nodules by up to 50%, and has increased the yield of cancers in surgical specimens from 10–15% up to 20–50% [1]. However, FNA is not yet the norm, and the proportion of patients having FNA varies in different centers. Recent studies from the USA and UK suggest that FNA is used as the initial procedure in only 52–84% of patients with thyroid nodules [2].

In dealing with the surgical specimen the pathologist should provide a definitive diagnosis and try to identify features that correlate with a more aggressive pattern of behavior. For example, distinguishing minimally from widely invasive follicular carcinoma and defining certain variants of papillary carcinoma. Pathology also contributes to the staging by defining the maximum dimension of the tumor, the presence or absence of extrathyroidal spread, the presence of ipsilateral or contralateral lymph node involvement, and sometimes the presence of metastases.

Fine-Needle Aspiration Cytology

Fine-needle aspiration should be performed on any solitary or dominant nodule more than 10 mm in diameter or in nodules as small as 8 mm with highly suspicious ultrasonographic characteristics. Where the nodule is palpable it can be aspirated under direct palpation in the first instance. In some places in Europe and the USA and in Japan, ultrasound guidance is used for all lesions. However, in view of the additional resource required, many centers would reserve its use for cases where standard FNA yields non-diagnostic material. It is also especially useful in complex cysts, in lesions that are difficult to palpate or are impalpable, and in targeting the dominant nodule(s) in multinodular goiter. Aspiration should be carried out by a clinician with an interest in thyroid disease, trained in good practice and performing aspirates regularly. This can be a cytopathologist, surgeon, endocrinologist, or radiologist. The cytopathologist reporting the FNA should also have an interest in thyroid disease and report sufficient cases to maintain expertise. There should be the opportunity for cytology review, and correlation with any subsequent histology is essential as part of audit. In most centers, a combination of wet and air-dried preparations is used. Additional material may be processed as cytospin slides, cell blocks or Millipore filter preparations for immunohistochemistry where appropriate, or processed for molecular genetic analysis. However, in most instances, the diagnosis is made on standard smears. The few publications on the use of liquid-based cytology for thyroid suggest that it is not as good as conventional smears [3,4].

Aspirates are usually divided into five categories: nondiagnostic; benign; follicular lesions (usually neoplasms); suspicious of malignancy (papillary, medullary or anaplastic carcinoma, or lymphoma); and diagnostic of malignancy (in the same range of tumors). A numerical grading system of Thy1 to Thy5 has recently been proposed in the British Thyroid Association guidelines [5]. This should be coupled with a descriptive report. Published figures would suggest that inadequate/nondiagnostic (Thy1) FNA cytology should be about 5–15% of the total, the figure being lower in ultrasound-guided lesions. Aspirates in this category include those with insufficient thyroid epithelial cells and those that cannot be interpreted because of technical artifact. Specimens are usually considered adequate when they contain at least six groups of 10 to 20 cells each on slides from two different passes [6]. This is especially important when making a benign diagnosis. A diagnosis of malignancy may be made with fewer cells where the characteristic features are pronounced (e.g. papillary carcinoma).

The aspirate from nodular goiter usually shows abundant thin colloid, sometimes with a "cracking" artifact. The follicular cells lie in sheets, in follicles or singly. Foamy and hemosiderin-laden macrophages are usually present, but their numbers will vary with the extent of degeneration. This will be classified as Thy2. Hyperplastic nodules may give rise to smears resembling those from follicular neoplasms (Thy3). Some would advocate that a benign diagnosis should be made confidently only on the basis of two aspirates, 3 to 6 months apart. However, others would not recommend a repeat if the first aspirate is adequate, the nodule is <20 mm in diameter, and is not increasing in size.

The third category (Thy3) comprises mainly follicular neoplasms. Follicular Hürthle cell tumors are included in this group. It is not possible to make the distinction between benign and malignant follicular tumors on cytology alone, and all cases in this group require lobectomy for definitive diagnosis. The majority of these lesions are follicular adenomas, with up to 15% reported as follicular carcinomas. These are cellular aspirates, comprising follicular or Hürthle cells arranged in microfollicles or three-dimensional groups, with little colloid (Figure 9.1). Nuclear atypia may be seen, but is not important in defining the behavior of the lesion, as atypical adenomas may show pleomorphism. There has been recent interest in the application of immunohistochemical markers for the preoperative diagnosis of follicular carcinoma, particularly galectin-3. A large European study suggested a positive predictive value of 92% and a diagnostic accuracy of 99% for galectin-3 positivity in predicting malignancy [7]. However, more recent investigations have demonstrated focal expression of galectin-3 in follicular adenomas and in nodular goiter and a number of follicular carcinomas have been reported as negative [8,9]. This might lead to erroneous diagnosis on cytology preparations.

Oncocytic follicular lesions also fall into the Thy3 category. Galectin 3 immunostaining has been reported as less specific in assessing malignant potential in oncocytic tumors [10]. Aspi-

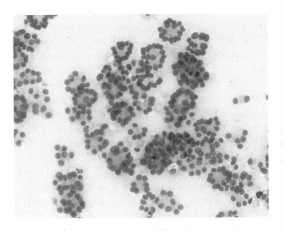

Figure 9.1 Fine-needle aspirate of a follicular neoplasm. The follicular epithelial cells are arranged in microfollicles and there is almost no colloid. It is not possible to distinguish adenoma from carcinoma on cytological examination. Histologically this was a minimally invasive follicular carcinoma.

rates from Hashimoto's thyroiditis will also contain oncocytes, but will also have a chronic inflammatory cell population.

Smears from classical papillary carcinoma are usually highly cellular, and may contain branching papillary tissue fragments and cell clusters. The tissue fragments often have a regular outline and show nuclear palisading. The nuclei are usually large and irregular and have grooves and pseudoinclusions. Thick colloid (chewing gum or ropy) is characteristic and multinucleate giant cells and psammoma bodies may also be found. Depending on how marked the changes are, these smears will be Thy4 (suspicious for malignancy) or Thy5 (definite for malignancy).

Follicular variant of papillary carcinoma (FVPC) may be recognized on cytology if the nuclear changes are pronounced. The smears show cells lying in sheets, cellular groups, or microfollicles. Colloid is usually thin, with thick "chewing gum" colloid less common than in the classic variant. The nuclei are elongated and show clearing of chromatin and thickening of the nuclear membrane, but nuclear grooves and inclusions are said to be less common than in the classic variant. The presence of mulinucleate giant cells is a factor in favor of the diagnosis of FVPC [11] and psammoma bodies may occasionally be found. In the cases where a confident diagnosis can be made, these smears would be classified as Thy5. However, where the nuclear features are not prominent, the smear may be interpreted as a follicular neoplasm (Thy3) or as Thy4 if there is some clearing of chromatin and a thick nuclear membrane. Distinction of microfollicular and macrofollicular variants has been attempted [12]. Attempts have also been made to identify tall cell [13] and columnar cell [14] variants on cytological examination. To increase the overall sensitivity of detection of papillary carcinoma on FNA, one group has used reverse-transcription polymerase chain reaction (RT-PCR) for the specific *RET/PTC* gene rearrangements that characterize a subset of these tumors and has identified tumor in specimens deemed inadequate for standard cytological assessment [15]. However, the *RET/PTC* gene may be found in benign tumors [16].

A cellular smear comprising small to intermediate sized cells with frequent mitotic

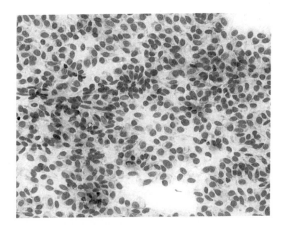

Figure 9.2 Fine-needle aspirate of medullary carcinoma. The cells are rather dys-cohesive. They have ovoid nuclei and a plasmacytoid appearance in places.

figures, little colloid, and evidence of necrosis raises the possibility of poorly differentiated carcinoma. However, specific diagnosis requires examination of the surgical specimen.

Anaplastic or undifferentiated carcinomas are usually cellular and often show significant pleomorphism and high mitotic activity. There is often evidence of necrosis and polymorphonuclear leukocytes. Osteoclast-like giant cells may be present.

Medullary carcinoma also gives a hypercellular smear (Figure 9.2). The cells may be polygonal or spindle-shaped and often have a plasmacytoid appearance. They tend to be poorly cohesive. Amyloid is present in up to 70% of cases. The diagnosis can be confirmed by immunostaining for calcitonin. These cases will be Thy4 or Thy5.

Thyroid lymphoma needs to be distinguished from chronic thyroiditis and is usually characterized on the immunophenotype of the lymphoid cells. This may be achieved by immunostaining of cell blocks or cytospins or by fluorescence activated cell sorting (FACS) analysis.

Follicular Lesions

Following on a cytology diagnosis of follicular lesion, the patient will undergo lobectomy. It is then the role of the pathologist to distinguish follicular carcinoma from follicular adenoma and a dominant nodule in nodular goiter. Frozen section should not be performed.

Nodular Goiter

This disease develops as the result of absolute or relative deficiency of iodine intake. Goiter is defined as endemic in areas where more than 10% of the population is affected and sporadic when the incidence is less than that. Endemic goiter occurs in areas of iodine deficiency. Increased requirement for thyroid hormones, individual dietary insufficiency of iodine, ingestion of goitrogens, and subclinical levels of dyshormonogenesis may be important in the pathogenesis of the sporadic form. The pathological features are a combination of hyperplastic and involutional change and nodule formation. The initial change is related to stimulation of secretion of thyroid hormones by pituitary thyroid-stimulating hormone (TSH) in response to an increased demand for thyroxine. This results in thyroid hyperplasia, with the development of increased numbers of small follicles with little storage of colloid. The follicular cells are columnar and may show pleomorphism and mitotic activity. When the thyroid hormone levels reach normal, the gland undergoes a process of involution. The follicular cells become flattened and there is accumulation of colloid within the follicles. Eventually, after periods of stimulation and involution the thyroid comprises a mixture of hyperplastic and involutional change with areas of degeneration, hemorrhage, and fibrosis. Some nodules may appear larger – dominant nodules. These may be nodules with extensive colloid accumulation and degeneration that are easily recognized on FNA, or hyperplastic nodules that histologically resemble follicular neoplasms. Some may be encapsulated. The question is whether to define them as adenomas or as nodules. In the context of overall nodularity, many pathologists would use the term "adenomatoid nodule." However, molecular analysis has shown that up to 70% of dominant nodules in nodular goiter are monoclonal, suggesting that they are neoplastic, while the remainder show a polyclonal pattern [17]. The specific classification is not important, as long as after appropriate examination there are no features to indicate malignancy. Any nodules within a goiter that have a thick capsule should be processed as for a follicular neoplasm.

Follicular Adenoma

Follicular adenoma is the most common thyroid tumor. It most often presents between 30 and 50 years of age with a female to male ratio of 20:1. It is usually a single nodule, with an expansile pattern of growth. Although they are described as encapsulated, the extent of capsule formation can vary. In some lesions there is a well-formed fibrous capsule, although it is usually thin. Sometimes, the normal thyroid follicles adjacent to the tumor undergo atrophy, and the stroma condenses to form a pseudocapsule. In some cases tumor cells can abut directly onto normal thyroid parenchyma. However, even where they are in close contact with the normal follicles, an expansile pattern of growth is maintained, and they do not infiltrate between follicles. A thick capsule is more often seen in follicular carcinoma. Follicles may become entrapped within the capsule in adenomas, but there is no penetration through the capsule. In order to make the diagnosis a proper assessment of the interface between the tumor and the normal gland is essential to rule out capsular or vascular invasion. It is suggested that lesions <3 cm in diameter be processed in their entirety, and that larger lesions should have 8 to 10 blocks processed [18,19].

Follicular adenomas show a range of histological appearances. In some a microfollicular pattern predominates, while in others there are mainly large colloid-filled follicles. Some tumors have a more solid or trabecular architecture. A mixed pattern may also be seen. These are of no clinical relevance. Most comprise small, fairly uniform cells with round nuclei and evenly dispersed chromatin. There may be central degenerative change with hyalinization or calcification, but these changes are more frequent in hyperplastic nodules. Mitotic activity is uncommon. In cases with marked nuclear atypia or mitotic activity, great care should be taken to rule out capsular or vascular invasion. Tumors with these features, but no evidence of invasion, are referred to as atypical adenomas. Most behave in a benign fashion. Areas of degeneration are often associated with pseudopapillary architecture, not to be confused with papillary carcinoma. There may also be some focal clearing of nuclei and this may cause the pathologist to consider a diagnosis of FVPC. In most cases it should be possible to make the distinction. The characteristic prominence of the nuclear membrane is not present, and nuclear grooves and inclusions are not usually seen. Immunostaining for cytokeratin (CK) 19 may show focal positivity, in contrast to the more widespread staining in FVPC. However, it should be noted that the threshold for interpreting nuclear features as characteristic of FVPC differs with individual pathologists. Changes associated with FNA are discussed below.

Rare variants include adenolipoma, where the tumor cells are interspersed with mature adipose tissue. This probably represents adipose metaplasia. Clear cell and signet ring cell tumors are also described. An origin from thyroid follicular cells can be confirmed by immunopositivity for thyroglobulin and thyroid transcription factor-1 (TTF-1) [20], a nuclear protein important in regulating the transcription of the thyroglobulin gene. It is preferable to use non-biotin immunohisto-chemical techniques as thyroid follicular cells may contain significant amounts of endogenous biotin, thus leading to false-positive staining.

Follicular Carcinoma

Follicular carcinoma accounts for 5–15% of all thyroid cancers in iodine-sufficient areas. It is more common in women and presents on average about 10 years later than papillary carcinoma. It is usually a single "cold" nodule. Occasional cases present as distant metastases, particularly in bone. On the basis of the extent of invasion, the tumor is subdivided into two categories – minimally and widely invasive. Minimally invasive tumors are more common. These are diagnosed on the presence of microscopic capsular and/or vascular invasion. Widely invasive tumors can often be seen infiltrating the normal gland by naked eye examination. This diagnosis may also be applied when extensive vascular invasion is identified at microscopic level. It is important to make the distinction between the two, as the outcome varies significantly. The 10-year survival rate for minimally invasive disease is 70–100% and for the widely invasive type, 25–45% [21]. Tumor-related deaths are more common in the widely invasive group, reported in 20–50% of cases, but in minimally invasive disease may only account for 3% of deaths [19,22].

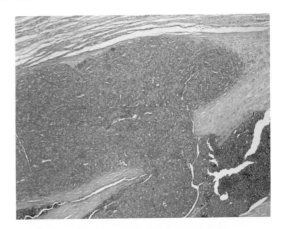

Figure 9.3 Minimally invasive follicular carcinoma showing capsular invasion. The tumor can be seen extending in mushroom-like fashion through the fibrous capsule, which shows "blunt ended" breaks. Compressed normal thyroid is seen to the top left of the figure.

Grossly, minimally invasive follicular carcinoma resembles follicular adenoma, although it often has a thicker capsule. Diagnosis depends on the identification of capsular (Figure 9.3) and/or vascular (Figure 9.4) invasion on histological examination. There has been debate over the years as to the definitions of these two features. It is now generally accepted that tumor cells must penetrate the entire thickness of the capsule to diagnose capsular invasion. This is usually associated with "blunt end" breaks in

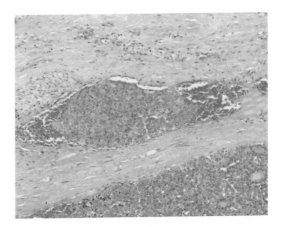

Figure 9.4 Minimally invasive follicular carcinoma showing vascular invasion. Tumor is seen within an intracapsular vessel. It is attached to the wall of the vessel in the lower part and is covered by endothelium.

the capsule and a "streaming" or mushroom pattern of growth of tumor through the capsule. This is in contrast to the entrapment of follicles within the capsule of an adenoma where there is no impression of an active process of cell movement. It is important to realize that the penetrating tumor mass often stimulates the formation of a new capsule. This means that the tumor may have a dumbbell appearance, or that there is the impression of subdivision of a follicular tumor by a fragmented fibrous band.

These appearances can be extremely difficult to interpret. Historically, some pathologists argued that malignant potential could not be diagnosed on the basis of capsular invasion alone and defined these tumors as "follicular neoplasms of undetermined malignant potential." However, metastases have occurred in tumors where only capsular invasion has been identified.

Vascular invasion is diagnosed only when tumor thrombi are attached to the wall of a medium sized or large vessel, either within or outside the capsule, and are covered by endothelium. It should be noted that tumor cells and vessels are often intermingled within the capsule, and it can sometimes be difficult to assess whether this is true invasion. It may be necessary to use immunohistochemistry for an endothelial marker such as CD31 or CD34 to define this. Factor VIII-related antigen is not generally useful, as it can be negative in vessels invaded by tumor. An unusual feature that might also be misinterpreted as invasion is endothelial hyperplasia in capsular vessels. However, if this is seen, it should prompt a search for vascular invasion, as it has usually been reported in carcinomas [23].

Immunohistochemistry has been applied in an attempt to distinguish benign and malignant lesions. Widespread strong positivity for galectin-3 would support a malignant diagnosis, but more focal staining can be found in benign follicular lesions and not all carcinomas are positive [8,24]. HBME-1 also stains malignant lesions more commonly than benign [25]. Ancillary techniques such as ploidy analysis have no role in making the distinction between adenoma and carcinoma.

Widely invasive tumors are usually easy to define. Grossly, the tumor can be seen infiltrating the normal gland. Some have no evidence of

a capsule, while others have a capsule with extensive capsular and vascular invasion.

Hürthle Cell (Oncocytic) Follicular Tumors

Follicular tumors are defined as Hürthle cell when more than 75% of the tumor cells are oncocytic. Grossly, these are usually single nodules with a deep brown cut surface. They often undergo infarction following FNA, and it has been suggested that this may be related to their microvasculature, which is different from other thyroid tumors. A higher proportion of Hürthle cell tumors are malignant (35%) than in follicular lesions. A variety of growth patterns is seen in both benign and malignant tumors including microfollicular, macrofollicular, trabecular, solid and pseudopapillary architecture. Trabecular and solid architecture are more common in Hürthle cell carcinomas. Nuclear atypia and mitotic activity are not uncommon. Some have suggested that where these features are marked, they signify malignant potential, but follow-up studies have refuted this. A category of atypical Hürthle cell adenoma has been proposed for such tumors or for those with spontaneous infarction or necrosis. The diagnosis of malignancy should be made solely on the basis of capsular and/or vascular invasion. Immunohistochemistry is not generally useful. The tumors stain positively for thyroglobulin, but the staining is usually weaker than in follicular lesions. Positivity for TTF-1 is variable [26]. Galectin-3 has been reported to stain up to 60% of carcinomas, but also gives positive staining of some adenomas [27]. A recent study has suggested that Hürthle cell carcinomas with a Ki-67 index >5% show a more aggressive pattern of behavior [28].

Although the pathologist should approach the diagnosis in the same manner as follicular tumors, there is some evidence that the molecular pathogenesis of Hürthle cell tumors differs from that of follicular tumors [29,30]. This may help explain the differences in behavior. Hürthle cell tumors rarely take up radioiodine, and lymph node and distant metastases are usually thought to be more common than in follicular carcinoma. However, one study has suggested that when patients are stratified according to the extent of tumor invasion at the time of presentation, there are no differences in outcome between the two [31].

Histological Changes Following Preoperative Fine-Needle Aspiration Cytology

Alterations in histology caused by preoperative FNA are increasingly recognized by pathologists in surgical specimens. Some of these cause problems in diagnosis. Sometimes, a needle track is obvious, with hemorrhage, granulation tissue, and hemosiderin-laden macrophages. Cholesterol crystals may also be present. The cells in the adjacent follicles may show some enlargement and atypia. There may be distortion or disruption of the capsule where the needle has passed through. The capsular changes may raise the question of invasion, particularly when there is active fibrogenesis associated with follicles in the capsule. The pattern is linear, however, in contrast to the "mushroom" pattern of growth usually seen with true invasion and the breaks in the capsule do not show the characteristic blunt ends. Hemosiderin-laden macrophages are common in the vicinity. Several weeks to months after FNA small foci of squamous metaplasia may be seen in the capsular area. It is important not to interpret these as squamous carcinoma. Spindle cell nodules have also been described [32] and these should not be confused with a dedifferentiated component of the tumor.

Tumor infarction can also be seen, and Hürthle cell tumors are particularly susceptible to this change. In cases where the whole tumor is infarcted, it can be difficult to make a diagnosis. Papillary endothelial hyperplasia has been described in the center of aspirated nodules. This may be related to thrombosis and recanalization of vessels following FNA.

Papillary Carcinoma

When a definite diagnosis of papillary carcinoma has been made on FNA, the surgeon may proceed to total thyroidectomy with or without lymph node dissection. In cases with a suspi-

cious FNA, preoperative core biopsy or intraoperative frozen section may be used to confirm the diagnosis.

Grossly, the tumor may range in size from less than 1 mm to several centimeters. Most are irregular in shape and infiltrate the gland. They are often associated with scarring. Some are encapsulated and others show cystic change. The diagnosis depends to a great extent on the characteristic nuclear features (Figure 9.5). These are nuclear enlargement and irregularity, nuclear clearing (or ground glass appearance), prominence of the nuclear membrane, grooves, and pseudoinclusions. There is heaping up of nuclei, with what has been described as a "basket of eggs" appearance. Most show a mixture of papillary and follicular structures and trabecular and solid areas may be found. Some show squamous metaplasia. This has no implications for tumor behavior. It is important not to confuse it with squamous carcinoma, which has an aggressive course. Psammoma bodies are often found. Indeed, they may be the only intrathyroidal evidence of tumor in some patients who present with nodal metastases and in whom the primary tumor has regressed. Multicentric tumors are common. Some of these may represent intrathyroidal lymphatic spread, but there is also evidence to suggest that some may be multiple primary tumors in that individual tumors within a gland showed different *RET/PTC* translocations [33].

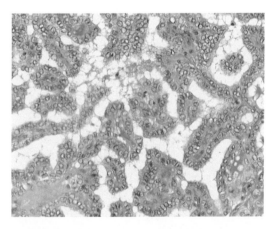

Figure 9.5 Papillary carcinoma of thyroid showing the typical nuclear features. There is nuclear clearing and heaping up and some cells show grooves and intranuclear pseudoinclusions.

Follicular Variant of Papillary Carcinoma

This is the next commonest variant to the classic variant of papillary carcinoma. It is characterized by follicular architecture, but the cells lining the follicles have the cytological features of papillary carcinoma. Where a mixed pattern of classic papillary and follicular architecture is present, the tumor should be classified as a classic variant. Most of these tumors are not encapsulated or have a poorly formed capsule. Prominent fibrous bands may extend between the tumor cells. The follicles are often of irregular shape with abortive attempts to produce papillae. There may also be interconnections between neighboring follicles [34]. The presence of multinucleate cells within the lumen of the follicles is another clue to diagnosis. These have a histiocytic phenotype [35]. Where these features are pronounced and present throughout the tumor, the diagnosis can be easy. However, in some tumors, the changes are more focal in distribution and distinction has to be made from follicular tumors or hyperplastic nodules. This can be difficult. A panel of antibodies has been proposed. These include cytokeratin 19 (CK19) (Figure 9.6), HBME-1, and RET. In a series of 84 cases of papillary carcinoma, 57% were positive for CK19, 45% for HBME-1, and 63% for RET protein. Only seven cases were negative with all three proteins [36].

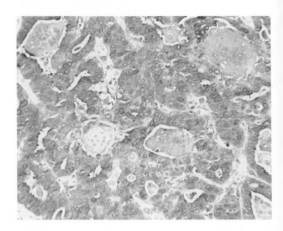

Figure 9.7 A follicular variant of papillary carcinoma showing widespread positivity for galectin-3. The follicles contain multinucleated histiocytic giant cells, which are associated with papillary carcinoma.

Strong diffuse staining for cytokeratin 19 is usually seen in the areas with nuclear changes, with weaker staining in the rest of the tumor. This contrasts with the focal reactivity that can be seen in follicular tumors. Papillary carcinomas are often positive for galectin-3 (Figure 9.7) [37,38]. Immunostaining with the antibodies to RET protein is an alternative approach, but there are no robust antibodies currently available commercially. In a few cases, it is extremely difficult to be sure of the diagnosis, and even endocrine pathologists will disagree as to how to categorize the lesion. It may be appropriate to say that the diagnosis of FVPC cannot be fully excluded. The development of multidisciplinary teams will allow discussion of how to proceed in these cases.

There are a number of patterns of growth of FVPC within the gland and it is important to recognize these as the behavior may differ. About 30% are encapsulated and have a good prognosis. Some tumors invade widely – the diffuse type [39]. These form multiple nodules throughout the gland and are commonly associated with lymph node and distant metastases Another group is the macrofollicular variant [40]. On low power, foci of tumor resemble hyperplastic nodules and the differential diagnosis may include macrofollicular adenoma or nodular goiter. The recognition of the nuclear features is important in making these distinc-

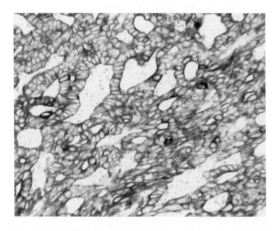

Figure 9.6 A follicular area in a papillary carcinoma of thyroid showing positivity for cytokeratin 19.

tions. This tumor has a low rate of lymph node metastases.

Other Variants of Papillary Carcinoma

An oncocytic variant is recognized [41] and the "Warthin-like" tumor is an oncocytic tumor with an extensive chronic inflammatory infiltrate [42] that resembles the tumor of the salivary gland. Clear cells may be admixed with oncocytic cells in some lesions, or may predominate. Immunopositivity for thyroid transcription factor 1 (TTF-1) [19] and thyroglobulin will confirm them as of thyroid origin. These patterns have no behavioral significance.

The diffuse sclerosing variant occurs in young people and shows multiple foci of tumor within lymphatics with marked squamous metaplasia, stromal fibrosis, prominent psammoma bodies, and a lymphocytic infiltrate [43,44]. Lymph node metastases are common and lung metastases are present in about a quarter of patients at presentation. The rare tall cell variant [45] occurs in older patients, usually men, and is often a large tumor with extrathyroidal extension and an aggressive course. The cells are oncocytic and are two to three times as tall as they are wide and the nuclei show marked grooves and pseudoinclusions. Columnar cell variant [46] is also rare and comprises pseudostratified columnar cells, some with sub- and supranuclear vacuoles. In general these also have a more aggressive course, unless they are encapsulated and confined to the thyroid [47,48]. Combined forms of these two have been described [49].

Solid variants have been more commonly described in the childhood tumors following on Chernobyl and may be associated with the *RET/PTC3* translocation and a short latent period before development [50]. A cribriform pattern is associated with familial adenomatous polyposis (FAP) or Gardner syndrome, usually in young females, but is occasionally seen in sporadic tumors. Papillary carcinoma with fasciitis-like stroma has no behavioral significance. In the very rare combined papillary and squamous carcinoma, the latter component has an aggressive course. It is important to distinguish this from the squamous metaplasia seen in some papillary carcinomas, as discussed above.

Papillary Microcarcinoma

This is a term that should be applied only to papillary carcinomas measuring <10 mm in maximum dimension found incidentally in a thyroid examined for other reasons. They are found in about 30% of thyroids sampled by step section at autopsy and in up to 24% of thyroids removed for other reasons. Most are probably of no clinical significance. The debate continues therefore as to how to deal with these lesions. Many would advise that, if there is no evidence of disease in the other lobe, they are of little risk, and should be defined as "microtumors" rather than "microcarcinomas" [51], with no need for further treatment. However, lesions of this size that present clinically, or are associated with metastases, should be treated in the same way as larger lesions.

Medullary Carcinoma

Medullary carcinoma (MTC) accounts for 5–10% of thyroid cancer and about one quarter are familial, in the context of multiple endocrine neoplasia type 2A and 2B and familial MTC. Sporadic tumors are usually single, while familial disease is multiple and bilateral and arises on a background of C-cell hyperplasia.

A variety of histological patterns can be seen and these are similar in both sporadic and familial disease. The most common is the alveolar and trabecular arrangement. The cells are polygonal or spindle-shaped with regular nuclei and coarse chromatin. They sometimes have a plasmacytoid appearance. There may be a prominent stromal component and amyloid is present in about 80% of cases. This can be demonstrated by Congo red or Sirius red stains and apple green birefringence on polarized light. The neuroendocrine nature of the tumor can be confirmed by immunopositivity for the general neuroendocrine markers synaptophysin and chromogranin A. There is specific positivity for calcitonin, although the extent and intensity of staining varies in individual tumors. Initial evidence that the proportion of cells staining for calcitonin had prognostic value [52] has not been substantiated in recent studies. In less well-differentiated tumors, where calcitonin immunoreactivity is lost, positivity for carcinoembryonic antigen (CEA) may serve as a surrogate marker [53].

Lymphatic invasion is common and around half of the patients have nodal metastases at time of presentation. Up to 15% may have distant metastases. A number of variants are described, but these do not have prognostic relevance.

Medullary carcinomas not infrequently contain scattered follicular structures. Some of these are formed by tumor cells, while others may represent entrapped normal follicles. Rarely, the predominant pattern is follicular. Immunostaining will show positivity for calcitonin within the cells in the follicular structures if they are tumor cells, with negative staining for thyroglobulin. In contrast, normal follicles can be identified by positivity for thyroglobulin.

C-Cell Hyperplasia

Familial disease develops on a background of C-cell hyperplasia [54,55]. This can be seen in the thyroid tissue surrounding medullary carcinoma and in thyroid glands removed from family members at risk of the disease. C cells naturally occur in the upper two-thirds of the thyroid lobes and this is what the pathologist must sample to look for it. Some would refer to this type of hyperplasia as medullary carcinoma in situ. The C cells are greatly increased in number and show atypia. They may obliterate follicular spaces. In cases of sporadic tumor an attempt should be made to look for C cells where possible, to identify a potential familial case. However, this is now less important with the advent of genetic testing for mutations in the *RET* gene.

Reactive C-cell hyperplasia has been reported in a number of situations, including hyperparathyroidism, adjacent to follicular tumors and in hypergastrinemia. The exact definition is unclear, but more than 50 C cells per low power field ($\times100$) in the normal C-cell areas is a criterion used by some. In contrast to the neoplastic type, the C cells are of normal appearance.

Mixed Follicular or Papillary and Medullary Carcinoma

This is a rare group of tumors in which there is evidence of both follicular and C-cell differentiation. They have been referred to as mixed, composite, or intermediate tumors. In some, the tumor cells show immunopositivity for both calcitonin and thyroglobulin [56], while in others there seem to be two individual populations. It has been suggested that they may arise from stem cells of the ultimobranchial body, or alternatively that they represent collision tumors. The latter explanation would be a possibility where two individual tumor components are identified (composite tumors) and recent molecular studies lend support to this concept [57]. However, this theory does not adequately explain the expression of calcitonin and thyroglobulin in the same tumor cell.

Hyalinizing Trabecular Tumor

This is a rare tumor that was first defined by Carney as hyalinizing trabecular adenoma [58] although it had been described earlier. The clinical behavior of the original series was benign, thus the term adenoma. However, more recent reports suggest that there is a malignant counterpart and these lesions are now defined as hyalinizing trabecular tumors, and the behavior is defined on the basis of capsular and vascular invasion. It is an encapsulated lesion derived from follicular cells comprising trabeculae of elongated cells around vascular channels, surrounded by matrix. The matrix may be hyalinized or may show calcification. The nuclei are elongated and show nuclear grooves and inclusions. Psammoma bodies may be present. Yellow intracytoplasmic inclusions have been described. These contain lipid, glycosaminoglycan, and proteoglycan and are consistent with giant lysosomes. They are present in most hyalinizing trabecular tumors, but are not specific as they may occasionally be found in follicular adenomas. Similar foci can be seen in some follicular adenomas and hyperplastic nodules.

Their histogenesis has been unclear. The overall arrangement of the cells resembles medullary carcinoma and paraganglioma and the lesion has also been defined as "paraganglioma-like adenoma of thyroid (PLAT)." However, none express calcitonin and all show immunopositivity for thyroglobulin, implying an origin from follicular cells. Focal positivity for general neuroendocrine markers has been described in a minority, raising the possibility of dual differentiation. The relationship to papillary carcinoma has been most widely debated. The nuclear features resemble those of papillary carcinoma and psammoma bodies are sometimes present. Papillary carcinomas can be found in the thyroid gland in about one third of cases of hyalinizing trabecular tumor and both appearances may coexist within the same nodule. Immunohistochemical data are inconsistent. Some have reported positivity for CK19 while others have found them negative. Recent studies have shown RET/PTC arrangements in some of these lesions, suggesting that they are a variant of papillary carcinoma [57,59]. However, not all cases show these changes and they may represent a spectrum of tumors.

Other Tumors

Thyroid lymphomas are usually extranodal B-cell lymphoma arising on a background of Hashimoto's thyroiditis. These should be diagnosed in conjunction with a specialist hematopathologist.

Occasional lesions arise from the stromal component including angiosarcoma and smooth muscle tumors. Metastases to the thyroid are infrequent in clinical practice, although they may be found at autopsy in about 25% of patients with carcinomatosis. Kidney is the most common primary site in clinical practice, followed by lung and uterus.

Conclusion

Molecular analysis is now clarifying the pathways in the development of the various types of thyroid tumor [60]. Interestingly, unlike other solid tumors, translocations occur in both follicular tumors and papillary carcinoma. Follicular carcinoma shows a PAX8-PPARγ fusion [61], while papillary carcinoma has a range of RET [62] and TRK rearrangements. Mutations in BRAF characterize a subset of papillary carcinoma without RET translocation [63,64]. RAS mutations have been reported in follicular tumors and more recently in papillary. A recent study suggests some links with aggressive behavior [65]. However, these findings are not yet translating into useful diagnostic tests, although this will almost certainly change in the next few years. The mainstay of pathological diagnosis remains the histological examination of adequately sampled tissue with appropriate immunohistochemistry.

References

1. Hamberger B, Gharib H, Melton LJ, 3rd, et al. Fine-needle aspiration biopsy of thyroid nodules. Impact on thyroid practice and cost of care. Am J Med 1982; 73:381–384.
2. Chen H, Dudley NE, Westra WH, et al. Utilization of fine-needle aspiration in patients undergoing thyroidectomy at two academic centers across the Atlantic. World J Surg 2003; 27:208–211.
3. Nasuti JF, Tam D, Gupta PK. Diagnostic value of liquid-based (Thinprep) preparations in nongynecologic cases. Diagn Cytopathol 2001; 24:137–141.
4. Cochand-Priollet B, Prat JJ, Polivka M, et al. Thyroid fine needle aspiration: the morphological features on Thin-Prep slide preparations. Eighty cases with histological control. Cytopathology 2003; 14:343–349.
5. British Thyroid Association. Guidelines for the management of thyroid cancer in adults. London: Royal College of Physicians, 2002.
6. Goellner JR. Problems and pitfalls in thyroid cytology. Monogr Pathol 1997; 39:75–93.
7. Bartolazzi A, Gasbarri A, Papotti M, et al. Application of an immunodiagnostic method for improving preoperative diagnosis of nodular thyroid lesions. Lancet 2001; 357:1644–1650.
8. Kovacs RB, Foldes J, Winkler G, et al. The investigation of galectin-3 in diseases of the thyroid gland. Eur J Endocrinol 2003; 149:449–453.
9. Herrmann ME, LiVolsi VA, Pasha TL, et al. Immunohistochemical expression of galectin-3 in benign and malignant thyroid lesions. Arch Pathol Lab Med 2002; 126:710–713.
10. Volante M, Bozzalla-Cassione F, DePompa R, et al. Galectin-3 and HBME-1 expression in oncocytic cell tumors of the thyroid. Virchows Arch 2004; 445:183–188.
11. Tsou PL, Hsiao YL, Chang TC. Multinucleated giant cells in fine needle aspirates. Can they help differentiate papillary thyroid cancer from benign nodular goiter? Acta Cytol 2002; 46:823–827.
12. Mesonero CE, Jugle JE, Wilbur DC, et al. Fine-needle aspiration of the macrofollicular and microfollicular subtypes of the follicular variant of papillary carcinoma of the thyroid. Cancer 1998; 84:235–244.
13. Solomon A, Gupta PK, LiVolsi VA, et al. Distinguishing tall cell variant of papillary thyroid carcinoma from usual variant of papillary thyroid carcinoma in cytologic specimens. Diagn Cytopathol 2002;27:143–148.

14. Jayaram G. Cytology of columnar-cell variant of papillary thyroid carcinoma. Diagn Cytopathol 2000; 22:227–229.

15. Cheung CC, Carydis B, Ezzat S, et al. Analysis of ret/PTC gene rearrangements refines the fine needle aspiration diagnosis of thyroid cancer. J Clin Endocrinol Metab 2001; 86:2187–2190.

16. Elisei R, Romei C, Vorontsova T, et al. Ret/ptc rearrangements in thyroid nodules: studies in irradiated and not irradiated, malignant and benign thyroid lesions in children and adults. J Clin Endocrinol Metab 2001; 86(7):3211–3216.

17. Baloch ZW, LiVolsi VA. Clonality in thyroid nodules: the hyperplasia-neoplasia sequence. Endocr Pathol 1998; 9: 287–292.

18. Franssila KO, Ackerman LV, Brown CL, et al. Follicular carcinoma. Semin Diagn Pathol 1985; 2:101–122.

19. Lang W, Choritz H, Hundeshagen H. Risk factors in follicular thyroid carcinomas. A retrospective follow-up study covering a 14-year period with emphasis on morphological findings. Am J Surg Pathol 1986; 10:246–255.

20. Katoh R, Kawaoi A, Miyagi E, et al. Thyroid transcription factor-1 in normal, hyperplastic, and neoplastic follicular thyroid cells examined by immunohistochemistry and nonradioactive in situ hybridization. Mod Pathol 2000; 13:570–576.

21. Rosai J, Carcangiu ML, DeLellis RA. Tumors of the thyroid gland. Third Series ed. Washington, DC: Armed Forces Institute of Pathology, 1992.

22. Woolner LB. Thyroid carcinoma: pathologic classification with data on prognosis. Semin Nucl Med 1971; 1:481–502.

23. Tse LL, Chan I, Chan JK. Capsular intravascular endothelial hyperplasia: a peculiar form of vasoproliferative lesion associated with thyroid carcinoma. Histopathology 2001,39:463–8.

24. Cvejic D, Savin S, Paunovic I, et al. Immunohistochemical localization of galectin-3 in malignant and benign human thyroid tissue. Anticancer Res 1998; 18:2637–2641.

25. Miettinen M, Karkkainen P. Differential reactivity of HBME-1 and CD15 antibodies in benign and malignant thyroid tumours. Preferential reactivity with malignant tumours. Virchows Arch 1996; 429:213–219.

26. Bejarano PA, Nikiforov YE, Swenson ES, et al. Thyroid transcription factor-1, thyroglobulin, cytokeratin 7, and cytokeratin 20 in thyroid neoplasms. Appl Immunohistochem Mol Morphol 2000; 8:189–194.

27. Costa SC, Nascimento LS, Ferreira FJ, et al. Lack of mutations of exon 2 of the MEN1 gene in endocrine and nonendocrine sporadic tumors. Braz J Med Biol Res 2001; 34:861–865.

28. Hoos A, Stojadinovic A, Singh B, et al. Clinical significance of molecular expression profiles of hurthle cell tumors of the thyroid gland analyzed via tissue microarrays. Am J Pathol 2002; 160:175–183.

29. Masood S, Auguste LJ, Westerband A, et al. Differential oncogenic expression in thyroid follicular and Hurthle cell carcinomas. Am J Surg 1993; 166:366–368.

30. Wada N, Duh QY, Miura D, et al. Chromosomal aberrations by comparative genomic hybridization in hurthle cell thyroid carcinomas are associated with tumor recurrence. J Clin Endocrinol Metab 2002; 87:4595–601.

31. Evans HL, Vassilopoulou-Sellin R. Follicular and Hurthle cell carcinomas of the thyroid: a comparative study. Am J Surg Pathol 1998; 22:1512–1520.

32. Baloch ZW, Abraham S, Roberts S, et al. Differential expression of cytokeratins in follicular variant of papillary carcinoma: an immunohistochemical study and its diagnostic utility. Hum Pathol 1999; 30:1166–1171.

33. Sugg SL, Ezzat S, Rosen IB, et al. Distinct multiple RET/PTC gene rearrangements in multifocal papillary thyroid neoplasia. J Clin Endocrinol Metab 1998; 83: 4116–4122.

34. Ambrosiani L, Declich P, Bellone S, et al. Thyroid metastases from renal clear cell carcinoma: a cytohistological study of two cases. Adv Clin Pathol 2001; 5:11–16.

35. Tabbara SO, Acoury N, Sidawy MK. Multinucleated giant cells in thyroid neoplasms. A cytologic, histologic and immunohistochemical study. Acta Cytol 1996; 40:1184–1188.

36. Asa SL, Cheung CC. The mind's eye. Am J Clin Pathol 2001; 116:635–636.

37. Rosai J. Immunohistochemical markers of thyroid tumors: significance and diagnostic applications. Tumori 2003; 89:517–519.

38. Casey MB, Lohse CM, Lloyd RV. Distinction between papillary thyroid hyperplasia and papillary thyroid carcinoma by immunohistochemical staining for cytokeratin 19, galectin-3, and HBME-1. Endocr Pathol 2003; 14:55–60.

39. Ivanova R, Soares P, Castro P, et al. Diffuse (or multinodular) follicular variant of papillary thyroid carcinoma: a clinicopathologic and immunohistochemical analysis of ten cases of an aggressive form of differentiated thyroid carcinoma. Virchows Arch 2002; 440:418–424.

40. Albores-Saavedra J, Gould E, Vardaman C, et al. The macrofollicular variant of papillary thyroid carcinoma: a study of 17 cases. Hum Pathol 1991; 22:1195–1205.

41. Berho M, Suster S. The oncocytic variant of papillary carcinoma of the thyroid: a clinicopathologic study of 15 cases. Hum Pathol 1997; 28:47–53.

42. Baloch ZW, LiVolsi VA. Warthin-like papillary carcinoma of the thyroid. Arch Pathol Lab Med 2000; 124:1192–1195.

43. Vickery AL, Jr., Carcangiu ML, Johannessen JV, et al. Papillary carcinoma. Semin Diagn Pathol 1985; 2:90–100.

44. Nishiyama RH. Overview of surgical pathology of the thyroid gland. World J Surg 2000; 24:898–906.

45. Prendiville S, Burman KD, Ringel MD, et al. Tall cell variant: an aggressive form of papillary thyroid carcinoma. Otolaryngol Head Neck Surg 2000; 122:352–357.

46. Evans HL. Columnar-cell carcinoma of the thyroid. A report of two cases of an aggressive variant of thyroid carcinoma. Am J Clin Pathol 1986; 85:77–80.

47. Wenig BM, Thompson LD, Adair CF, et al. Thyroid papillary carcinoma of columnar cell type: a clinicopathologic study of 16 cases [see comments]. Cancer 1998; 82:740–753.

48. Evans HL. Encapsulated papillary neoplasms of the thyroid. A study of 14 cases followed for a minimum of 10 years. Am J Surg Pathol 1987; 11:592–597.

49. Putti TC, Bhuiya TA. Mixed columnar cell and tall cell variant of papillary carcinoma of thyroid: a case report and review of the literature. Pathology 2000; 32:286–289.

50. Williams ED, Abrosimov A, Bogdanova T, et al. Thyroid carcinoma after Chernobyl latent period, morphology and aggressiveness. Br J Cancer 2004; 90:2219–2224.

51. Rosai J, LiVolsi VA, Sobrinho-Simoes M, et al. Renaming papillary microcarcinoma of the thyroid gland: the Porto proposal. Int J Surg Pathol 2003; 11:249–251.

52. Saad MF, Ordonez NG, Guido JJ, et al. The prognostic value of calcitonin immunostaining in medullary carcinoma of the thyroid. J Clin Endocrinol Metab 1984; 59:850–856.

53. Kakudo K, Takami H, Katayama S, et al. Carcinoembryonic antigen and nonspecific cross-reacting antigen in medullary carcinoma of the thyroid. Acta Pathol Jpn 1990; 40:261–266.

54. LiVolsi VA. C cell hyperplasia/neoplasia. J Clin Endocrinol Metab 1997; 82:39–41.

55. Williams ED. C cell hyperplasia. Bull Cancer 1984; 71:122–124.

56. Holm R, Sobrinho-Simoes M, Nesland JM, et al. Concurrent production of calcitonin and thyroglobulin by the same neoplastic cells. Ultrastruct Pathol 1986; 10:241–248.

57. Papotti M, Volante M, Giuliano A, et al. RET/PTC activation in hyalinizing trabecular tumors of the thyroid. Am J Surg Pathol 2000; 24:1615–1621.

58. Carney JA. Unusual tumefactive spindle cell lesions in the adrenal glands. Hum Pathol 1987; 18:980–985.

59. Cheung CC, Boerner SL, MacMillan CM, et al. Hyalinizing trabecular tumor of the thyroid: a variant of papillary carcinoma proved by molecular genetics. Am J Surg Pathol 2000; 24:1622–1626.

60. Kroll TG. Molecular rearrangements and morphology in thyroid cancer. Am J Pathol 2002; 160:1941–1944.

61. Knauf JA, Ward LS, Nikiforov YE, et al. Isozyme-specific abnormalities of PKC in thyroid cancer: evidence for post-transcriptional changes in PKC epsilon. J Clin Endocrinol Metab 2002; 87:2150–2159.

62. Tallini G, Asa SL. RET oncogene activation in papillary thyroid carcinoma. Adv Anat Pathol 2001; 8:345–354.

63. Xu X, Quiros RM, Gattuso P, et al. High prevalence of BRAF gene mutation in papillary thyroid carcinomas and thyroid tumor cell lines. Cancer Res 2003; 63:4561–4567.

64. Soares P, Trovisco V, Rocha AS, et al. BRAF mutations and RET/PTC rearrangements are alternative events in the etiopathogenesis of PTC. Oncogene 2003; 22:4578–4580.

65. Garcia-Rostan G, Zhao H, Camp RL, et al. ras mutations are associated with aggressive tumor phenotypes and poor prognosis in thyroid cancer. J Clin Oncol 2003; 21:3226–3235.

10

Thyroid Cancer and the Endocrinologist

Wilmar M. Wiersinga

The long-term outcome of treatment for papillary and follicular thyroid cancer is generally good: the overall 10-year survival for adult patients with differentiated thyroid carcinoma is 80–90%. However, local or regional recurrences develop in up to 30% of patients, distant metastases in up to 20%, and 8–10% of patients die of their disease [1,2]. Thyroid cancer patients thus require a very long-term follow-up.

Adequacy of surgical treatment and ^{131}I ablation apparently have an important influence on the long-term outcome [1,3,4]. Nevertheless, audits on existing clinical practices identified several shortcomings from what might be considered optimum management of thyroid cancer [5–7]. In one particular study, adequacy of surgery was considered deficient in 20%, adequacy of T_4 suppression in 22%, monitoring by serum thyroglobulin in 15%, and use of ^{131}I therapy in 12% [7]. Deficiencies were observed more often where patients were seen by a number of generalists (probably related to poor communications between disciplines) as compared to patients seen in multidisciplinary specialist clinics. This is not too surprising as thyroid cancer, although being the most common of all malignant endocrine tumours, is quite rare. Thus the experience of individual physicians with thyroid cancer is limited if they do not work in specialized centers. These issues have led to several specific recommendations. For instance, that thyroid malignancy "will only be managed effectively by multidisciplinary teams in units familiar with the condition," and that designated specialists work together in multidisciplinary teams and that "decisions regarding diagnosis, treatment and care of individual patients . . . are multidisciplinary decisions" [8].

Bringing together the expertise available in various disciplines provides added value, and institution of multidisciplinary teams is likely to improve the outcome of the illness. Specialists involved in the management of thyroid cancer are usually the internist-endocrinologist, the pathologist, the surgeon, and the nuclear medicine physician; in addition, consultations might be needed from the ear-nose-throat physician, the radiologist, or the oncologist. The more people and disciplines are involved in the multidisciplinary team, the greater the need for a coordinating person. Although the multidisciplinary team has a shared responsibility for the management plan, this is not to say that there is no need for the patient to have a single doctor who is primarily responsible for his health and charged with the continuous delivery of care during the long-term follow-up. In my experience the patient appreciates the group effort and deliberations in the multidisciplinary team, but still likes to have his own doctor who is directly accountable for his overall treatment. It is probably optimal if the coordinator of the multidisciplinary team and the doctor primarily in charge of the patient is one and the same person. Which person is the most appropriate one for this role will depend heavily on the local situation. However, it appears that the internist-endocrinologist is most suited for this role in view of his continuing relationship with the patient during all stages of the disease. It is against this background that the present chapter is written: the role of the endocrinologist as the patient's own doctor who is responsible for continuity in the care and as the coordinator of treatments given by other care providers.

Role of the Endocrinologist in the Presurgical (Diagnostic) Phase of Thyroid Cancer

The presenting symptom of thyroid cancer is usually a visible and/or palpable thyroid nodule. The patient will be referred to an internist-endocrinologist or surgeon to rule out malignancy. The main tasks of the physician in this diagnostic phase are outlined in (Table 10.1) and described below.

Evaluation of Clinical Risk Factors for Thyroid Cancer

The history and physical examination of the patient may give important clues with regard to the nature of a thyroid nodule. Features suggesting malignancy are external neck irradiation during childhood, family history of thyroid cancer, male sex, age <25 years or >60 years, hoarseness, dysphagia, rapid increase of nodule size over weeks or months, nodules that are firm in consistency and irregular or attached to surrounding tissues, and palpable neck lymph nodes. If there is a very high clinical suspicion of thyroid cancer, one may already conclude that thyroid surgery is necessary irrespective of the fine-needle aspiration cytology (FNAC) results [9].

Table 10.1 Role of the endocrinologist in the presurgical (diagnostic) phase of thyroid cancer

1. Evaluation of clinical risk factors (including family history) for thyroid cancer
2. Evaluation of FNAC results
3. Outline of the management plan, in consultation with the multidisciplinary team and the patient

A family history of benign thyroid disease will decrease and a family history of thyroid cancer will increase the suspicion of malignancy. Medullary thyroid cancer in the family will of course require measurement of serum calcitonin and DNA mutation analysis in the patient. Routine measurement of serum calcitonin in every patient with a thyroid nodule has been advocated as it detects about one case of medullary thyroid cancer in every 200 thyroid nodules [10,11]. The cost-effectiveness of this approach is, however, debated. A careful family history is furthermore important to discover rare syndromes associated with papillary or follicular thyroid cancer, which may have consequences for the patient and his family (Table 10.2). Familial clustering of differentiated thyroid cancer may not be as exotic as previously thought: it accounts for approximately 5–10% of all papillary and follicular thyroid carcinomas [12]. A study among first degree relatives of cases (unselected nonmedullary thyroid cancer patients) and controls reports that the relative risk for thyroid cancer is 10-fold higher in relatives of cancer patients than in controls (incidence rate ratio 10.3, 95% CI 2.2–47.6), and the incidence of any type of cancer is 38% higher in thyroid cancer relatives than in control relatives [13].

The workup of the patient with a thyroid nodule should also include measurement of serum thyroid-stimulating hormone (TSH). Virtually all patients with thyroid cancer have a normal serum TSH and are euthyroid, although thyrotoxicosis resulting from a very large tumor load of thyroid cancer can occur. The presence of a suppressed TSH qualifies for thyroid scintigraphy. Thyroid nodules in patients with Graves' disease are more likely to be malignant than nodules in euthyroid patients [14]. In patients with Hashimoto's thyroiditis the risk of malignancy in thyroid nodules is not increased, but the rare thyroid lymphoma almost always develops against the background of chronic lymphocytic thyroiditis [15].

Evaluation of the FNAC Results

Fine-needle aspiration cytology is presently the most accurate test for determining the nature of the thyroid nodule. Its sensitivity and specificity for the diagnosis of thyroid cancer approximates 95%. However, the procedure is not

Table 10.2 Familial syndromes associated with thyroid cancer

Familial syndrome	Thyroid cancer	Other manifestations	Gene/chromosomal location
MEN2A	MTC	Pheochromocytoma	*RET*/10q11.2
		Hyperparathyroidism	
MEN2B	MTC	Pheochromocytoma	*RET*/10q11.2
		Mucosal neuromas	
Familial MTC	MTC	None	*RET*/10q.11.2
Familial PTC	PTC	None	Unknown
Famital PTC	PTC	Renal cell carcinoma	Unknown/1q21
Familial polyposis coli	PTC	Intestinal polyps	*APC*/5q21
Gardner syndrome	PTC	Intestinal polyps	*APC*/5q21
		Osteomas, fibromas, lipomas	
Cowden syndrome	FTC	Multiple hamartomas	*PTEN*/10q22.23
		Breast tumors	
Carney syndrome	FTC	Spotty skin pigmentation	Unknown, *PRKARIA*
		Myxoma, schwannoma	2p16,17q23
		Pigmented adrenal nodules	
		Pituitary adenomas	
		Testicular endocrine tumors	

MEN, multiple endocrine neoplasia; MTC, medullary thyroid carcinoma; PTC, papillary thyroid carcinoma; FTC, follicular thyroid carcinoma.

without pitfalls. It is the task of the treating clinician/endocrinologist to check the adequacy and representativeness of the FNAC.

The report of the pathologist evaluating the FNAC should be written in a way that is meaningful to the clinician: that is, the clinician must be able to judge from the report if the obtained sample allows an accurate cytological diagnosis (in other words there must be adequate cellularity) and in which diagnostic category the sample falls. Preferably the FNAC report should end with one of the four following conclusions:

1. Inadequate cytology. The clinician then knows the FNAC has to be repeated, possibly under guidance of ultrasound. Quantitative criteria are helpful to judge the adequacy of the sample.
2. Benign cytology. Unless there is a compelling reason to still suspect thyroid cancer, the patient can be reassured. But it is up to the endocrinologist to decide whether or not a repeat FNAC after 6–12 months is in order in view of the few false-negative FNAC results [16]. After having ruled out malignancy, the patient still is in the possession of a lump in the neck and may ask that something is done in view of cosmetic or mechanic complaints. To

answer questions on the natural history and to advise on the most appropriate treatment, if any, suits the endocrinologist very well.

3. Suspicious cytology. FNAC can not discriminate between follicular adenomas and follicular carcinomas, and a diagnostic (hemi)thyroidectomy is indicated. The multidisciplinary team may decide to study the usefulness in their institution of new molecular markers in cytological specimens allowing better discrimination between benign and malignant follicular lesions.

4. Malignant cytology. Thyroidectomy is indicated.

Description of the adequacy of the obtained sample and classification in one of the four above-mentioned categories renders the FNAC report a valid one. However, it does not answer the question whether or not the cytological aspirate is representative for the nodule. Performing multiple aspirates in the same session will increase the likelihood of a representative sample. Ideally the FNAC report should also mention how many aspirates were done and in which lesion the needle was located. Especially in mixed cystic/solid nodules the position of the needle can be critical, as the cancer may reside in a particular area of the wall of the lesion, only visible during ultrasound. Indeed centers may decide to perform FNAC routinely under echographic guidance, because this procedure increases the diagnostic accuracy of FNAC [17]. The problem of obtaining a representative sample can be even greater in multinodular goiter. The current recommendation is to do FNAC of only the dominant (largest) nodule. Indeed thyroid cancer in multinodular goiter is most often unifocal (61%) and present in the dominant nodule (71%). However, 29% of thyroid malignancies arise in the nondominant nodule and thus would be missed with the current strategy [18].

Outline of the Management Plan

Based on the clinical evaluation and the FNAC report a management plan should be designed, preferably by the multidisciplinary team and in consultation with the patient. In most cases thyroid surgery is the first procedure in the treatment plan, for diagnostic reasons in case of follicular lesions and otherwise for removal of tumor. The presence of the nuclear medicine physician in the team at this stage is helpful for logistic reasons to plan future ^{131}I ablative therapy. The extent of the thyroidectomy, and whether or not lymph node dissection should be done, should be discussed. The decision to operate may not be straightforward with papillary microcarcinomas ($\leq$1 cm in diameter), especially when the nodule is not palpable and incidentally detected by ultrasonography. One study found that during a mean follow-up of 46 months the size of the microcarcinoma did not change in 65%, increased by $\geq$2 mm in 25% and decreased by $\geq$2 mm in 10% [19]. In such cases a common policy supported by all members of the team can avoid confusion.

Role of the Endocrinologist in the Postsurgical Phase Prior to ^{131}I Ablation

The role of the endocrinologist in this phase is outlined in (Table 10.3).

Table 10.3 Role of the endocrinologist in the postsurgical phase prior to ^{131}I ablation

1. Management plan for postoperative complications
2. Evaluation of prognosis according to TNM or other classification systems
3. Preparation for ablative ^{131}I therapy
4. DNA mutation analysis in patient and family members if indicated

Management Plan for Postoperative Complications

Direct postoperative complications are mostly managed by the surgeon. Shortness of breath or stridor may indicate neck hematoma, bilateral recurrent laryngeal nerve injury, or vocal cord edema; it requires immediate investigation and appropriate treatment. Laryngeal nerve injury is rare but not completely avoidable, occurring in about 2% of cases; it may resolve spontaneously within a few weeks; its sequelae in persistent cases can be lessened by speech rehabilitation therapy. The ear-nose-throat physician should be involved in such cases.

Serum calcium and albumin should be routinely measured, for example 5 h and 24 h after surgery. Postoperative hypocalcemia occurs in about 30% depending on the extent of surgery and the experience of the surgeon. Asymptomatic moderate hypocalcemia can be observed, but symptomatic hypocalcemia should be treated with calcium supplementation either orally (1–2 g every 4 to 8 h) or intravenously (20 ml of 10% calcium gluconate, diluted in saline or glucose, over 10 minutes). Postoperative hypoparathyroidism may be due to ischemic parathyroid damage; it usually reverts to normal in about 6 weeks. Hypoparathyroidism after parathyroid autotransplantation is not infrequent; it also resolves mostly in a few months, but may require temporary treatment with calcium and vitamin D derivatives. Permanent hypoparathyroidism due to ablation or necrosis of parathyroid glands occurs in about 2%, and requires administration of calcium salts (1–2 g daily as calcium carbonate, gluconate, citrate, or lactate) and vitamin D derivatives (usually 0.5–1.0 μg of calcitriol or 1–2 μg of alfacalcidol daily). At the start of treatment weekly measurement of serum and urinary calcium and phosphate is indicated, especially to avoid overtreatment and significant hypercalciuria. Once the right dose has been obtained, controls every 6 months or so suffices. Requirements usually remain stable with time, but reduction of the extracellular volume (e.g. by acute diarrhea or the use of diuretics) increases the risk of hypercalcemia. The long-term surveillance of calcium metabolism is mostly done by the endocrinologist.

Evaluation of Prognosis According to TNM or Other Classification Systems

Prognostic factors associated with poor survival are older age, male sex, family history, histology (particular variants of papillary and follicular cancers, capsular invasion), large tumor size, and lymph node and distant metastases. Multivariate analysis reveals three independent prognostic factors: age, histological type, and tumor extent. The preoperative evaluation, the findings during surgery and the pathology of the surgical specimen will usually allow correct classification of the cancer in a prognostic scoring system in the immediate direct postoperative period. Several prognostic scores have been developed for use in thyroid cancer. The multidisciplinary term should decide which scoring system is to be used in their institution. Which score is selected will depend more on local preference than on superiority of one score over the others: predictability of patient outcome is very similar for different staging systems (including TNM, EORTC, ASES, AMES, and MACIS scores) in comparison studies [20,21]. Whatever system is used, it is very important in planning further management (e.g. [131]I therapy) and subsequent follow-up (e.g. extent of TSH suppression). The prognostic score also facilitates informing the patient on the most likely outcome of his disease.

Preparation for Ablative [131]I Therapy

The multidisciplinary team has to decide whether or not ablative ^{131}I therapy will be given, and if so, at which time. If there is only a low risk of cancer-specific mortality and a low risk of relapse according to the prognostic score, there may be no indication. However,

ablative ^{131}I therapy may still be favored in that it improves the diagnostic accuracy of serum thyroglobulin and ^{131}I total body scan for remaining tumor tissue after total ablation of the thyroid gland [22]. The internist-endocrinologist can play an important role in the preparation for ^{131}I treatment. For the efficacy of ^{131}I ablation depends on how much of the administered ^{131}I dose is taken up by remaining thyroid tissue, which is greatly stimulated by high serum TSH and low serum inorganic iodide concentrations. The endocrinologist should see to it that at the time of ^{131}I ablation the serum TSH is elevated (arbitrarily up to at least 25–30 mU/L) and the serum iodide is definitely not high but preferably low. After (near) total thyroidectomy simply withholding T_4 treatment will ensure high TSH levels after 4–6 weeks, the usual time for ^{131}I ablation. If for any reason the interval between surgery and planned ^{131}I treatment is longer, it is prudent to start T_4 treatment in order to avoid severe hypothyroidism in the patient. In such cases, T_4 treatment should be discontinued 4 weeks before the planned ^{131}I therapy. Alternatively, after discontinuation of T_4 treatment one may administer T_3 for 3 weeks (25 µg daily in week 1, 2×25 µg daily in week 2, 3×25 µg daily in week 3), then stop T_3 for 2 weeks and administer the therapeutic dose of ^{131}I in week 6. The advantage of this alternative scheme is that the patient may suffer less from hypothyroid symptoms and signs. A recent study, however, questions the benefits from using T_3 in preparing patients for ^{131}I therapy [23]. Serum TSH concentrations of more than 30 mU/L were reached 18 days after thyroidectomy and 22 days after withdrawal of suppressive thyroxine treatment in more than 95% of patients, with minimal symptoms of hypothyroidism. These authors recommend serum TSH measurements twice weekly, starting 10 days after thyroidectomy or T_4 withdrawal.

With regard to iodine intake, patients are usually instructed to avoid iodine-containing medications and iodine-rich foods for 10 days prior to ^{131}I therapy. The value of a stringent low iodine diet has been questioned as similar ablation rates were observed in patients on a low iodine diet and on a regular diet [24]. However, a recent study reports a significantly higher successful ablation rate after a low iodine diet than in controls (65% versus 48%) [25]. A 2-week low iodine diet will also induce iodine deficiency in patients who continue their levothyroxine medication [26].

The patient should be informed of possible damage of ^{131}I therapy to radiation-sensitive tissues. Usually this is done by the nuclear medicine physician, but the endocrinologist may play a role as well. Many patients in their reproductive years are concerned with gonadal damage. The standard advice is to refrain from pregnancy and not father a child during the first 4 to 6 months after ^{131}I therapy. About 20–30% of women experience transient amenorrhea or menstrual irregularities in the first year after treatment [27,28]. Apart from a greater miscarriage rate in the first year ^{131}I therapy seems to have no effect on fertility or the outcome of subsequent pregnancies, but menopause occurs on average 1.5 year earlier [29]. In men, spermatogenesis can be transiently suppressed associated with a rise of serum FSH, related to the total amount of [131]I [30]. The risk of permanent male infertility is very low; in men likely to receive a cumulative dose of >17 GBq sperm banking may be considered.

DNA Mutation Analysis

About 25% of medullary thyroid carcinomas are hereditary, and it is important to recognize the heritable form because of the risk of other tumors in the patient and in the family. Lack of family history does not exclude heritable medullary thyroid cancer: the disease may not be apparent in relatives because of skipped generations or an isolated case may be the start of a new family. Consequently, every case of medullary thyroid carcinoma should be offered genetic testing to look for genomic mutations in the RET proto-oncogene. Particular mutations in the RET proto-oncogene have been linked with a particularly good or bad prognosis [31]. However, before DNA mutation analysis is done, a clear explanation should be given about the nature of the test and the possible implications of a positive or negative test result for the patient and the family. The postoperative period might be the appropriate time to start such discussions, and it is up to the endocrinologist of the team to conduct investigation of family members if the index patient has the genomic mutation.

Role of the Endocrinologist in the Postsurgical Postablative Stage

The role of the endocrinologist in this phase is outlined in Table 10.4.

Administration of TSH-Suppressive Doses of L-Thyroxine

After thyroidectomy and ^{131}I ablation there is a need for life-long T_4 replacement therapy. In patients with nonmedullary thyroid cancer the prescribed daily T_4 dose is usually higher than the replacement dose in order to reach suppression and not just normalization of serum TSH values. For a number of studies have shown that TSH suppression is associated with a longer disease-free interval [4]. A French study reports a longer relapse-free survival in patients with constantly suppressed TSH (all values ≤0.05 mU/ L) than in patients with nonsuppressed TSH (all values ≥1 mU/L); the degree of TSH suppression predicted relapse-free survival independently of other factors [32]. In a US cooperative study the degree of TSH suppression was an independent predictor of disease progression in high risk patients with papillary carcinoma, but not in low risk patients or when radioiodine treatment was included in the model [3]. A Finnish study reports that a nonsuppressed TSH is an independent predictor for recurrence in multivariate analysis [33]. A study from Taiwan suggests stratification: TSH should be suppressed in patients with active disease, but might be kept within the normal range in patients who are clinically disease free [34].

The question thus arises which degree of TSH suppression is most appropriate (<0.4, <0.1 or

Table 10.4 Role of the endocrinologist in the postsurgical postablative phase

1. Administration of TSH-suppressive doses of L-thyroxine
2. Long-term follow-up with search for residual thyroid cancer at regular intervals
3. Management plan for recurrent or metastatic thyroid cancer
4. Attention to quality of life

<0.01 mU/L?) and for how long should TSH suppression be maintained. This should be discussed in the multidisciplinary team. The endocrinologist seems best suited to monitor the required TSH level by adjusting the daily T_4 dose. A suppressed TSH effectively means induction of subclinical hyperthyroidism, a condition with potential adverse side effects notably on the heart and the bones. It also befits the endocrinologist to evaluate these risks in the individual patient and to take preventive measures if indicated.

There is no doubt that subclinical hyperthyroidism increases the risk of atrial fibrillation [35]. Careful investigations, however, have also shown subtle cardiac dysfunction in these patients as evident from an increased left ventricular mass, impaired ventricular relaxation, and reduced exercise performance [36]. The long-term consequences of this cardiac dysfunction are unknown, but β-blockade improves cardiac function [36,37]. If there is a clear indication for marked TSH suppression, it may be prudent to prescribe β-blockers. This may be especially worthwhile if the patient does not tolerate the high doses of thyroxine.

Subclinical hyperthyroidism is also associated with high bone turnover [38], and may induce bone loss according to meta-analyses, especially in postmenopausal women [39,40]. It has not been demonstrated that this results in a higher fracture rate [41], but again it seems prudent that the endocrinologist monitors the risk in individual patients (by taking a history with respect to the well-known risk factors for osteoporosis, and performing bone densimetry in selected cases) and takes appropriate action in high risk patients (ensuring sufficient calcium intake, and considering supplementation with vitamin D).

Long-Term Follow-up with Search for Residual Thyroid Cancer at Regular Intervals

In view of the long natural history of the disease, thyroid cancer patients require life-long follow-up. For medullary thyroid cancer, serum calcitonin and CEA can be used as tumor markers; a progressive rise in their serum concentrations will demand imaging studies, but otherwise appropriate time intervals for follow-up visits are 6–12 months.

For papillary and follicular thyroid carcinoma, the long-term follow-up is important in view of (a) late recurrences which can be successfully treated, (b) monitoring of the consequences of suppressed TSH, and (c) evaluation of late side effects of ^{131}I such as leukemia or second tumours, although fortunately these are very rare. Most important is the measurement of serum thyroglobulin (Tg) as a tumor marker, but for a valid interpretation of the Tg test results the endocrinologist should make sure TgAbs are absent in the sample under investigation; close collaboration with the clinical chemistry laboratory is helpful in this respect, and the endocrinologist should be familiar with the characteristics of the Tg assay used in his institution and which methods are used to exclude the presence of TgAb. The multidisciplinary team should decide on their policy on follow-up in low risk patients [42], and whether or not to rely on Tg measurements after thyroxine withdrawal or after recombinant human TSH (rhTSH) administration. Control visits should be rather frequent in the first 2 years (e.g. every 3 months); thereafter the frequency can be reduced to once every 6 months for 3 years, and finally once a year in uncomplicated cases.

Management Plan for Recurrent or Metastatic Thyroid Cancer

Once recurrent or metastatic cancer has been diagnosed, consultations within the multidisciplinary team should lead to the most appropriate management plan. For recurrence in the thyroid bed or cervical lymph nodes, surgical re-exploration usually followed by ^{131}I therapy is mostly preferred. Bone metastases can be treated with ^{131}I, external radiotherapy, embolization, or orthopedic intervention. Metastases in the lungs and elsewhere not amenable to surgery can be treated with [131]I. In otherwise uncontrolled end-stage disease chemotherapy with doxorubicin and cisplatinum has been tried, with limited success.

The internist-endocrinologist should clearly act as the coordinator in the management of the disease at this stage. He is likely well informed on new developments and may propose innovative, still experimental treatment strategies in advanced cases. He may also deliver palliative care when needed. The immediate causes of death in 106 fatal cases of thyroid carcinoma were respiratory insufficiency (43%), circulatory failure (15%), hemorrhage (15%), and airway obstruction (13%) [43].

Attention to Quality of Life

The physician in charge of the continuity in care of the thyroid cancer patient (likely the endocrinologist) is instrumental in promoting compliance with the long-term follow-up and the required repeat investigations. Compliance can be enhanced by giving attention to many details which – although not determining the main outcome of the disease – may severely affect the patient's life. The cost of care should not be forgotten, as patients may have no or insufficient insurance [44]. The incidence of chronic xerostomia as a result of ^{131}I-induced sialadenitis may decrease considerably with amifostine pretreatment [45]. During thyroid hormone withdrawal, hypothyroid symptoms are common such as fatigue, weight gain, peripheral edema, muscle cramps, skin dryness, anxiety, constipation, cold, depression, and impairment of memory and concentration; these complaints are more pronounced in the elderly than in younger patients [45]. It is thus not surprising that quality-of-life questionnaires indicate significant reduction in physical, psychosocial, and social wellbeing in this period. Whereas troublesome physical symptoms relating to thyroid hormone withdrawal are readily appreciated, the negative psychological, family, and work sequelae are less apparent [46]. The professional consequences of the hypothyroid period should not easily be dismissed: 11 to 14 days of missed work are on average associated with T_4 withdrawal [42]. Adequate information to the patient and reassurance of the relatively good prognosis may greatly enhance compliance. It is often helpful to give addresses of patient support groups and of websites with useful information. Nevertheless, it is not unusual that patients refuse to undergo another period of T_4 withdrawal in view of their past experience with this procedure; the fear of another depressive episode can be quite realistic. In such cases the use of rhTSH greatly promotes compliance [47]. A much wider use of rhTSH replacing T_4 withdrawal is foreseen in the near future, and this will certainly increase the quality of life of thyroid cancer patients and decrease the number of days of missed work [42].

References

1. Mazzaferri EL, Jhiang SM. Long-term impact of initial surgical and medical therapy on papillary and follicular thyroid cancer. Am J Med 1994; 97:418–428.
2. Schlumberger MJ. Papillary and follicular thyroid carcinoma. N Engl J Med 1998; 338:297–306.
3. Cooper DS, Specker B, Ho M, et al. Thyrotropin suppression and disease progression in patients with differentiated thyroid cancer; results from the National Thyroid Cancer Treatment Cooperative Registry. Thyroid 1998; 8:737–744.
4. Mazzaferri EL. An overview of the management of papillary and follicular thyroid carcinoma. Thyroid 1999; 9:421–427.
5. Hardy KJ, Walker BR, Lindsay RS, et al. Thyroid cancer management. Clin Endocrinol 1995; 42:651–655.
6. Vanderpump MPJ, Alexander L, Scarpello JHB, et al. An audit of the management of thyroid cancer in a district general hospital. Clin Endocrinol 1998; 48:419–424.
7. Kumar H, Daykin J, Holder R, et al. An audit of management of differentiated thyroid cancer in specialist and non-specialist clinic settings. Clin Endocrinol 2001; 54:719–723.
8. Kendall-Taylor P. Thyroid cancer in the UK: can we do it better? Clin Endocrinol 2001; 54:705–706.
9. Hamming JF, Goslings BM, van Steenis GJ, et al. The value of fine-needle aspiration biopsy in patients with nodular thyroid disease divided into groups of suspicion of malignant neoplasm on clinical grounds. Arch Intern Med 1990; 150:113.
10. Elisei R, Bottici V, Luchetti F, et al. Impact of routine measurement of serum calcitonin on the diagnosis and outcome of medullary thyroid cancer: experience in 10,864 patients with nodular thyroid disorders. J Clin Endocrinol Metab 2004; 89:163–168.
11. Vierhapper H, Raber W, Bieglmayer C, et al. Routine measurement of plasma calcitonin in nodular thyroid diseases. J Clin Endocrinol Metab 1997; 89:1589–1593.
12. Eng C. Familial papillary thyroid cancer – many syndromes, too many genes? J Clin Endocrinol Metab 2000; 85:1755–1757
13. Pal T, Vogl FD, Chappuis PO, et al. Increased risk for non-medullary thyroid cancer in the first degree relatives of prevalent cases of nonmedullary thyroid cancer: a hospital-based study. J Clin Endocrinol Metab 2001; 85:5307–5312.
14. Belfiore A, Russo D, Vigneri R, Filetti S. Graves' disease, thyroid nodules and thyroid cancer. Clin Endocrinol 2001; 55:711–718.
15. Kossev P, Livolsi V. Lymphoid lesions of the thyroid: review in light of the revised European-American lymphoma classification and upcoming World Health Organization classification. Thyroid 1999; 9:1273–1280.
16. Wiersinga WM. Is repeated fine-needle aspiration cytology indicated in (benign) thyroid nodules? Eur J Endocrinol 1995; 132:661–662.
17. Danese D, Seiaochitano S, Farsetti A, Andreoli M, Pontecorvi A. Diagnostic accuracy of conventional

versus sonography–guided fine-needle aspiration biopsy of thyroid nodules. Thyroid 1998; 8:15–21.

18. Kunreuther E, Orcutt J, Benson CB, et al. The predictive value of FNAC from the dominant (largest) nodule thyroid nodule in a multinodular goiter (abstract). Thyroid 2004; 14:760.

19. Ito Y, Urono T, Nakano K, et al. An observation trial without surgical treatment in patients with papillary microcarcinoma of the thyroid. Thyroid 2003; 13:381–387.

20. Brierly JD, Panzarella T, Tsang RW, Gospodarowicz MK, O'Sullivan B. A comparison of different staging systems' predictability of patient outcome: thyroid carcinoma as an example. Cancer 1997; 79:2414–2423.

21. D'Avanzo A, Ituarte P, Treseler P, et al. Prognostic scoring systems in patients with follicular thyroid cancer: a comparison of different staging systems in predicting the patient outcome. Thyroid 2004; 14:453–458.

22. Mazzaferri E. A randomized trial of remnant ablation – in search of an impossible dream? J Clin Endocrinol Metab 2004; 89:3662–3664.

23. Serhal DI, Nasrallah MP, Arafah BM. Rapid rise in serum thyrotropin concentrations after thyroidectomy or withdrawal of suppressive thyroxine therapy in preparation for radioactive iodine administration to patients with differentiated thyroid cancer. J Clin Endocrinol Metab 2004; 89:3285–3289.

24. Morris LF, Wilder MS, Waxman AD, Braunstein GD. Reevaluation of the impact of a stringent low-iodine diet on ablation rates in radioiodine treatment of thyroid carcinoma. Thyroid 2001; 11:749–755.

25. Pluymen MJHM, Eustatia-Rutten C, Goslings BM, et al. Effects of low-iodide diet on postsurgical radioiodide ablation therapy in patients with differentiated thyroid carcinoma. Clin Endocrinol 2003; 58:428–435.

26. Park II JT, Hennessey JV. Two-week low iodine diet is necessary for adequate outpatient preparation for radioiodine rhTSH scanning in patient taking levothyroxine. Thyroid 2004; 14:57–63.

27. Mazzaferri EL. Gonadal damage from ^{131}I therapy for thyroid cancer. Clin Endocrinol 2002; 57:313–314.

28. Vini L, Hyer S, Al-Sandi A, Pratt B, Harmer C. Prognosis for fertility and ovarian function after treatment with radioiodine for thyroid cancer. Postgrad Med J 2002; 78:92–93.

29. Ceccarelli C, Bencivelli W, Morciano D, Pinchera A, Pacini F. [131]I therapy for differentiated thyroid cancer leads to an earlier onset of menopause: results of a retrospective study. J Clin Endocrinol Metab 2001; 86:3512–3515.

30. Hyer S, Vini L, O'Connell M, Pratt B, Harmer C. Testicular dose and fertility in men following I[131] therapy for thyroid cancer. Clin Endocrinol 2002; 56:755–758.

31. Machens A, Niccoli-Sire P, Hoegel J, et al. Early malignant progression of hereditary medullary thyroid cancer. N Engl J Med 2003; 349:1517–1525.

32. Pujol P, Daures J-P, Nsakala N, et al. Degree of thyrotropin suppression as a prognostic determinant in differentiated thyroid cancer. J Clin Endocrinol Metab 1996; 81:4318–4323.

33. Böhm J, Kosma V-M, Eskelinen M, et al. Non-suppressed thyrotropin and elevated thyroglobulin are independent predictors of recurrence in differentiated thyroid carcinoma. Eur J Endocrinol 1999; 141:460–467.

34. Wang P-W, Wang S-T, Liu R-T, et al. Levothyroxine suppression of thyroglobulin in patients with differentiated thyroid carcinoma. J Clin Endocrinol Metab 1999; 84:4549–4553.

35. Sawin CT, Geller A, Wolf PA, et al. Low serum thyrotropin concentrations as a risk factor for atrial fibrillation in older persons. N Engl J Med 1994; 331:1249–1252.

36. Fazio S, Palmieri EA, Lombardi G, Biondi B. Effect of thyroid hormone on the cardiovascular system. Recent Prog Horm Res 2004; 59:31–50.

37. Gullus S, Altuntas F, Dinzer I, Erol C, Kamel N. Effect of TSH-suppressive therapy on cardiac morphology and function: beneficial effects of the addition of β-blockade on cardiac function. Eur J Endocrinol 2004; 150:655–661.

38. Toivonen J, Tähtelä R, Laitinen K, Risteli J, Välimäki MJ. Markers of bone turnover in patients with differentiated thyroid cancer with and following withdrawal of thyroxine suppressive therapy. Eur J Endocrinol 1998; 138:667–673.

39. Faber J, Galloe AM. Changes in bone mass during prolonged subclinical hyperthyroidism due to L-thyroxine treatment: a meta-analysis. Eur J Endocrinol 1994; 130:350–356.

40. Uzzan B, Campos J, Cucherat M, et al. Effect on bone mass of long-term treatment with thyroid hormones: a meta-analysis. J Clin Endocrinol Metab 1996; 81:4278–4289.

41. Surks MI, Ortin E, Daniels GH, et al. Subclinical thyroid disease: scientific review and guidelines for diagnosis and management. JAMA 2004; 291:228–238.

42. Schlumberger M, Berg G, Cohen O, et al. Follow-up of low-risk patients with differentiated thyroid carcinoma: a European perspective. Eur J Endocrinol 2004; 150:105–112.

43. Kitamura Y, Shimazu K, Nagahama M, et al. Immediate causes of death in thyroid carcinoma: clinicopathological analysis of 161 fatal cases. J Clin Endocrinol Metab 1999; 84:4043–4049.

44. Levy EG. Cost of care. Thyroid 2000; 10:1119–1121.

45. Mendoza A, Shaffer B, Karakla D, et al. Quality-of-life with well-differentiated thyroid cancer: treatment toxicities and their reduction. Thyroid 2004; 14:133–140.

46. Dow KH, Ferrell BR, Anello C. Quality-of-life changes in patients with thyroid cancer after withdrawal of thyroid hormone therapy. Thyroid 1997; 7:613–619.

47. Cohen O, Dabhi S, Karasik A, Zwas SZ. Compliance with follow-up and the informative value of diagnostic whole-body scan in patients with differentiated thyroid carcinoma given recombinant human TSH. Eur J Endocrinol 2004; 150:285–290.

Section III

Initial Thyroid Surgery

11

The Specialist Endocrine Surgeon

Nadine R. Caron, Cord Sturgeon, and Orlo H. Clark

Introduction

Surgeons who treat patients with thyroid cancer and other endocrine diseases have varied clinical backgrounds. Their training or clinical practice may be based in general surgery, otolaryngology, head and neck surgery, surgical oncology, urology (for adrenal tumors), or endocrine surgery. Regardless of the surgeon's title, a surgeon specializing in endocrine disease has a role and responsibility far beyond the operating room. This chapter examines the general surgeon and the specialist endocrine surgeon in the context of thyroid and other endocrine surgery.

Historically, endocrine disease was a prominent aspect of the general surgeon's practice. Indeed, some of the greatest names in the history of surgery have left their mark within endocrine surgery. General surgeons including Kocher, Halsted, Lahey, Mayo, Crile, and Cope played dominant roles in the development of the surgical treatment of endocrine disease [1,2]. Before the role of iodine deficiency in endemic goiter was understood, this was a common disease treated with thyroidectomy performed by general surgeons [3]. Before the 1940s, when therapeutic radioiodine and antithyroid medications were first introduced, surgery was also the only available treatment for hyperthyroid states such as diffuse goiter (Graves' disease), toxic multinodular goiter (Plummer's disease), and toxic adenomas [2]. Although Kocher

(1841–1917) is well known as the first surgeon to perform a high volume of endocrine (thyroid) procedures (Figure 11.1) [2], it was not until the 1950s that surgeons in several countries embraced the philosophy that an understanding of the physiology, embryology, and pathology of the endocrine system was an important companion to technical expertise in the operating room. Realizing that advances in knowledge and skill would accompany increased clinical experience, these early "endocrine surgeons" focused their practice on endocrine surgery as a separate subspecialty within general surgery [2].

This relatively informal stance essentially still applies today. The "specialist endocrine surgeon" remains a loosely defined term that, in the USA, has no formal definition or requirements. Although often defined by the scope of the surgeon's clinical practice, it simultaneously refers to the level of training, the extent of clinical practice for the ongoing development and maintenance of skills, the advancement of knowledge in surgical endocrinology through clinical and basic science research, and the role in educating medical students, surgical residents, and endocrine surgery fellows. The specialist surgeon exchanges knowledge and opinions at national and international medical meetings to help develop improved and evidence-based treatments as well as guidelines for the surgical treatment of benign and malignant endocrine disease. Specialist surgeons recognize the importance of a multidisciplinary approach

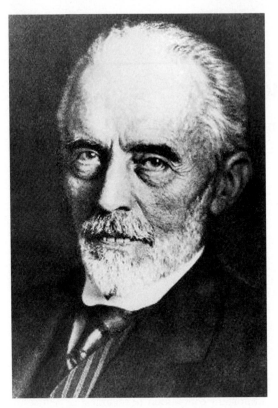

Figure 11.1 Theodore Emil Kocher (1841–1917); a pioneer "endocrine" surgeon. (Reproduced with permission from Welbourn [2], page 16.)

and should serve as leaders in fostering relationships between the surgeon, endocrinologist, oncologist, radiologist, nuclear medicine physician, pathologist, primary care physician, and allied healthcare professionals.

Exponential growth in medical knowledge and technology has fueled the demand for advanced knowledge and skills for every disease process that general surgeons treat, regardless of what subspecialty umbrella it falls under. This advanced level of expertise is becoming increasingly difficult for a general surgeon to obtain and maintain. This chapter will evaluate thyroid and other endocrine surgery training, analyze clinical practice profiles of those practicing endocrine surgery in the USA, and depict professional aspects of endocrine surgery that separate the general surgeon or otolaryngologist who performs endocrine surgery from the endocrine surgeon who specializes in the treatment of endocrine diseases. The successful

surgical management of thyroid and other endocrine diseases requires the cooperation of both general and endocrine surgeons.

Training in Endocrine Surgery – Obtaining the Skills and Knowledge

Two levels of endocrine surgery training now exist: surgical residency and endocrine surgery fellowship training. The baseline level of training for thyroid surgery is received in surgical residency and is a mandatory component of general surgery and otolaryngology programs. This chapter will focus on the general surgery perspective. Additional surgical endocrinology fellowship training remains an informal process at present, but discussion regarding the standardization of formal fellowship training is under way within many associations, including the American Association of Endocrine Surgeons (AAES).

General Surgery Residency Training

According to the Accreditation Council for Graduate Medical Education (ACGME) Residency Review Committee (RRC) for Surgery, a standard general surgery residency program is expected to provide the training to enable its graduates to perform endocrine surgery safely, efficiently, and with appropriate indications, preoperative preparation and postoperative care [4,5]. The majority of surgeons in the USA who perform endocrine operations rely on this level of training.

Harness et al. evaluated the operative experience of graduating general surgery residents in the USA in an attempt to characterize what baseline level of training general surgeons have obtained for thyroid, parathyroid, and adrenal surgery [5]. They found extremely varied levels of experience for all three endocrine glands, including the thyroid (Figure 11.2) [1,5]. The average number of thyroidectomies performed by graduating chief residents ranged from 10.8 (1986–1987) up to 15.2 (1998–1999). Despite the limited experience treating thyroid disease, it still made up an average of two thirds of the total operative endocrine experience in resi-

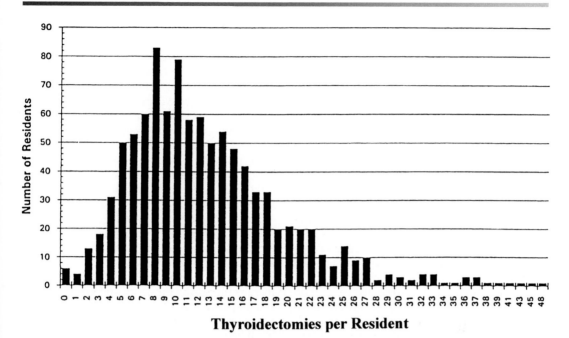

Thyroidectomies per Resident

Figure 11.2 Distribution of thyroidectomies performed by residents (1993–1994). (Reproduced from Harness K, Organ CH Jr, Thompson NW. Operative experience of U.S. general surgery residents in thyroid and parathyroid disease. Surgery. 1995 Dec; 118(6):1065. Copyright 1995, with permission from Elsevier.)

dency [5]. The average number of parathyroidectomies ranged from 4.1 to 5.1 per year, and even fewer adrenalectomies (0.98 per year) were performed [5,6]. While an increasing trend was seen, this study questioned whether this relatively small volume of cases provided adequate exposure to the broad array of thyroid disorders that surgeons may encounter in an active clinical practice. Less common clinical entities such as large substernal goiters, invasive malignancies, large distorting neoplasms, locally recurrent tumors, and anaplastic or medullary thyroid cancer all add complexity and difficulty to thyroid operations and are unlikely to have been encountered to any great degree during residency training. It is probable that experience with the lymph node dissections often required for appropriate treatment of patients with thyroid cancer is equally limited, although no data, to our knowledge, are currently available.

Since residency remains the endpoint in training for most surgeons who perform thyroidectomies and other endocrine procedures, it is important to consider how many operative procedures should be performed during residency in order for a trainee to be considered competent and qualified. The Residency Review

Committee (RRC) for Surgery in the USA defines the minimum number of operations required in training for each category of general surgery, and has established that only eight endocrine operations are required. The minimum for the "head and neck" category is 24, but this criterion can be fulfilled by operations such as neck exploration for trauma, carotid endarterectomy, superficial parotidectomy, as well as thyroid, parathyroid, and lymph node resections [5]. The endocrine requirements do not specify criteria for each specific endocrine gland (thyroid, parathyroid, adrenal or endocrine pancreas) or for specific disease processes (benign or malignant). Strictly from an accreditation point of view, the average general surgery resident in the USA easily meets the current caseload criteria for endocrine surgery training; however, when the Accreditation Council for Graduate Medical Education requirements were established, they did not take into consideration the range of pathology treated within surgical endocrinology.

Some residents receive appreciable experience in endocrine surgery during their residency. Harness et al. found that the maximum number of thyroid operations (either partial or complete thyroidectomies) performed by a single resident was 102 [5]. The maximum number of parathyroidectomies and adrenalectomies performed were 60 and 15, respectively [5,6]. These numbers are significantly above the average resident's experience, and indeed, some residents will perform more thyroid operations in their residency than many general surgeons will in their entire career [1,5,7]. This variability suggests that the level of skill, knowledge, and understanding of endocrine diseases to achieve the successful practice of endocrine surgery within a general surgery career can be acceptable for many residents, and even exceptional for some. Whereas minimal experience in residency coupled with an occasional thyroidectomy in practice is not an optimal situation. Currently, evidence-derived recommendations for minimum training volume do not exist. Because of the large variations in exposure to endocrine operations among residency programs and general surgery practices, carefully controlled studies are needed to shed light on this controversial issue.

Some residency programs and residents have difficulty meeting the RRC minimum standards for training in endocrine surgery. Although the mean values from the Harness study could be influenced by case volume outliers, the modal values for thyroidectomy (8 to 10 cases per graduating resident) and parathyroidectomy (2 to 3 per graduating resident) continue to reflect a concerning paucity of exposure [5]. A limited residency case volume is likely indicative of a limited endocrine practice of the faculty members within such programs.

The majority of general surgery residency programs do not have specialist endocrine surgeons on their faculty. A study of the 268 general surgery residency programs in the USA in 1993–1994 discovered that only 70 programs (26%) had an endocrine surgeon (defined as a member of the American Association of Endocrine Surgeons) on staff [4]. This proved to be an important factor. Those programs with an endocrine surgeon had greater numbers of thyroidectomies, parathyroidectomies, and overall endocrine cases than those without one. In addition, residents from programs with an endocrine surgeon tended to score higher on the endocrine section of the qualifying examination of the American Board of Surgery in 1994, and this difference was statistically significant in 1995 [4]. While the value of having

endocrine surgeons teach the corresponding clinical workup, operative procedures, and post operative follow-up was statistically evident by standardized test results, whether the test results and case volume differences noted in this previous study were clinically relevant is debatable. The presence of an endocrine surgeon on the teaching faculty did not affect the paucity of residents' exposure to uncommon endocrine procedures, such as those involving the endocrine pancreas [4]. This is likely due to the lack of power to detect such a difference, as the overall number of these cases is low.

There are other probable advantages to having an endocrine surgeon on the teaching faculty that were not evaluated in the Harness study. These surgeons tend to operate on greater numbers of patients with endocrine disease, thereby increasing the depth and breadth of the resident's exposure. This not only provides additional training in the clinic and operating room, but it helps create an understanding of the complexity of cases that this discipline can entail. This understanding stems from the uncommon and challenging clinical endocrine scenarios that have a low incidence in the general population, but an increased incidence in the referral practice of the specialist faculty. Respect for the amount of experience and knowledge required to provide optimal patient care can be garnered from an endocrine surgeon – perhaps better than it can be from a nonreferral-based and nonspecialized surgeon. This view is supported by Cheadle et al., who demonstrated an increase in the volume and complexity of chief resident cases when specialty faculty from other areas of general surgery joined the department [8]. New faculty members specializing in surgical oncology, hepatobiliary, colorectal, and vascular surgery developed major referral practices that exposed residents to a wider, more challenging range of cases in their fields [8]. The greater volume and complexity of a surgical referral center may be accompanied by an increased multidisciplinary involvement of colleagues in radiology, nuclear medicine, pathology, and endocrinology and this also contributes to the residents' clinical exposure.

An Australian study of complications from total thyroidectomy demonstrated that appropriately trained general surgeons performed this operation with complication rates comparable to their endocrine surgeon counterparts, despite the significant difference in practice volume (146 versus 2–16 thyroidectomies per year) [9]. The general surgeons were former trainees in an endocrine surgery specialty unit during their residencies and at the time of their graduation were thought to be proficient in thyroid surgery. This study suggests that well-trained general surgeons who are proficient and safe in endocrine surgery when they complete their residency training can continue to be once they are in practice in the community.

Perhaps the most important influence an endocrine surgeon has in a general surgery training program is on the recruitment of future endocrine surgeons by exposing residents to the opportunities in the field. Endocrine surgeons may serve as mentors for medical students and residents who have an interest in this field of surgery or who will develop such an interest because of their mentorship. A survey of senior surgeons at regional and national surgical societies found that their "role models" were the number one influence on their choice of career specialty [10]. A separate survey found that two thirds of general surgery graduates chose the same career as their mentor [11]. With the declining number of medical students pursuing careers in surgery and the high attrition rates of those who begin general surgery programs [12], the general surgery profession and its specialties need more role models to encourage and support young surgeons [13,14].

General surgery residencies should provide adequate experience in thyroid surgery so that their graduates can perform uncomplicated thyroid operations with minimal morbidity [4,15,16]. With this solid baseline training, and by staying on top of emerging and changing treatment options and guidelines, these graduates can continue to safely and effectively treat most endocrine diseases that require surgery. Recognition of personal and institutional limitations will result in appropriate referrals to colleagues who have additional training and experience [15].

Endocrine Surgery Fellowship Training

Although most surgeons in the USA who perform endocrine operations do so in the context of a broad general surgery practice, many believe that additional training in endocrine surgery is required for those who will serve as experts in the field. Endocrine surgery fellowships of variable duration add clinical, operative, and research experiences onto the standard surgical residency training. The duration and curriculum for such programs have not been formally established. Current fellowships in the USA, Canada, Australia, Europe, and Asia range from 3 months to 4 years in duration and may include clinical practice, clinical research, basic science research or combinations thereof. As per the International Association of Endocrine Surgeons (IAES) website [17], there are 85 centers that have or are planning to create endocrine surgery fellowships and this number will continue to increase. No formal certification process currently accompanies this fellowship training in the USA, but it is generally agreed that an endocrine surgery fellowship should prepare the surgeon for all elements of a career in this subspecialty. To date, there have been no specific studies on the impact of endocrine surgery fellowship programs on clinical outcomes.

Surgical endocrinology does not merely involve technical skill. The additional clinical experience of a fellowship program builds in-depth knowledge in the areas of prevention, diagnosis, natural history, treatment options, preoperative preparation, operative technique, and management of surgical complications in patients with a broad range of endocrine disorders. A firm understanding of endocrine biology and pathophysiology is mandatory. Knowledge of investigative options, including their indications and limitations, allows accurate and timely diagnosis while minimizing invasiveness and cost. The use of novel and experimental treatment options not yet found in textbooks is an important aspect of fellowship training because these future endocrine surgeons will help dictate the ultimate role these therapeutic options will play. Surgical technique, including preoperative and intraoperative decision-making, must be taught by those who are experienced in the field. Appropriate postoperative and long-term follow-up care including hormone substitution therapy and surveillance for disease recurrence are vital aspects of patient management. Knowledge of the indications for and potential complications of adjuvant oncological treatment is also required. Because of advances in molecular genetics, screening for familial disease or detecting genetic markers to predict tumor behavior will play an increasing role in patient evaluation, treatment, and follow-up care. A key element of fellowship training involves achieving greater clinical and operative experience while under the guidance of endocrine surgeon mentors.

The emerging specialist should be competent in the operative and nonoperative components of surgical endocrinology. For this reason, it has been suggested that the clinical aspect of a fellowship program include nonsurgical skills such as neck ultrasonography, fine-needle aspiration biopsy, and direct laryngoscopy. Clinical experience should include nonoperative rotations in endocrinology, endocrine pathology, and related radiology and nuclear medicine investigations and treatments. Achieving this competency is an important component of specialty training.

Endocrine surgery fellowships should include a research component – basic science, clinical or both. Regardless of the type of research, development of the associated skills is a vital tool that the graduating endocrine surgeon takes from their fellowship to their professional practice. The contributions from original research are one of the yardsticks by which academic surgeons are measured. More importantly, such contributions are mandatory for the continued improvement in patient care, because advances and innovations in technique and knowledge are the products of these research efforts. In addition to the increased volume and depth of clinical experience, the research element of an endocrine surgery fellowship also differentiates it from the residency training on which they are building.

With the range and depth of clinical and research experience an endocrine fellowship program can provide, it is possible to visualize how one begins to make the transformation from general surgery graduate to specialized endocrine surgeon.

Clinical Practice – Maintaining the Skills and Knowledge and Building on Them

Surgeons who perform endocrine surgery must ensure that they maintain their level of practice at an acceptable standard, regardless of whether they have additional fellowship training or not.

The maintenance of these standards should include a critical self-appraisal of patient outcomes as they relate to clinical decision-making, timing and accuracy of diagnosis, indications for and choice of operation, postoperative follow-up care and adjuvant treatment. Since medicine is a dynamic profession, this clinical competency must reflect past training and experience while incorporating any changes in clinical practice guidelines and treatment modalities. Any surgeon caring for patients with endocrine disorders such as thyroid cancer must remain up to date on the advances in the multidisciplinary care (operative and nonoperative) that these diseases require. The specialist surgeon should play an active role in the development of these advances and in the promotion of the multidisciplinary approach.

Maintenance of Technical Surgical Skills: the Volume–Outcome Relationship

Perhaps the most widely quoted perspective for the role that specialist surgeons play in treating endocrine diseases stems from studies correlating surgical and hospital volume to patient outcomes. Low surgeon case-volume has been associated with higher complication rates in studies involving a vast array of specialties such as vascular, pediatric, colorectal, pancreatic, and endocrine surgery [18–24]. These studies suggest that surgeons who perform either a greater number of specific procedures or who dedicate a greater percentage of their overall practice to a specific procedure have better outcomes than surgeons whose practice is less active or focused. This association has held true with respect to mortality rates, complication rates, successful cure rates, length of hospital stay and healthcare charges in several studies, and endocrine surgery is no exception.

However, the studies that demonstrate this volume–outcome relationship have some limitations [22]. Although associations may be statistically significant, proving causality is much more difficult. For example, to prove a causal relationship, one must determine if high volume surgeons truly have better results or if they are simply drawing more referrals because they excel at those procedures [25]. In addition, despite efforts of case-mix adjustments in these studies, there may be selective referral of patients to high volume surgeons or centers. It is possible that the lower volume surgeons are actually performing more difficult procedures on sicker patients, but at this point there is no evidence to suggest this within endocrine surgery. The surgeon's volume–outcome association may be confounded by hospital volume, which may, in turn, be related to patient outcomes. This association between patient outcomes and hospital volume has been demonstrated in studies of pancreatico-duodenectomy, cholecystectomy, and coronary angioplasty [22,26–28], but has not been found for thyroid surgery. This may be due to the relatively young and otherwise healthy patient population that most commonly undergoes thyroid surgery; these patients are not heavily reliant on subspecialty care, complex equipment or monitoring [22]. Publication bias may also be an issue, because investigators in academic centers who conduct volume–outcome research may be more likely to publish results that support their role as referral centers.

Most volume–outcome studies that include results for community surgeons are based on large administrative databases that permit statistically valid estimates of associations between patient outcomes and surgeon volume [29]. While these databases offer powerful information, they have their limitations. They are often not set up to answer specific research questions. The information available may not include key variables that permit the most appropriate statistical assessment of study endpoints. An example is the extrapolation of treatment complications from hospital database "length of stay" information for patients who have had thyroid surgery. The main complications and endpoints in thyroid surgery studies are often confirmed after discharge – and after data collection has been completed. Complications such as recurrent or superior laryngeal nerve injury, persistent or recurrent hyperparathyroidism, permanent hypoparathyroidism, or wound infection may develop or be diagnosed after discharge, and therefore may not be accurately reflected in a discharge database. In addition, confounding issues, such as previous neck surgery or locally invasive malignancies, are significant risk factors for complications in thyroid operations that are often not available in databases not constructed specifically for analy-

sis of surgical outcome and complications. Other important patient information that allows accurate case-mix adjustment may not be optimal and is database dependent.

Two studies that used discharge databases examined the volume–outcome relationship in endocrine surgery. Chen et al. [30] used the Maryland inpatient discharge database to evaluate the state's experience with parathyroidectomy between 1990 and 1994. Their study confirmed the high cure rates and low morbidity and mortality rates associated with specialist surgeons that have been reported in previous studies. Database limitations did not permit the evaluation of cure rates or complication rates of the patients whose operations were performed outside of the endocrine center, but the analysis did show a significantly longer length of stay at these other hospitals (3.1 versus 1.3 days). The authors speculated that length of stay may be a proxy for operative complications, but although plausible, this is an assumption that has been both supported and criticized in the literature on surgical outcome. Sosa et al. used hospital discharge data from nonfederal acute care hospitals in Maryland to compare the results of endocrine surgeons with those of lower volume surgeons [22]. They found an association between high volume surgeons and decreased complication rates and shorter lengths of stay, which seemed strongest for the subgroups of patients who had more complex diagnoses or procedures, such as malignancies and total thyroidectomies.

Although many studies suggest that increased surgical volume is associated with better clinical outcome, the concentration of endocrine surgery into the hands of specialist surgeons has not been widely adopted in the USA. When evaluating who was performing endocrine procedures (thyroid, parathyroid, and adrenal) in the USA, Saunders et al. evaluated surgeons based on the number of endocrine cases they performed and the percentage of each surgeon's practice that was endocrine in nature [7]. Surgeons whose endocrine experience comprised 25% or less of their practice performed 78% of all parathyroidectomies, 94% of all adrenalectomies, and 82% of all thyroidectomies (Figure 11.3) completed in the USA in the years 1988 through 2000 [7]. Surgeons for whom endocrine procedures comprised 75% or more of their practice performed only 5% of all parathy-

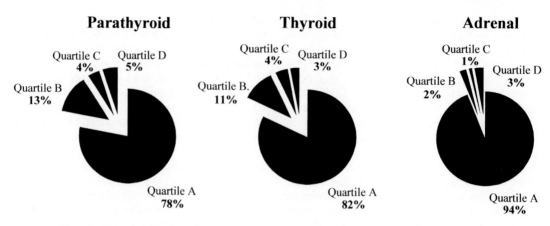

Figure 11.3 Contribution of individual surgeon quartiles to the total number of patients who underwent operation (calculated on percentage of practice calculation: quartile A: 0–25%; quartile B: 26–50%; quartile C: 51–75%; quartile D: 76–100%). (Reproduced from Saunders BD, Nainess RM, Dimick JB, et al. Who performs endocrine operations in the United States? Surgery. 2003 Dec; 134(6):928. Copyright 2003, with permission from Elsevier.)

roidectomies, 3% of all adrenalectomies, and 3% of all thyroidectomies in this same time period. In a study of thyroidectomies, 78.6% of surgeons who perform these procedures did fewer than ten thyroid operations per year (Figure 11.4) [22].

There are, however, geographic regions in the USA where the bulk of endocrine surgeries are performed in specialist centers. In Maryland, between the years 1990 and 1994, an increasing percentage (8% to 21%) of the state's parathyroidectomies were being performed by a single

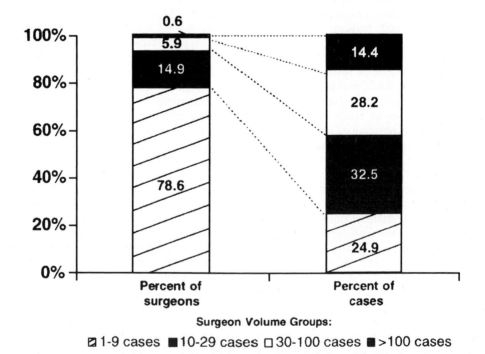

Figure 11.4 Summary of the distribution of thyroid surgeons and cases by the four surgeon volume groups. (Reproduced with permission from Sosa et al. [22], page 323.)

endocrine surgeon [30]. Similarly, between 1991 and 1996, the highest volume thyroid surgeons in Maryland (those performing over 100 cases per year) noted an increased referral pattern as their share of thyroidectomies increased from 11.9% (1991–1993) to 17.6% (1994–1996) [22]. Overall, those surgeons performing 30 or more thyroidectomies completed 42.6% of the total thyroidectomies in the state, while comprising only 6.5% of the surgeons (Figure 11.4) [22].

Some studies do not support the "volume–outcome" relationship in endocrine surgery. These looked at smaller series, at trainees' experience, and at general surgeons in community practices [9,25,31–33]. Even studies that find an association between surgical volume and clinical outcome must be interpreted with caution. Sosa et al. showed there was no significant difference for rates of hypoparathyroidism between any of the surgeon volume categories, but did find an increased rate (1.5% versus 0.4%) of recurrent laryngeal nerve injury after thyroidectomy in the lowest volume group (fewer than 10 thyroidectomies per year) as compared to the highest volume group (over 100 thyroidectomies per year) [22]. There was, however, no significant difference in nerve injury rates between the mid-volume groups who performed between 10 and 100 thyroid operations per year and those who performed over 100 (0.5–0.8% versus 0.4%). Perhaps this is suggestive of a threshold annual number of cases where the volume–outcome relationship exists and above which the relationship weakens.

The results from Sosa et al. must be considered in light of the differences in the patient populations. Surgeons who operated on more than 100 patients with thyroid disease per year were performing more total thyroidectomies (versus lobectomy), treating more malignant (versus benign) conditions and had a significantly younger patient population than the lower volume surgeons [22]. The finding that the highest volume group treated the more challenging and complex patient population may support one of two views: First, that the small difference in recurrent laryngeal nerve injury rates and the absence of difference in the hypoparathyroidism rates are biased towards the null, that is, that the difference in complication rates would be greater if the lower volume surgeons performed more complex cases.

Second, and conversely, that appropriate selection of thyroid cases based on the surgeon's training and experience (and appropriate referrals based on case complexity) enables safe endocrine surgery to be performed by all surgeons who maintain their skills with an adequate number of cases. Both are probably true to some extent, although more definitive conclusions cannot be made without clinical evidence.

The threshold at which one becomes a "high volume" surgeon is variable and to some extent, arbitrary. Some published thresholds for "high volume" surgeons reflect this variability: parathyroidectomy, over 50 cases per year [34], carotid endarterectomy, 30 or more cases per year [35], thyroid surgery, over 20 cases per year (P. Haigh, 2004, personal communication), colorectal procedures, over 10 per year [36]. This variability in case number suggests that it may be more than just pure annual volume of cases that determines surgical expertise and subsequent clinical outcome for patients. Clinical outcomes are a multifactorial entity with patient selection, appropriate choice of procedure, referral pattern, institutional impact, and surgical skill all part of this surgical outcome puzzle.

Maintenance of Surgical Decision-Making

Integral to surgical success and often entwined in the volume–outcome relationship is the ability of the surgeon to use clinical information, diagnostic study results, and professional judgment to determine treatment recommendations. How the operative approach and treatment guidelines should be modified for each individual patient are challenging aspects of endocrine surgery that are taught in residency, refined in fellowship and remain a dynamic challenge in clinical practice.

As the optimal surgical treatment for thyroid disease is often debated, it provides an excellent example of how clinical decision-making requires sound knowledge of accepted guidelines, as well as an understanding of the controversies and the study results which support or refute the various treatment options. This allows one to tailor treatment for individual patients. Although controversial, the current trend for treatment of selected benign and most malignant thyroid disease is towards more extensive surgery, such as near-total or total thyroidectomy [37–39]. When used to treat thyroid malignancies, these operations may involve central and/or lateral lymph node dissections, the indications for which are also a source of controversy. With an active clinical practice and ongoing hands-on research in this field, specialist surgeons treating thyroid disease are most adept at making these difficult clinical decisions.

Total thyroidectomy has many proposed advantages [40]. It facilitates the subsequent use of radioactive iodine for thyroid remnant ablation, diagnostic scanning, and treatment of locally recurrent and metastatic disease. Serum thyroglobulin level is a more sensitive tumor marker for early detection of disease recurrence and metastases when no normal thyroid cells remain. Up to 85% of patients with papillary thyroid cancer have occult multicentric disease that would be eliminated as possible sites of local recurrence if total thyroidectomy were performed [41]. When tumor foci are left in situ, about 7% of such patients will develop local recurrence in the contralateral lobe and 50% of those will die from their disease [40]. Total thyroidectomy decreases the risk of local recurrence, decreases the 1% risk of dedifferentiation of papillary and follicular thyroid cancer and improves survival for patients with high risk papillary thyroid cancers [37,40,42,43].

At the University of California, San Francisco, total thyroidectomy is recommended for most patients with pathology proven well-differentiated thyroid cancer. Total thyroidectomy is especially recommended for higher risk patients such as those under 15 or older than 45, those with a previous history of exposure to low dose therapeutic irradiation to the cervical region, those with a family history of well-differentiated thyroid cancer, those for whom preoperative assessment demonstrates papillary thyroid cancer one centimeter or greater, and those with bilateral disease, extrathyroidal extension, or the presence of lymphatic or systemic metastases. In addition, for patients who did not meet any of the preoperative criteria for total thyroidectomy, a completion thyroidectomy would be recommended for positive margins, multifocal disease, non-minimally invasive follicular cancer or aggressive histology (tall cell, columnar cell, insular or poorly differentiated). Many

other surgeons use all or some of these indications to determine the extent of thyroidectomy and other centers support this liberal approach to total thyroidectomy for papillary and follicular thyroid cancer when the complication rate is low [40,44–50].

Others do not advocate total thyroidectomy, and cite various reasons for a less aggressive surgical approach [40,42]. Local recurrence in the contralateral lobe would be diagnosed with standard patient follow-up and 50% are cured with surgery. Fewer than 5% of recurrences actually occur in the thyroid bed. Potential contralateral occult papillary thyroid cancers are of questionable clinical significance, and have an excellent prognosis when treated with less than a total thyroidectomy. Indeed, some studies have not found a survival benefit for total thyroidectomy in either low risk or high risk differentiated thyroid cancer patients and advocate against using an aggressive surgical approach in all but the most select patient population [51,52]. There are currently no prospective studies to help end this controversy.

Oncological endpoints such as recurrence and survival are the pillars of the debate over the extent of resection for thyroid cancer, but the potential for complications has also been evaluated. Some think that lobectomy with isthmusectomy is associated with fewer complications than a total thyroidectomy because dissection is limited to one side, theoretically decreasing the incidence of hypoparathyroidism and recurrent laryngeal nerve injury [22]. Others think the risks of operative complications with total thyroidectomy are not significantly greater than with lobectomy and isthmusectomy [53,54]. Most larger, robust series document comparable complication rates for the two procedures [40], findings which are true for total resections at the time of initial procedure as well as for completion thyroidectomies [55,56].

Despite evidence supporting the safety and efficacy of total thyroidectomy for malignant and benign disease, there are some reports that total thyroidectomies make up a significantly smaller percentage of all thyroid procedures in the lower volume general surgeon's practice than in the higher volume endocrine surgeon's practice [22,37,57,58]. Given that the extent of resection is a controversial topic, this difference between general and endocrine surgeons may reflect an honest underlying difference of opinion regarding total thyroidectomy versus lobectomy. It may also reflect a referral bias if patients who are more likely to require total resection are referred to specialists. Operative indications should not be influenced by the surgeon's level of training, practice volume, or comfort level with extensive thyroid resection – these are on no one's "list of indications" for cancer treatment. If these are an issue and the patient would benefit from a more complex or extensive surgical approach, then this patient requires referral to a more experienced surgeon – not a change in the operative approach.

Who should be performing thyroid surgery? One does not need to be an endocrine surgeon to treat thyroid cancer. Considering that there were an estimated 18 400 thyroid cancers diagnosed in the USA in the year 2000 (not including thyroid operations for nodules eventually diagnosed as benign) [59] and there are only 298 current members in the AAES (237 practicing in the USA) (J. Pasieka, 2004, personal communication), it would not be possible for thyroid surgery to remain solely in the hands of endocrine surgeons. Therefore, there should be a concerted effort to determine whether a particular case should be managed by a well-trained general surgeon or by a specialized endocrine surgeon.

The decision to assume the surgical care for a patient with thyroid cancer or to refer the patient to a more experienced colleague who specializes in this area should be based on patient, surgeon, and institutional factors. A surgeon's level of training, endocrine knowledge, operative skills, and clinical acumen determine if one can safely and effectively provide the surgical care required. The institution's strengths and limitations should be considered in terms of operative equipment, medical resources, and colleague support. While the surgeon and institutional factors remain fairly constant, the patient factors make each decision unique. Table 11.1 refers to clinical scenarios we generally consider to be within the specialist's domain, because of the technical challenge of the surgical procedure or the anticipated complexity of multidisciplinary treatment and follow-up care. It is the responsibility of each surgeon to maintain a personal audit of his or her procedures, complications, and clinical outcomes so that these decisions can be as objective as possible.

Table 11.1 Potential indications for referral to a specialist surgeon[a]

Recurrent disease: reoperative procedures
Anaplastic thyroid cancer
Medullary thyroid cancer, including central lymph node dissection
Multiple endocrine neoplasia syndromes
Advanced malignancies
Modified radical neck dissection
Symptoms: airway obstruction, dysphagia, hoarse voice, substernal extension
Goiters
WHO classification, stage III, possibly stage II
Substernal goiters
Graves' disease
Patient factors that increase complexity or difficulty of procedure
Large body habitus
Comorbidities that add significant technical and medical challenges
Documented recurrent laryngeal nerve injury
Coexisting endocrine disease, i.e. hyperparathyroidism
Previous exposure to low dose therapeutic radiation
Pediatric thyroid surgery
Patient request for specialist surgeon

[a] Indications may be based on technical challenge of required surgical procedure or anticipated complexity of multidisciplinary care.

Maintenance of "Points of Good Practice"

The final component in the treatment of thyroid cancer is the clinical follow-up of the patient. This demands a full understanding of the disease process and the indications for elements such as postoperative radioiodine ablation, chronic thyroid-stimulating hormone suppression, and the clinical, radiological, and biochemical monitoring of the patient for recurrent disease. Surgeons operating on the thyroid gland must be active in these treatment decisions and not succumb to the simple role of "technician."

Kumar et al. assessed the degree to which "points of good practice" were met by groups of specialists with an interest in thyroid cancer compared to physicians and surgeons outside of a specialist clinic setting [60]. The specialist group included endocrine surgeons, endocrinologists, and oncologists. The points of good practice evaluated were defined in conservative terms to highlight patterns of practice that departed from acceptable standards based on review of the literature and national guidelines. Ninety percent of specialist surgeons performed the more extensive total or near-total thyroidectomy when it was deemed appropriate, but only 62% in the nonspecialist setting met such treatment recommendations. It is noteworthy that complication rates were similar in both groups. In addition, in both groups, postoperative L-thyroxine administration was inadequate for greater than 20% of the patients (goal of thyroid-stimulating hormone <0.1 mU/L) and surveillance thyroglobulin levels were not monitored in almost 15% of patients. Inadequate postoperative L-thyroxine administration and thyroglobulin monitoring tended to occur more commonly in the nonspecialist group, but the differences were not statistically significant. The recommended approach to rising thyroglobulin levels and the use of radioiodine were achieved more commonly in the specialist clinics than outside them, and this difference was statistically significant. This study highlights a volume–outcome relationship by comparing important aspects in the clinical treatment of thyroid cancer, rather than comparing surgical outcome. Overall, patients received more comprehensive, complete care in specialist clinics than in nonspecialist environments [60].

Postoperative management and long-term follow-up of patients with thyroid cancer are not technically demanding aspects of patient care, but require attention to detail and knowledge of changes in the dynamic field of endocrine oncology. Specialists in thyroid cancer need not direct this care, but patients should always receive the same standard of care as these specialists provide. While a general surgeon treating thyroid cancer must stay abreast of advances in diagnostic and treatment elements, it is the extensive clinical experience and research efforts of endocrine specialists that drive these advances.

Conclusion: The Endocrine Surgeon

The endocrine surgeon provides clinical expertise in the management of endocrine disease. This clinical role extends beyond the operating theater to ensure provision of quality preoperative preparation, postoperative care, and long-term follow-up. Academic endocrine surgeons may conduct clinical research, basic science research, or both, and through their contributions to the fields of surgical endocrinology, molecular genetics, and clinical outcomes, they continue to improve the care of patients with endocrine disease. Advances in operative techniques and intraoperative equipment are developed and scrutinized in efforts to decrease the morbidity of a procedure while improving the outcome for the patient. Through extensive professional experience and original research projects, these specialists formulate treatment recommendations and guidelines that become the yardsticks by which all practitioners of endocrine surgery are measured. Attendance at national and international meetings and membership in specialty associations are important educational and professional elements of a specialist's career. Specialist surgeons provide tertiary care for the more complex and challenging cases, while also treating a broad range of general endocrine diseases. With surgery being a central component of thyroid cancer treatment (and many other endocrine diseases), endocrine surgeons must occupy a central role in the multidisciplinary approach to these diseases.

The endocrine surgeon serves as educator, mentor, and role model for surgical trainees. Specialist surgeons serving on surgical faculties enhance the clinical experience of residents in terms of the volume and the breadth of clinical exposure to ensure that the graduates have developed competency in endocrine surgery. Their impact as role models or mentors for medical students and residents is less quantifiable but equally as important – especially when it influences career choice. In addition, the presence of one or more specialist surgeons is required for fellowship training in endocrine surgery, which is becoming the hallmark for entry into the specialty community.

The endocrine surgeon should provide leadership in the academic, clinical, and administrative domains to promote and protect the discipline of endocrine surgery. For example, adequate exposure of general surgery residents to endocrine surgery should be ensured, novel operative equipment and resources should be available if they will benefit the patient's outcome, and funding for fellowship and research positions is essential if the best health-care is to be provided for our population.

Endocrine surgeons are not meant to replace general surgeons. Rather, they extend the role of surgical care, education, research, and influence by virtue of their focus and dedication to this field.

References

1. Harness JK. Presidential address: Interdisciplinary care – the future of endocrine surgery. Surgery 2000; 128:873–880.
2. Welbourn R. Highlights from endocrine surgical history. World J Surg 1996; 20:603–612.
3. Harness JK, van Heerden JA, Lennquist S, et al. Future of thyroid surgery and training surgeons to meet the expectations of 2000 and beyond. World J Surg 2000; 24:976–982.
4. Prinz RA. Endocrine surgical training – some ABC measures. Surgery 1996; 120:905–912.
5. Harness JK, Organ CH Jr, Thompson NW. Operative experience of US general surgery residents in thyroid and parathyroid disease. Surgery 1995; 118:1063–1070.
6. Harness JK, Organ CH Jr, Thompson NW. Operative experience of US general surgery residents with diseases of the adrenal glands, endocrine pancreas, and other less common endocrine organs. World J Surg 1996; 20: 885–890; discussion 890–891.
7. Saunders BD, Wainess RM, Dimick JB, et al. Who performs endocrine operations in the United States? Surgery 2003; 134:924–931.
8. Cheadle WG, Franklin GA, Richardson JD, Polk HC Jr. Broad-based general surgery training is a model of continued utility for the future. Ann Surg 2004; 239:627–632; discussion 632–636.
9. Reeve TS, Curtin A, Fingleton L, et al. Can total thyroidectomy be performed as safely by general surgeons in provincial centers as by surgeons in specialized endocrine surgical units? Making the case for surgical training. Arch Surg 1994; 129:834–836.
10. Ko CY, Whang EE, Karamanoukian R, Longmire WP, McFadden DW. What is the best method of surgical training? A report of America's leading senior surgeons. Arch Surg 1998; 133:900–905.
11. Thakur A, Fedorka P, Ko C, et al. Impact of mentor guidance in surgical career selection. J Pediatr Surg 2001; 36:1802–1804.
12. Wolfson PJ, Robeson MR, Veloski JJ. Medical students who enter general surgery residency programs: a follow-up between 1972 and 1986. Am J Surg 1991; 162:491–494.
13. Kwakwa F, Biester TW, Ritchie WP Jr, Jonasson O. Career pathways of graduates of general surgery residency programs: an analysis of graduates from 1983 to 1990. J Am Coll Surg 2002; 194:48–53.
14. Neumayer L. Mentoring: the VA experience. Am J Surg 2003; 186:417–419.
15. Pasieka JL. The surgeon as a prognostic factor in endocrine surgical diseases. Surg Oncol Clin North Am 2000; 9:13–20, v–vi.
16. Pasieka JL, Rotstein LE. Consensus conference on well-differentiated thyroid cancer: a summary. Can J Surg 1993; 36:298–301.
17. International Association of Endocrine Surgeons Website. http://www.iaes-endocrine-surgeons.com/. Accessed: 1 May 2004.
18. Feasby TE, Quan H, Ghali WA. Hospital and surgeon determinants of carotid endarterectomy outcomes. Arch Neurol 2002; 59:1877–1881.
19. Pearce WH, Parker MA, Feinglass J, Ujiki M, Manheim LM. The importance of surgeon volume and training in outcomes for vascular surgical procedures. J Vasc Surg 1999; 29:768–776; discussion 777–778.
20. Pranikoff T, Campbell BT, Travis J, Hirschl RB. Differences in outcome with subspecialty care: pyloromyotomy in North Carolina. J Pediatr Surg 2002; 37: 352–356.
21. Porter GA, Soskolne CL, Yakimets WW, Newman SC. Surgeon-related factors and outcome in rectal cancer. Ann Surg 1998; 227:157–167.
22. Sosa JA, Bowman HM, Tielsch JM, et al. The importance of surgeon experience for clinical and economic outcomes from thyroidectomy. Ann Surg 1998; 228:320–330.
23. Birkmeyer JD, Stukel TA, Siewers AE, et al. Surgeon volume and operative mortality in the United States. N Engl J Med 2003; 349:2117–2127.
24. Bachmann MO, Alderson D, Peters TJ, et al. Influence of specialization on the management and outcome of patients with pancreatic cancer. Br J Surg 2003; 90:171–177.
25. Harris S. Thyroid and parathyroid surgical complications. Am J Surg 1992; 163:476–478.
26. Lieberman MD, Kilburn H, Lindsey M, Brennan MF. Relation of perioperative deaths to hospital volume among patients undergoing pancreatic resection for malignancy. Ann Surg 1995; 222:638–645.
27. Hannan EL, O'Donnell JF, Kilburn H Jr, Bernard HR, Yazici A. Investigation of the relationship between volume and mortality for surgical procedures performed in New York State hospitals. JAMA 1989; 262: 503–510.
28. Jollis JG, Peterson ED, DeLong ER, et al. The relation between the volume of coronary angioplasty procedures at hospitals treating Medicare beneficiaries and short-term mortality. N Engl J Med 1994; 331:1625–1629.
29. Rosenberg L, Joseph L, Barkun A. Surgical Arithmetic: epidemiological, statistical and outcome-based approach to surgical practice. Georgetown, TX: Landes Bioscience, 2000.
30. Chen H, Zeiger MA, Gordon TA, Udelsman R. Parathyroidectomy in Maryland: effects of an endocrine center. Surgery 1996; 120:948–952; discussion 952–953.
31. Mishra A, Agarwal G, Agarwal A, Mishra SK. Safety and efficacy of total thyroidectomy in hands of endocrine surgery trainees. Am J Surg 1999; 178:377–380.
32. Shindo M, Sinha U, Rice D. Safety of thyroidectomy in residency: a review of 186 consecutive cases. Laryngoscope 1995; 105:1173–1175.
33. Bergamaschi R, Becouarn G, Ronceray J, Arnaud JP. Morbidity of thyroid surgery. Am J Surg 1998; 176:71–75.
34. Sosa JA, Powe NR, Levine MA, Udelsman R, Zeiger MA. Profile of a clinical practice: Thresholds for surgery and surgical outcomes for patients with primary hyperparathyroidism: a national survey of endocrine surgeons. J Clin Endocrinol Metab 1998; 83:2658–2665.

35. Cowan JA Jr, Dimick JB, Thompson BG, Stanley JC, Upchurch GR Jr. Surgeon volume as an indicator of outcomes after carotid endarterectomy: an effect independent of specialty practice and hospital volume. J Am Coll Surg 2002; 195:814–821.

36. Harmon JW, Tang DG, Gordon TA, et al. Hospital volume can serve as a surrogate for surgeon volume for achieving excellent outcomes in colorectal resection. Ann Surg 1999; 230:404–411; discussion 411–413.

37. Gough IR, Wilkinson D. Total thyroidectomy for management of thyroid disease. World J Surg 2000; 24:962–965.

38. Hay ID, Thompson GB, Grant CS, et al. Papillary thyroid carcinoma managed at the Mayo Clinic during six decades (1940–1999): temporal trends in initial therapy and long-term outcome in 2444 consecutively treated patients. World J Surg 2002; 26:879–885.

39. Liu Q, Djuricin G, Prinz RA. Total thyroidectomy for benign thyroid disease. Surgery 1998; 123:2–7.

40. Kebebew E, Clark OH. Differentiated thyroid cancer: "complete" rational approach. World J Surg 2000; 24:942–951.

41. Witterick IJ, Abel SM, Noyek AM, Freeman JL, Chapnik JS. Nonpalpable occult and metastatic papillary thyroid carcinoma. Laryngoscope 1993; 103:149–155.

42. Jossart G, Clark OH. Well differentiated thyroid cancer. Curr Probl Surg 1994; 31:939.

43. Grant CS, Hay ID, Gough IR, et al. Local recurrence in papillary thyroid carcinoma: is extent of surgical resection important? Surgery 1988; 104:954–962.

44. Santini J, Haddad A. Total thyroidectomy is the recommended treatment for all papillary thyroid carcinoma (PTC). Acta Otorhinolaryngol Belg 1999; 53:161–164.

45. Mazzaferri EL. An overview of the management of papillary and follicular thyroid carcinoma. Thyroid 1999; 9:421–427.

46. Ardito G, Revelli L, Tosti F, et al. Surgery of differentiated thyroid carcinoma, lymph node metastases and locoregional recurrence. Rays 2000; 25:199–206.

47. Hay ID, Grant CS, Bergstralh EJ, et al. Unilateral total lobectomy: is it sufficient surgical treatment for patients with AMES low-risk papillary thyroid carcinoma? Surgery 1998; 124:958–964; discussion 964–966.

48. Welch Dinauer CA, Tuttle RM, Robie DK, McClellan DR, Francis GL. Extensive surgery improves recurrence-free survival for children and young patients with class I papillary thyroid carcinoma. J Pediatr Surg 1999; 34:1799–1804.

49. Beenken S, Roye D, Weiss H, et al. Extent of surgery for intermediate-risk well-differentiated thyroid cancer. Am J Surg 2000; 179:51–56.

50. Hay ID, Bergstralh EJ, Grant CS, et al. Impact of primary surgery on outcome in 300 patients with pathologic tumor-node-metastasis stage III papillary thyroid carcinoma treated at one institution from 1940 through 1989. Surgery 1999; 126:1173–1181; discussion 1181–1182.

51. Shaha AR, Shah JP, Loree TR. Low-risk differentiated thyroid cancer: the need for selective treatment. Ann Surg Oncol 1997; 4:328–333.

52. Wanebo H, Coburn M, Teates D, Cole B. Total thyroidectomy does not enhance disease control or survival even in high-risk patients with differentiated thyroid cancer. Ann Surg 1998; 227:912–921.

53. Sand J, Palkola K, Salmi J. Surgical complications after total thyroidectomy and resections for differentiated thyroid carcinoma. Ann Chir Gynaecol 1996; 85:305–308.

54. Hines JR, Winchester DJ. Total lobectomy and total thyroidectomy in the management of thyroid lesions. Arch Surg 1993; 128:1060–1063; discussion 1064.

55. DeGroot LJ, Kaplan EL. Second operations for "completion" of thyroidectomy in treatment of differentiated thyroid cancer. Surgery 1991; 110:936–939; discussion 939–940.

56. Agarwal A, Mishra SK. Completion total thyroidectomy in the management of differentiated thyroid carcinoma. Aust N Z J Surg 1996; 66:358–360.

57. Thompson G. Thyroid surgery survey report. RACS Bull 1997; 17:56.

58. O'Brien CJ. Complications of thyroidectomy: the benefits of personal audit. Aust N Z J Surg 1997; 67:A25.

59. Jean M, Termuhlen P, Grau A. Carcinoma of the thyroid and parathyroid glands. In: Feig B, Berger D, Fuhrman G (eds) The M.D. Anderson surgical oncology handbook. Philadelphia, PA: Lippincott Williams & Wilkins, 2003: 370–387.

60. Kumar H, Daykin J, Holder R, et al. An audit of management of differentiated thyroid cancer in specialist and non-specialist clinic settings. Clin Endocrinol (Oxf) 2001; 54:719–723.

12

Initial Thyroid Surgery for Patient with Differentiated Thyroid Carcinoma

Douglas B. Villaret and Ernest L. Mazzaferri

Introduction

Prognosis of differentiated thyroid carcinoma (DTC) is typically so favorable that it is difficult to demonstrate an effect of therapy unless very large cohorts are studied for several decades. Moreover, analysis of therapy based only upon cancer-specific mortality rates fails to take into account the large number of patients, about 20% in most series [1], who experience locoregional recurrence and distant metastases that often occur decades after initial treatment [2]. No prospective randomized clinical trials of therapy have been done. Thus, all contemporary views of the efficacy of therapy are based upon retrospective studies, which often have been performed on small cohorts of patients in whom follow-up is very limited. To get a complete picture of the impact of therapy, follow-up must span virtually the entire lifespan of the patient [3]. It is accordingly not surprising that the optimal extent of initial thyroid surgery for DTC continues to generate some controversy, mainly in the USA where a few surgeons argue that lobectomy is sufficient treatment for the majority of patients with this disease [4,5]. It must be emphasized that surgery and ^{131}I therapy have complementary but differing effects on outcome, and the assumption that subtotal thyroidectomy can be rectified by ^{131}I ablation is incorrect (Figure 12.1).

Staging and Prognostic Scoring Systems

The debate surrounding the extent of initial thyroid resection centers mainly on the use of prognostic scoring systems to select the extent of surgery based upon the patient's "risk," for dying of the disease and relates directly to the differing effects of age on recurrence and mortality rates. Young patients have a low risk of mortality but experience high tumor relapse rates, whereas cancer-specific mortality rates rise sharply after 45 years of age.

Current Tumor Staging Systems

Nine staging and tumor scoring systems have been proposed over the years (Table 12.1). The sheer number of staging systems underscores their lack of general acceptance. Most use patient age at the time of initial therapy and tumor factors to discriminate patients at high risk of dying from thyroid cancer (Table 12.1) [6–13]. In one study [11], four of the schemes that use age (EORTC, TNM, AMES, AGES) when applied to the papillary carcinoma survival data from the Mayo Clinic, were effective in separating low risk patients in whom cancer-specific mortality was 1% at 20 years from high risk

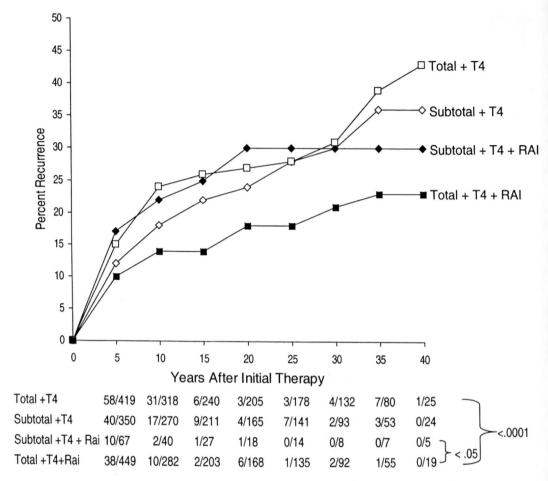

Total +T4	58/419	31/318	6/240	3/205	3/178	4/132	7/80	1/25
Subtotal +T4	40/350	17/270	9/211	4/165	7/141	2/93	3/53	0/24
Subtotal +T4 + Rai	10/67	2/40	1/27	1/18	0/14	0/8	0/7	0/5
Total +T4+Rai	38/449	10/282	2/203	6/168	1/135	2/92	1/55	0/19

<.0001
< .05

Figure 12.1 Tumor recurrence 40 years (median 16.7 years) after thyroid surgery and thyroid hormone therapy with and without ^{131}I ablation of uptake in the thyroid bed. Total thyroidectomy includes ipsilateral lobectomy, isthmusectomy, and near-total contralateral thyroidectomy; subtotal thyroidectomy is lobectomy with or without isthmusectomy. Patients undergoing total thyroidectomy had more advanced tumor stage than those undergoing subtotal thyroidectomy (ANOVA, $P < 0.001$). (Reproduced with permission from Mazzaferri EL, Kloos RT. Current approaches to primary therapy for papillary and follicular thyroid cancer. J Clin Endocrinol Metab 2001; 86(4):1447–1463. Copyright 2001, The Endocrine Society.)

patients in whom it was 30% to 40% at 20 years [10]. Twenty-year survival rates for patients with MACIS scores less than 6, 6 to 6.99, 7 to 7.99, and 8+ were 99%, 89%, 56%, and 24%, respectively. Another study, however, that categorized 269 patients with papillary carcinoma according to five different prognostic scoring schemes found that some patients in the lowest risk group for each scheme died of cancer [7]. This is particularly true of the schemes that simply categorize risk dichotomously as low or high [6,14]. Moreover, these schemes do not consider tumor recurrence and are inaccurate

in predicting disease-free survival. The latest American Joint Committee (AJCC) TNM staging system [13] for thyroid cancer (Table 12.2) classifies even more patients as being at low risk than did the former version. Staging systems derived from multivariate analyses that do not take into account the effects of therapy assume that treatment does not alter outcome. This is very likely incorrect. Treatment is not factored into the multivariate analyses that underpin most of the prognostic scoring systems, a weakness highlighted by the authors of the first thyroid cancer scoring system ever to be devised

Table 12.1 Components of staging systems and rating schemes for defining risk category in patients with differentiated thyroid carcinoma

Variable at time of diagnosis	TNM[a,b]	EORTC[b]	AMES[b]	AGES[c]	MACIS[c]	NTCTCS[b]	MSK[a,b]	University of Chicago[c]	Ohio State University[b]
Patient characteristics									
Age	X	X	X	X	X	X	X		
Sex	X	X	X						
Tumor characteristics									
Cell type	X	X							
Size	X		X	X	X	X		X	X
Grade (histological)				X			X		
Extrathyroidal extension	X	X	X	X	X	X	X	X	X
Lymph node metastases	X[d]					X		X	X
Distant metastases	X	X	X	X	X	X	X	X	X
Therapy characteristics									
Incomplete resection						X			

[a] T, primary tumor, T1, ≤2 cm; T2, >2 cm to 4 cm; T3, >4 cm; T4a, any size tumor to invade subcutaneous soft tissues, larynx, trachea, esophagus, or recurrent laryngeal nerve; T4b, tumor invades prevertebral fascia or encases carotid artery or mediastinal vessels; all anaplastic tumors are considered T4: T4a intrathyroidal anaplastic carcinoma surgically resectable, T4b extrathyroidal anaplastic carcinoma surgically unresectable; regional lymph nodes are the central compartment, lateral cervical and upper mediastinal lymph nodes, N1a, metastases to level IV (pretracheal, paratracheal, and prelaryngeal/Delphian lymph nodes), N1b metastases to unilateral, bilateral, or contralateral cervical or superior mediastinal lymph nodes; M0 distant metastases absent, M1 distant metastases present.

[b] Both papillary and follicular carcinoma.

[c] Only papillary carcinoma.

[d] Not applied to patients with papillary or follicular carcinoma under 45 years.

See footnote to Table 12.2. for definitions of study abbreviations.

Table 12.2 Scoring methods. TNM (American Joint Committee on Cancer [13]) staging varies with cell type and age. Undifferentiated (anaplastic) carcinomas are stage IV.

Stage	Papillary or follicular		Medullary
	<45 years	**≥45 years**	**Medullary**
I	M0	T1+N0+M0	T1+N0+M0
II	M1	T2+N0+M0	T2+N0+M0
	None	T3+N0+M0	T3+N0+M0
III		T1-3+N1a	T1+N1a+M0
			T2+N1a+M0
			T3+N1a+M0
	None	T4a+N0+M0	T4a+N0+M0
		T4a+N1a+M0	T4a+N1a+M0
IVA		T1+N1b+M0	T1+N1b+M0
		T2+N1b+M0	T2+N1b+M0
		T3+N1b+M0	T3+N1b+M0
		T4a+N1b+M0	T4a+N1b+M0
IVB	None	T4b+Any N+M0	T4b+Any N+M0
IVC	None	Any T+Any N+M1	Any T+Any N+M1

EORTC (European Organization for Research and Treatment of Cancer) [9]. Age in years + 12 if male, +10 if medullary, +10 if poorly differentiated follicular, +45 if anaplastic, +10 if extending beyond thyroid, +15 if one distant metastases + 30 if multiple distant metastases.

AMES (Age-Metastasis-Extent-Size) [6]. High risk is female > 50 years, male > 40 years, tumor > 5 cm (if older age), distant metastases, substantial extension beyond tumor capsule (follicular) or gland capsule (papillary).

AGES (Age-Grade-Extent-Size) [10]. Calculated from $0.5 \times$ age in years (if >40), +1 (if grade 2), +3 (if grade 3 or 4), +1 (if extrathyroidal), +3 (if distant spread), $+0.2 \times$ maximum tumor diameter.

MACIS (Metastasis-Age-Completeness of resection, Invasion-Size) [11]. MACIS = 3.1 (if aged ≤39 years) or $0.08 \times$ age (if aged ≥40 years), $+0.3 \times$ tumor size (in centimeters), +1 (if incompletely resected), +3 (if distant metastases present).

NTCTCS (National Thyroid Cancer Treatment Cooperative Study) [8]. Staging variables not scored quantitatively.

University of Chicago system for papillary carcinoma [15]. Staging variables (part A) not scored quantitatively.

MSK is Memorial Sloan Kettering system [16,5] for papillary and follicular thyroid carcinoma, not scored quantitatively. Low risk: age <45, tumor <1–4 cm, M0, low grade histology. Intermediate risk: age < 45, tumor <1–4 cm, M0 low grade. Intermediate age ≥ 45, tumor >4 cm or invasive, M1 and/or high grade. High risk: age ≥45, tumor >4 cm or invasive, M1 and/or high grade.

The Ohio State system for papillary or follicular carcinoma [3]. Staging not scored quantitatively.

[9]. This explains why none of the risk strati-fication schemas provide sufficient information to make therapeutic decisions for individual patients regarding the extent of surgery. Their main use lies in stratifying patients in epidemi-ological studies to permit comparisons of dif-ferent patient cohorts.

Survival and Relapse Rates Using Scoring Systems

Mortality rates from DTC are so low for patients under 45 years of age that thousands of patients must be studied to get a clear picture of the fea-tures that affect cancer-specific mortality rates [17]. Conversely, tumor relapse is so common as to provide a clear endpoint with which to analyze therapeutic efficacy. For example, Hay et al. [18] reported in 1987 that patients treated at the Mayo Clinic for low risk papillary thyroid cancers (MACIS score ≤3.99) had no improve-ment in survival rates after undergoing more than ipsilateral lobectomy and accordingly con-cluded that more extensive surgery was indi-cated only for those with higher MACIS scores. In 1998, however, Hay et al. [19] reported the results of a study designed to compare cancer-specific mortality and recurrence rates after unilateral or bilateral lobectomy for patients with papillary cancer considered to be low risk by AMES criteria. In this analysis, although there were no significant differences in cancer-specific mortality or distant metastasis rates between the two groups, the 20-year rates for local recurrence and nodal metastasis after unilateral lobectomy were 14% and 19%, significantly higher ($P = 0.0001$) than the 2% and 6% rates seen after bilateral thyroid lobe resection. On the basis of these observations, Hay et al. [19] recommended bilateral thyroid resection as the preferable initial surgical approach to patients with low risk papillary cancer. Some [4,20] do not concur with this view, justifying lobectomy alone for nearly all patients with papillary and follicular thyroid cancer on the basis of the low mortality rates of these tumors and high complication rates with more extensive thyroidectomy [4,21]. The vast majority of patients are categorized as being at "low risk" by the AMES, MSK, TNM, and MACIS classifications systems in which age is used to stratify risk.

Further insight into this issue comes from analyzing a recent large DTC outcome study [17] in which the 10-year relative survival rates for 53 856 patients with thyroid carcinoma treated in the USA between 1985 and 1995 were 93% for papillary carcinoma, 85% for follicular carcinoma, and 76% for Hürthle cell carcinoma. Still, over half the deaths from thyroid cancer were caused by papillary carcinoma, the tumor with the best long-term prognosis [17]. It is difficult to predict who will die from these tumors.

Aggressive disease may occur in patients who appear to be at low risk at the time of diagnosis [14,17]. Hundahl et al. [17] reported 96% and 68% relative 10-year survival rates for patients with papillary carcinoma. However, when 9369 of the patients with papillary thyroid carcinoma in this series were stratified according to the AMES criteria (Age, Metastases, Extent, Size, Table 12.1) [12], almost 94% of them (8770) were categorized as "low risk" while only 599 were classified as "high risk." Ten-year relative survival rates in the two groups, respectively, were 96% and 68%; however, almost *two thirds of the cancer deaths occurred in the "low-risk" group* – patients who are expected to survive – because they outnumbered high risk patients by 16:1 [17]. This is true of virtually all the scoring systems that use patient age as a principal factor to predict prognosis. It underscores how difficult it is to know a patient's potential for an adverse outcome and the tumor status before there has been a careful assessment of the response to initial surgery and thyroid ^{131}I remnant ablation. The rigid application of staging systems in support of conservative treatment for low risk patients thus may lead to inadequate initial therapy in a relatively large number of patients.

Current Opinion Concerning Initial Therapy

When such great emphasis is assigned to the patient's age, the relative importance of tumor stage is substantially diminished. This concept, however, does not appear to be widely accepted among practicing physicians because young patients with low prognostic scores often have tumor recurrence [22]. At an international consensus conference in 1987, only five of 160 participants treated younger patients more conservatively [23]. Similarly, in an international survey of thyroid specialists done in 1988 [24], and in a survey of clinical members of the American Thyroid Association done in 1996 [25], age was not used by the majority of respondents in their therapeutic decisions. Current recommendations for the treatment of children now suggest the same therapy – total thyroidectomy and ^{131}I remnant ablation – as that given to adults with similarly staged tumors [22].

Practice in US and European Hospitals

Two large clinical studies shed even more light upon the current practice. A study of 5583 cases of thyroid carcinoma treated in over 1500 hospitals in the USA during 1996 found that total or near-total thyroidectomy was performed in the vast majority (~75%) of patients with DTC [26], almost all of whom were at low risk according to their TNM status. After surgery at least half were treated with ^{131}I and were given thyroid hormone to suppress thyroid-stimulating hormone (TSH), although the rates of these medical treatments were underreported in the study. A report from Germany [27] of 2376 patients with DTC treated in 1996 indicated that total thyroidectomy was performed in about 90% of the patients and that ^{131}I was almost always administered postoperatively (74% papillary, over 90% follicular). Lymph node dissection was performed in 22% of those with papillary carcinoma.

The Efficacy of Total or Near-Total Thyroidectomy in the Treatment of DTC

Many surgeons perform an operation called near-total thyroidectomy, but its definition is open-ended, leaving much doubt as to the actual extent of surgery and the amount of thyroid tissue left behind. For this reason, the National Cancer Center Network guidelines [28] on the treatment of thyroid cancer avoid this term. In practice, many patients have substantial thyroid remnants when evaluated by thyroid ultrasonography and thyroglobulin (Tg) determina-

tions even after reportedly undergoing total thyroidectomy. Thyroid ultrasound may be useful when the extent of surgery is in question, since leaving a thyroid remnant smaller than 2 g facilitates postoperative ^{131}I ablation.

Relapse Rates and the Extent of Initial Thyroid Surgery

Recurrence rates are high with large thyroid gland remnants. Some find that patients treated by lobectomy alone have a 5% to 10% recurrence rate in the opposite thyroid lobe [16,29] and an overall long-term recurrence rate over 30% (versus 1% after total thyroidectomy and ^{131}I therapy [3]) and the highest frequency (11%) of subsequent pulmonary metastases [30]. Higher recurrence rates are also observed with cervical lymph node metastases and multicentric tumors, which also provide justification for more complete initial thyroid resection [3].

In one study from the Mayo Clinic [31] of patients with papillary carcinoma, tumor recurrence rates during the first 2 years after surgery were about fourfold greater after unilateral lobectomy than after total or near-total thyroidectomy (26% versus 6%, $P = 0.01$). In a subsequent report from the same institution, patients with papillary carcinoma whose AGES score was 4 or more had a 25-year cancer mortality rate almost twice as high after lobectomy than after bilateral thyroid resection (65% versus 35%, $P = 0.06$) [18]. In a study of AMES low risk patients from the same institution, 20-year rates for local recurrence and nodal metastases were, respectively, 14% and 19% after unilateral lobectomy, and 2% and 6% after bilateral lobar resection ($P = 0.001$), leading the authors to conclude that bilateral lobar resection represents the preferable initial surgical approach to patients with low risk papillary thyroid carcinoma [19]. In another study of patients with papillary carcinoma [15], near-total thyroidectomy decreased the risk of death from tumors larger than 1 cm and decreased the risk of recurrence as compared with lobectomy or bilateral subtotal thyroidectomy.

We found recurrence and cancer death rates were both about 50% lower after near-total or total thyroidectomy as compared with less surgery in patients with stage II and III tumors

(Figures 12.2 and 12.3) [3], and that surgery more extensive than lobectomy was an independent variable that by multivariate analysis reduced the mortality rate of thyroid carcinoma by 50%. Moreover, the differences in outcome between total thyroidectomy and lobectomy cannot be resolved by ^{131}I therapy (Figure 12.1). Thus, there is abundant evidence that microscopic residual disease remaining after initial surgery leads to high recurrence and carcinoma mortality rates.

Current Guidelines for Surgery

Current guidelines on the treatment of DTC from the USA [32] and Europe [33] advise total

or near-total thyroidectomy followed by ^{131}I ablation of the thyroid remnant for most patients. Although the treatment of children has been more controversial, many now recommend that they be treated the same as adults [22]. Thus, when the diagnosis of thyroid cancer is known preoperatively total or near-total thyroidectomy should be done for nearly all patients [34] because it improves disease-free survival, even in children and adults with low risk tumors [19,35–37]. Lobectomy alone is adequate surgery for papillary microcarcinomas provided the patient has not been exposed to radiation and has no other risk factors, including a familial predisposition to the tumor, and the papillary carcinoma is smaller than 1 cm

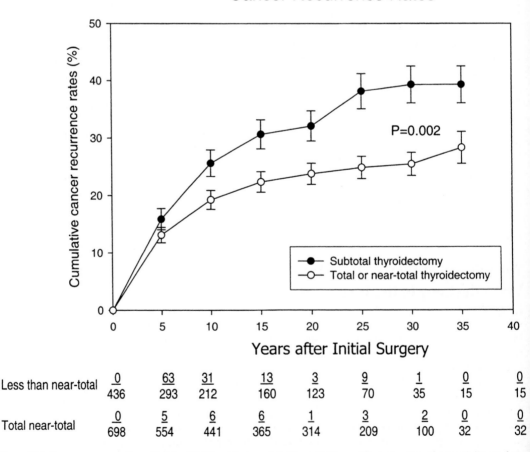

Figure 12.2 Tumor recurrence after subtotal or total thyroidectomy (see Figure 12.1 legend for explanation of surgery). (Drawn from the data of Mazzaferri and Kloos [2].)

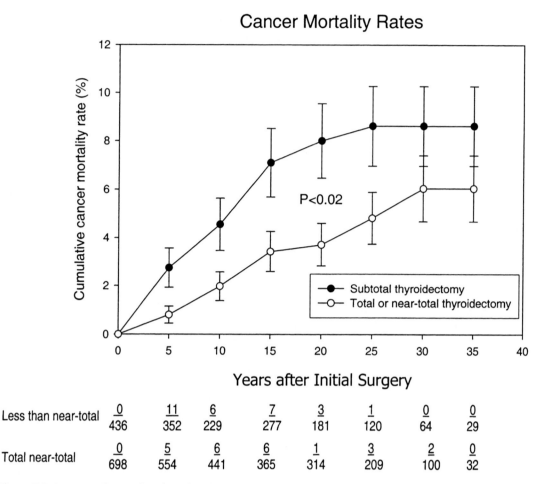

Figure 12.3 Cancer-specific mortality after subtotal or total thyroidectomy (see Figure 12.1 legend for explanation of surgery). (Drawn from the data of Mazzaferri and Kloos [2].)

and is unifocal and confined to the thyroid without vascular invasion (see Chapter 29) [3,38,39]. The same is true for minimally invasive follicular cancers smaller than about 2 cm. A large thyroid remnant, however, hampers follow-up with serum Tg determinations and whole-body ^{131}I scans and the decision to forgo complete thyroidectomy should be made in consultation with the patient, who must be informed of the difficulty in follow-up when lobectomy alone is performed.

Thyroglossal Duct Cyst Carcinomas

Small papillary carcinomas that arise in a thyroglossal duct remnant are typically encapsu-

lated by the cyst and usually are not recognized until the permanent histological sections are reviewed [40]. When the clinical diagnosis of a thyroglossal duct cyst is made, the workup should include an ultrasound examination and fine-needle aspiration cytology in order to plan the correct surgery for a possible carcinoma [41]. Dissection of the tract and removal of the hyoid bone (Sistrunk operation) is adequate for most patients because these tumors rarely metastasize [42]. However, one study found a high incidence of intrathyroidal carcinomas in such cases, some with aggressive behavior, suggesting that total thyroidectomy may be justified [43]. Treatment must be tempered by the patient's age and the size and extent of the tumor [44]. It is difficult to justify anything more than a Sistrunk procedure for a young person with a small (<1 cm) tumor confined to a thyroglossal cyst and an ultrasonographically normal thyroid. On the other hand, with older patients and those with invasive or metastatic tumor or histological features that portend a poor prognosis, or following head and neck irradiation, or with a malignant tumor in the thyroid gland, the more classic approach of total thyroidectomy and ^{131}I therapy seems warranted [44].

Completion Thyroidectomy

Residual tumor is common in the contralateral thyroid lobe but cannot be predicted on the basis of the tumor size in the ipsilateral lobe or the presence of regional lymph node metastases [45] but is more likely if there are multiple tumors in the ipsilateral thyroid lobe and if the serum thyroglobulin level is very high [46]. Completion thyroidectomy should be considered for tumors that have the potential for recurrence because large thyroid remnants are difficult to ablate with [131]I [47] and almost always leave the serum thyroglobulin detectable [48]. Completion thyroidectomy has a low complication rate and is appropriate to perform routinely for tumors 1 cm or larger because about half the patients have residual cancer in the contralateral thyroid lobe [49–53]. This is more common when the tumor is familial, or when it is associated with head and neck irradiation or other familial syndromes (see Chapter 1).

When there has been a local or distant tumor recurrence after lobectomy, residual cancer is found in over 60% of the excised contralateral lobes. A study of irradiated children from Chernobyl with thyroid cancer that had been treated by lobectomy found that 61% had unrecognized lung or lymph node metastases that could only be identified after completion thyroidectomy had been performed [37]. In another study, patients who underwent completion thyroidectomy within 6 months of their primary operation developed significantly fewer lymph node and hematogenous recurrences and survived significantly longer than those in whom the second operation was delayed for longer than 6 months [53].

What the Internist Should Know about Thyroidectomy

Preoperative Assessment

The preceding part of the chapter explains the rationale for partial versus total thyroidectomy. Essentially, a total thyroidectomy is performed for all cases of known cancer, for bilateral enlarged goiter with compressive symptoms or severe problems with cosmesis, and for certain cases of hyperthyroidism. Hemithyroidectomies are performed for thyroid nodules of indeterminate cytology with negative frozen sections intraoperatively and for unilateral goiters.

The new patient visit starts with the history. While almost all patients with thyroid cancer are euthyroid, surgery is performed on patients with large goiters who might be hypothyroid and occasionally on patients with hyperthyroidism who are not amenable to medical control. Any previous neck operations must be understood in detail to elucidate the altered anatomy the surgeon will encounter. Important questions are used to delineate their clinical thyroid status (heat/cold intolerance, skin changes, hair changes, cardiovascular status, and bowel changes) and also to investigate for possible multiple endocrine neoplasia (MEN) syndrome with vasoactive tumors of the adrenal glands. For cancer patients, a 1-year history of any excess iodine exposure, especially computed tomography (CT) scans, is obtained to assess how long postoperative radioactive iodine may need to be delayed. This will be checked with 24-hour urine iodine levels prior to administration of [131]I. Present medications are checked for drugs influencing thyroid metabolism such as Synthroid, PTU, lithium, and for anticoagulants. Anesthesia risk factors are searched for such as significant cardiopulmonary history/symptoms, history of thyrotoxic storm, previous or family reactions to anesthesia.

The physical examination centers on any compressive symptoms such as dysphagia and dysphonia, the function of the recurrent laryngeal nerve (RLN), the lymph nodes in the neck, and the parathyroid function. The low anterior neck is palpated first to evaluate the thyroid and any nodules, their nature as to fixation of the gland, and any substernal component. The lateral neck is palpated to evaluate for any clinically obvious lymph nodes. We prefer to do this from behind the patient so as to feel beneath the sternocleidomastoid muscle and to be able to compare both sides of the neck simultaneously. The vocal cords are then evaluated either by indirect laryngoscopy or directly by using the flexible laryngoscope. The vocal cords may have either diminished mobility or complete paralysis from compression of the RLN (less common) or direct invasion of the nerve. Even if the patient has no hoarseness, it is imperative that the cords are visualized as slow compression of the RLN may have allowed the contralateral cord to compensate for the paretic cord. Finally, a rough estimate of the patient's calcium level is obtained by performing Chvostek's test by tapping in the pretragal area; a positive test is an involuntary twitch of the lips. Up to 10% of patients who are normocalcemic will have a positive Chvostek's test. Trousseau's test is more specific and is performed by occluding the brachial artery with a blood pressure cuff for 3 minutes. A positive test is carpopedal spasm.

Diagnostic tests include an ultrasound performed by an endocrinologist or someone equally skilled in this examination, thyroid function tests, calcium level, and a hematocrit and chest X-ray if appropriate for surgery. CT scans are avoided if cancer is suspected due to the heavy iodine load in the contrast agent.

Primary Thyroidectomy

An incision is made in a skin crease about 2 cm cephalad to the clavicles. Once a surgeon gains more experience with this procedure, the transverse incision decreases in length from about 8 cm to about 4–5 cm. This generally results in an imperceptible scar, and negates the benefits of endoscopic assisted thyroidectomy, a much more complex and lengthy procedure. Superior and inferior flaps are raised in a subplatysmal plane. These really only need to be done in between the sternocleidomastoid muscles as more lateral dissection does not improve visualization. This is the basis for reducing the size of the incision to 4 cm in primary cases.

The strap muscles are separated in the midline and elevated off of the thyroid gland. Only in rare circumstances (extremely enlarged goiter, direct cancer invasion) are the strap

muscles divided. These muscles assist in swallowing and so are preserved intact when possible. The thyroid gland is now exposed. We prefer to divide the superior pole vessels primarily, as this allows improved mobilization of the thyroid gland and facilitates dissection of the RLN. The initial step is to separate the thyrotracheal fascia between the medial aspect of the superior pole and the upper trachea and larynx. Blunt dissection forms a plane between these structures that allows mobilization of the superior pole, allowing it to be brought inferiorly into the surgical field. This mobilization is another method that permits the use of small incisions. The external branch of the superior laryngeal nerve can usually be seen entering the cricothyroid muscle. Blunt dissection ensures that it is free of the superior thyroid artery and veins as they enter the thyroid gland. The vascular bundle is divided and ligated, allowing the superior pole to be mobilized inferiorly and medially.

Dissection on the thyroid capsule inferiorly encounters the middle thyroid vein, which is now divided. The gland is now freely mobile in its superior half, facilitating further dissection. Medial retraction on the gland exposes the fibrofatty plane between the carotid artery and the trachea. Blunt dissection just above the most inferior aspect of the gland and at approximately a 60-degree angle referenced to the trachea will quickly expose the pulsating inferior thyroid artery. This can be followed medially. Just lateral to the tracheoesophageal groove, the RLN follows a course of variable reference to the artery: generally deep but it can also intertwine or be superficial to it. At this time the parathyroid glands can usually be identified. As long as meticulous dissection has freed all tissue of the thyroid capsule, the parathyroid glands are generally found within a 2 cm circumference based at the junction of the inferior thyroid artery and the RLN. The nerve is then followed to its entry into the larynx near the cricothyroid joint. During this dissection, it is imperative to make sure the parathyroid glands retain their vascular supply. It is quite easy to expose the nerve and leave the parathyroid glands medially, thus robbing them of their blood supply resulting in hypoparathyroidism.

As the nerve enters the larynx, there is routinely a fine tongue of thyroid tissue that is intimately involved with the nerve. Careful dissection in this area will reduce the amount of residual uptake seen in posttreatment ^{131}I scans. Also, there are several thin-walled vessels that accompany the nerve and gland in this area which bleed persistently until controlled. It is important to use bipolar cautery in this region to prevent damage to the RLN by the dissipated energy from a unipolar cautery. Once the nerve has been dissected free, the inferior thyroid veins are ligated and unipolar cautery is used to free the gland from the trachea (separate Berry's ligament). If a cancer operation is to be performed, the contralateral lobe is dissected similarly. If there is doubt as to the pathology of the lesion, it is sent for frozen section. If cancer cannot be confirmed, then the isthmus is dissected free and a right angle clamp is passed between the isthmus and the contralateral lobe. The ipsilateral lobe and isthmus is then removed and the stump of thyroid is suture ligated.

The wound is copiously irrigated and meticulous hemostasis is achieved. Small suction drains can be placed with no deleterious effects to the RLN, but they are not always necessary. We now close our wounds with 4-0 Vicryl sutures to reapproximate the platysmal layer and then 4-0 Biosyn subcuticular sutures. This allows the patient to have no sutures removed, reduces the chances of hypertrophic scar, and once a Tegaderm dressing is applied, lets the patient shower in the first postoperative day.

Enlarged Thyroid Goiters

Depending upon how massive the enlargement is, various techniques may need to be employed to obtain access and deliver the gland. The patient must be placed in as much cervical extension as is safe to passively pull the thyroid out of the chest and into the neck as far as possible. The skin incision is generally larger, and extends at least from the medial aspects of the sternocleidomastoid muscle on each side of the neck. The subplatysmal flaps are sometimes raised to the level of the hyoid bone. Removing the strap muscles can be difficult as they are stretched, thin, and overlie engorged veins. Careful dissection is a must to prevent bleeding. If the superior aspect of the gland is enlarged, then the strap muscles are separated as superiorly as possible (they are innervated via the ansa hypoglossi which enters inferiorly). The superior laryngeal nerve is at great risk in massively

enlarged goiters, as the nerve has been found even lateral to the superior pedicle in normal size glands. Careful dissection will normally find the nerve in the cricothyroid space, but it can run intramuscularly 20% of the time and not be easily identified. Once the superior pole is mobilized and access to the lateral and then posterior aspect of the gland is achieved, the lower pole of the gland is finger-dissected and literally pulled out of the chest. Once it is delivered into the neck, the RLN is then found in the usual manner. We have dissected goiters abutting the aortic arch in this manner. It is extremely unlikely that a sternal split will be needed to remove the gland in these cases. Thyroid cancers with a substernal component are a different case; they often have extrathyroidal spread and do not bluntly dissect easily.

Revision Thyroidectomy

This operation is one of the most difficult of the thyroid operations. To one degree or another, the pristine surgical planes have been violated, which greatly increases the odds of damage to vital structures: RLN, parathyroid glands, trachea, and esophagus. The first step is to get a clear understanding of the previous operation. If the contralateral lobe was resected for a nodule of indeterminate pathology and returned as cancer, returning to the operating room within the week is imperative so as to access the remaining lobe before the scarring sets in. If a different surgeon operated on the first side, then the details of the operation are needed, especially to ascertain if the RLN and parathyroids were already dissected on the remaining side. Even through scar, the important structures may once again be dissected free, but a wider exposure is needed and the surgeon must prepare for a longer, more tedious dissection. Also, active monitoring of the RLN with a specialized probe on the endotracheal tube must be considered to increase the likelihood of safely finding the nerve.

Recurrent Cancer

Whether it has been 6 months or 50 years, recurrent thyroid cancer poses a special problem. If an adequate operation was performed at the initial setting, then the RLN and the parathyroids have been dissected and now are incorporated into a scar of varying thickness. The recurrences most often show up in the tracheoesophageal groove from the level of the thyroid cartilage (level III) to the thoracic inlet (level VI). Often it is unclear if the tumor has obliterated a lymph node or if it has recurred in the soft tissue. The distinction is important as the soft tissue recurrence may need external beam radiotherapy for ultimate cure and the lymph node recurrence will need an ipsilateral neck dissection. The surgery can be as technically challenging as the revision thyroid case, but is more consistently difficult as the nerve on both sides has almost always been previously dissected. Tumor can reappear in the superior mediastinum also, and as long as it does not have significant extracapsular spread, this can be removed via a transcervical approach by cleaning the root of the carotid arteries to the innominate artery.

Lymph Node Metastases

There is much debate about the need for neck dissections in well-differentiated thyroid cancer. Some retrospective reviews have reported that lymph node metastases do not impact on the overall survival of this disease (with one older report showing an improvement in survival in patients with lymph node metastases, though this was not controlled for patient age). Other prospective reports have shown a slight survival benefit in bilateral neck dissections for papillary cancer. Common practice lies somewhere in between these extremes. The days of the "lumpectomy" are fading away, being replaced by the functional neck dissection for any patient with a node-positive neck. The functional neck dissection usually includes all of the node-bearing tissue in the anterior neck except for the submandibular triangle (level I). Most important to dissect is level VI, or that area between the omohyoid muscles, inferior to the thyroid cartilage, and superior to the thoracic inlet. All major neurovascular structures and muscles are left intact. The difference from the classic "radical neck dissection" is that the latter sacrifices the sternocleidomastoid muscle, internal jugular vein, and the spinal accessory nerve while dissecting levels I through V.

Dissecting level VI in the functional neck carries with it the high possibility of devascularizing the parathyroid glands. When possible, an intact parathyroid should have its distal pole biopsied while leaving the rest attached to the vascular stalk. Once this is confirmed as parathyroid tissue, then it may be safely preserved while the rest of level VI is removed.

Our incision for these cases has changed from the "hockey-stick" design (mastoid to posterior border of the inferior sternocleidomastoid muscle (SCM), then horizontally across to midline) to just taking the standard thyroid incision and extending it laterally in a skin crease. Subplatysmal flaps are raised to above the hyoid bone and the digastric muscle is exposed. The hypoglossal nerve is then identified lateral to the digastric muscle and followed toward the skull base. The fascia overlying the SCM is then incised and is removed from this muscle. During this maneuver, the spinal accessory nerve (cranial nerve (CN) XI) is identified and freed of all soft tissue in between the digastric muscle and the SCM. Level IIB, or that tissue posterosuperior to CN XI, anterior to the trapezius, and lateral to the internal jugular, is freed and passed underneath CN XI. The lymphatic tissues in levels II to V are then removed off the deep cervical fascia, leaving the cervical sensory nerves intact and taken anteriorly over the internal jugular vein. The tissues are then taken off of the vagus and carotid, then brought anteriorly to the level of the omohyoid and removed. Level VI is dissected separately with the warnings as noted above.

Tracheoesophageal Invasion

Well-differentiated thyroid cancer is often thought of as an indolent cancer that rarely results in death. While this is mostly true, this disease can present in a serious manner. With symptoms of pain, dysphagia, dyspnea, hoarseness, and occasionally hemoptysis, aggressive local invasion can be very hard to resect, reconstruct and cure. A basic tenet of surgery for tracheoesophageal invasion is that if there is no penetration into the lumen of either structure, then the tumor should be "shaved off" the external surface. For the esophagus, this usually means dissecting deep to the pharyngeal constrictor muscles. For the trachea, it is often necessary to remove a partial thickness of the tracheal rings. Usually in these cases the RLN must be sacrificed to remove as much of the gross tumor as possible. If all gross tumor has been removed, reasonable cure rates may be obtained with the use of postoperative radioactive iodine and external beam therapy.

For those tumors that perforate a viscus, every attempt must be made to do a full-thickness resection. Tracheal resections (after mobilization of the RLN if possible) can be repaired by either auricular cartilage or costochondral grafts or sometimes by direct reapproximation. Laryngeal invasion can be resected by either a partial or total laryngectomy with anything from direct closure to a radial forearm free flap reconstruction to make a functional neo-larynx. A tracheotomy is usually required for postoperative ventilation, but decannulation is attempted as soon as possible to allow for a return to their premorbid status. Finally, esophageal invasion sometimes must be resected with a partial or total pharyngectomy and closure with a myocutaneous (pectoralis major) flap or vascularized fasciocutaneous flap (anterolateral thigh, lateral arm, or radial forearm) or vascularized jejunum flap. Reconstruction usually permits a normal or near normal diet after extensive swallowing therapy.

References

1. Mazzaferri EL, Robbins RJ, Spencer CA, et al. A consensus report of the role of serum thyroglobulin as a monitoring method for low-risk patients with papillary thyroid carcinoma. J Clin Endocrinol Metab 2003; 88(4): 1433–1441.

2. Mazzaferri EL, Kloos RT. Current approaches to primary therapy for papillary and follicular thyroid cancer. J Clin Endocrinol Metab 2001; 86(4):1447–1463.

3. Mazzaferri EL, Jhiang SM. Long-term impact of initial surgical and medical therapy on papillary and follicular thyroid cancer. Am J Med 1994; 97:418–428.

4. Cady B. Our AMES is true: How an old concept still hits the mark: or, risk group assignment points the arrow to rational therapy selection in differentiated thyroid cancer. Am J Surg 1997; 174:462–468.

5. Shaha AR, Shah JP, Loree TR. Low-risk differentiated thyroid cancer: the need for selective treatment. Ann Surg Oncol 1997; 4(4):328–333.

6. Cady B, Sedgwick CE, Meissner WA, Wool MS, Salzman FA, Werber J. Risk factor analysis in differentiated thyroid cancer. Cancer 1979; 43:810–820.

7. DeGroot LJ, Kaplan EL, Straus FH, Shukla MS. Does the method of management of papillary thyroid carcinoma make a difference in outcome? World J Surg 1994; 18: 123–130.

8. Sherman SI, Brierley JD, Sperling M, et al. Prospective multicenter study of thyroid carcinoma treatment –

9. Byar DP, Green SB, Dor P, et al. A prognostic index for thyroid carcinoma. A study of the EORTC Thyroid Cancer Cooperative Group. Eur J Cancer 1979; 15:1033–1041.

10. Hay ID. Papillary thyroid carcinoma. Endocrinol Metab Clin North Am 1990; 19(3):545–576.

11. Hay ID, Bergstralh EJ, Goellner JR, Ebersold JR, Grant CS. Predicting outcome in papillary thyroid carcinoma: Development of a reliable prognostic scoring system in a cohort of 1779 patients surgically treated at one institution during 1940 through 1989. Surgery 1993; 114: 1050–1058.

12. Cady B, Rossi R. An expanded view of risk-group definition in differentiated thyroid carcinoma. Surgery 1988; 104:947–953.

13. Greene FL, Page DL, Fleming ID, Fritz A, Balch CM. AJCC cancer staging manual, 6 edn. Chicago: Springer Verlag, 2003.

14. American Joint Committee on Cancer. Head and Neck Tumors. Thyroid gland. In: Beahrs OH, Henson DE, Hutter RVP, Myers MH (eds) Manual for staging of cancer. Philadelphia: JB Lippincott, 1992: 53–54.

15. DeGroot LJ, Kaplan EL, McCormick M, Straus FH. Natural history, treatment, and course of papillary thyroid carcinoma. J Clin Endocrinol Metab 1990; 71: 414–424.

16. Shaha AR, Shah JP, Loree TR. Risk group stratification and prognostic factors in papillary carcinoma of thyroid. Ann Surg Oncol 1996; 3(6):534–538.

17. Hundahl SA, Fleming ID, Fremgen AM, Menck HR. A National Cancer Data Base report on 53 856 cases of thyroid carcinoma treated in the US, 1985–1995. Cancer 1998; 83:2638–2648.

18. Hay ID, Grant CS, Taylor WF, McConahey WM. Ipsilateral lobectomy versus bilateral lobar resection in papillary thyroid carcinoma: a retrospective analysis of surgical outcome using a novel prognostic scoring system. Surgery 1987; 102:1088–1095.

19. Hay ID, Grant CS, Bergstralh EJ, Thompson GB, van Heerden JA. Unilateral total lobectomy: Is it sufficient surgical treatment for patients with AMES low-risk papillary thyroid carcinoma? Surgery 1998; 124:958–966.

20. Shaha AR. Thyroid carcinoma – implications of prognostic factors. Cancer 1998; 83:401–402.

21. Shaha AR, Loree TR, Shah JP. Prognostic factors and risk group analysis in follicular carcinoma of the thyroid. Surgery 1995; 118:1131–1138.

22. Hung W, Sarlis NJ. Current controversies in the management of pediatric patients with well-differentiated non-medullary thyroid cancer: A review. Thyroid 2002; 12:683–702.

23. Van De Velde CJH, Hamming JF, Goslings BM, et al. Report of the consensus development conference on the management of differentiated thyroid cancer in the Netherlands. Eur J Cancer Clin Oncol 1988; 24:287–292.

24. Baldet L, Manderscheid JC, Glinoer D, Jaffiol C, Coste Seignovert B, Percheron C. The management of differentiated thyroid cancer in Europe in 1988. Results of an international survey. Acta Endocrinol (Copenh) 1989; 120:547–558.

25. Solomon BL, Wartofsky L, Burman KD. Current trends in the management of well differentiated papillary thyroid carcinoma. J Clin Endocrinol Metab 1996; 81: 333–339.

26. Hundahl SA, Cady B, Cunningham MP, et al. Initial results from a prospective cohort study of 5583 cases of thyroid carcinoma treated in the united states during 1996. US and German Thyroid Cancer Study Group. An American College of Surgeons Commission on Cancer Patient Care Evaluation study. Cancer 2000; 89(1):202–217.

27. Holzer S, Reiners C, Mann K, et al. Patterns of care for patients with primary differentiated carcinoma of the thyroid gland treated in Germany during 1996. US and German Thyroid Cancer Group. Cancer 2000; 89(1):192–201.

28. Mazzaferri EL. NCCN Thyroid cancer practice guidelines. Oncology 13 Supplement 11A, NCCN Proceedings http://www.nccn.org/physician_gls/f_guidelines.html. 1999.

29. Mazzaferri EL. Thyroid carcinoma: Papillary and follicular. In: Mazzaferri EL, Samaan N (eds) Endocrine tumors. Cambridge: Blackwell Scientific Publications, 1993: 278–333.

30. Massin JP, Savoie JC, Garnier H, Guiraudon G, Leger FA, Bacourt F. Pulmonary metastases in differentiated thyroid carcinoma. Study of 58 cases with implications for the primary tumor treatment. Cancer 1984; 53:982–992.

31. McConahey WM, Hay ID, Woolner LB, van Heerden JA, Taylor WF. Papillary thyroid cancer treated at the Mayo Clinic, 1946 through 1970: Initial manifestations, pathologic findings, therapy and outcome. Mayo Clin Proc 1986; 61:978–996.

32. Mazzaferri EL. NCCN thyroid carcinoma practice guidelines. Oncology 1999; 13 Supplement 11A, NCCN Proceedings http://www.nccn.org/physician_gls/f_guidelines.html:391–442.

33. British Thyroid Association. Guidelines for the Management of differentiated thyroid cancer in adults. http://www.british-thyroid-association.org/guidelines.htm. 2002.

34. Schlumberger MJ. Medical progress – papillary and follicular thyroid carcinoma. N Engl J Med 1998; 338:297–306.

35. Mazzaferri EL. Treating differentiated thyroid carcinoma: where do we draw the line? Mayo Clin Proc 1991; 66:105–111.

36. Newman KD, Black T, Heller G, et al. Differentiated thyroid cancer: Determinants of disease progression in patients <21 years of age at diagnosis – a report from the Surgical Discipline Committee of the Children's Cancer Group. Ann Surg 1998; 227:533–541.

37. Miccoli P, Antonelli A, Spinelli C, Ferdeghini M, Fallahi P, Baschieri L. Completion total thyroidectomy in children with thyroid cancer secondary to the Chernobyl accident. Arch Surg 1998; 133:89–93.

38. Baudin E, Travagli JP, Ropers J, et al. Microcarcinoma of the thyroid gland – the Gustave-Roussy Institute Experience. Cancer 1998; 83:553–559.

39. Moosa M, Mazzaferri EL. Occult thyroid carcinoma. Cancer J 1997; 10:180–188.

40. Luna-Ortiz K, Hurtado-Lopez LM, Valderrama-Landaeta JL, Ruiz-Vega A. Thyroglossal duct cyst with papillary carcinoma: what must be done? Thyroid 2004; 14(5):363–366.

41. Miccoli P, Minuto MN, Galleri D, Puccini M, Berti P. Extent of surgery in thyroglossal duct carcinoma: reflections on a series of eighteen cases. Thyroid 2004; 14(2):121–123.

42. Patel SG, Escrig M, Shaha AR, Singh B, Shah JP. Management of well-differentiated thyroid carcinoma presenting within a thyroglossal duct cyst. J Surg Oncol 2002; 79(3):134–139.

43. Miccoli P, Pacini F, Basolo S, Iacconi P, Puccini M, Pinchera A. [Thyroid carcinoma in a thyroglossal duct cyst: tumor resection alone or a total thyroidectomy?]. Ann Chir 1998; 52(5):452–454.

44. Mazzaferri EL. Thyroid cancer in thyroglossal duct remnants: a diagnostic and therapeutic dilemma. Thyroid 2004; 14(5):335–336.

45. Pacini F, Elisei R, Capezzone M, et al. Contralateral papillary thyroid cancer is frequent at completion thyroidectomy with no difference in low- and high-risk patients. Thyroid 2001; 11(9):877–881.

46. Alzahrani AS, Al Mandil M, Chaudhary MA, Ahmed M, Mohammed GE. Frequency and predictive factors of malignancy in residual thyroid tissue and cervical lymph nodes after partial thyroidectomy for differentiated thyroid cancer. Surgery 2002; 131(4):443–449.

47. Maxon HR, Englaro EE, Thomas SR, et al. Radioiodine-131 therapy for well-differentiated thyroid cancer – a quantitative radiation dosimetric approach: outcome and validation in 85 patients. J Nucl Med 1992; 33:1132–1136.

48. Randolph GW, Daniels GH. Radioactive iodine lobe ablation as an alternative to completion thyroidectomy for follicular carcinoma of the thyroid. Thyroid 2002; 12(11):989–996.

49. Chao TC, Jeng LB, Lin JD, Chen MF. Completion thyroidectomy for differentiated thyroid carcinoma. Otolaryngol Head Neck Surg 1998; 118:896–899.

50. DeGroot LJ, Kaplan EL. Second operations for "completion" of thyroidectomy in treatment of differentiated thyroid cancer. Surgery 1991; 110:936–940.

51. Emerick GT, Duh Q-Y, Siperstein AE, Burrow GN, Clark OH. Diagnosis, treatment, and outcome of follicular thyroid carcinoma. Cancer 1993; 72:3287–3295.

52. Mettlin C, Lee F, Drago J, Murphy GP. The American Cancer Society National Prostate Cancer Detection Project. Cancer 1991; 67(12):2929–2958.

53. Scheumann GFW, Seeliger H, Musholt TJ, et al. Completion thyroidectomy in 131 patients with differentiated thyroid carcinoma. Eur J Surg 1996; 162:677–684.

13

Management of Cervical Lymph Nodes in Differentiated Thyroid Cancer

John C. Watkinson

Introduction

The majority of patients with differentiated thyroid cancer have papillary carcinoma and most are treated by total thyroidectomy. Metastases to the regional cervical lymph nodes are relatively common and occur early on. It has been reported that the incidence of palpable neck metastases in papillary carcinoma is between 15% and 40%, and up to 90% have occult disease [1–4]. The incidence of neck metastases is higher in children [2]. Of those patients who have total thyroidectomy, between 10% and 15% subsequently develop palpable neck disease over the next 5 to 10 years [1,5,6] and recurrent disease in lymph nodes accounts for 60–75% of all neck recurrences [7]. Lymph node metastases from follicular carcinoma are less common and occur in less than 20% of cases [2].

Although the incidence of occult neck disease is high in papillary carcinoma, its prognostic significance is unclear. This is because its natural history is not known as many patients are treated with radioactive iodine [1], and

Search strategy: A Medline search was carried out from 1970 to 2003 supplemented by searches on the Cochrane Library and a number of Worldwide Web resources which included cancerlit and cancernet. The following key words were used: Differentiated Thyroid Cancer, Cervical Lymph Nodes, Surgery.
Levels of evidence: Levels of evidence are mainly II/III and the clinical recommendations are predominantly B/C.

there is no rationale for elective neck dissection as there is with head and neck squamous carcinoma [8]. The prognostic factors in differentiated thyroid cancer are shown below. Physicians and surgeons have no control over patient and tumor factors but can influence the management (Table 13.1) [9].

The presence of palpable regional cervical lymphadenopathy is a poor prognosis in elderly patients, and in those with bilateral and mediastinal disease [1]. Some studies have shown no difference in survival between node-positive and node-negative patients [10] but fail to acknowledge that palpable disease occurs more commonly in younger patients. In addition, in those studies that showed unfavorable outcomes for patients with metastatic neck disease, age and regional recurrence were not taken into account and such variables should be included in further studies [11–13]. Another problem is distinguishing between local recurrence at the primary site and that in a level VI lymph node within the central compartment of the neck.

Palpable cervical metastases can occur at any age and are not related to the size of the primary tumor [1,14,15] and in one series, 32% of patients with papillary microcarcinoma had cervical nodal metastases at presentation [14]. Follicular carcinoma usually metastasizes by the blood route and lymph node metastases occur in less than 20% of patients [2]. It is the more aggressive, widely invasive follicular carcinomas that tend to spread, not only locoregionally but

Table 13.1 Prognostic factors associated with thyroid cancer

Patient factors	Tumor factors	Management factors
Age	Tumor size	Delay in therapy
Sex	Tumor histology	Extent of surgery
	Nodal metastases (in elderly patients)	Experience of the surgeon
	Local invasion	Thyroid hormone therapy
	Distant metastases	Treatment with postoperative radioiodine
No control	*No control*	*Control*

Source: Adapted from Moosa and Mazzaferri [9].

Table 13.2 The main controversies in the management of cervical lymph nodes in patients with differentiated thyroid cancer

- Assessment and staging
- Surgical management and extent of neck dissection
- Management of invasive and recurrent disease
- Mode of follow-up

also to distant sites, and they are associated with a worse prognosis.

The main controversies in the management of cervical lymph nodes in differentiated thyroid cancer are listed in Table 13.2.

Lymph Nodes

There are 500 lymph nodes in the body and of these, 200 are in the head and neck region [16]. In the lateral compartment of the neck, these lymph nodes are divided into a superficial lymph node system (Waldeyer's external ring) and a deep system (the cervical lymph nodes proper). These cervical lymph nodes proper are further divided into levels I to V [17,18] and within the central compartment of the neck there is an anterior visceral compartment group (level VI) and a group within the upper anterior mediastinum (level VII).

Superficial Lymph Node System (Waldeyer's External Ring)

The lymphatic drainage of head and neck tissue is divided into superficial and deep systems and usually, but not always, the passage of lymph is lateralized and sequential and follows a predefined route from superficial to deep. The superficial nodal system, which drains the superficial tissues, consists of two circles of nodes, one in the head and the other in the neck. In the head, the nodes are situated around the skull base and are known as the occipital, postauricular, parotid or preauricular and then buccal or facial nodes. They are in continuity with the superficial nodes in the upper neck consisting of the superficial cervical, submandibular, and submental nodes, along with the anterior cervical nodes. These latter nodes are situated along the external jugular vein and the anterior jugular veins, respectively. This superficial system receives drainage from the skin and underlying tissues of the scalp, eyelids and face, along with Waldeyer's internal ring (lymphatic oropharyngeal tissue consisting of the pharyngeal, tubal, and lingual tonsils), nasal sinuses, and oral cavity.

Deep System (Cervical Lymph Nodes Proper)

The deeper fascial structures of the head and neck drain either directly into the deep cervical lymph nodes or through the superficial system first and then into the deep system. These superficial nodes have already been described. The deep cervical lymph nodes proper (Figure 13.1) consist of the junctional nodes, the upper, middle, and lower cervical nodal groups which are situated along the internal jugular vein, the spinal accessory group which accompanies the accessory nerve in the posterior triangle, the nuchal nodes, the visceral nodes in the midline of the neck, and nodes in the upper mediastinum. The junctional nodes represent the confluence of nodes at the junction of the posterior part of the submandibular triangle with the retropharyngeal nodes where they meet at the junction of the upper and middle deep cervical nodes.

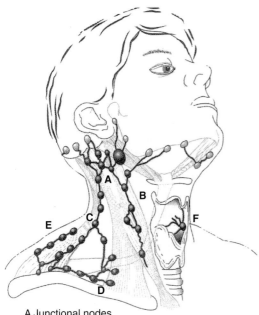

A Junctional nodes
B Internal Jugular nodes
C Spinal accessory nodes
D Supraclavicular nodes
E Nuchal nodes
F Deep medial visceral nodes

Figure 13.1 The Deep Cervical Lymph Nodes. (From Watkinson JC, Gaze MN and Wilson JA. Stell & Maran's Head & Neck Surgery, page 200, Butterworth Heinemann 2000. Reproduced by permission of Hodder Arnold.)

In general, the passage of lymph within these systems has been well documented using lymphography and follows a sequential pattern from superficial to deep, and from the upper to lower parts of the neck [16]. These lower confluent vessels form into a jugular trunk which on the right side ends at the junction of the jugular vein, the brachiocephalic vein or joins the right lymphatic duct. On the left side, the trunk will usually join the thoracic duct as it arches behind the lower part of the carotid sheath and in front of the subclavian artery to enter the junction of the internal jugular vein with the brachiocephalic vein.

Lymph Node Levels

Level I: Submental and Submandibular Groups

This consists of the submental group of lymph nodes within the triangle bounded by the ante-rior belly of digastric and hyoid bone, and the submandibular group of nodes bounded by the posterior belly of digastric and body of the mandible.

Level II: Upper Jugular Group

This consists of the lymph nodes located around the upper third of the internal jugular vein and adjacent spinal accessory nodes extending from the skull base down to the level of the carotid bifurcation where the digastric muscle crosses the internal jugular vein. This point relates to level of the hyoid bone on a computed tomographic (CT) scan. It contains the junctional and sometimes the jugulodigastric nodes. Level II is further subdivided into level II_A, which is in front of the accessory nerve, and level II_B, which is behind. This is known as Suarez's triangle and contains Suarez's fat pad [19].

Level III: Middle Jugular Group

This consists of lymph nodes located around the middle third of the internal jugular vein extending from the carotid bifurcation superiorly (bottom of level II) down to the upper part of the cricoid cartilage (seen on a CT scan) and represents the level where the omohyoid muscle crosses the internal jugular vein. It usually contains the jugulo-omohyoid nodes and may contain the jugulodigastric node.

Level IV: Lower Jugular Group

This consists of lymph nodes located around the lower third of the internal jugular vein extending from the cricoid cartilage down to the clavicle inferiorly. It may contain some jugulo-omohyoid nodes.

Level V: Posterior Triangle Group

These nodes are located along the lower half of the spinal accessory nerve and the transverse cervical artery. Supraclavicular nodes are also included in this group. The posterior limit is the anterior border of the trapezius and the anterior border is the anterior border of sternomastoid. Level V is further subdivided into level V_A above the omohyoid muscle and level V_B below.

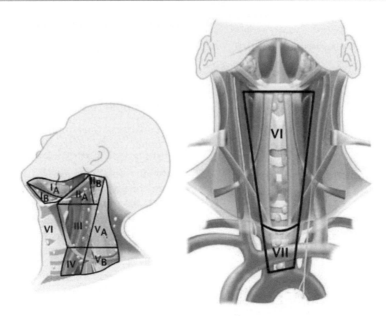

Figure 13.2 Lymph node levels in the head and neck. (From Watkinson JC, Gaze MN and Wilson JA. Stell & Maran's Head & Neck Sugery, page 201, Butterworth Heineman 2000. Reproduced by permission of Hodder Arnold.)

Level VI: Anterior Compartment Group (Visceral Group)

This consists of lymph nodes surrounding the midline visceral structures of the neck extending from the hyoid bone superiorly to the suprasternal notch inferiorly. The lateral border on each side is the medial border of the sternomastoid muscle. It contains the parathyroids, the paratracheal and pretracheal, and the perilaryngeal and precricoid lymph nodes.

Level VII

This contains the lymph nodes in the upper anterior mediastinum as well as the thymus gland. The lymph node levels are shown in Figure 13.2.

The above drainage patterns apply only to the non-violated neck. Once the natural history of the disease is altered, lymph node metastases can occur anywhere. This explains why the operation of selective neck dissection is only applicable in the previously untreated neck. An incision in the neck for a nodal biopsy can alter patterns of lymphatic drainage for up to 1 year following surgery. Further shunting of lymph with opening up of abnormal channels

occurs when more extensive surgery and radiotherapy are undertaken, and once a malignant lymph node is palpable, there may be shunting of cells to the contralateral neck. All of these factors play a part in the management of neck disease and need to be borne in mind when assessing anatomical images following previous surgery.

Patterns of Spread

The thyroid gland contains a dense network of intrathyroidal lymphatics which surround the thyroid follicles and facilitate direct communication across the isthmus between the two lobes of the gland. This explains the multifocality of papillary thyroid cancer and forms one of the rationales for total thyroidectomy. This intrathyroidal lymphatic network then joins collecting and draining lymphatic trunks within the subcapsular region of the gland that run alongside the extensive vascular network within the thyroid and leave the gland together with the venous drainage. This results not only in early multifocal thyroid carcinoma, but also in significant locoregional spread [1–4]. It is not uncommon to have an occult thyroid

Table 13.3 Patterns of lymphatic drainage of the thyroid gland

Major
- Middle jugular nodes – level III
- Lower jugular nodes – level IV
- Posterior triangle nodes – level V$_B$

Minor
- Pretracheal and paratracheal nodes – level VI
- Superior mediastinal nodes – level VII

The lymph node groups at the highest risk of metastases from differentiated thyroid cancer are in the central compartment (level VI), lower jugular chain (levels III and IV), and the posterior triangle (level V$_B$) (Figure 13.3)

microcarcinoma with palpable neck disease [14,15], but it is uncommon to have a tumor in one lobe of the thyroid gland and contralateral neck disease without palpable unilateral neck nodes [20].

The primary lymphatic drainage from the thyroid (Table 13.3) can travel in a superior, lateral, and inferior direction and follows the vascular pedicles of both the superior and inferior thyroid vessels as well as the middle thyroid vein. The upper poles of the gland together with the isthmus and the pyramidal lobe drain superiorly, terminating in the lateral neck in levels II/III while the lateral aspect of each lobe drains into level III and IV. The lower pole of the gland drains into the peri- and paratracheal nodes in level VI, and then onto both level IV and level VII nodes. Lymphatic drainage

may also pass to nodes within the parapharyngeal and retropharyngeal spaces, but this usually tends to occur when other nodes are involved and shunting occurs, or when there has been previous treatment with either surgery or irradiation. It is very uncommon for differentiated thyroid malignancy to present with an isolated metastasis in the parapharyngeal space [21]. There are also extensive communications between the lateral cervical lymph nodes in levels II, III, and IV and the superior mediastinum via level VI.

Tumors in the upper pole tend to metastasize to levels II/III; tumors in the middle third of the gland spread to the paraglandular and paratracheal nodes while those in the lower third spread predominately to the paratracheal nodes. Isthmus tumors spread most often to the pretracheal nodes [20].

The thyroid gland occupies the central compartment of the neck and overlies the second to fourth tracheal rings. There are a number of lymph nodes that are not only attached to the inferior surface of the gland, but also lie within the perithyroidal region, which includes the para – and pretracheal regions, and this whole area is called level VI. It runs from the hyoid bone down to the suprasternal notch and lies between the medial borders of the sternomastoid muscle and carotid sheath. It contains the parathyroid glands, as well as the paratracheal and pretracheal, perilaryngeal and precricoid lymph nodes. It also contains the recurrent laryngeal nerves.

Assessment and Staging

The majority of patients with differentiated thyroid cancer will present with a palpable goiter and a clinically negative neck (within both the central and lateral compartments). The treatment rationale for such patients is discussed later but in general, since there is no evidence that elective surgery for the N0 (no nodes palpable) neck improves survival, there are currently few indications for elective imaging. In the future, increased use of ultrasound at the primary site may involve lymph node assessment in level VI and while it provides a guide to which patients need elective surgery, more of these patients are now being treated by total thyroidectomy and level VI neck dissection.

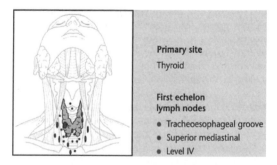

Primary site
Thyroid

First echelon lymph nodes
- Tracheoesophageal groove
- Superior mediastinal
- Level IV

Figure 13.3 First echelon thyroid lymph nodes. (Reprinted from Shah JP, Head and Neck Surgery & Oncology, 3rd Edition, page 358, Copyright 2003, with permission from Elsevier.)

Table 13.4 Modalities used to evaluate patients with differentiated thyroid cancer

- Clinical examination
- CT scan
- MRI scan
- Ultrasound
- Positron emission tomography (PET)

The evaluation of patients with differentiated thyroid cancer involves several modalities (Table 13.4). Clinical examination of the neck has a variable reliability with inevitable false-positive and false-negative rates of around 20–30% [22]. This is compounded by the fact that many patients have micrometastases which are often small and therefore impalpable. The central and lateral compartments of the neck may be evaluated using the modalities listed in Table 13.4.

The range of normal or nonpathological cervical neck nodes is from 3 mm to 3 cm, but for squamous cell carcinoma of the neck, nodes greater than a centimeter in size on CT scanning usually contain metastatic disease. However, for papillary thyroid cancer, the size criteria are different and metastatic nodes are usually smaller [23]. There is little evidence in the literature to justify routine elective imaging of the N0 neck. Levels I to VII should be clinically evaluated and, those patients with either palpable or suspected neck disease, as well as those with proven recurrence, should be imaged anatomically. When assessing recurrent disease, it is important to evaluate both the retropharyngeal and parapharyngeal spaces since patterns of drainage can be altered by previous treatment with either surgery or external beam radiotherapy.

The CT criteria for malignancy include cystic and hemorrhagic change, calcification, contrast enhancement, and a hypoplastic appearance [21]. Imaging can be done with or without contrast, but the iodine load from the former will interfere with subsequent treatment with radioactive iodine for up to 3 months or sometimes longer. MRI uses similar staging characteristics to CT with regard to malignancy but usually takes longer and is inferior to CT when imaging the chest.

Ultrasound is becoming more important in the primary evaluation of lymph node metastases and in the follow-up of patients treated with differentiated thyroid cancer. Lymph node metastases as small as 2 to 3 mm can now be detected when ultrasonography is performed with a high frequency probe [24]. Some units suggest that neck ultrasonography should be routinely performed in all patients with differentiated thyroid carcinoma at presentation [25] and this not only includes level VI, but the "at risk levels" in the lateral compartments (levels III, IV, and V).

Suspicious nodes tend to be round, hypoechoic, and devoid of an echoic central line, with microcalcifications or cystic components, and are hypervascular on Doppler ultrasonography [25].

Following initial treatment, patients are followed up with TSH suppression and sequential thyroglobulin monitoring. In the presence of a truly positive elevated thyroglobulin, recurrent disease is assessed with whole-body ^{131}I scanning and anatomical imaging with either CT or ultrasound. The role of PET in the evaluation of cervical lymphadenopathy in differentiated thyroid cancer is controversial. There is currently no role in using PET to detect occult metastases in the N0 neck but it maybe useful in detecting recurrent neck disease in the presence of an elevated serum thyroglobulin with negative ^{131}I scans and anatomical images.

All tumors should be TNM staged. In the past, the UIIC-AJCC *TNM Classification of Malignant Tumours* (5th edn) staged the regional lymph nodes as described in Table 13.5.

The latest UICC-AJCC TNM classification of malignant tumors (6th edn) has amended this as shown in Table 13.6.

Reasons for these changes are that in the past, little prognostic significance was given to level VI regional lymphadenopathy, and an emphasis was placed on prognostic differences between unilateral and bilateral neck disease, for which there is now thought to be little evidence (Professor J. Shah, personal communication).

Table 13.5 Lymph node staging according to the 5th edition of the UICC-AJCC TNM classification [26]

N	Regional lymph nodes
NX	Regional lymph nodes cannot be assessed
N0	No regional lymph node metastasis
N1	Regional lymph node metastasis

Source: UICC-AJCC [26].

Table 13.6 Lymph node staging according to the 6th edition of the UICC-AJCC TNM classification [27]

N	Regional nodes
NX	Regional lymph nodes cannot be assessed
N0	No regional lymph node metastasis
N1	Regional lymph node metastasis
N1a	Metastasis in level VI (pretracheal and paratracheal, including prelaryngeal and Delphin lymph nodes)
N1b	Metastasis in other unilateral, bilateral, or contralateral cervical or upper/superior mediastinal lymph nodes

Source: UICC-AJCC [27].

Treatment Philosophy

Many patients with differentiated thyroid cancer have metastatic spread within the regional lymph nodes and for the majority, this usually represents occult disease [1–4]. Its frequency is related to histology (more common in papillary thyroid cancer) and to the size of the primary tumor. The chances of having regional lymph node metastases with follicular carcinoma is much lower and occurs in less than 20% of cases [2].

Lymph node metastases in differentiated thyroid cancer are often multiple, and of variable size and this is one of the arguments for selective neck dissection of "at risk levels" rather than "berry picking" (selective removal of isolated lymph nodes) [20,25]. The latter procedure has now been shown to have a less favorable prognosis than formal neck dissection [28]. The spread of disease is usually ipsilateral [20,25], and involves progression in an orderly defined manner from level VI either laterally to levels III and IV or inferiorly into the mediastinum (level VII). Spread into level II either occurs from the superior pole of the thyroid or directly from levels III and IV. Spread into level I and the retropharyngeal and parapharyngeal spaces tends to occur when other levels are involved, or in the previously treated neck.

Many studies show that lymph node involvement is associated with a significantly higher risk of both local and regional recurrences and of distant metastases [1]. It is not clear whether its presence has an impact on survival because other prognostic factors are involved. There does appear to be an increased risk of cancer-related mortality when lymph node metastases are extensive, bilateral, located in the mediastinum, associated with extensive primary disease, or when they occur in elderly patients [1].

In the past, there has been a trend not to perform elective lateral neck dissection in patients with differentiated thyroid cancer but to perform a "berry picking" procedure for palpable disease. There is now strong evidence to support a formal selective neck/modified radical neck dissection (dissecting at least levels III, IV, and V_B) in the lateral compartment for palpable or suspected disease [20,25,28]. This is on the basis of the high incidence of nodal involvement, and that formal lymph node dissection facilitates accurate workup of the initial extent of the disease. Furthermore, a number of studies have shown improved outcomes with formal lymph node dissection [25] and in one series, the 20-year recurrence rate was significantly reduced after formal lymph node dissection [29]. In one study, recurrent disease after lymph node spread from papillary thyroid cancer was associated with a significant increase in the risk of death [30]. Surgery is the most effective way of treating lymph node metastases, and in particular those nodes in the so-called "coffin corners" where detection is difficult such as the retropharyngeal and parapharyngeal spaces, pre- and paratracheal grooves, and Chaissaignac's triangle (Figure 13.4).

The majority of patients have a palpable goiter and are clinically N0 in both level VI and

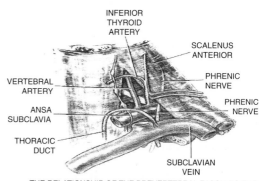

THE RELATIONSHIP OF THE PREVERTEBRAL FASCIA TO THE SCALENE MUSCLES AND THE STRUCTURES OVER THE APEX OF THE LEFT LUNG.

Figure 13.4 The relationship of the prevertebral fascia to the scalene muscles and the structures over the apex of the left lung (Chaissaignac's triangle). (Reproduced from Last RJ, *Anatomy Regional and Applied*, 6th edn, London: Churchill Livingstone, 1978, page 377.)

the lateral neck compartment (levels II–V). Some workers now argue strongly that at the time of initial thyroidectomy, level VI should be routinely dissected [25,31,32], particularly for high risk disease, although its exact role awaits clarification [33]. Its use is justified on the basis that recurrence and reoperation rates may be reduced and overall survival improved although there is no prospective evidence to support this. Indeed, some surgeons extend the dissection to the ipsilateral supraclavicular area, thereby allowing elective dissection of the retrovascular and external part of the jugulocarotid chain, as well as the transverse superficial chain along the accessory nerve in level V [25]. This dissection is performed through a transverse incision and the operative specimen submitted to frozen section. Morbidity is said to be low [25] but the same authors acknowledge that level VI dissection increases the risk of hypoparathyroidism and recurrent laryngeal nerve palsy [25]. Although there are no prospective studies looking at whether there is any increase in complication rates following elective lymphadenectomy of the central compartment, one study showed that the rates of temporary and permanent hypoparathyroidism following level VII dissection were 70% and 50%, respectively [34]. In a personal series of 363 total thyroidectomies from 1993 to 2003 (of whom 147 had a routine level VI neck dissection for differentiated thyroid cancer), the incidence of temporary and permanent hypoparathyroidism was 19% and 1.9%, respectively. In those patients having lobectomy or total thyroidectomy for malignancy ($n = 353$), the incidence of temporary and permanent recurrent laryngeal nerve palsy was 1.4% and 0.9%, respectively. The wound infection rate was 0.9% and hematoma rate 1.4%.

Patients with differentiated thyroid cancer (particularly papillary) are at high risk of occult cervical metastases. The central compartment (level VI) can be evaluated by both palpation and elective imaging, and high risk patients considered for elective neck dissection. Another alternative would be to consider sentinel node biopsy. This involves intraoperative surgical mapping of the first echelon lymph nodes using an injection of 1% isosulfan blue dye into the thyroid nodule. Within seconds, the dye can be seen to pass to the sentinel lymph node. One study looked at 12 malignant cases (11 papillary, 1 follicular), all of whom had an N0 central compartment. Of these, only 5 out of 12 had positive sentinel nodes and there was one false-negative and one false-positive result. The problem is this technique involves injecting the nodule and violates an oncologically significant area (level VI). It may also highlight the parathyroids, sometimes leading to their inadvertent removal. Further studies are awaited but currently elective neck dissection in high risk patients is probably safer and more cost-effective than sentinel node biopsy, and proceed to central neck dissection if the node is positive [35].

How then should we manage our patients? Several different types of lymph node dissection may be done in patients with differentiated thyroid carcinoma (Table 13.7). For those undergoing a unilateral lobectomy for a suspicious fine-needle aspiration cytology (FNAC) for a papillary carcinoma, a unilateral level VI neck dissection may be performed in high risk patients (those with T3/T4 tumors, children, males >45 years) which removes the soft tissue and lymph nodes in that area with preservation of both recurrent laryngeal nerves, the external branches of the superior laryngeal nerves and all the parathyroid glands (Table 13.7). For a suspected or proven malignancy when a near-total or total thyroidectomy is being performed, this procedure is carried out bilaterally. Large nodules in the isthmus (T3/T4 lesions) require

Table 13.7 Neck dissections performed for differentiated thyroid carcinoma

- Level VI neck dissection
- Level VII neck dissection
- Selective neck dissection (usually levels II$_A$ to V$_B$; or levels III and IV, levels III to V$_B$, or levels IV to V$_B$)
- Modified radical neck dissection (type 1) preserving the accessory nerve (levels I–V dissected)
- Modified radical neck dissection (type 2) preserving the accessory nerve and the internal jugular vein (levels I–V dissected)
- Modified radical neck dissection (type 3) preserving the accessory nerve, internal jugular vein, and sternomastoid muscle (levels I–V dissected). Sometimes called a comprehensive neck dissection.
- Radical neck dissection (levels I–V dissected). The accessory nerve, internal jugular vein, and sternomastoid muscle are all sacrificed.
- Extended radical neck dissection (levels I–V dissected). This involves a radical neck dissection with sacrifice of other structures such as external skin, digastric muscle, etc.

bilateral dissection. At the time of surgery for near-total or total thyroidectomy, levels II, III, and IV should be palpated. If there is any suggestion of metastatic spread, a frozen section should be performed and the presence of metastatic disease indicates the need for an elective selective dissection of the lateral neck compartment. There is confusion in the literature about which levels should be routinely dissected. One study has shown that in the presence of palpable disease, nodal involvement is at a single level in 39% of cases, while 14% of cases involved four or more levels [36]. The majority of surgeons will always dissect at least levels III and IV [31,36; Professor J. Shah, personal communication; Professor C. O'Brien, personal communication] and some also routinely dissect levels II_A to V_B (Professor P. Gullane, personal communication). In the presence of gross disease in level II_A, level II_B should be dissected as recurrent disease at this site is difficult to treat surgically (Professor J. Shah, personal communication). The author's preference for palpable neck disease is to dissect at least levels IIA to V_B (below the accessory nerve) with preservation of the sternomastoid muscle, internal jugular vein, and the accessory nerve [37]. This falls just short of a modified radical neck dissection type three (comprehensive neck dissection) since level I is not usually routinely dissected, although in one series, approximately 12% of cases had disease at this level [20]. This procedure may be extended to include level I, and then one or other of the accessory nerve, internal jugular vein, or sternomastoid muscle may need to be sacrificed for more advanced disease (modified or radical neck dissection). This is discussed below. Palpable disease in level VI is treated with a level VI neck dissection.

Treatment of lymph node metastases for follicular carcinoma is treated in a similar way to the papillary cancer, although there seems little justification to perform a level VI neck dissection in the N0 neck as the chance of occult disease is less than 20%.

Surgical Management

A level VI neck dissection can be done through a formal thyroid incision and simply involves an extended total thyroidectomy with removal of the soft tissue bearing areas of level VI that con-

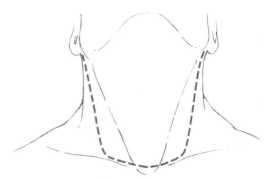

Figure 13.5 Standard thyroidectomy incision with bilateral thyroid utility extensions. A "W" plasty can be incorporated at the upper end of the utility incision in order to achieve a better scar.

tains the lymph nodes. The parathyroid glands are preserved together with the recurrent laryngeal nerves and external branches of the superior laryngeal nerves. The dissection may be facilitated by the use of operating loupes and can be extended using the cervical approach to remove the lymph node bearing areas of level VII down to the brachiocephalic vein [30]. This is usually facilitated by cervical thymectomy. For extensive disease with possible vascular involvement, a formal approach to the mediastinum is required using either a limited or full sternotomy.

The incision for a standard selective lateral compartment neck dissection is usually best done with an extended thyroid incision (thyroid utility: Figure 13.5). This facilitates formal access to levels II to V (Figures 13.6 and 13.7). Further access to levels II to IV can be achieved either by lifting sternomastoid up to dissect beneath the muscle or (in the author's preference) by dividing the sternomastoid at its lower end and

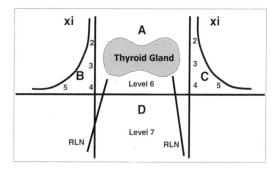

Figure 13.6 Schematic outline of central compartment dissection and a lateral neck dissection, dissecting levels II, III, IV, and V below the accessory nerve. RLN = recurrent laryngeal nerve.

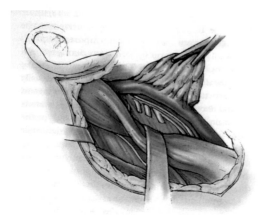

Figure 13.7 As part of a selective neck dissection, the lymph node bearing tissue of level V is removed followed by access to levels II, III, and IV obtained by either retracting or dividing the sternomastoid muscle. The internal jugular vein and accessory nerve are also preserved. The cervical plexus is usually divided. (Reproduced with permission from Johnson JT and Gluckman JL (eds), *Carcinoma of the Thyroid*, Oxford: Isis Medical Media, 1999, page 79.)

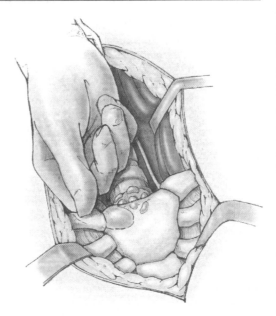

Figure 13.8 During a formal total thyroidectomy with level VI neck dissection, access to level VII can usually be achieved by a cervical approach. (Reproduced with permission from Johnson JT and Gluckman JL (eds), *Carcinoma of the Thyroid*, Oxford: Isis Medical Media, 1999, page 78.)

elevating it up to improve the exposure. Access to level VII can easily be achieved with a cervical approach (Figure 13.8). The accessory nerve is formally identified in the posterior triangle at Erb's point (which is 1 cm above where the greater auricular nerve winds around the posterior border of sternomastoid) and in the untreated neck there is no need to dissect above the nerve. Lymph node bearing tissue of the posterior triangle below the accessory nerve (essentially level V_B) is removed together with tissue in levels IIA, III, and IV to include the omohyoid muscle. Special care is taken to access Chaissaignac's triangle, which lies behind the posterior part of the lower end of the internal jugular vein (Figure 13.4) and which often contains occult metastases from differentiated thyroid cancer.

The dissection proceeds in an upward and medial direction clearing levels II_A to V_B with every attempt made to preserve the sensory branches of the cervical plexus, although it is difficult to carry out an adequate selective neck dissection without sometimes dividing some or all of these branches. This is the author's practice and the technique of routinely taking the cervical plexus with a selective neck dissection is well described [38]. For more extensive disease, level I may have to be dissected and one or all of the internal jugular vein, sternoma-

stoid muscle, and accessory nerve sacrificed (modified radical or radical neck dissection). Very occasionally, other structures have to be removed (i.e. the digastric muscle, external skin) and this is an extended radical neck dissection. The areas dissected and key steps of a selective neck dissection (levels II_A–V_B) are shown in Figures 13.9–13.15. In a personal

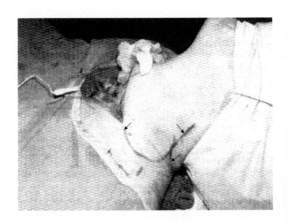

Figure 13.9 Lateral utility incision marked out on the skin.

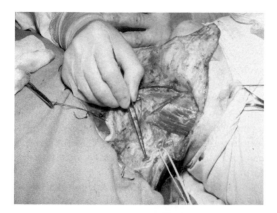

Figure 13.10 Posterior triangle identified with the accessory nerve having been isolated with a sloop.

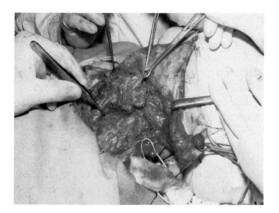

Figure 13.11 The sternomastoid muscle has been divided and retracted superiorly. The accessory nerve is identified with a sloop and the lymphoid bearing tissue in level V below the nerve is removed; the dissection is carried forward to remove the lymph node bearing area in level IV together with the scalene nodes behind the lower end of the internal jugular vein (Chaissaignac's triangle – this area is being pointed to with a pair of forceps).

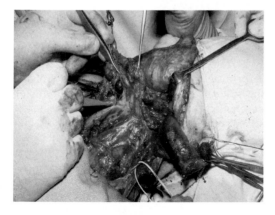

Figure 13.12 The dissection is continued superiorly removing the lymph node bearing tissue in levels III and II$_A$. The mass is dissected from the internal jugular vein.

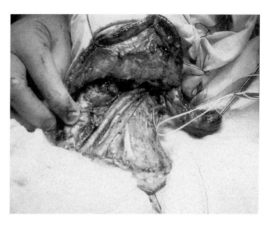

Figure 13.13 The dissection is completed showing from lateral to medial, the divided lower end of the sternomastoid muscle, accessory nerve with a sloop around it, the brachial plexus, Chaissaignac's triangle, the internal jugular vein, the vagus nerve and the common carotid artery. The author's index finger is retracting the trachea medially and the recurrent laryngeal nerve can be seen between it and the common carotid.

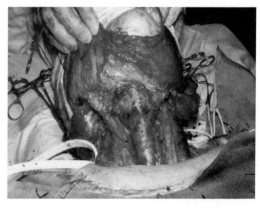

Figure 13.14 Final result following total thyroidectomy and bilateral selective neck dissection (levels II$_A$–V$_B$).

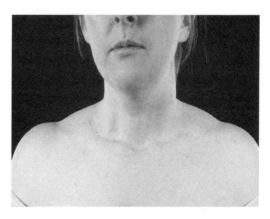

Figure 13.15 Final result following total thyroidectomy and bilateral selective neck dissection in the same patient.

Table 13.8 Author's personal series of patients undergoing lateral neck dissection for differentiated thyroid cancer (1994–2004)

Extended radical neck dissection	3
Radical neck dissection	3
Modified radical neck dissection	17
Selective neck dissection levels II to V	44
Selective neck dissection levels III to V	6
Selective neck dissection levels II to IV	4
Total	77

Table 13.9 The key steps for performing a selective neck dissection in patients with differentiated thyroid carcinoma

- Adequate incision
- Identify levels II, III, IV, and V
- Clearly identify the accessory nerve
- Deal with the sternomastoid muscle
- Dissect corners one and two
- Preserve the internal jugular vein, phrenic nerve and brachial plexus
- Access Chaissaignac's triangle
- Finally dissect levels II$_A$ to V$_B$

series of 77 neck dissections (Table 13.8), the hematoma and infection rates were 0.8%. One patient had an accessory nerve palsy (the nerve was deliberately divided), and another had a chyle leak which required re-exploration.

The key steps for performing a selective neck dissection in differentiated thyroid carcinoma are shown in Table 13.9.

Complications

Complications relating to neck dissection for differentiated thyroid cancer can be divided into early, intermediate and late, local and general. Important complications of neck dissection are listed in Table 13.10.

Table 13.10 The major complications of neck dissections performed for differentiated thyroid carcinoma

- Temporary and permanent hypoparathyroidism
- Bleeding
- Chyle leak
- Nerve injury
- Wound infection
- Poor scar

Although bleeding is uncommon following neck dissection, it can be dramatic. It is usually either reactionary or secondary and tends to occur in the first 6 hours following surgery. It can be kept to a minimum by meticulous technique, doubly ligating or ligating and transfixing named vessels and with the routine use of drains. Significant bleeding requires return to theater.

A chyle leak can occur when operating on the left side of the neck. The thoracic duct is particularly vulnerable when dissecting Chaissaignac's triangle. Low volume leaks may be treated conservatively using a low fat diet and low suction drainage. It may be possible to inject a sclerosant into the wound (such as tetracycline or talc) to promote a seal. For those leaks that are of high volume (greater than 500 ml a day) or for those that do not settle conservatively, surgical re-exploration is required. This can be done through the neck by reopening the wound when the duct is identified and ligated. The use of loupes can facilitate the dissection. Alternatively the thoracic duct can be ligated in the chest by a thoracic surgeon. For those leaks that are high volume, early exploration is advisable rather than adopting a conservative approach. Damage to the jugular lymph ducts can give rise to lymphatic leaks which generally settle conservatively. This can occur bilaterally. A chyle leak from the right lower neck is very uncommon but can occur. Seromas occur later on in the postoperative period (usually following drain removal) and are generally treated conservatively. Some, however, may require aspiration.

Nerve Injury

There are several nerves that are at risk during the performance of a neck dissection (Table 13.11). The accessory nerve should be identified early on as part of the neck dissection. Probably the best way to find it is at Erb's point, which is one centimeter above where the greater auricular nerve winds round the posterior border of the sternomastoid. Once identified, it can be isolated with a sloop, and the dissection proceeds caudal to the nerve. In a certain proportion of cases, the main nerve supply to trapezius comes

Table 13.11 The nerves at risk during neck dissection for differentiated thyroid carcinoma

- Accessory nerve
- Hypoglossal nerve
- Vagus nerve
- Phrenic nerve
- Brachial plexus
- Cervical plexus

Level VI neck dissection only:
- Recurrent laryngeal nerve
- External branch of the superior laryngeal nerve

from the contribution to the accessory nerve from the cervical plexus. In addition, preservation of the nerve does not guarantee it functions postoperatively, presumably due to devascularization. Damage to the phrenic nerve and brachial plexus can be avoided by clear identification of the prevertebral fascia and not allowing the dissection to proceed below that structure. The vagus is identified in the carotid sheath and should not be damaged unless it is invaded by tumor. The same applies to the hypoglossal nerve.

It is extremely difficult to carry out a proper neck dissection without damaging branches of the cervical plexus, and this includes the greater auricular nerve. While it may be possible in some cases to preserve these nerves, given the need for oncological clearance, and removal of all involved lymph nodes, it is better to sacrifice them since this results in minimal morbidity (loss of sensation over the side of neck and shoulder).

In general, incisions in the neck that are correctly placed heal well. Like fine wine, scars mature but if they are wrongly sited they can have disastrous results. One of the problems with using a thyroid utility incision is that in the upper posterior neck, there is a lack of platysma so that some of the scars can become hypertrophic (Figure 13.16). This can be kept to a minimum by meticulous surgical technique, a two-layer closure, keeping the sutures in for 7 to 10 days, and incorporating a "W" plasty in the upper end of the incision. Generally the scar (particularly in women) can be hidden within the hairline but when patients are unhappy with the final result, scar revision may be performed.

The use of triamcinolone given subcutaneously can help. Alternatively, a different incision can be used which involves a higher than usual collar thyroidectomy incision that is simply extended across the posterior triangle without any significant upward extension. This is particularly useful when access only to levels III, VI, and V_B is required.

The Difficult Neck

In patients with differentiated thyroid cancer, the management of the neck can be difficult for a number of reasons. Patients can be difficult to examine and assess, as well as being difficult to operate on and follow up. Necks can be difficult to examine and assess because of either obesity or previous treatment with surgery or irradiation. Difficult necks to operate on include those with extensive disease, bilateral disease, those with mediastinal extension and residual and recurrent disease following previous treatment. All the above situations can be difficult to follow up. Where there is any difficulty arising regarding clinical assessment, anatomical imaging is mandatory.

Follow-up

The majority of necks are followed up routinely by clinical examination. The thyroid bed is examined along with both lateral neck compartments (to include levels I to V). Previous surgery can alter patterns of lymphatic drainage, so it is not uncommon that lymph nodes may be detected after treatment. Some are benign and regress over time but those patients whose lesions persist, or who are at high risk of recurrence or have an elevated thyroglobulin will need further investigation. Some institutions recommend routine ultrasonography for post-treatment neck evaluation [7,39] and if a metastasis is suspected, FNAC can be performed (under ultrasound guidance if indicated) and the liquid can also be analyzed for thyroglobulin [7,39]. There should be an agreed protocol for the investigation of those patients who have a difficult neck to examine and who are ^{131}I negative and serum thyroglobulin positive.

Recurrent disease in the treated neck should be dealt with, where possible, with further surgery. If a formal neck dissection has not been previously performed, then this should be completed. If it has been done, local resection suffices with recourse then to further treatment with radioactive iodine ablation/therapy and consideration for external beam radiotherapy when residual macroscopic disease is present.

Conclusion

The majority of patients with differentiated thyroid cancer have papillary carcinoma and most will be treated by a near-total or total thyroidectomy. Regional metastases to the cervical lymph nodes are relatively common, occur early on and are more frequent in children. The incidence of palpable neck metastases in papillary carcinoma is between 15% and 40% and up to 90% have occult disease. The first echelon lymph nodes for drainage occur commonly in levels III, IV, V_B, VI, and VII and in the untreated neck, patterns of lymph node drainage occur in a recognized, predictable, and systematic manner so as to facilitate selective neck surgery.

In the N0 neck within the central compartment (level VI), routine dissection should be considered as part of a total thyroidectomy, particularly in high risk patients. There is no role for routine elective surgery in the lateral compartment in the N0 neck, and for palpable (or suspected) disease, a selective neck dissection should be carried out of at least levels III, IV, and V_B preserving the sternomastoid muscle, the accessory nerve, and the internal jugular vein. This operation can be performed with low morbidity, and there is no role for "berry picking."

Key Points

- The majority of patients with differentiated thyroid cancer have papillary carcinoma and most are treated by total thyroidectomy.
- Metastases to the regional cervical lymph nodes are relatively common and occur early on.
- The incidence of palpable neck metastases in papillary carcinoma is between 15% and 40%, and up to 90% have occult disease.

- In the untreated neck, patterns of lymph node drainage occur in a recognized and systematic manner, which facilitates selective neck surgery.
- Lymph node metastases occur commonly in levels III, IV, V_B, VI, and VII.

In the N0 neck in level VI, routine dissection should be considered as part of a total thyroidectomy in high risk patients.

- There is no role for routine elective surgery in the N0 lateral compartment neck.
- When there is palpable (or suspected) disease within the lateral neck compartment, a selective neck dissection should be carried out including at least levels III, IV, and V_B preserving wherever possible, the sternomastoid muscle, accessory nerve, and internal jugular vein.
- Selective neck surgery for differentiated thyroid cancer can be performed with low morbidity.
- There is no role for "berry picking."
- Follow-up is for life.

References

1. Mazzaferri EL, Kloos RT. Current approaches to primary therapy for papillary and follicular thyroid cancer. J Clin Endocrinol Metab 2001; 86(4):1447–1463.
2. Grebe SKG, Hay ID. Thyroid cancer nodal metastases: biologic significance and therapeutic considerations. Surg Oncol Clin N Am 1996; 5:43–63.
3. Noguchim S, Noguchi N, Murakami N. Papillary carcinoma of the thyroid. The value of prophylactic lymph node excision. Cancer 1970; 26:1061–1064.
4. Attie JN, Khafif RA, Steckler RM. Elective neck dissection in papillary carcinoma of the thyroid. Am J Surg 1971; 22:464–471.
5. McConahey WM, Hay ID, Woolner LB, et al. Papillary thyroid cancer treated at Mayo Clinic, 1946 through 1970: initial manifestations, pathologic findings, therapy and outcome. Mayo Clin Proc 1986; 61:978–996.
6. Noguchi M, Kinami S, Kinoshita K, et al. Risk of bilateral cervical lymph node metastasis in papillary thyroid cancer. J Surg Oncol 1993; 52:155–159.
7. Schlumberger M, Pacini F. Local and regional recurrences. Thyroid tumors, 2nd edn. Paris: Editions Nucleon, 2003: 181–192.
8. Watkinson JC, Mastronikolis N, Glaholm J, Fitzgerald DA, MaGuire, D, Neary, Z. The management of squamous cell carcinoma of the neck. The Birmingham UK Experience. Eur J Surg Oncol 2005 (in press).
9. Moosa M, Mazzaferri E. Management of thyroid neoplasms. In: Cummings CW, Fredrickson JM, Harker LA,

Krause CJ, Richardson MA, Schuller DE (eds) Otolaryngology head and neck surgery, 3rd edn, Vol 3. St Louis: Mosby, 1998: 2480–2518.

10. Cady B, Sedgwick L, Meissner W, et al. Changing clinical pathologic, therapeutic and surgical patterns in differentiated thyroid carcinoma. Am J Surg 1976; 184: 541–553.

11. Tubiana M, Schlumgerger M, Rougier P. Long-term results and prognostic factors in patients with differentiated thyroid carcinoma. Cancer 1985; 55:794–804.

12. McGregor GI, Luoma A, Jackson SM. Lymph node metastases from well-differentiated thyroid cancer. Am J Surg 1985; 149:610–612.

13. Harwood J, Clark OH, Dunphy JE. Significance of lymph node metastasis in differentiated thyroid cancer. Am J Surg 1978; 136:107–112.

14. Hay ID, Grant CS, Van Heerden JA, Goellner JR, Ebersold JR, Bergstralh EJ. Papillary thyroid microcarcinoma: a study of 535 cases observed in a 50 year period. Surgery 1992; 112:1139–1147.

15. Baudin E, Travagli JP, Ropers J, et al. Microcarcinoma of the thyroid gland: The Gustave-Roussy Institute experience. Cancer 1998; 83:553–559.

16. Watkinson JC, Gaze MN, Wilson JA. Metastatic neck disease. In: Stell and Maran's Head and Neck Surgery, 4th edn. Oxford: Butterworth Heinemann, 2000:197–214.

17. Shah JP, Strong E, Spiro RH, Vikram B. Neck dissection: current status and future possibilities. Clin Bull 1981; 11:25–33.

18. Shah JP. Cervical lymph nodes. In: Head and neck: surgery and oncology, 3rd edn Edinburgh: Mosby, 2003: 353–394.

19. Gavilan J, Gavilan C, Herranz J. Functional neck dissection; three decades of controversy. Ann Otol Rhinol Laryngol 1992; 101:339–341.

20. Quabain SM, Nakano S, Baba, M, Takao S, Aikou T. Distribution of lymph node micrometastasis in pN0 well differentiated thyroid cancer. Surgery 2002; 131(3): 249–255.

21. Thomas G, Pandey M, Jayasree K, et al. Parapharyngeal metastasis from papillary microcarcinoma of thyroid: report of a case diagnosed by peroral fine needle aspiration. Br J Oral Maxillofac Surg 2002; 40:229–231.

22. Ali S, Tiwari R, Snow GB. False-positive and false-negative neck nodes. Head Neck Surg 1985; 8:78–82.

23. Watkinson JC, Gaze MN, Wilson JA. Radiology. In: Stell and Maran's Head and Neck Surgery, 4th edn. Oxford: Butterworth Heinemann, 2000: 29–47.

24. Frasoldati A, Pesenti M, Gallo M, Caroggio A, Salvo D, Valcavi R. Diagnosis of neck recurrences in patients with differentiated thyroid carcinoma. Cancer 2003; 97: 90–96.

25. Schlumberger M, Pacini F. Initial treatment. In: Thyroid tumours, 2nd edn. Paris: Editions Nucleon, 2003: 127–146.

26. UICC–AJCC. TNM classification of malignant tumours, 5th edn. Head and neck tumours, thyroid gland. New York: Wiley, 1997: 48.

27. UICC–AJCC. TNM classification of malignant tumours, 6th edn. Head and neck tumours, thyroid gland. New York: Wiley, 2003: 52.

28. Rhys E, Pracy JP, Vini L, A'Hern, Harmer C. Selective neck dissection or simple nodal excision in the management of cervical metastases from differentiated carcinoma of the thyroid. Presented at 5th International Conference on Head and Neck Cancer, San Francisco 2000. Abstract Book. Sponsored by the American Head and Neck Society; p. 67.

29. Hay ID, Bergstrahl EJ, Grant CS, et al. Impact of surgery on outcome in 300 patients with pathologic tumour-node-metastasis stage III papillary thyroid carcinoma treated at one institution from 1940 through 1989. Surgery 1999; 126:1173–1181.

30. Vassilopoulou-Sellin R, Schultz M, Haynie TP. Clinical outcome of patients with papillary thyroid carcinoma who have recurrence after initial radioactive iodine therapy. Cancer 1996; 78:493–501.

31. British Thyroid Association and Royal College of Physicians. Guidelines for the management of thyroid cancer in adults. 2002. www.british-thyroid-association.org.

32. Shah JP. Thyroid and parathyroid glands. Head and neck surgery and oncology, 3rd edn. Edinburgh: Mosby, 2003: 395–437.

33. Vini L, Harmer C. Management of thyroid cancer. Lancet Oncol 2002; 3:407–414.

34. Khoo ML, Freeman JL. Transcervical superior mediastinal lymphadenectomy in the management of papillary thyroid carcinoma. Head Neck 2003; 25:10–14.

35. Kelemen PR, Van Herle AJ, Giuliano AE. Sentinel lymphadenectomy in thyroid malignant neoplasms. Arch Surg 1998; 133:288–292.

36. Pingpank JF, Sasson AR, Hanlon AL, Friedman CD, Ridge JA. Tumour above the spinal accessory nerve in papillary thyroid cancer that involves lateral neck nodes. A common occurrence. Arch Otol Head Neck Surg 2002; 128:1275–1278.

37. Watkinson JC, Gaze MN, Wilson JA. Thyroid. Tumours of the thyroid and parathyroid glands. In: Stell and Maran's head and neck surgery, 4th edn. Oxford: Butterworth Heinemann, 2000: 459–485.

38. Zaja JM, Gluckman JL. Lymphadenectomy for thyroid cancer. In: Johnson JT, Gluckman JL (eds) Carcinoma of the Thyroid. Oxford: Isis Medical Media, 1999: 75–80.

39. Schlumberger M, Pacini F. Follow up: Lessons from the past. In: Thyroid tumours, 2nd edn. Paris: Editions Nucleon, 2003: 147–164.

14

Complications of Thyroid Surgery

Thomas W.J. Lennard

The concept of patient choice, informed consent, and risk management is now embedded in surgical practice. The greater availability of information for patients through use of the internet and the wider acceptance and recognition by surgeons of the need to have careful discussions about the pros and cons of surgery for each patient, coupled with the ever increasing threat of medicolegal action, have meant that potential complications from surgery receive much greater prominence in the 21st century than they did in the 20th century.

Through audit, clinical governance, and risk management information, the complications and consequences of surgery have gained increased prominence and now assume equal importance alongside the intended benefits of an operation.

Complication rates associated with thyroid surgery and the consequences of thyroid surgery can be evaluated through follow-up data, local and national audit initiatives (e.g. the British Association of Endocrine Surgeons Audit), and analyses of case series. When obtaining consent for a procedure and in the approach to the final decision to move to an operation, patients should be given information about commonly occurring complications, which enables them to make their decision as to whether or not to proceed based upon a realistic understanding of the complications and the likely outcome of the operation.

Cosmetic Implications

Patients should be advised about the scar, which will usually be a transverse cervicotomy performed in a skin crease, either with subcuticular absorbable stitches or with metal clips [1]. In most patients the scar will leave a fine line similar to a crease in the neck, but in some cases broadening of the scar and keloid formation can occur. There may be some local reduction in sensation in the upper or lower skin flaps, which will gradually improve over the first 9 months postoperatively, and there may be redundant skin if there has been an extremely large goiter. Wound infection following thyroid surgery is very uncommon [2]. Tethering of the skin of the neck to the underlying laryngeal cartilage or trachea can occur, resulting in movement of the neck skin on swallowing or talking, but this is an uncommon complication and can be minimized by anatomical closure of the wound at the end of the operation.

Replacement Therapy

Patients undergoing total thyroidectomy should be aware that they will need thyroid hormone replacement therapy. This life-long therapy may alternate between the use of triiodothyronine (T_3) and levothyroxine (T_4) depending on the need for postoperative scans in the follow-up period. Patients need to be warned that cessation of thyroid hormone replacement therapy will result in hypothyroidism in approximately 10 days in the case of T_3 and approximately 1 month in the case of T_4.

Further Surgery and General Complications

Patients who are undergoing a diagnostic thyroid lobectomy for a suspicious lesion should be advised if the diagnosis of carcinoma is confirmed that a contralateral lobectomy will almost certainly be required. The above may be considered consequences of thyroid surgery rather than true complications but nevertheless these are important issues that should be discussed with the patient prior to consent and operation. In addition, the general complications or consequences of any operation should be explained: namely risks associated with general anesthesia, the already mentioned very small risk of wound infection, chest infections, deep vein thrombosis, and pulmonary emboli.

Specific complications related to surgery on the thyroid include the risks of bleeding and the specific consequences of this in the neck, changes to the voice after thyroid surgery, and hypoparathyroidism.

Hemorrhage

Bleeding in the neck after thyroid surgery can lead to compromise of the airway and it is therefore a potentially very serious complication. The overall incidence of bleeding in the neck reported in the literature is around 1.2% of cases [2] and although thyroid surgeons would probably feel that patients with thyrotoxicosis and large multinodular goiters are more likely to bleed postoperatively than those with thyroid carcinoma, this is not borne out in the literature [3].

Meticulous attention to detail at the operation with careful identification and control of the main vessels supplying and draining the thyroid will minimize the risk of bleeding. The placement of drains into the operative site will not influence the risk of bleeding, will not always ensure that bleeding is declared by blood passing into the drain before it becomes clinically critical, and may mislead the surgeon and nursing staff into thinking that bleeding is not happening if the drain is empty. On the other hand, occasionally drains will allow a prompt diagnosis of bleeding in the neck and will relieve pressure within the neck around the airway if the blood preferentially passes into the drain. A large dead space left in the neck following the removal of a large goiter would be a common indication for leaving a drain in place, usually a closed suction drain. It is important that the postoperative reception areas and wards are alert to the possibility of bleeding in the neck and its early signs and symptoms. Swelling in the neck, restlessness, stridor or noisy breathing should all be promptly reported to the medical staff. The early recognition and management of bleeding in the neck is essential. Airway compromise from laryngotracheal compression from wound bleeding requires surgical evacuation of the hematoma in the neck as a matter of urgency. The incidence of bleeding in the neck does not seem to be related to the number of operations performed by a surgeon on a regular basis, but is more closely related to the surgeon's training in thyroid surgery [4].

It is not known whether the accepted increased risk of bleeding consequent upon the use of low dose anticoagulants as part of thrombo prophylaxis is an added risk in neck surgery but some thyroid surgeons will avoid any medication which may interfere with blood clotting whilst others are not concerned by this. Prospective data on this important question are required.

Postoperative Calcium Changes

Malfunction of the parathyroid glands following thyroid surgery is explained on the basis of their anatomical and vascular relationship with the thyroid gland. The parathyroid glands are most commonly close to the posterior and lateral aspect of the thyroid gland and share their blood supply with the thyroid. It is therefore incumbent upon the thyroid surgeon to accurately identify the parathyroid glands at the time of the operation and to preserve and protect them when possible. When the parathyroid glands are not closely adherent to the thyroid they can by gently swept away from it laterally, allowing them to maintain their blood supply and be left in situ in the neck. If the glands are lying high up the thyroid or have been displaced by a grossly enlarged thyroid and they cannot be preserved with their blood supply, then it may be necessary to autotransplant them, most commonly into the sternomastoid muscle to preserve parathyroid function [5]. The technique of capsular dissection of the thyroid, whereby the blood supply to the thyroid gland is secured very close to the edge of the gland, as opposed to the main trunk of the superior or inferior thyroid arteries, should minimize devascularization of the parathyroid glands [6]. Extensive lymph node involvement secondary to thyroid carcinoma, very large goiters, and parathyroid glands that are intimately attached to or associated with the thyroid gland can all make preservation of parathyroid function more difficult. Nevertheless it is estimated that normal parathyroid function can be achieved by one third of one normal parathyroid gland alone [7], so if it is impossible to preserve all of the parathyroids every effort should be made to protect and preserve at least one.

Hypoparathyroidism after total thyroidectomy is an important complication and it can be treated by replacement therapy (calcium supplements orally or intravenously and/or the use of 1α-colecalciferol). Permanent hypoparathyroidism rates quoted in the literature range from 0.7% to 3% of operations [2] but the incidence of temporary hypoparathyroidism may be as high as 15% of patients when total thyroidectomy has been performed. All patients should therefore be warned that low serum calcium may occur after total thyroidectomy and that this complication will be monitored from the first day after operation onwards until such time as the calcium is stable and in the normal range. In some units there is a policy of immediately starting calcium supplements postoperatively on all patients to facilitate early discharge and avoid the distressing symptoms of hypocalcemia. In the postoperative period the calcium supplements and cholecalciferol are gradually withdrawn and the vast majority of patients will not require them within 3 months.

Postoperative Voice Change

Voice change and dysphagia can occur after surgery to the thyroid gland. Dysphagia is reported in up to 1.4% of patients and should be mentioned in the preoperative discussions [2]. Voice change is reported in the literature and through national audits as being permanent in about 1% of the patients due to recurrent laryngeal nerve damage on one side and in approximately 3.7% due to damage to the superior laryngeal nerve [8]. Careful voice studies demonstrate both improvement and deficiencies in voice quality after thyroid surgery and the more sophisticated the investigative tools used to analyze voice change after thyroidectomy the more disturbance in function can be found (albeit usually subclinical) [9]. Overall, though, patients should be told and warned that permanent voice hoarseness and change in voice quality will occur in approximately 1% of first time thyroid operations due to recurrent laryngeal nerve damage. There is an often quoted transient voice change at double this rate but spontaneous improvement does occur and this is presumably due to neurapraxia of the recurrent laryngeal nerve. In roughly 0.4% of patients bilateral recurrent nerve damage will occur, resulting in the need for tracheostomy and security of the airway beneath the vocal cords. While unilateral recurrent laryngeal nerve or superior laryngeal nerve damage may lead to a significant reduction in the quality of voice, bilateral damage is of course far more consequential. A variety of procedures can be performed to fix and attempt to correct vocal cord position, but generally speaking these should not be attempted for 6 months after the operation in order to allow time for spontaneous improvement. It is, however, important to start voice rehabilitation early (within 2–3 weeks) in all cases of vocal cord paralysis.

Damage from nerve injuries can be reduced to a minimum if the nerves are routinely located during the operation and traced to the inlet of the lower pharyngeal constrictor muscle. Unipolar diathermy should be avoided in close proximity to the nerve and care should be taken to look for evidence of a non-recurrent laryngeal nerve, particularly on the right side of the neck where it may occur in 1% of individuals, taking an abnormal route through the neck and thereby being more vulnerable to misidentification and damage [10]. In some centers direct stimulation of the nerve and monitoring of vocal cord activity by an electrode placed in the endotracheal tube is used but this is not a widely employed application at the present time [11].

Superior laryngeal nerve injuries are often underestimated, as the clinical effects of damage to this nerve are more difficult to distinguish both for the patient and for the clinician. A lowered voice tone, early fatigue of the voice, and in singers difficulty in reaching the same notes as before operation may be observed. Minimizing damage to the superior laryngeal nerve can be achieved by retracting the upper pole of the thyroid laterally before isolating its vascular pedicle and by securing the vascular pedicle very close to the thyroid gland.

Reoperations

The above complications with their quoted incidence and etiology are all significantly increased in revision surgery where scarring and recurrent pathology will significantly hinder the careful anatomical identification of structures within the neck [12]. Few if any accurate data exist regarding complications in this setting and each individual case will of course be different depending upon the patient's previous surgery and pathology.

Audit

Each surgeon should critically evaluate his or her own complication rates and compare these to those reported by national and international specialist associations and societies. An informed discussion can then take place with the patient preoperatively so that all parties have a realistic expectation of the outcome and risks involved [13].

References

1. Reed MR, Lennard TWJ. Prospective randomized trial of clips versus subcuticular polydioxanone for neck wound closure. Br J Surg 1997; 84:118.
2. Rosato L, Avenia N, Bernante P, et al. Complications of thyroid surgery: Analysis of a multi centric study on 14,934 patients operated on in Italy over 5 years. World J Surg 2004; 28:271–276.
3. Bron LP, O'Brien CJ. Total thyroidectomy for clinically benign disease of the thyroid. Br J Surg 2004; 91:569–574.
4. Gough IR. Total thyroidectomy: indications, technique and training. Aust N Z J Surg 1992; 62:87–89.
5. Henry JF, Denizot A, Audiffret J. Autotransplantation parathyroidienne de nécessité en chirurgie thyroidienne. Ann Chir 1990; 44:378–381.
6. Reeve T, Thompson NW. Complications of thyroid surgery: how to avoid them, how to manage them and observations on their possible effect on the whole patient. World J Surg 2000; 24:971–975.
7. Sasson AR, Pingpank JF, Wetherington RW, et al. Incidental parathyroidectomy during thyroid surgery does not cause transient symptomatic hypocalcaemia. Arch Otolaryngol Head Neck Surg 2001; 127:304–308.
8. Cernea CR, Ferraz AR, Furlani J, et al. Identification of the external branch of the superior laryngeal nerve during thyroidectomy. Am J Surg 1992; 164:634–639.
9. Carding PN. Voice pathology in the UK. BMJ 2003; 327:514–515.
10. Henry JF, Audiffret J, Denizot A. The non recurrent inferior laryngeal nerve: review of 33 cases including 2 on the left side. Surgery 1988; 104:977–984.
11. Hemmerling TM, Schmidt J, Bosert C, et al. Intraoperative monitoring of the recurrent laryngeal nerve in 151 consecutive patients undergoing thyroid surgery. Anesth Analg 2001; 93:396–399.
12. Reeve TS, Delbridge L, Cohen A, Crummer P. Total thyroidectomy: the preferred option for multi nodular goitre. Ann Surg 1987; 106:782–786.
13. Lennard TWJ. Surgery for thyroid cancer. Surg Oncol 1996; 5:103–105.

Section IV

Non-surgical Management of Differentiated Thyroid Cancer

15

Non-surgical Management of Thyroid Cancer

Masud S. Haq and Clive Harmer

Ablation of Residual Normal Thyroid Tissue

In the management of differentiated thyroid cancer (DTC) ablation of thyroid remnants with ^{131}I aims to destroy all residual normal thyroid tissue. Total (or near-total) thyroidectomy will permit this to be achieved with a modest administered activity. Remnant ablation after lobectomy is more difficult and a repeat administration may be required. Ablation of a large remnant may cause radiation thyroiditis with neck pain and swelling. Furthermore thyroid-stimulating hormone (TSH) levels may fail to rise above 30 mU/L following hormone withdrawal, resulting in suboptimal ^{131}I uptake.

The advantages of remnant ablation are that it permits subsequent identification by iodine whole-body scan (WBS) of any residual or metastatic carcinoma and facilitates interpretation of serial serum thyroglobulin (Tg) monitoring [1] (Figure 15.1). A large remnant may show a star burst artifact on WBS, obscuring tumor uptake in abnormal cervical nodes. Measurement of stimulated Tg is also facilitated following remnant ablation, and represents the most sensitive method of detecting recurrence [2–4]. Remnant ablation also destroys microscopic metastases; several retrospective studies have documented decreases in both local recurrence and death from thyroid cancer [5,6]. The benefit of ^{131}I ablation is seen mainly in patients who are at high risk of recurrence, including those with larger tumors, extrathyroidal extension, involved lymph nodes, and residual disease [7,8]. However, in low risk patients and especially in those with microcarcinoma, prognosis is so favorable after surgery alone that little further benefit is achieved [9].

Mazzaferri and Kloos retrospectively studied 1510 patients without distant metastases. Remnant ablation was found to be an independent variable that reduced cancer recurrence, distant recurrence, and cancer death rates [10,11]. Other studies have demonstrated similar results [12].

Total (or near-total) thyroidectomy followed by radioiodine ablation is considered to be the ideal treatment for high risk tumors. However, ^{131}I ablation remains possible following hemithyroidectomy. Bal et al. studied 93 patients with DTC and evaluated the role of radioiodine ablation in patients following hemithyroidectomy [13]. They were evaluated with a diagnostic ^{131}I WBS, 48-hour neck uptake, and Tg measurement following 4–6 weeks withdrawal of thyroxine. The thyroid lobe was successfully ablated in 57% of patients after one ablation dose of [131]I (mean activity 1.18 ± 0.4 GBq, 31.8 ± 11.7 mCi) and 92% after two ablation doses (mean activity 1.5 ± 0.51 GBq, 40.5 ± 13.8 mCi). Hoyes et al. have also demonstrated successful lobar ablation following 3.5 GBq [131]I (95 mCi): 98% of patients treated by total thyroidectomy were successfully ablated by one ^{131}I treatment, compared with 90% after lobectomy ($P < 0.05$) [14]. Ablation of an intact

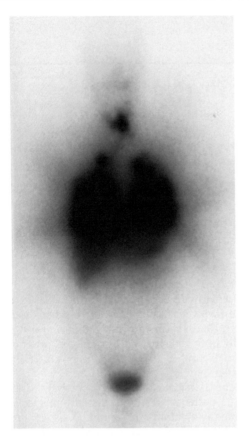

Figure 15.1 Postablation whole-body ^{131}I scan (anterior image). Focal uptake is displayed in the left side of neck. Additional uptake is visible in the apices but more diffusely in both lung fields compatible with extensive pulmonary metastases.

lobe therefore remains possible and can be achieved with moderate activities of radioiodine. It remains an alternative for patients refusing completion thyroidectomy or for those in whom a second operation is contraindicated.

The optimal activity of ^{131}I required to achieve successful ablation is controversial, with doses ranging from 0.85 to 9.5 GBq (23 to 257 mCi) having been advocated. Many centers in North America previously used 1.1 GBq (30 mCi) to ablate small thyroid remnants in order to avoid hospital admission. Administration of a lesser activity has the advantage of lower whole-body radiation exposure, lower cost, and patient convenience. Beierwaltes' philosophy of high dose ablation was based on the premise that it not only ablates normal remnants but also treats possible micrometastatic

deposits [15]. He also stressed the importance of delivering a high radiation dose from the first iodine administration because the biological half-life of subsequent administrations falls, therefore reducing the radiation dose delivered. Samuel and Rajashekharrao also support high initial dose rates to achieve successful ablation [16] but there has been no prospective randomized trial to substantiate these proposals. Proponents of high activity ablation argue that lesser activities are less effective at treating micrometastases, leading to higher recurrence rates. However, Mazzaferri and Jhiang found no difference in long-term recurrence rates (7% versus 9% after median follow-up of 14.7 years) between low dose (29–50 mCi) and high dose (51–200 mCi) ^{131}I remnant ablation [10].

In 1976, McCowen et al. first reported that doses of 3–3.7 GBq were no more effective than 1.1 GBq and this has been confirmed by other retrospective analyses [17]. Despite numerous studies evaluating low dose ablation, one meta-analysis found that a single administered activity of 1074–1110 MBq (29–30 mCi) was more likely to be unsuccessful in fully ablating thyroid remnants compared to higher activities of 2775–3700 MBq [18]. Of 13 studies evaluated, 518 patients were low dose and 449 were high dose. The average failure of a single low dose was 46% versus 27% for high dose ablation ($P < 0.01$).

Bal et al. performed the first prospective randomized clinical trial to evaluate the optimal ^{131}I ablation dose in 149 patients and demonstrated that increasing the administered activity beyond 1.85 GBq (50 mCi) resulted in plateauing of the dose–response curve; a radiation absorbed dose greater than 300 Gy to the thyroid remnant did not appear to yield a higher ablation rate [19]. Successful ablation was defined as the absence of any detectable radioiodine-concentrating tissue in a diagnostic 5 mCi ^{131}I scan at 6 to 12 months (following discontinuation of thyroxine 4–6 weeks before), neck uptake of less than 0.2%, and a Tg level of less than 10 µg/L. Overall successful ablation was achieved in 78% of thyroid remnants. Their more recent study assessed the smallest possible effective dose for remnant ablation [20] in a randomized prospective trial with different ablation activities between 15 mCi up to 50 mCi. In 509 eligible patients the overall ablation rate was 77.6%. The successful ablation rate was statistically different in patients receiving less than 25 mCi ^{131}I compared with those receiving at least 25 mCi (63 of 102, 61.8%, versus 332 of 407, 81.6%, $P = 0.006$). There was no significant inter-group difference in outcome among patients receiving 25–50 mCi of [131]I. However, patients receiving at least 25 mCi ^{131}I had a three times better chance of remnant ablation than patients receiving lesser activities.

Maxon et al. individualized administered activity to deliver a radiation dose of 300 Gy to the thyroid remnants and reported an 81% ablation rate, with no apparent gain from using a dose greater than 300 Gy. Further evaluation of different administered activities with a large randomized prospective trial is required with ablation success rates and recurrence as the main outcome measures (Table 15.1) [21,22].

Sodium iodide ^{131}I is available in the form of a capsule, liquid preparation, or intravenous injection. The capsule is most commonly used due to safety and ease of handling. Four weeks after total thyroidectomy, by which time the TSH level will be above 30 mU/L, we recommend an ablation dose of 3 to 3.7 GBq (111 to 137 mCi) [131]I to all patients after total thyroidectomy except for children over 10 years of age with small node-negative tumors and young patients with unifocal microcarcinoma [6,23] (Figure 15.2). This delivers a mean absorbed dose of 410 Gy and ablates 75% of remnants [24]. An ^{131}I WBS is obtained after 3 days, when the patient is usually allowed to return home, subject to the total body radioactivity having fallen below the permitted level. In the USA, patients treated with ^{131}I are usually permitted to go home, providing certain conditions are met. Replacement thyroid hormone is then commenced in the form of triiodothyronine (liothyronine, T_3) 20 mcg three times a day. A blood sample is taken on the day of iodine

administration to confirm TSH elevation and also on day 6 to measure the protein bound (PBI) [131]I level [25].

Regulations for use of radioiodine remain extremely variable throughout the world, although there is general acceptance of the basic protection measures. Treatment must be carried out in a protected environment (single-bedded shielded room with ensuite bathroom and toilet) approved for this purpose by the local radiation protection advisor. Written and oral information should be given to patients before treatment. Prior to therapy, pregnancy must be excluded in women of childbearing age. Because the concentration of ^{131}I in maternal milk is significant, breastfeeding is strictly contraindicated for 4 months after administration.

Patients are reviewed 6 weeks after ablation with results of hematology, biochemistry, TSH, Tg, and ablation WBS. Provided the latter demonstrates uptake in only a small thyroid remnant, a stimulated Tg obtained either following withdrawal of T_3 for 10–14 days or following use of recombinant TSH injections while continuing suppression therapy is measured 4 to 6 months postablation [26,27]. If this stimulated Tg level is ≤2 μg/L, patients can be reviewed annually and the patient switched to thyroxine at an average daily dose of 200 mcg in order to suppress TSH secretion to a level of less than 0.1 mU/L [2,28]. Follow-up assessment comprises clinical examination and monitoring of free T_3, TSH, and Tg levels but we do not perform diagnostic iodine scans routinely except in patients with anti-Tg antibodies [29]. In the past, a diagnostic WBS with 150–185 MBq (4–5 mCi) [131]I was performed at 4–6 months to determine the success of remnant ablation but this is no longer standard practice. If the postablation scan demonstrates significant uptake in the thyroid bed or elsewhere (cervical node or

Table 15.1 Summary results of a systematic review of randomized trials of radioiodine ablation. Percentage of patients who had successful ablation according to administered activity (patient number in parentheses)

Study	30 mCi (1.1 GBq)	50 mCi (1.8 GBq)	90 or 100 mCi (3.7 GBq)
Creutzig 1987 [124]	50 (5/10)		60 (6/10)
Johansen 1991 [125]	58 (21/36)		52 (14/27)
Bal et al. 1996 [19]	63 (17/27)	78 (42/54)	74 (28/38)
Sirisalipoch 2004 [126]		65 (41/63)	89 (67/75)
Bal et al. 2004 [20]	83 (61/73)	82 (63/77)	
Combined	71 (104/146)	75 (146/194)	77 (115/150)
Test for difference between the percentages	$P = 0.01$	$P = 0.06$	$P < 0.001$

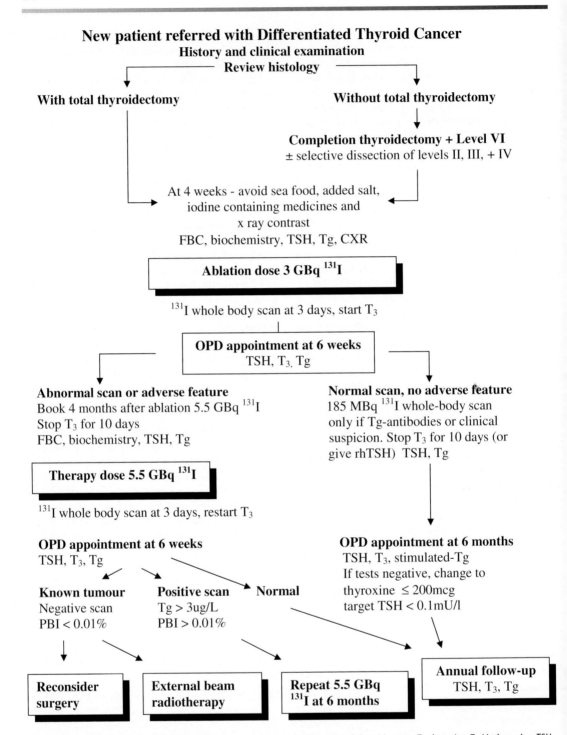

Figure 15.2 Royal Marsden Hospital policy for the management of differentiated thyroid cancer. T_4, thyroxine; T_3, Liothyronine; TSH, thyroid-stimulating hormone; CXR, chest radiograph; FBC, full blood count; Tg, thyroglobulin; PBI, protein-bound radioactive iodine concentration; rhTSH, recombinant TSH (thyrogen).

distant metastasis) further investigation is required. A CT scan without contrast or preferably an enhanced MRI of the neck plus mediastinum ± CT of the lungs ± bone scintigraphy will clarify the extent and distribution of disease suitable for further neck surgery, metastasectomy, or radioiodine therapy.

Typical postablation scans demonstrate normal physiological uptake of iodine within the salivary glands, gastrointestinal tract, and bladder. Occasionally, false-positive ^{131}I wholebody scans may occur [30]. These may be seen with esophageal retention of salivary secretions, gut motility disorders such as Meckel's diverticulum, malformations of the urinary tract, pathological transudates or exudates, inflammatory or infectious lesions, specific organ uptake such as in breast, liver or thymus, tumors containing thyroid tissue such as struma ovarii or teratoma, and lung or abdominal adenocarcinoma.

To optimize radioiodine uptake by both residual normal thyroid and cancer, TSH stimulation is mandatory and dietary iodine should be restricted for one month before and for several days after ablation. Dietary restriction of iodine intake to 50 µg per day can increase the ^{131}I uptake twofold after ablation [31]. Iodized salt, dairy products, eggs, and seafood should be avoided [32]. Iodine-rich contrast media must also be avoided and T_3 tablets omitted for 2 weeks; any patient on thyroxine would need to discontinue these tablets 4 weeks prior to ablation. As an alternative to thyroid hormone withdrawal patients may be prepared for remnant ablation with recombinant TSH (rhTSH, Thyrogen, Genzyme). Robbins et al. reported that successful remnant ablation can be achieved after two injections of 0.9 mg of rhTSH [33]. Their retrospective study compared the rate of complete ablation in 42 patients prepared with thyroid hormone withdrawal and 45 patients with rhTSH. Successful ablation was comparable in both groups (81% versus 84%, no statistical difference). However, Pacini et al. demonstrated contrasting results [34] in a prospective study using 30 mCi ^{131}I during thyroid hormone therapy. Patients were treated while hypothyroid ($n = 50$), hypothyroid with rhTSH stimulation ($n = 42$), or euthyroid on thyroid hormone therapy with rhTSH stimulation ($n = 70$). Outcome was assessed by a 4 mCi diagnostic ^{131}I WBS following conventional thyroid

hormone withdrawal. The rate of successful ablation was similar in the hypothyroid and hypothyroid plus rhTSH groups (84% and 78.5%, respectively) but significantly lower (54%) in the euthyroid plus rhTSH group.

Recombinant TSH remains unlicensed in the UK for ablation or therapy but is available for diagnostic iodine WBS and stimulated Tg. It remains expensive but markedly improves patient quality of life, which is otherwise severely impaired during the prolonged period of hypothyroidism [35]. We recommend its routine use for diagnostic purposes and for ablation or therapy in patients unable to produce TSH, and especially those in whom thyroid hormone withdrawal is medically contraindicated. This includes patients with cardiac disease, psychiatric disorders, postpartum, hypopituitarism, and patients unable to tolerate prolonged hypothyroidism [36,37]. Patient groups are campaigning for its routine use in diagnosis and therapy but cost and licensing restriction currently make wider availability impracticable in the UK. Thyrogen is well tolerated but may occasionally cause nausea or transient headache. Contraindications to its use are brain or spinal metastases as cerebral edema or cord compression may occur.

Differentiated thyroid cancer is common in women of childbearing age. Population-based studies have suggested that up to 10% of thyroid cancers occurring in women during their reproductive years are diagnosed in pregnancy or in the first year after giving birth. Outcome remains favorable with prognosis of DTC discovered in pregnancy similar to that occurring in nonpregnant women of similar age [38]. A small retrospective study of nine patients from the Royal Marsden Hospital assessed outcome during pregnancy [39]. Four were discovered at antenatal assessment to have a thyroid nodule; the reminder had a thyroid lump in the neck. In all cases, the thyroid nodule was reported to double in size during pregnancy. One patient had a subtotal thyroidectomy during the second trimester; eight were operated on within 3–10 months from delivery (five total thyroidectomy, 4 subtotal thyroidectomy). Eight patients remained disease free but one patient who had radioiodine treatment delayed due to a further pregnancy died 7 years later from distant metastases. For tumors discovered early in pregnancy, total thyroidectomy can be performed safely during the mid-trimester, while those found later can be managed after delivery. Radioiodine ablation can be deferred until after the pregnancy and breastfeeding, although should not be delayed for more than a year.

Thyroid cancer is discovered in 1–4% of patients undergoing surgery for hyperthyroidism due to Graves' disease or multinodular goiter [40]. In most patients the tumors are small or microscopic and no further treatment is required. For larger tumors, multiple foci, or involved lymph nodes, completion thyroidectomy plus ablation should be considered.

Carcinoma of the thyroid is rare in children, although the incidence in Europe has increased as a result of exposure to radioactive fallout from Chernobyl [41]. Tumors are usually papillary and often of advanced local stage. More have metastatic disease at presentation and a higher proportion of disease-related deaths occur on prolonged follow-up, compared with adults [42]. Children under the age of 10 years are at higher risk of recurrence and should be treated with total thyroidectomy, paratracheal node dissection ± selective neck dissection, and radioiodine.

TSH Suppression

Following successful ablation, life-long thyroxine at a dose adequate to suppress TSH levels to <0.1 mU/L is recommended. Recurrence rates including distant relapse are significantly reduced with TSH suppression [10,43]. There is no evidence that undetectable TSH levels offer any advantage over low but detectable levels. Monitoring the free thyroxine level in the athyroid patient receiving exogenous thyroxine will give a false high value because of binding and can be confusing. We therefore favor monitoring of the free T_3 level, in order to avoid hyperthyroidism. The long-term effects of subclinical thyrotoxicosis on the heart and bone are of greater importance in elderly patients as a low TSH maybe associated with arrhythmias [44]. However, prognosis is worse in older patients, such that TSH suppression is usually advisable. When the diagnosis has been made many years previously and the recurrence-free interval is long, relaxation of the need for TSH suppression is permissible.

Follow-up

The aim of follow-up is early detection of residual tumor or recurrence, which affects 20% of patients. Following total thyroidectomy and remnant ablation, serum Tg measurement has become the gold standard for early detection of recurrent DTC [45]. Thyroglobulin is a glycoprotein produced by normal and neoplastic follicular cells. Modern immunoradiometric assays based on monoclonal antibodies offer a functional sensitivity of 1 μg/L or even lower. Provided there is no residual or recurrent disease, in most patients the Tg concentration will be below the limit of detection under thyrotropin suppression. However, 2–7% of patients have a detectable but low concentration (<3 μg/L); the concentration maybe up to 10 μg/L if iodine ablation has been omitted. Provided that it remains low and no rising trend is noted, recurrence is unlikely [46]. An undetectable serum Tg that does not rise in response to TSH stimulation is found in patients who are disease free, whereas a rising Tg is associated with the presence of residual normal thyroid or tumor recurrence [47]. Persistent disease is unlikely when serum Tg values are less than 2 μg/L after rhTSH stimulation or thyroxine withdrawal [2]. However, serum Tg concentrations are more difficult to interpret when there is a large thyroid remnant as values will be raised. In cases of very high Tg concentrations, a "hook effect" may occur; the sample should be diluted and reassayed to give a true value.

The major limitation of serial Tg monitoring is potential interference from antibodies to thyroglobulin (TgAbs); an undetectable concentration in the presence of antibodies is not reliable [48]. Antibodies are present in up to 25% of patients with DTC compared to 10% of the general population. They must be measured in the same serum sample used for the Tg assay. A recovery test should be performed in all samples that have a positive TgAb titer. The recovery of Tg in the test sample can indicate the possible degree of interference. A value less than 70% suggests definite interference. Studies have demonstrated the correlation of a rising TgAb level with tumor recurrence and disappearance of TgAb with successful treatment [49]. In the absence of TgAbs, serial Tg monitoring provides an invaluable guide for early detection of recurrent or metastatic carcinoma. A diagnostic ^{131}I WBS (following thyroid hormone withdrawal or under rhTSH stimulation) and neck ultrasonography may be helpful if recurrence is suspected. Because recurrence may occur more than 40 years after initial treatment, follow-up must be life-long, with annual clinical examination and measurement of Tg.

Treatment of Recurrent and Metastatic Disease

Recurrence in the thyroid bed or cervical lymph nodes develops in 5–20% of patients with DTC. Surgery is the dominant treatment for locoregional recurrence and complete resection should be attempted. Selective dissection is preferable to single lymph node excision. Even if tumor cannot be completely removed, surgical debulking is beneficial and facilitates subsequent use of therapeutic radioiodine [5]. External beam radiotherapy (EBRT) can control local disease but the full potential of iodine treatment should first be exploited. Repeat doses of radioiodine may be required with each administered activity ranging from 3.7 to 10.1 GBq (100 to 270 mCi) at 3–12-month intervals. There is no maximum limit to the cumulative ^{131}I dose that can be given to patients with persistent disease if benefit can be documented, providing that individual doses do not exceed 2 Gy total body exposure and there is at least a 6-month interval between doses. A normal blood count must be confirmed prior to each administration and impairment of renal function would demand a lower dose.

The British Thyroid Association recommends withdrawal of thyroxine (T$_4$) 4 weeks before radioiodine, or triiodothyronine (T$_3$) 2 weeks before so that endogenous TSH levels rise to above 30 mU/L, thereby optimizing iodine uptake [50]. This will induce symptomatic hypothyroidism, which may result in lethargy, cognitive impairment, or depression. Quality of life may be significantly impaired and many patients are unable to drive or work. This symptomatic period may be shortened by substitution of T$_3$ for T$_4$ 4 weeks with discontinuation of T$_3$ 14 days prior to admission. If patients are unable to tolerate hypothyroidism, ^{131}I may be given following rhTSH stimulation, with continuation of thyroid hormone replacement, although it remains unlicensed for this purpose. Retention of radioiodine is reduced due to rapid clearance in the euthyroid state, whereas renal excretion is reduced when thyroid hormone withdrawal is performed [51]. This may result in higher activities of radioiodine being necessary for therapy with rhTSH[34].

A retrospective audit of Royal Marsden Hospital practice of thyroid hormone withdrawal prior to ^{131}I administration has recently been performed as we normally discontinue T$_4$ for only 21 days and T$_3$ for only 10 days. Of 95 patients who stopped thyroid hormone as we advised, 80/95 (84%) had TSH levels above 30 mU/L and uptake appeared to be adequate in the remainder. Based on these results our current practice remains unchanged, although a prospective study to assess the optimal period of withdrawal is required.

A whole-body scan 2–6 days after iodine administration provides scintigraphic assessment of disease and response to treatment. Diagnostic scans using a tracer dose of ^{131}I are not required prior to therapy and may have an adverse effect by causing tumor stunning and reducing the uptake of therapeutic [131]I [52]. Furthermore, in a significant proportion of patients with residual tumor as evidenced by an elevated Tg level, uptake has been documented in the posttherapy scan despite a prior negative diagnostic scan. The use of ^{123}I as a scanning agent has been suggested to prevent stunning because of its short half-life [53]. However, it remains expensive and not widely available.

The real benefit of iodine ablation is well documented. Mazzaferri and Kloos demonstrated the beneficial effects of ablation in 1510 patients without distant metastases [11]. Radioiodine was an independent variable that favored lower local recurrence ($P < 0.0005$), distant recurrence ($P < 0.0001$) and death ($P < 0.0001$) in patients over 40 with tumors greater than 1.5 cm in diameter. In 1998, a Canadian study of 382 patients with DTC demonstrated total thyroidectomy and ablation to be associated with a significantly lower rate of local relapse independent of tumor stage [12].

The benefit from ^{131}I therapy is more difficult to quantify. Younger patients who have limited volume metastases mainly in the lungs, and who achieve a complete response to ^{131}I, have been shown consistently to have the best prognosis, with a 15-year survival of 89% [54]. In contrast, older patients and those with large metastases or bone involvement are less likely to respond [55]. Although distant metastases may remain stable for years, there is evidence that early treatment benefits outcome. Microscopic foci are more radioresponsive; complete response was reported in 82% of patients with uptake in lung metastases not seen on chest radiography but in only 15% of those with visible micro- or macronodules [21]. The radioresistance of large deposits may be due to poor vascularity, resulting in limited and inhomogeneous iodine distribution, or to the appearance of radioresistance clones. Bone lesions are associated with a low response rate; surgical excision when possible, or external beam radiotherapy should be added [56,57]. We recommend surgical resection with curative intent for patients with a solitary deposit that does not concentrate iodine adequately [58].

Therapeutic efficacy of ^{131}I therapy is related to the ability of tumor to concentrate and retain iodine [59]. The sodium iodide symporter (NIS) is a plasma glycoprotein that actively transports iodide into thyroid follicular cells as the first step in thyroid hormone biosynthesis. Cloning of the gene and the development of specific NIS antibodies have allowed the characterization of the pathogenic role of NIS in thyroid cancer [60]. In tumors that no longer have the capacity to concentrate iodine, reduced NIS expression has been demonstrated. Up to 80% of differentiated thyroid cancers have the ability to concentrate iodine but when tumors are non-iodine avid, despite meticulous patient preparation, further ^{131}I should be avoided [61]. This is more commonly seen in older male patients with poorly differentiated tumors, Hürthle cell variant, and tall cell or insular subtypes [62] (Figure 15.3). Reduced ability to concentrate iodine is often associated with more aggressive growth and metastatic spread (Figure 15.4).

Retinoic acid, a derivative of vitamin A, can enhance NIS expression in vitro [63]. In cell cultures, redifferentiation of thyroid follicular cancer results in increased iodine uptake. Grunwald et al. [64] treated 12 patients with

non-iodine avid tumors with retinoic acid for 2 months prior to radioiodine therapy. In two patients a significant increase in radioiodine uptake was seen, with a further three patients demonstrating faint uptake; seven patients did not benefit. Response was associated with a significant rise in Tg levels, suggesting restoration of Tg synthesis. A more recent study of 25 patients [65] administered retinoic acid (1 mg/kg) for 3 months prior to ^{131}I therapy. Only five patients demonstrated slight increase in ^{131}I uptake but Tg failed to correlate with either success or failure of treatment. Side effects occurred in two thirds of patients comprising sunburn, cheilitis, mucositis, conjunctivitis, and raised transaminases, although all were reversible. The Royal Marsden Hospital prospective trial results were equally disappointing. The initial promise of redifferentiation therapy has therefore not been fulfilled and is no longer recommended.

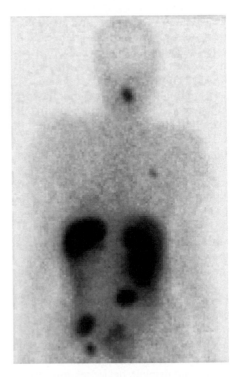

Figure 15.3 Diagnostic indium octreotide scan (posterior view): patient with non-iodine avid Hürthle cell carcinoma previously treated with total thyroidectomy. Octreotide uptake is seen in the neck, right chest, right of midline at L5 level and left pelvis. Pelvic radiotherapy was followed by 4 treatments with yttrium-90 octreotide labeled DOTATOC with good response.

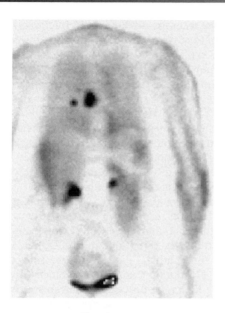

Figure 15.4 Stimulated ^{18}FDG-PET scan: patient with differentiated thyroid cancer and elevated serum thyroglobulin but no demonstrable disease despite ^{131}I whole-body scan, ^{111}In-octreotide scan, and CT neck and chest. A stimulated ^{18}FDG-PET following recombinant TSH demonstrated subcarinal and right hilar uptake.

True Hürthle cell carcinoma (consisting of at least 75% Hürthle cells) is usually differentiated and expresses Tg. In our retrospective series of 50 patients, none of the 20 with recurrent or metastatic disease showed uptake at sites of known disease; alternative treatment comprising further surgery or EBRT was therefore necessary. However, because of its worse prognosis, follow-up of Hürthle carcinoma needs to be diligent and initial ^{131}I ablation is beneficial in rendering Tg monitoring more accurate. In the more recently published series of 89 patients with Hürthle cell carcinoma from the M.D. Anderson Cancer Center [66] those who received ^{131}I ablation had better outcomes. Of the 37 patients with known metastases, 38% showed radioiodine uptake in lymph nodes, bone, or lung.

The effectiveness of ^{131}I therapy could theoretically be improved by increasing radioiodine uptake by tumor or altering tumor metabolism so that iodine retention is prolonged. Administration of a higher activity is the simplest approach but repeated activities greater than the empirical standard of 5.5 GBq are associated with an increased risk of bone marrow suppression, leukemia, lung fibrosis (for patients with miliary metastases), and salivary gland damage; benefit remains unproven. A retrospective study of 38 patients with advanced DTC treated with 9 GBq (243 mCi) ^{131}I, who had previously failed to respond to standard activities of 5.5 GBq (150 mCi) [67], was not advantageous. Complete response was observed in 18% (7/38), stable disease in 11% (4/38), and progressive disease in 71% (27/38). Grade 3 (9.7%) and grade 4 (3.2%) hematological toxicity was limited based on WHO criteria but significant salivary gland morbidity was identified. A persistent dry mouth was present in 30% of individuals with a further 27% complaining of salivary gland swelling and discomfort.

Metastatic tumor may persist despite administration and uptake of repeated doses of ^{131}I. This may be the consequence of rapid turnover of radioiodine (short effective half-life) with discharge before adequate energy has been deposited. The effective half-life in metastases responding to therapy has been shown to be longer than in those not responding: 5.5 days compared with 3.2 days [68].

Lithium carbonate reduces the release rate of radioiodine from normal thyroid as well as from thyroid tumors. Its administration in doses that produce blood levels of 0.8–1.2 mmol/L prolonged the biological half-life in 10 of 12 thyroid tumors, without increasing the radiation dose received by the whole body [69]. However, lithium blood levels need to be monitored closely to avoid toxicity and psychiatric expertise is valuable such that its routine use is often impracticable in many hospitals, although a number of centers in the USA use this tactic, without psychiatric consultation, to increase tumor retention of ^{131}I.

Metastasectomy

Distant metastases develop in 5–23% of patients with DTC and another 1–4% demonstrate distant metastases at presentation [70–72]. Most commonly affected are the lung and bone, with the liver and brain rarely being involved. Despite improved outcome compared with other cancers, at least half of thyroid cancer patients will die of metastatic disease. We have reported overall survival at 5 and 10 years of

63% and 44% [73]. Schlumberger et al. reported similar overall figures of 53% and 38% at 5 and 10 years, respectively [70].

Age has been shown to be a strong predictor of cause-specific survival in numerous retrospective studies, with age less than 40 years associated with improved survival. Age has also been shown to be an independent predictor of survival for metastatic disease, with older age associated with a worse prognosis. Samaan et al. [61] demonstrated a cause-specific survival of 71% versus 16% when comparing patients younger than 40 with those older than 40 ($P < 0.01$) Radioiodine uptake in distant metastases has also been shown to affect prognosis. Schlumberger et al. [74] demonstrated a 10-year survival of 54% and 9% in patients with and without iodine uptake ($P < 0.0001$).

Site and extent of metastatic disease also influence outcome. A 10-year survival of 57% and 27% ($P < 0.0001$) has been reported in lung only and bone only metastases, respectively [70]. Our retrospective study of 111 patients with distant metastases has demonstrated a 10-year cause-specific survival of 42% and 26% for lung only and bone only metastases [75]; tumor involving multiple sites carried a very poor prognosis with none alive at 10 years. In 1979 a 10-year survival rate of 80% was reported in young patients with micronodular disease visible on chest radiograph [76]. More recent data describe a 10-year cause-specific survival of 95% compared to 8% for iodine-avid and non-iodine-avid lung metastases [77].

Less favorable responses are seen in patients with bone metastases [56,57]. Our recent results analysis demonstrates 5- and 10-year cause-specific survivals of 32% and 25%; for patients with isolated bone metastases, for which surgical resection is recommended [78] and orthopedic manipulation may prove beneficial in cases of vertebral collapse. Radioiodine alone is rarely curative as metastases are often bulky and widespread but repeated high activity radioiodine may be of benefit. Petrich et al. described complete remission with high activity therapy (11.1 GBq, 300 mCi ^{131}I) in three out of four patients with up to three bone metastases under the age of 45 years; older subjects with more numerous metastases fared less well [79]. External beam radiotherapy offers significant palliation for bone pain in unresectable lesions. They respond poorly to low dose irradiation

and we recommend 35 Gy in 15 fractions over 3 weeks (or 6 Gy once weekly for up to 4 weeks if brain and spinal cord are not in the target volume). Continuing care and adequate analgesia remain paramount in these patients.

The option of surgery for distant metastases in DTC should not be neglected. Stojadinovic et al. reviewed 260 patients with distant metastases of whom 59 underwent surgery [80]. Those who underwent complete metastasectomy survived longer than those having incomplete resection or no surgical intervention (5-year cause-specific survival 78% versus 43% versus 46%, $P = 0.03$). Our experience of 16 patients with intrathoracic metastases undergoing surgical resection described one postoperative death [58]. Nine patients died of disease (mean survival 37 months) and six remained alive, of whom four were disease free (mean survival 52 months). Five-year cause-specific survival was 32.5%. Surgery should therefore be considered for patients with metastases at any site who fail to benefit from radioiodine therapy because of large size or lack of iodine avidity. An attempt at complete resection is recommended.

Dosimetry

Radioiodine administration has been based on three different approaches: empirical fixed activity, dose limited by safe upper limits of blood dosimetry, and quantitative absorbed tumor dosimetry.

Fixed activities of 1.1–3.7 GBq for remnant ablation and 3.7–7.4 GBq for therapy are based on experience. They are known to be safe and this is the most widely used system but insufficient ^{131}I may be delivered to eradicate tumor [22]. To overcome this problem some centers administer up to 11.1 GBq (300 mCi) in patients with distant metastases [79]. This may be associated with greater toxicity and unnecessary whole-body radiation exposure.

Activities administered within a safe upper limit of blood dose is an alternative method. Radioiodine administration is limited by bone marrow reserve with excessive doses resulting in hematological depression. Benua et al. recommended a maximum upper limit of 2 Gy blood dose [81]. Serious hematological complications were more common when blood doses exceeded 2 Gy compared to administrations below these limits (28% versus 6%, respectively). A number of centers perform this routinely to assist safe ^{131}I administration.

Quantitative tumor dosimetry is the third alternative [68]. The rationale is that tumors have different biological behavior in different individuals which merits ^{131}I treatment on a calculated patient-specific basis (Figure 15.5). Measurement of the absorbed dose in tumor has several advantages. Firstly, overtreatment and overall radiation exposure is kept to a minimum; an absorbed dose can vary widely with fixed activities, from ineffective to excessive. Secondly, it is the best way to determine whether future ^{131}I therapy will be effective, so that treatment can be optimized and unnecessary treatment avoided. The greatest advantage is that adequate doses can be calculated to give the highest probability that tumor will be successfully eradicated [21,22].

Since the early 1970s, many attempts have been made to calculate the radiation dose absorbed by thyroid remnants and metastatic deposits [24]. Three parameters must first be determined: the initial activity (A_o) in the target tissue, the effective half-life of the radioiodine (T_e), and the mass of tissue (m). We use single photon emission computed tomography (SPECT) or positron emission tomography

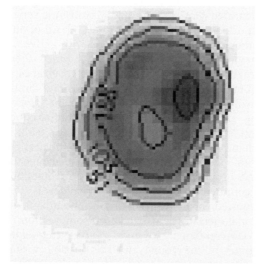

Figure 15.5 Dose map displaying absorbed dose within shoulder metastases from a patient with differentiated thyroid cancer calculated from voxel-based quantitative dosimetry using RMDP (Radionuclide Multimodality Dosimetry Package). Isobars represent varying absorbed doses.

imaging to measure the volume (mass) of metabolically active thyroid tissue or tumor and, after iodine treatment, perform sequential quantitative scans from which activity–time curves can be produced. By fitting the data and extrapolating to the time of administration, the initial activity in the target tissue and the effective half-life of iodine are determined. Calculations are then performed using the medical internal radiation dosimetry (MIRD) formula: D (absorbed dose) = $0.16A_oT_e/m$.

Preliminary analysis of 25 dosimetric studies in patients with metastatic lesions has shown a wide variation of 5 to 621 Gy in the radiation absorbed dose from a fixed administered ^{131}I activity of 5.5 GBq [82]. There was evidence of a dose–response relationship, clearly explaining the spectrum of clinical response. Unfortunately, MIRD calculations are based on several assumptions, in particular that radioactivity is uniformly distributed throughout tumor and that washout of ^{131}I from these tissues is governed by a single exponential function. If these assumptions are inaccurate, errors will be introduced into dosimetry estimates. In addition, errors in each of the other parameters (percentage uptake, target activity, effective half-life, and organ mass) will contribute to a combined error of absorbed dose [83]. Given all the problems with dosimetry and the potential for large errors, it could be questioned whether trying to perform dose calculations is worthwhile. However, with current efforts to produce accurate sequential registered three-dimensional SPECT images and dose–volume histograms of therapy distributions, a greater level of accuracy should be achieved, eventually resulting in improved effectiveness of treatment [84–89].

Complications of Radioiodine Treatment

Radioiodine therapy is well tolerated and usually lacks serious complications. Patients may experience nausea and vomiting, especially during the first 24 hours after administration; prophylactic use of metoclopramide 10 mg 30 minutes prior to ^{131}I is therefore recommended [90]. Radiation thyroiditis may occur within the first week and last for several days after ablation of a large remnant; this is characterized by local discomfort, pain on swallowing, neck swelling, and even transient thyrotoxicosis [91]. Non-steroidal anti-inflammatory drugs such as aspirin are usually effective but corticosteroid treatment with prednisolone 30 mg daily may be required. Very rarely edema of the neck may threaten upper airway obstruction.

The salivary glands accumulate radioiodine and are thereby prone to damage. Salivary dysfunction (xerostomia and sialadenitis) following radioiodine may occur in up to a third of patients and is related to the cumulative activity of ^{131}I administered [92]. Acute sialadenitis affecting the parotid or submandibular salivary glands occurs within 48 hours of administration and may last for a few days but may be protracted. This is more commonly seen with higher administered activities. Chronic symptoms include recurrent salivary tenderness, swelling, dry mouth, and altered (metallic or chemical) taste sensation [93]. Lack of saliva can result in dental caries and teeth may require extraction (Figure 15.6). Several studies have quantified salivary damage by technetium scintigraphy and shown a direct relationship between administered cumulative radioiodine dose and severity of salivary gland dysfunction [92].

A liberal fluid intake, frequent use of sodium citrate containing lozenges and massage over the parotid areas will reduce salivary radiation. Intravenous administration of amifostine, an organic thiophosphate, has been reported to reduce salivary uptake of [131]I. A double-blind placebo-controlled trial comparing 25 patients treated with amifostine to 25 controls identified preservation of salivary gland function in the treated group but knowledge is limited regarding the effects of amifostine on tumor uptake [94]. Further study is therefore required to assess potential benefit before widespread use can be recommended. Sialadenitis of the parotid may progress to a chronic phase with recurrent episodes over several years and a persistent painful salivary mass may require evaluation for surgical removal.

Radiation pneumonitis (acute) and pulmonary fibrosis (chronic) have been reported in patients with diffuse pulmonary metastases following therapeutic radioiodine [95]. Benua et al. reported 5 of 59 patients developing radiation pneumonitis which resulted in two deaths [81]. Single administrations exceeding 9 GBq (243 mCi) may cause both pneumonitis and fibrosis. By limiting individual doses and increasing the interval between administrations to 9–12 months pulmonary complications can be minimized. In all patients with diffuse pulmonary metastases serial lung function testing should be performed and if deterioration occurs, the size of further ^{131}I doses can be reduced. Wide-field external beam therapy should be avoided.

Brain and spinal cord metastases are rare in DTC. In our retrospective series of 649 patients with DTC treated between 1936 and 1991, only six patients with brain metastases were identified (0.92%) [96]. The Mayo Clinic series reported an incidence of 0.75% [97]. All of our patients were papillary tumors with active or previously treated metastases at other sites. Prognosis was poor with median survival of 4 months from the time of diagnosis of brain involvement. Multimodality treatment involving external beam radiotherapy, radioiodine, and surgery should be considered. Cerebral edema may follow radioiodine administration with potential life-threatening consequences and prophylactic dexamethasone is therefore recommended. Similarly, prophylaxis is required prior to radioiodine treatment of spinal metastases to avoid cord compression.

Differentiated thyroid cancer frequently occurs in the young and the possibility that iodine treatment may affect fertility has created significant concern [98]. We have previously reported a study of 496 women under the age of 40 who received radioiodine [99]. Of these, 322 had a single 3 GBq (81 mCi) ablation dose while

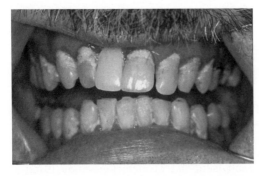

Figure 15.6 Dental caries: multiple radioiodine treatments resulted in severe xerostomia and dental caries. Further radioiodine was refused due to these unwanted side effects.

the remainder received subsequent treatment for residual, recurrent, or metastatic disease (8.5–59 GBq, 230–1591 mCi, cumulative dose). Transient amenorrhea or menstrual irregularities lasting up to 10 months were experienced in 83 patients (17%). No case of permanent ovarian failure was recorded. In patients with amenorrhea, there was a temporary increase in both follicle-stimulating hormone (FSH) and luteinizing hormone (LH) levels indicating transient ovarian dysfunction. Patients experiencing menstrual disturbance had received greater cumulative activities compared to those with normal menses (median cumulative dose 14 GBq versus 3 GBq).

Male patients also develop transient elevation of FSH levels following ^{131}I treatment. In our study of 93 patients, 106 children were fathered by 59 patients; the remainder had no wish to have children [100]. Of these 59, 12 had received a single 3 GBq ablation dose, 19 had been treated with up to 14 GBq, and 28 had received up to 44 GBq. No major malformations were reported. In 14 patients followed prospectively with determination of dose to the testes using thermoluminescent dosimetry, the median dose to each testis was 6.4 cGy following 3 GBq, 14.1 cGy following 5.5 GBq, and 21.2 cGy following 9.2 GBq. There was transient elevation in serum FSH after radioiodine which normalized within 9 months from the last administration. LH levels rose transiently in only two patients. Serum testosterone did not change significantly. The germinal epithelium of the testes is more sensitive to radiation damage than the ovary and male patients likely to require repeated doses of radioiodine should be offered sperm banking because of the potential risk of permanent sterility [101]. A reduction in sperm count proportional to the administered activity may occur but permanent testicular damage with azoospermia appears to be rare.

There is no significant difference in observed fertility rates, birth rates, or premature delivery among women treated with radioiodine compared with those who have not received [131]I. In our series of 496 patients, temporary amenorrhea and minor menstrual irregularities were seen in 20%; 427 normal children were born to 276 women and only one patient was unable to conceive [99]. On the basis of these data there is no reason for patients who are treated with radioiodine to avoid subsequent pregnancy.

However, it is recommended to avoid conception (for both males and females) for at least 4 months after ^{131}I administration, by which time all radiation-induced chromosomal alterations should have been eliminated or repaired. During pregnancy thyroid hormonal levels should be monitored every 2 months and thyroxine replacement increased only if required [39]. Thyroxine requirement may increase during the antenatal period but complete TSH suppression is unnecessary and levels can be permitted to rise into the normal range.

Patients may develop a transient slight reduction in platelet and white cell counts (mainly lymphopenia) after ^{131}I therapy [90], which is of no practical importance. These effects reach a nadir at 5–9 weeks after therapy with recovery in the majority within 6 months. Bloods counts should be monitored before each therapy dose, which is withheld if significant depression is present. Patients with multiple bone metastases, the elderly, and patients previously exposed to external beam irradiation are more prone to bone marrow suppression and demonstrate a more protracted recovery. Myelodysplasia leading to aplastic anemia is rare and likely to occur only in those who have received a very high cumulative blood dose in excess of 2 Gy per treatment [81]. Use of autologous stem cell transplantation may have a potential role in the future prior to planned high activity treatment.

The carcinogenic hazard of ^{131}I in the treatment of thyroid cancer has been the subject of several reports [102]. An increased risk of acute myeloid leukemia was seen in the past, especially in patients receiving a cumulative activity in excess of 40 GBq (1081 mCi), although patient numbers were small [103]. In more recent series the incidence of leukemia is much lower, probably owing to efforts to limit the total blood dose to 2 Gy per treatment and the longer interval of 6–12 months between doses. A recently published multicenter study involving 6841 thyroid cancer patients from Sweden, Italy, and France has quantified the risk of subsequent second primary malignancy [104]. Compared to the general population an increased risk of 27% was seen. It was estimated that 3.7 GBq (100 mCi) of ^{131}I would induce an excess of 53 solid malignant tumors and 3 leukemias in 10000 patients during 10 years of follow-up. In addition, a strong correlation existed between the cumulative activity of radioiodine and the risk of bone, soft-tissue, colorectal, and salivary gland cancers. These results highlight the need to restrict radioiodine treatment to those likely to benefit.

The radiation dose delivered by ^{131}I to each organ is difficult to estimate from established mathematical models; uptake by metastases may modify the dose delivered to a given organ and the hypothyroid status at the time of iodine administration decreases renal clearance of ^{131}I, thereby increasing the body retention of iodine by a factor of 2–4. Liberal fluid intake, frequent micturition, and use of laxatives will promote iodine excretion and reduce radiation exposure.

External Beam Radiotherapy

The value of external beam radiotherapy (EBRT) in the management of differentiated thyroid cancer remains controversial because published data are conflicting. In many reports, results are presented with no distinction between prophylactic (adjuvant) postoperative EBRT and treatment of microscopic or macroscopic residual disease. Due to the rarity of the disease and its long natural history there are no prospective randomized controlled trials.

EBRT does not prevent simultaneous administration of radioiodine, although ^{131}I should be given first whenever possible as uptake may be diminished after radiotherapy and, if there is good uptake by tumor, EBRT may become unnecessary. However, 20% of tumors fail to concentrate iodine. Radiotherapy is not indicated in patients with favorable prognostic features, nor in young patients with residual disease demonstrating avid iodine uptake [105]. Patients at higher risk for locoregional recurrence benefit from treatment similar to those with squamous carcinoma of the head and neck [106]. Indications include macroscopic unre-

sectable residual tumor and microscopic disease or involved excision margins. Adjuvant irradiation is required only in older patients with less differentiated cancers unlikely to concentrate radioiodine, especially those with extensive extrathyroidal spread, extracapsular lymph node extension, or recurrent disease (Table 15.2).

Farahati et al. suggest that adjuvant EBRT should be restricted to patients older than 40 years with locally advanced tumors (pT_4) which are non-iodine avid [107]. Treatment improved local control in those aged over 40 years with invasive papillary cancer and lymph node involvement from 22% to 90% at 10 years ($P = 0.01$). A similar group of patients with follicular cancer did not show any significant benefit. Since locoregional recurrence is infrequent in patients without lymph node disease, the addition of EBRT should be discouraged.

In 1985 Tubiana et al. reported on 97 patients treated with EBRT after incomplete surgery [108]: local recurrence at 15 years was 11% in the irradiated group compared to 23% for those treated with surgery alone. More recently Tsang et al. reported on 207 patients (155 papillary, 52 follicular) with residual microscopic disease postoperatively [12]. In the subgroup of papillary cancers, those irradiated had a 10-year cause-specific survival (CSS) of 100% and a local relapse-free rate (LRFR) of 93%; in comparison, the non-irradiated group had a CSS of 95% ($P = 0.038$) and LRFR of 78% ($P = 0.01$). EBRT did not significantly affect CSS or LRFR for follicular tumors. The most plausible explanation is that patients with follicular tumors have a worse survival due to hematogenous spread and any effects of local treatment may be obscured by this biological pattern of behavior.

The presence of gross inoperable macroscopic disease is another indication for EBRT. In our retrospective study, EBRT achieved com-

Table 15.2 Indications for external beam radiotherapy in differentiated thyroid cancer

Postoperative:	
High dose:	3D conformal plan for phase II or intensity modulated radiotherapy (IMRT)
Known macroscopic disease:	^{131}I + 66 Gy + ^{131}I
Known microscopic disease:	Age > 45, poor differentiation, Hürthle cell carcinoma
No known residual tumor:	Extensive pT_4, extracapsular node extension, recurrent disease
Palliative irradiation:	
35 Gy 15# over 3 weeks or 6 Gy once weekly	

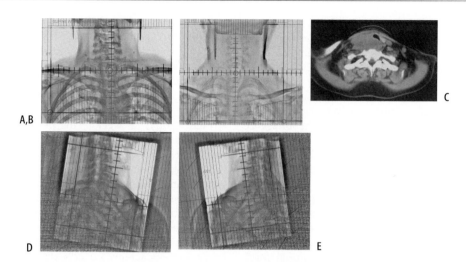

Figure 15.7 A and **B** Phase I: routine phase I comprising anterior and undercouched fields extending from hyoid to carina excluding parotid and submandibular salivary glands. Multileaf collimator protects infraclavicular portions of lungs. Chinstrap immobilization as an alternative to a Perspex shell avoids build-up to the skin and reduces skin toxicity. Occasionally, the upper deep cervical level II nodes must be treated, with the beam extending to the mastoid tips. The mandible and submandibular salivary glands still deserve protection. **C** Therapy CT scan for planning: large inoperable tumor displacing and compressing trachea. **D** and **E** Phase II: right anterior oblique beam encompasses residual tumor and also covers spinal cord. Left anterior oblique beam avoids spinal cord by use of multileaf collimator, limiting total dose to 46 Gy.

plete regression in 37.5% and partial regression in 25% [109]. Similarly, Chow et al. [110] reported the beneficial effects of EBRT in patients with gross macroscopic residual disease with an improvement in local control from 24% to 56% at 10 years ($P < 0.001$). EBRT is also effective for advanced and recurrent inoperable Hürthle cell carcinoma, claiming a relatively more important role because this tumor takes up iodine less frequently [111].

Despite the small study size, the 5-year local recurrence rates from Birmingham indicate a possible dose response [112]. These were 63% following a dose of less than 50 Gy but only 15% and 18% for doses of 50–54 Gy and more than 54 Gy.

Our policy is to use EBRT infrequently because high dose is required and side effects, especially oesophagitis, are unavoidable. The phase I target volume comprises both sides of the neck (bilateral deep cervical plus supraclavicular nodes), thyroid bed and superior mediastinum from the level of the hyoid down to the carina, with shielding of the subapical portions of the lungs (Figure 15.7A and B). Anterior and undercouched fields ensure comprehensive coverage, with the patient su-

pine and neck maximally extended. Lead protection of the submandibular salivary glands is required if the treatment volume needs to extend proximally to the tips of the mastoid. A Perspex shell is then fashioned for the phase II volume which includes sites of micro- or macroscopic tumor. We recommend three-dimensional planning and conformal beam shaping assisted by a multileaf collimator (Figure 15.7C, D, and E). The aim is to deliver 60 Gy in 30 daily fractions over 6 weeks using 4–6 MV photons. The phase I prescription should be a dose of 46 Gy in 2 Gy daily fractions (maximum spinal cord tolerance) with phase II delivering 14 Gy in seven fractions. Known residual tumor in the region of the thyroid bed or neck nodes may be treated with a small phase III volume, adding 6 Gy in three fractions, provided there is no additional dose to the spinal cord. Intensity-modulated radiotherapy can improve the dose distribution by minimizing dose to the spinal cord and thus permit dose escalation [113].

A brisk cutaneous erythema is invariable with acute radiation esophagitis, which develops during the third week of radiotherapy. Liquid analgesics, liberal hydration, and adequate dietary intake are required. Symptoms resolve within 2 weeks after completion of treatment. Acute laryngitis and dysphonia also resolve completely. Late effects include dysphagia, which may occur months or years later caused by stricture or motility changes as a result of muscle or nerve damage. Reduction in the length of the esophagus in the phase II volume minimizes such risks. Due to shielding of the subapical portions of the lungs, apical fibrosis may be visible on chest radiograph but is of no clinical significance.

Palliative radiotherapy is indicated for fungating nodes, bleeding, stridor, dysphagia, and superior vena caval obstruction due to progressive disease. Bone metastases causing pain, vertebral involvement threatening the spinal cord, long bone involvement if there is a potential for fracture, and brain metastases should also be treated with palliative radiotherapy. Tumor in the lung or mediastinum can be treated if unresectable. Low dose treatment is inadequate; 35 Gy in 15 fractions is required, or 6 Gy once weekly for up to four fractions when the central nervous system is not in field.

Chemotherapy

Experience with chemotherapy in DTC is limited by the rarity of tumors not controlled by surgery, radioiodine, or external beam radiotherapy. However, a minority of patients who do not respond to conventional therapy may survive with minimal symptoms. Because presently available drugs are of limited benefit and cause significant morbidity our practice is to reserve chemotherapy for patients with progressive and symptomatic disease that fails to concentrate radioiodine [114].

Doxorubicin (Adriamycin) is the anthracycline cytotoxic most extensively used with response rates of 30–40%. It is rapidly metabolized by the liver but is myelosuppressive and causes gastrointestinal toxicity. Long-term administration is limited by dose-dependent cardiotoxicity. Irreversible cardiomyopathy may occur in patients who have received total doses in excess of 500–550 mg/m^2. However, cardiac toxicity may also be induced by lower cumulative doses. Doxorubicin is therefore contraindicated in patients with major cardiac disease and patients with impaired liver function.

In 1975 Gottlieb and Stratton Hill reported a series of 43 patients treated with doxorubicin 75 mg/m^2 every 3 weeks: complete or partial response was seen in 35% [115]. In 1987 a review of all published data estimated the overall response rate to be 38% [116], with the usual effective dose 60–90 mg/m^2 every 3 weeks or 10 mg/m^2 once a week. The best responses were observed in patients with pulmonary metastases, followed by bone metastases, and locoregional disease. A prolonged median survival from 3–5 months (nonresponders) to 15–20 months (responders) was reported [116].

Aclarubicin, a newer agent less cardiotoxic than doxorubicin, has also been assessed [117]: 25–30 mg/m^2 given daily for 4 days and repeated every 3 weeks achieved a 22% response rate in a series of 24 patients. The challenge remains, however, to find a suitable and effective agent with minimal cardiac toxicity. This may be possible with the introduction of polyethylene glycol-coated (pegylated) liposomal doxorubicin (Caelyx). A multicenter prospective study is ongoing in the UK (Newcastle, U. Mallick) with the administration of liposomal doxorubicin to any advanced metastatic thyroid cancer. Other agents including bleomycin, cisplatin, somatostatin analogues, interferon-α, and interleukin-2 used as monotherapy have failed to demonstrate significant clinical benefit.

Combination therapy which includes doxorubicin has been assessed in the hope of additional tumor response. Doxorubicin with cisplatin has been compared with doxorubicin alone. Shimaoka et al. described 41 patients who received doxorubicin (60 mg/m^2 every 3 weeks) as monotherapy [118]: partial response was seen in only 7 (17%). Forty-three patients received combination treatment (doxorubicin 60 mg/m^2 3-weekly and cisplatin 40 mg/m^2), of whom 11 had either a partial or complete response (26%). Overall response rates were not significantly different between the two groups but complete response was seen only in the combination therapy group and lasted more than 2 years in four of five patients. A second prospective study with doxorubicin and cisplatin was carried out in 22 patients with all types of advanced thyroid cancer [119]: only brief partial response was seen in two cases (10%). Similarly, the combination was found to be ineffective in a series from the Institut Gustave-Roussy [120]. In all studies, serious toxicity occurred more often in patients treated with combination therapy. Chemotherapy may be beneficial in patients with advanced non-iodine avid thyroid cancer by inducing uptake of subsequent radioiodine therapy. Morris et al. reported on a patient treated with cisplatin and doxorubicin in whom repeat ^{131}I imaging after three cycles showed significant uptake in previously non-iodine avid lesions [121].

Other combination protocols including doxorubicin have failed to show a therapeutic effect superior to doxorubicin monotherapy. This includes combination with bleomycin, etoposide, 5-fluorouracil, and cyclophosphamide.

Doxorubicin in combination with EBRT may be effective in treating unresectable locally advanced disease refractory to radioiodine. Kim and Leeper reported on 22 patients with DTC given doxorubicin ($10\,mg/m^2$ per week) with concomitant radiation at doses of $2\,Gy/day$ for 5 days each week to a total of $56\,Gy$ [122]. The results revealed a 91% complete response rate, 77% long-term local control, and overall survival of 50% at 5 years. Significant toxicity was observed, with all patients developing esophagitis and tracheitis within 4 weeks, but none demanded discontinuation of treatment.

In conclusion, doxorubicin monotherapy still provides the best clinical results with overall response rates of 30–40% and combination therapy is not superior. Chemotherapy should be given only to patients with unresectable symptomatic progressive disease which is non-iodine avid and not amenable to external irradiation. Even in these patients, the possible benefit from chemotherapy should be weighed against quality of life without systemic treatment.

Conclusions

There has been substantial progress in our understanding of thyroid cancer over the past few decades [123]. Despite the lack of randomized studies, there have been improvements in overall management and through information derived from retrospective series, treatment policies have become evidence based.

Surgery remains the initial and potentially curative treatment. After total thyroidectomy and paratracheal lymph node sampling ± selective node dissection, ablation of thyroid remnants with radioactive iodine reduces the risk of locoregional recurrence and death from cancer in patients with poor prognostic factors. Radioiodine therapy is the mainstay of treatment for disseminated thyroid cancer; a worthwhile proportion of patients can be cured and in others durable palliation can be achieved. Treatment is well tolerated and serious long-term complications are rare. Management of all patients by a multidisciplinary team in a specialized unit, publication of national guidelines by the British Thyroid Association, registration of all new cases with prospective data collection, and regular audit of outcomes are guaranteed to further improve patient outcome.

References

1. Schlumberger M, Fragu P, Parmentier C, Tubiana M. Thyroglobulin assay in the follow-up of patients with differentiated thyroid carcinomas: comparison of its value in patients with or without normal residual tissue. Acta Endocrinol (Copenh) 1981; 98(2):215–221.
2. Mazzaferri EL, Robbins RJ, Spencer CA, et al. A consensus report of the role of serum thyroglobulin as a monitoring method for low-risk patients with papillary thyroid carcinoma. J Clin Endocrinol Metab 2003; 88(4):1433–1441.
3. Pacini F, Molinaro E, Lippi F, et al. Prediction of disease status by recombinant human TSH-stimulated serum Tg in the postsurgical follow-up of differentiated thyroid carcinoma. J Clin Endocrinol Metab 2001; 86(12):5686–5690.
4. Pacini F, Molinaro E, Castagna MG, et al. Recombinant human thyrotropin-stimulated serum thyroglobulin combined with neck ultrasonography has the highest sensitivity in monitoring differentiated thyroid carcinoma. J Clin Endocrinol Metab 2003; 88(8):3668–3673.
5. Mazzaferri EL, Jhiang SM. Long-term impact of initial surgical and medical therapy on papillary and follicular thyroid cancer. Am J Med 1994; 97(5):418–428.
6. Vini L, Harmer C. Radioiodine treatment for differentiated thyroid cancer. Clin Oncol (R Coll Radiol) 2000; 12(6):365–372.
7. Taylor T, Specker B, Robbins J, et al. Outcome after treatment of high-risk papillary and non-Hurthle-cell follicular thyroid carcinoma. Ann Intern Med 1998; 129(8):622–627.
8. Samaan NA, Schultz PN, Hickey RC, et al. The results of various modalities of treatment of well differentiated thyroid carcinomas: a retrospective review of 1599 patients. J Clin Endocrinol Metab 1992; 75(3):714–720.
9. Hay ID, Grant CS, van Heerden JA, Goellner JR, Ebersold JR, Bergstrahl EJ. Papillary thyroid microcarcinoma: a study of 535 cases observed in a 50-year period. Surgery 1992; 112(6):1139–1146.
10. Mazzaferri EL. Thyroid remnant ^{131}I ablation for papillary and follicular thyroid carcinoma. Thyroid 1997; 7(2):265–271.

11. Mazzaferri EL, Kloos RT. Clinical review 128: Current approaches to primary therapy for papillary and follicular thyroid cancer. J Clin Endocrinol Metab 2001; 86(4):1447–1463.

12. Tsang RW, Brierley JD, Simpson WJ, Panzarella T, Gospodarowicz MK, Sutcliffe SB. The effects of surgery, radioiodine, and external radiation therapy on the clinical outcome of patients with differentiated thyroid carcinoma. Cancer 1998; 82(2):375–388.

13. Bal CS, Kumar A, Pant GS. Radioiodine lobar ablation as an alternative to completion thyroidectomy in patients with differentiated thyroid cancer. Nucl Med Commun 2003; 24(2):203–208.

14. Hoyes KP, Owens SE, Millns MM, Allan E. Differentiated thyroid cancer: radioiodine following lobectomy – a clinical feasibility study. Nucl Med Commun 2004; 25(3):245–251.

15. Beierwaltes WH, Rabbani R, Dmuchowski C, Lloyd RV, Eyre P, Mallette S. An analysis of "ablation of thyroid remnants" with I-131 in 511 patients from 1947–1984: experience at University of Michigan. J Nucl Med 1984; 25(12):1287–1293.

16. Samuel AM, Rajashekharrao B. Radioiodine therapy for well-differentiated thyroid cancer: a quantitative dosimetric evaluation for remnant thyroid ablation after surgery. J Nucl Med 1994; 35(12): 1944–1950.

17. McCowen KD, Adler RA, Ghaed N, Verdon T, Hofeldt FD. Low dose radioiodide thyroid ablation in postsurgical patients with thyroid cancer. Am J Med 1976; 61(1):52–58.

18. Doi SA, Woodhouse NJ. Ablation of the thyroid remnant and ^{131}I dose in differentiated thyroid cancer. Clin Endocrinol (Oxf) 2000; 52(6):765–773.

19. Bal C, Padhy AK, Jana S, Pant GS, Basu AK. Prospective randomized clinical trial to evaluate the optimal dose of ^{131}I for remnant ablation in patients with differentiated thyroid carcinoma. Cancer 1996; 77(12):2574–2580.

20. Bal CS, Kumar A, Pant GS. Radioiodine dose for remnant ablation in differentiated thyroid carcinoma: a randomized clinical trial in 509 patients. J Clin Endocrinol Metab 2004; 89(4):1666–1673.

21. Maxon HR, Thomas SR, Samaratunga RC. Dosimetric considerations in the radioiodine treatment of macrometastases and micrometastases from differentiated thyroid cancer. Thyroid 1997; 7(2):183–187.

22. Maxon HR, III, Englaro EE, Thomas SR, et al. Radioiodine-131 therapy for well-differentiated thyroid cancer – a quantitative radiation dosimetric approach: outcome and validation in 85 patients. J Nucl Med 1992; 33(6):1132–1136.

23. Vini L, Harmer C. Management of thyroid cancer. Lancet Oncol 2002; 3(7):407–414.

24. O'Connell ME, Flower MA, Hinton PJ, Harmer CL, McCready VR. Radiation dose assessment in radioiodine therapy. Dose-response relationships in differentiated thyroid carcinoma using quantitative scanning and PET. Radiother Oncol 1993; 28(1):16–26.

25. Hammersley PA, Al Saadi A, Chittenden S, Flux GD, McCready VR, Harmer CL. Value of protein-bound radioactive iodine measurements in the management of differentiated thyroid cancer treated with (131)I. Br J Radiol 2001; 74(881):429–433.

26. Pacini F. Follow-up of differentiated thyroid cancer. Eur J Nucl Med Mol Imaging 2002; 29(Suppl 2):S492–S496.

27. Robbins RJ, Chon JT, Fleisher M, Larson SM, Tuttle RM. Is the serum thyroglobulin response to recombinant human thyrotropin sufficient, by itself, to monitor for residual thyroid carcinoma? J Clin Endocrinol Metab 2002; 87(7):3242–3247.

28. Mazzaferri EL, Massoll N. Management of papillary and follicular (differentiated) thyroid cancer: new paradigms using recombinant human thyrotropin. Endocr Relat Cancer 2002; 9(4):227–247.

29. Taylor H, Hyer S, Vini L, Pratt B, Cook G, Harmer C. Diagnostic ^{131}I whole body scanning after thyroidectomy and ablation for differentiated thyroid cancer. Eur J Endocrinol 2004; 150(5):649–653.

30. Carlisle MR, Lu C, McDougall IR. The interpretation of ^{131}I scans in the evaluation of thyroid cancer, with an emphasis on false positive findings. Nucl Med Commun 2003; 24(6):715–735.

31. Maruca J, Santner S, Miller K, Santen RJ. Prolonged iodine clearance with a depletion regimen for thyroid carcinoma: concise communication. J Nucl Med 1984; 25(10):1089–1093.

32. Lakshmanan M, Schaffer A, Robbins J, Reynolds J, Norton J. A simplified low iodine diet in I-131 scanning and therapy of thyroid cancer. Clin Nucl Med 1988; 13(12):866–868.

33. Robbins RJ, Larson SM, Sinha N, et al. A retrospective review of the effectiveness of recombinant human TSH as a preparation for radioiodine thyroid remnant ablation. J Nucl Med 2002; 43(11):1482–1488.

34. Pacini F, Molinaro E, Castagna MG, et al. Ablation of thyroid residues with 30 mCi (131)I: a comparison in thyroid cancer patients prepared with recombinant human TSH or thyroid hormone withdrawal. J Clin Endocrinol Metab 2002; 87(9):4063–4068.

35. Dow KH, Ferrell BR, Anello C. Quality-of-life changes in patients with thyroid cancer after withdrawal of thyroid hormone therapy. Thyroid 1997; 7(4):613–619.

36. Mazzaferri EL, Kloos RT. Using recombinant human TSH in the management of well-differentiated thyroid cancer: current strategies and future directions. Thyroid 2000; 10(9):767–778.

37. Ladenson PW, Braverman LE, Mazzaferri EL, et al. Comparison of administration of recombinant human thyrotropin with withdrawal of thyroid hormone for radioactive iodine scanning in patients with thyroid carcinoma. N Engl J Med 1997; 337(13):888–896.

38. Schlumberger M, de Vathaire F, Ceccarelli C, Francese C, Pinchera A, Parmentier C. Outcome of pregnancy in women with thyroid carcinoma. J Endocrinol Invest 1995; 18(2):150–151.

39. Vini L, Hyer S, Pratt B, Harmer C. Management of differentiated thyroid cancer diagnosed during pregnancy. Eur J Endocrinol 1999; 140(5):404–406.

40. Vini L, Hyer S, Pratt B, Harmer C. Good prognosis in thyroid cancer found incidentally at surgery for thyrotoxicosis. Postgrad Med J 1999; 75(881):169–170.

41. Williams ED, Pacini F, Pinchera A. Thyroid cancer following Chernobyl. J Endocrinol Invest 1995; 18(2):144–146.

42. Landau D, Vini L, A'Hern R, Harmer C. Thyroid cancer in children: the Royal Marsden Hospital experience. Eur J Cancer 2000; 36(2):214–220.

43. Mazzaferri EL, Jhiang SM. Differentiated thyroid cancer: long-term impact of initial therapy. Trans Am Clin Climatol Assoc 1994; 106:151–168.

44. Toft AD. Clinical practice. Subclinical hyperthyroidism. N Engl J Med 2001; 345(7):512–516.

45. Black EG, Cassoni A, Gimlette TM, et al. Serum thyroglobulin in thyroid cancer. Lancet 1981; ii(8244): 443–445.

46. Schlumberger M, Baudin E. Serum thyroglobulin determination in the follow-up of patients with differentiated thyroid carcinoma. Eur J Endocrinol 1998; 138(3):249–252.

47. Cailleux AF, Baudin E, Travagli JP, Ricard M, Schlumberger M. Is diagnostic iodine-131 scanning useful after total thyroid ablation for differentiated thyroid cancer? J Clin Endocrinol Metab 2000; 85(1):175–178.

48. Mariotti S, Barbesino G, Caturegli P, et al. Assay of thyroglobulin in serum with thyroglobulin autoantibodies: an unobtainable goal? J Clin Endocrinol Metab 1995; 80(2):468–472.

49. Spencer CA, Takeuchi M, Kazarosyan M, et al. Serum thyroglobulin autoantibodies: prevalence, influence on serum thyroglobulin measurement, and prognostic significance in patients with differentiated thyroid carcinoma. J Clin Endocrinol Metab 1998; 83(4):1121–1127.

50. British Thyroid Association. Guidelines for the management of thyroid cancer in adults. London: Royal College of Physicians, 2002.

51. Luster M, Sherman SI, Skarulis MC, et al. Comparison of radioiodine biokinetics following the administration of recombinant human thyroid stimulating hormone and after thyroid hormone withdrawal in thyroid carcinoma. Eur J Nucl Med Mol Imaging 2003; 30(10):1371–1377.

52. Coakley AJ. Thyroid stunning. Eur J Nucl Med 1998; 25(3):203–204.

53. Cohen JB, Kalinyak JE, McDougall IR. Clinical implications of the differences between diagnostic ^{123}I and post-therapy ^{131}I scans. Nucl Med Commun 2004; 25(2):129–134.

54. Schlumberger M, Challeton C, de Vathaire F, et al. Radioactive iodine treatment and external radiotherapy for lung and bone metastases from thyroid carcinoma. J Nucl Med 1996; 37(4):598–605.

55. Vini L, Hyer SL, Marshall J, A'Hern R, Harmer C. Long-term results in elderly patients with differentiated thyroid carcinoma. Cancer 2003; 97(11):2736–2742.

56. Marcocci C, Pacini F, Elisei R, et al. Clinical and biologic behavior of bone metastases from differentiated thyroid carcinoma. Surgery 1989; 106(6):960–966.

57. Niederle B, Roka R, Schemper M, Fritsch A, Weissel M, Ramach W. Surgical treatment of distant metastases in differentiated thyroid cancer: indication and results. Surgery 1986; 100(6):1088–1097.

58. Protopapas AD, Nicholson AG, Vini L, Harmer CL, Goldstraw P. Thoracic metastasectomy in thyroid malignancies. Ann Thorac Surg 2001; 72(6):1906–1908.

59. Venkataraman GM, Yatin M, Marcinek R, Ain KB. Restoration of iodide uptake in dedifferentiated thyroid carcinoma: relationship to human Na$^+$/I-symporter gene methylation status. J Clin Endocrinol Metab 1999; 84(7):2449–2457.

60. Dai G, Levy O, Carrasco N. Cloning and characterization of the thyroid iodide transporter. Nature 1996; 379(6564):458–460.

61. Samaan NA, Schultz PN, Haynie TP, Ordonez NG. Pulmonary metastasis of differentiated thyroid carcinoma: treatment results in 101 patients. J Clin Endocrinol Metab 1985; 60(2):376–380.

62. Fatourechi V, Hay ID, Javedan H, Wiseman GA, Mullan BP, Gorman CA. Lack of impact of radioiodine therapy in Tg-positive, diagnostic whole-body scan-negative patients with follicular cell-derived thyroid cancer. J Clin Endocrinol Metab 2002; 87(4):1521–1526.

63. Van Herle AJ, Agatep ML, Padua DN, III, et al. Effects of 13 cis-retinoic acid on growth and differentiation of human follicular carcinoma cells (UCLA R0 82 W-1) in vitro. J Clin Endocrinol Metab 1990; 71(3):755–763.

64. Grunwald F, Menzel C, Bender H, et al. Redifferentiation therapy-induced radioiodine uptake in thyroid cancer. J Nucl Med 1998; 39(11):1903–1906.

65. Gruning T, Tiepolt C, Zophel K, Bredow J, Kropp J, Franke WG. Retinoic acid for redifferentiation of thyroid cancer – does it hold its promise? Eur J Endocrinol 2003; 148(4):395–402.

66. Lopez-Penabad L, Chiu AC, Hoff AO, et al. Prognostic factors in patients with Hurthle cell neoplasms of the thyroid. Cancer 2003; 97(5):1186–1194.

67. Haq MS, McCready RV, Harmer CL. Treatment of advanced differentiated thyroid carcinoma with high activity radioiodine therapy. Nucl Med Commun 2004; 25(8):799–805.

68. Maxon HR, Thomas SR, Hertzberg VS, et al. Relation between effective radiation dose and outcome of radioiodine therapy for thyroid cancer. N Engl J Med 1983; 309(16):937–941.

69. Koong SS, Reynolds JC, Movius EG, et al. Lithium as a potential adjuvant to ^{131}I therapy of metastatic, well differentiated thyroid carcinoma. J Clin Endocrinol Metab 1999; 84(3):912–916.

70. Schlumberger M, Tubiana M, de Vathaire F, et al. Long-term results of treatment of 283 patients with lung and bone metastases from differentiated thyroid carcinoma. J Clin Endocrinol Metab 1986; 63(4):960–967.

71. Schlumberger M, Challeton C, de Vathaire F, Parmentier C. Treatment of distant metastases of differentiated thyroid carcinoma. J Endocrinol Invest 1995; 18(2):170–172.

72. Shoup M, Stojadinovic A, Nissan A, et al. Prognostic indicators of outcomes in patients with distant metastases from differentiated thyroid carcinoma. J Am Coll Surg 2003; 197(2):191–197.

73. Brown AP, Greening WP, McCready VR, Shaw HJ, Harmer CL. Radioiodine treatment of metastatic thyroid carcinoma: the Royal Marsden Hospital experience. Br J Radiol 1984; 57(676):323–327.

74. Mazzaferri EL. Papillary and follicular thyroid cancer: selective therapy. Compr Ther 1981; 7(5):6–14.

75. Haq M, Harner C. Differentiated thyroid carcinoma with distant metastases at presentation: prognostic factors and outcome. Clin Endocrinol 2005(suppl); 63:87–93.

76. Nemec J, Zamrazil V, Pohunkova D, Rohling S. Radioiodide treatment of pulmonary metastases of differentiated thyroid cancer. Results and prognostic factors. Nuklearmedizin 1979; 18(2):86–90.

77. Casara D, Rubello D, Saladini G, et al. Different features of pulmonary metastases in differentiated thyroid cancer: natural history and multivariate statistical analysis of prognostic variables. J Nucl Med 1993; 34(10):1626–1631.

78. Vini L, Harmer C, Goldstraw P. The role of metastasectomy in differentiated thyroid cancer. Eur J Surg Oncol 1998; 24:348.

79. Petrich T, Widjaja A, Musholt TJ, et al. Outcome after radioiodine therapy in 107 patients with differentiated thyroid carcinoma and initial bone metastases: side-effects and influence of age. Eur J Nucl Med 2001; 28(2):203–208.

80. Stojadinovic A, Shoup M, Ghossein RA, et al. The role of operations for distantly metastatic well-differentiated thyroid carcinoma. Surgery 2002; 131(6): 636–643.

81. Benua S, Cicale NR, Sonenberg M, Rawson RW. The relation of radioiodine dosimetry to results and complications in the treatment of metastatic thyroid cancer. Am J Roentgenol Radium Ther Nucl Med 1962; 87:171–182.

82. Vini L, Chittenden S, Pratt B, Harmer C. In vivo dosimetry of radioiodine in patients with metastatic differentiated thyroid cancer. J Nucl Med 1998; 25: 904.

83. Flower MA, McCready VR. Radionuclide therapy dose calculations: what accuracy can be achieved? Eur J Nucl Med 1997; 24(12):1462–1464.

84. Bodey RK, Flux GD, Evans PM. Combining dosimetry for targeted radionuclide and external beam therapies using the biologically effective dose. Cancer Biother Radiopharm 2003; 18(1):89–97.

85. Guy MJ, Flux GD, Papavasileiou P, Flower MA, Ott RJ. RMDP: a dedicated package for ^{131}I SPECT quantification, registration and patient-specific dosimetry. Cancer Biother Radiopharm 2003; 18(1):61–69.

86. Flux GD, Guy MJ, Beddows R, Pryor M, Flower MA. Estimation and implications of random errors in whole-body dosimetry for targeted radionuclide therapy. Phys Med Biol 2002; 47(17):3211–3223.

87. Haq M, Gear J, Guy M, et al. Whole-body desimetry in the treatment of differentiated thyroid cancer. Eur J Med 2004(suppl 2); 877.

88. Papavasileiou P, Flux GD, Flower MA, Guy MJ. An automated technique for SPECT marker-based image registration in radionuclide therapy. Phys Med Biol 2001; 46(8):2085–2097.

89. Flux GD, Webb S, Ott RJ, Chittenden SJ, Thomas R. Three-dimensional dosimetry for intralesional radionuclide therapy using mathematical modeling and multimodality imaging. J Nucl Med 1997; 38(7):1059–1066.

90. Van Nostrand D, Neutze J, Atkins F. Side effects of "rational dose" iodine-131 therapy for metastatic well-differentiated thyroid carcinoma. J Nucl Med 1986; 27(10):1519–1527.

91. Burmeister LA, du Cret RP, Mariash CN. Local reactions to radioiodine in the treatment of thyroid cancer. Am J Med 1991; 90(2):217–222.

92. Bohuslavizki KH, Brenner W, Lassmann S, et al. Quantitative salivary gland scintigraphy in the diagnosis of parenchymal damage after treatment with radioiodine. Nucl Med Commun 1996; 17(8):681–686.

93. Alexander C, Bader JB, Schaefer A, Finke C, Kirsch CM. Intermediate and long-term side effects of high-dose radioiodine therapy for thyroid carcinoma. J Nucl Med 1998; 39(9):1551–1554.

94. Bohuslavizki KH, Klutmann S, Brenner W, Mester J, Henze E, Clausen M. Salivary gland protection by amifostine in high-dose radioiodine treatment: results of a double-blind placebo-controlled study. J Clin Oncol 1998; 16(11):3542–3549.

95. Leeper RD, Shimaoka K. Treatment of metastatic thyroid cancer. Clin Endocrinol Metab 1980; 9(2):383–404.

96. Hjiyiannakis P, Jefferies S, Harmer CL. Brain metastases in patients with differentiated thyroid carcinoma. Clin Oncol (R Coll Radiol) 1996; 8(5):327–330.

97. McConahey WM, Hay ID, Woolner LB, van Heerden JA, Taylor WF. Papillary thyroid cancer treated at the Mayo Clinic, 1946 through 1970: initial manifestations, pathologic findings, therapy, and outcome. Mayo Clin Proc 1986; 61(12):978–996.

98. Dottorini ME, Lomuscio G, Mazzucchelli L, Vignati A, Colombo L. Assessment of female fertility and carcinogenesis after iodine-131 therapy for differentiated thyroid carcinoma. J Nucl Med 1995; 36(1):21–27.

99. Vini L, Hyer S, Al Saadi A, Pratt B, Harmer C. Prognosis for fertility and ovarian function after treatment with radioiodine for thyroid cancer. Postgrad Med J 2002; 78(916):92–93.

100. Hyer S, Vini L, O'Connell M, Pratt B, Harmer C. Testicular dose and fertility in men following I(131) therapy for thyroid cancer. Clin Endocrinol (Oxf) 2002; 56(6): 755–758.

101. Pacini F, Gasperi M, Fugazzola L, et al. Testicular function in patients with differentiated thyroid carcinoma treated with radioiodine. J Nucl Med 1994; 35(9):1418–1422.

102. Edmonds CJ, Smith T. The long-term hazards of the treatment of thyroid cancer with radioiodine. Br J Radiol 1986; 59(697):45–51.

103. Maxon HR, III, Smith HS. Radioiodine-131 in the diagnosis and treatment of metastatic well differentiated thyroid cancer. Endocrinol Metab Clin North Am 1990; 19(3):685–718.

104. Rubino C, de Vathaire F, Dottorini ME, et al. Second primary malignancies in thyroid cancer patients. Br J Cancer 2003; 89(9):1638–1644.

105. Harmer C, Bidmead M, Shepherd S, Sharpe A, Vini L. Radiotherapy planning techniques for thyroid cancer. Br J Radiol 1998; 71(850):1069–1075.

106. Rhys-Evans P, See A, Harmer C. Cancer of the thyroid gland. In: Rhys-Evans P, Montgomery P, Gullane P (eds) Principles and practice of head and neck oncology. London: Martin Dunitz, 2003: 405–430.

107. Farahati J, Reiners C, Stuschke M, et al. Differentiated thyroid cancer. Impact of adjuvant external radiotherapy in patients with perithyroidal tumor infiltration (stage pT4). Cancer 1996; 77(1):172–180.

108. Tubiana M, Haddad E, Schlumberger M, Hill C, Rougier P, Sarrazin D. External radiotherapy in thyroid cancers. Cancer 1985; 55(9 Suppl):2062–2071.

109. O'Connell ME, A'Hern RP, Harmer CL. Results of external beam radiotherapy in differentiated thyroid carcinoma: a retrospective study from the Royal Marsden Hospital. Eur J Cancer 1994; 30A(6):733–739.

110. Chow SM, Law SC, Mendenhall WM, et al. Papillary thyroid carcinoma: prognostic factors and the role of radioiodine and external radiotherapy. Int J Radiat Oncol Biol Phys 2002; 52(3):784–795.
111. Vini L, Fisher C, A'Hern R, Harmer C. Hurthle cell cancer of the thyroid: the Royal Marsden experience. Thyroid 1998; 8(12):1228.
112. Ford D, Giridharan S, McConkey C, et al. External beam radiotherapy in the management of differentiated thyroid cancer. Clin Oncol (R Coll Radiol) 2003; 15(6):337–341.
113. Nutting CM, Convery DJ, Cosgrove VP, et al. Improvements in target coverage and reduced spinal cord irradiation using intensity-modulated radiotherapy (IMRT) in patients with carcinoma of the thyroid gland. Radiother Oncol 2001; 60(2):173–180.
114. Hoskin PJ, Harmer C. Chemotherapy for thyroid cancer. Radiother Oncol 1987; 10(3):187–194.
115. Gottlieb J, Stratton Hill C. Adriamycin therapy in thyroid carcinoma. Cancer Chemotherapy Reports 1975; 6:283–296.
116. Ahuja S, Ernst H. Chemotherapy of thyroid carcinoma. J Endocrinol Invest 1987; 10(3):303–310.
117. Samonigg H, Hossfeld DK, Spehn J, Fill H, Leb G. Aclarubicin in advanced thyroid cancer: a phase II study. Eur J Cancer Clin Oncol 1988; 24(8):1271–1275.
118. Shimaoka K, Schoenfeld DA, DeWys WD, Creech RH, DeConti R. A randomized trial of doxorubicin versus doxorubicin plus cisplatin in patients with advanced thyroid carcinoma. Cancer 1985; 56(9):2155–2160.
119. Williams SD, Birch R, Einhorn LH. Phase II evaluation of doxorubicin plus cisplatin in advanced thyroid cancer: a Southeastern Cancer Study Group Trial. Cancer Treat Rep 1986; 70(3):405–407.
120. Droz JP, Schlumberger M, Rougier P, Ghosn M, Gardet P, Parmentier C. Chemotherapy in metastatic nonanaplastic thyroid cancer: experience at the Institut Gustave-Roussy. Tumori 1990; 76(5):480–483.
121. Morris JC, Kim CK, Padilla ML, Mechanick JI. Conversion of non-iodine-concentrating differentiated thyroid carcinoma metastases into iodine-concentrating foci after anticancer chemotherapy. Thyroid 1997; 7(1):63–66.
122. Kim JH, Leeper RD. Treatment of locally advanced thyroid carcinoma with combination doxorubicin and radiation therapy. Cancer 1987; 60(10):2372–2375.
123. Kendall-Taylor P. Managing differentiated thyroid cancer. BMJ 2002; 324(7344):988–989.
124. Creutzig H. High or low dose radioiodine ablation of thyroid remnants? Eur J Nuc Med 1987; 12:500–502.
125. Johansen K, Woodhouse NJ, Odugbesan O. Comparison of 1073 MBq and 3700 MBq ^{131}I in postoperative ablation of residual thyroid tissue in patients with differentiated thyroid cancer. J Nuc Med 1991; 32:252–254.
126. Sirisalipoch S. Prospective randomised trial for the evaluation of the efficacy of low vs high dose ^{131}I for post-operative remnant ablation in differentiated thyroid cancer. World J Nuc Med 2004;3(Suppl 1):S36.

16

Fertility Following Treatment with Iodine-131 for Thyroid Cancer

Louiza Vini

Introduction

The earliest clinical use of radioiodine in the treatment of thyroid cancer was reported by Hamilton in 1940. Since those early days dramatic responses and cures have been documented even in disseminated tumors, establishing iodine as the most effective non-surgical treatment for thyroid cancer [1]. Most adult patients with tumors greater than 1 cm will be treated with an ablation dose (usually 3–3.7 GBq, 81–100 mCi) of ^{131}I while those with adverse prognostic factors or metastatic disease will need to receive several doses of radioiodine. The safety of ^{131}I is well documented [2]. Acute toxicity is mild – side effects include nausea, sialoadenitis, neck discomfort, and transient hematological depression. Late complications such as pulmonary fibrosis, myelodysplasia, leukemia, and second malignancies are rare. The risk of leukemia and possibly second cancers increases with high cumulative dose of ^{131}I [3].

Differentiated thyroid cancer is not uncommon in women of childbearing years or in young men, and can also affect children, particularly those previously exposed to radiotherapy to the head and neck. For this group of patients prognosis is excellent with a long-term survival of over 90% [1]. In recent years the possibility of long-term gonadal damage from radioactive iodine has become increasingly appreciated and the subject of several reports.

Effects on Female Fertility

In normally menstruating women, ovarian function depends on pituitary production of follicle-stimulating hormone (FSH), which stimulates the ovarian follicular granulosa cells to develop and produce estradiol. This causes feedback inhibition of the pituitary maintaining FSH at a low level. At puberty approximately 200 000 ovarian follicles are present and functioning in the ovary. This number progressively declines with age to approximately 400 at the time of menopause. Fertility in women can be assessed from the menstrual history and by measuring FSH levels. Persisting amenorrhea with FSH levels more than 30 IU/L implies the onset of menopause.

Radiation produces dose-related gonadal damage to both the germ cell and the endocrine component of ovarian tissue. Experience with external beam radiotherapy suggests that the probability of infertility for a given dose of radiation increases with age; treatment with 4 Gy will produce infertility in only 30% of young women but in 100% of those over the age of 40. In addition, resumption of menstruation has been seen in adolescents irradiated to doses as high as 20 Gy [4]. The same age effect is recognized following exposure to chemotherapy drugs.

Following administration of high activities of ^{131}I, menstrual irregularities have been reported in 20–30% of premenopausal female patients

[5]. Amenorrhea has been reported to occur within 6 months after treatment but lasted only for a short time (less than 6 months in most patients). In our retrospective analysis of 409 female patients under the age of 40 years, 8% developed amenorrhea lasting 4–10 months and 12% reported menstrual changes such as lighter menses and shorter or longer cycle but these reverted to normal within 6 months [6]. Patients who developed temporary amenorrhea were older (median age 36, range 29–40) compared with those who either had mild menstrual changes (median age 28 years) or no changes (median age 31 years). In our study only women under the age of 40 were included; however, we noticed four older patients (age 44–46 years) who became menopausal following radioiodine therapy. These observations possibly indicate a higher ovarian sensitivity to irradiation with older age.

High serum FSH/luteinizing hormone (LH) values in women with temporary amenorrhea following radioiodine therapy indicate temporary ovarian failure [5]. Contributing factors are not known. Both psychological stress leading to hypothalamic amenorrhea and hypothyroidism have been implicated. However, in most cases amenorrhea appears 1–3 months after treatment when the patient is on thyroxine replacement. This interval also excludes an action of radioactivity on the maturing follicle, possibly suggesting an effect on the oocytes involved in future cycles.

After radioiodine administration, sources of radiation to the ovaries are the blood, bladder, gut, and functioning metastases close to the ovaries. Based on the Medical Internal Radiation Dose (MIRD) estimate, the dose received by each ovary is 0.14 cGy/37 MBq (1 mCi) [7]. However, the "ideal MIRD model" subject is morphologically bigger than the average patient and the kinetic model used applies to euthyroid patients; iodine-treated patients are severely hypothyroid at the time of administration and renal clearance of iodine is decreased, resulting in a more prolonged gonadal exposure. Mathematical models taking into account individual patient morphology lead to ovarian dose estimates approximately threefold higher (0.4 cGy/37 MBq (1 mCi). Applying this model to a group of 50 patients with metastases treated with a dose of 10–11.1 GBq (300 mCi) [131]I, no difference was found

between the calculated dose to the ovary in 12 patients who developed amenorrhea (1.29 ± 0.33 Gy) and 33 who did not (1.08 ± 0.33 Gy) [8].

Despite the documented ovarian dysfunction following radioiodine therapy, there is no indication that this is correlated with lasting infertility. Several large studies have reported that exposure to radioiodine does not affect the outcome of subsequent pregnancy or offspring [6,9–12]. An early study in children and adolescents treated with a mean total dose of 196 mCi of radioiodine reported a 12% incidence of infertility, 1.4% incidence of miscarriage, 8% incidence of prematurity, and 1% incidence of congenital anomaly; these rates were not significantly different from those of the general population [11]. In our series, a total of 427 children were born to 276 women. Seven patients were advised against conception and 125 had no wish to have children. Four premature deaths and 14 spontaneous abortions were reported but no malformations [6]. In the Gustave-Roussy series an increased incidence of miscarriage (20%) was seen especially within the first year after ^{131}I administration. However, whether and to what extent this is related to gonadal irradiation rather than to suboptimal control of thyroid status could not be established. With the exception of miscarriages, there was no evidence that exposure to radioiodine affects the outcome of subsequent pregnancies and offspring [12]. ARSAC (Administration of Radioactive Substances Advisory Committee) recommends a minimum period of 4 months before conception as the dose to the fetus should not exceed 1 mGy [13]. Suppressive thyroxine therapy should continue during pregnancy and thyroid function tests should be monitored regularly to ensure that thyroid-stimulating hormone (TSH) remains suppressed as thyroxine requirements may increase during pregnancy.

Effects on Male Fertility

Sperm production in males is maintained by production of FSH by the pituitary and regulated by a negative feedback mechanism by inhibin produced by the seminiferous tubules within the testes. Androgen production is maintained by pituitary production of LH, also controlled by a negative feedback mechanism by production of testosterone by the testicular Leydig cells. Fertility in men is assessed by semen analysis with assessment of sperm concentration, motility, and percentage of abnormal forms. An alternative, although less accurate, method of assessing spermatogenesis is by measuring FSH levels; elevated levels are associated with poor spermatogenesis.

The spermatogonia (germinal epithelium) are very sensitive to radiation and unlike most tissues are not spared by fractionation [14]. Transient suppression of spermatogenesis occurs with doses as low as 0.5 Gy. Following a dose of 2–3 Gy there is a period of azoospermia, after which full recovery is expected by 3 years. At doses of 4–6 Gy recovery is not universal and may take up to 5 years [15]. After 6 Gy there is a high risk of permanent sterility. The Leydig cells are more resistant to irradiation but doses in excess of 15 Gy may affect their function and production of testosterone.

Following ^{131}I administration, sources of radiation to the testes are the blood, bladder, gut, and functioning metastases close to the testes. Another source of testicular irradiation is derived from organified ^{131}I, which is incorporated into a variety of iodoproteins. These have relatively long half-lives and produce continuous blood-borne irradiation for weeks [16]. The MIRD to the testes is 0.085 cGy/37 MBq (1 mCi) in euthyroid adults [7]. Theoretical models taking into account the hypothyroid status of the patients, which decreases renal clearance of iodine resulting in a more prolonged exposure, suggested a higher testicular dose in the order of 0.5–1 cGy/37 MBq [17]. Thus the cumulative radiation dose following a standard ablation iodine activity of 3 GBq (81 mCi) is approximately 40–80 cGy. Using thermoluminescent dosimetry (TLD) we measured the dose in 14 patients; the mean dose to each testis was 6.4 cGy, 14.1 cGy, and 21.2 cGy following administration of 3, 5.5 and 9.2 GBq (81, 149 and 249 mCi) of ^{131}I, respectively. Testicular dose was higher following administration of larger iodine activities but still smaller than that estimated [18]. All of our 14 patients had persistent uptake of ^{131}I only in the neck and excreted the iodine relatively quickly; both factors would have contributed to the low absorbed testicular dose. Obviously the measured dose on the surface of the scrotum is likely to be less than that absorbed by the testes.

The serum FSH level is the best marker of germinal cell failure and serial measurements have been suggested as a useful prognostic indicator for recovery of spermatogenic function, since falling values indicate stem cell repopulation. We noted an elevation in serum FSH level even with low absorbed testicular doses. Mean FSH levels were lower before than after ^{131}I administration: 6.3 ± 4.1 versus 16.3 ± 4.8, respectively (normal range 3–12 IU/L). However, the levels normalized in all patients within 9 months from the last administration. Similar results were reported by Pacini et al., who found an increase in FSH levels in 36.8% of patients treated with high activities of radioiodine, as well as a positive correlation between FSH levels and the cumulative dose of ^{131}I received [19]. They also noted that in most patients FSH levels returned to normal 6–12 months after treatment but remained constantly elevated in four who had been treated with several doses of iodine, indicating permanent damage to the germinal epithelium. In another study a threshold dose of 100 mCi (3.7 GBq) [131]I for testicular damage was suggested since no elevation in serum FSH was seen in men treated with a single dose up to 100 mCi [20].

Fifty-nine patients in our series fathered 106 children 3.5–18 years after iodine treatment and none of the others reported infertility. Because of these results, as well as the low testicular dose measured using TLD, we did not perform semen analysis. There is, however, some evidence that iodine therapy can cause oligo- and even azoospermia which is correlated with cumulative dose [21]. Postmortem findings of testicular atrophy with absent spermatogenesis have been reported in three men aged 53–75 years treated with cumulative ^{131}I doses of 17 to 30.4 GBq (459 to 820 mCi) and external beam radiotherapy [22]. It is not clear whether these postmortem changes were due only to iodine therapy since other factors such as age, hypothyroidism, and terminal disease might have contributed. The administration of therapeutic doses of ionic forms of longer-lived radionuclides is a possible source of concern because of the appearance of quantities of such radionuclides in ejaculate and in sperm. It may be prudent, therefore, to advise sexually active males who have been treated with ^{131}I to avoid fathering children for a period of 4 months (suggested as it is greater than the life of a sperm cell) [13].

Our data as well as those of others indicate that radioiodine treatment for differentiated thyroid cancer may cause a transient impairment of testicular function. For patients who are treated with a single ablation dose, testicular function recovers within months and the risk of infertility seems negligible. However, gonadal damage may be cumulative in those who require multiple administrations for persistent disease. In addition to efforts aimed at reducing radiation exposure such as generous hydration with frequent micturition and avoidance of constipation, sperm banking may need to be considered in these patients [23].

Conclusion

Efforts should be made to reduce at least some of the radiation sources to the gonads. These include generous hydration (2–3 liters per day) with frequent micturition and avoidance of constipation using regular laxatives prior and during iodine administration. As with any form of radiotherapy, careful appraisal of the risks and benefits of radioiodine treatment is mandatory, especially when advising repeated doses to young patients [23]. Since there is evidence of cumulative gonadal damage with repeated iodine administration, it is recommended that the total cumulative iodine activity should be kept as low as possible [24]. In vivo dosimetry, which measures the actual absorbed dose received by remnant thyroid tissue, functioning metastatic disease, and normal organs with a view to optimizing the administered iodine dose, may help in achieving this goal [25].

References

1. Mazzaferri EL, Jhiang S. Long-term impact of initial surgical and medical therapy on papillary and follicular cancer. Am J Med 1994; 97:418–429.
2. Freitas JE, Gross MD, Ripley S, Shapiro B. Radionuclide diagnosis and therapy of thyroid cancer: current status report. Semin Nucl Med 1985; 15:106–131.
3. Edmonds CJ, Smith T. The long-term hazards of the treatment of thyroid cancer with radioiodine. Br J Radiol 1986; 59:45–51.
4. Madsen BL, Giudice L, Donaldson SS. Radiation induced menopause: a misconception. Int J Radiat Oncol Biol Phys 1995; 30:1461–1464.
5. Raymond JP, Izembart M, Marliac V, et al. Temporary ovarian failure in thyroid cancer patients after thyroid remnant ablation with radioactive iodine. J Clin Endocrinol Metab 1989; 69:186–189.
6. Vini L, Hyer S, Al-Saadi A, Pratt B, Harmer C. Prognosis for fertility and ovarian function after treatment with radioiodine for thyroid cancer. Postgrad Med J 2002; 78:92–93.
7. MIRD. Dose estimate report no. 5. J Nucl Med 1975; 16:857–860.
8. Izembart M, Chavaudra J, Aubert B, Vallee G. Retrospective evaluation of the dose received by the ovary after iodine therapy for thyroid cancer. Eur J Nucl Med 1992; 19:243–247.
9. Casara D, Rubello D, Saladini G, et al. Pregnancy after high therapeutic doses of iodine-131 in differentiated thyroid cancer: potential risks and recommendations. Eur J Nucl Med 1993; 20:192–194.
10. Dottorini ME, Lomuscio G, Mazzucchelli L, Vignati A, Colombo L. Assessment of female fertility and carcinogenesis after iodine-131 therapy for differentiated thyroid carcinoma. J Nucl Med 1995; 36:21–27.
11. Sarkar SD, Beierwaltes WH, Gill SP, Cowley BJ. Subsequent fertility and birth histories of children and adolescents treated with ^{131}I for thyroid cancer. J Nucl Med 1976; 17:460–464.
12. Schlumberger M, De Vathaire F, Ceccarelli C, et al. Exposure to radioactive iodine-131 for scintigraphy or therapy does not preclude pregnancy in thyroid cancer patients. J Nucl Med 1996; 37:606–612.
13. Notes for Guidance on the Clinical Administration of Radiopharmaceuticals and use of Sealed Radioactive Sources. Administration of Radioactive Substances Advisory Committee. December 1998.
14. Ash P. The influence of radiation on fertility in man. Br J Radiol 1980; 53:271–278.
15. Shapiro E, Kinsella TJ, Makosh RW, et al. Effects of fractionated irradiation on endocrine aspects of testicular function. J Clin Oncol 1985; 3:1232–1239.
16. Jeevanram RK, Shah DH, Sharma SM, Ganatra RD. Disappearance rate of endogenously radioiodinated thyroglobulin and thyroxine after radioiodine treatment. Cancer 1982; 49:2281–2284.
17. Maxon HR, Smith HS. Radioiodine-131 in diagnosis and treatment of metastatic well differentiated thyroid cancer. Endocrinol Metab Clin North Am 1990; 19:685–718.
18. Hyer S, Vini L, O'Connell M, Pratt M, Harmer. Testicular dose and fertility in men following I-131 therapy for thyroid cancer. C. Clin Endocrinol (Oxf) 2002; 57:313–314.
19. Pacini F, Gasperi M, Fugazzola L, et al. Testicular function in patients with differentiated thyroid carcinoma treated with radioiodine. J Nucl Med 1994; 35:1418–1422.
20. Handelsman DJ, Turtle JR. Testicular damage after radioactive iodine therapy for thyroid cancer. Clin Endocrinol 1983; 18:465–472.
21. Handelsman DJ, Conway AJ, Donnelly PE, Turtle JR. Azoospermia after iodine-131 treatment for thyroid carcinoma. BMJ 1980; 281:1527.

22. Trunnell JB, Duffy DG, Godwin JT, et al. The distribution of radioactive iodine in human tissues: necropsy in nine patients. J Clin Endocrinol 1950; 10:1007–1021.

23. Vini L, Harmer C. Management of thyroid cancer. Lancet Oncol 2002; 3:407–414.

24. Guidelines for the management of thyroid cancer. British Thyroid Association, 2002.

25. Vini L, Chittenden S, Pratt B, et al. In vivo dosimetry of radioiodine in patients with metastatic differentiated thyroid cancer. Eur J Nucl Med 1998; 25:904(OS 272).

Section V

Follow-up Management of Differentiated
Thyroid Cancer

17

Recombinant Human TSH (rhTSH): Use in Papillary and Follicular Thyroid Cancer

Furio Pacini and Martin J. Schlumberger

Introduction

Thyrotropin (TSH), a specific and potent thyroid stimulator, is essential for normal thyroid function, promoting iodide uptake and thyroglobulin (Tg) synthesis and cell growth. Papillary and follicular thyroid carcinomas, and their metastases, retain some features of normal thyroid tissue, including iodine uptake and Tg synthesis, upon stimulation by TSH. These properties are suited for the postsurgical follow-up and for treatment of persistent and recurrent disease: ^{131}I whole-body scan (^{131}I-WBS) and serum Tg measurement at the diagnostic level and ^{131}I administration at the therapeutic level.

In the absence of TSH stimulation, radioiodine uptake is not elicited and serum Tg is suppressed to undetectable levels in at least 5% of patients with micronodular lung metastases and in 20% of patients with lymph node metastases.

Multiple metabolic defects being present in thyroid cancer tissue, both procedures to be effective require intensive TSH stimulation. This is typically achieved by withdrawing L-thyroxine therapy for 4 to 6 weeks to induce a transient state of hypothyroidism, under which high serum TSH (>25 mU/L) can stimulate iodine uptake and Tg secretion [1]. During this period, patients experience signs and symptoms of hypothyroidism which may be severe and may result in substantial impairment of the patient's quality of life and ability to work [2–4]. In addition, once L-T$_4$ treatment is resumed, it may take up to 10 weeks for serum TSH to normalize, and this prolongs the impact of hypothyroidism on the patient's life. Furthermore, prolonged periods of TSH hyperstimulation may be associated with increased growth of metastatic thyroid tissue. Also, hypothyroidism may induce changes in drug metabolism and may worsen concomitant pathological conditions.

To overcome the inconvenience of hypothyroidism, several procedures have been used, such as substituting the more rapidly metabolized triiodothyronine (L-T$_3$) for thyroxine for 3 weeks and then withdrawing it for 2 weeks. This procedure proved to be effective, and reduces but does not avoid signs and symptoms of hypothyroidism. Other authors have simply reduced the L-T$_4$ dose by 33–50%, but the effectiveness of this procedure as compared with withdrawal has not been documented.

In the past, exogenous administration of bovine TSH (bTSH) (10 U for 3 consecutive days) was successfully employed to stimulate radioiodine uptake in thyroid cancer patients, without the need for withdrawing thyroid hormone therapy. However, bTSH was less effective than endogenous TSH, was associated with adverse reactions, including urticaria and anaphylactic shock, and induced TSH antibodies. The potential use of human TSH (hTSH) purified from pooled pituitary glands obtained at autopsy is similarly unsuitable, due to the possible transmission of Creutzfeldt–Jakob disease, as observed in patients treated with human growth hormone (hGH).

Production of Recombinant Human TSH (rhTSH)

TSH is a pituitary heterodimeric glycoprotein composed of an α-subunit common to gonadotropins and a hormone-specific-β-subunit. Once the β-subunit of the human TSH gene had been cloned, the encoded protein could be overexpressed in a cell system, by transfection with the human α- and β-subunits of complementary or genomic DNA. With this technique, high quantities of highly purified rhTSH with biological properties similar to native TSH can be obtained.

In vitro studies have shown that rhTSH can effectively stimulate cAMP production in a rat thyroid cell line (FRTL-5 cells), and promote the growth of human fetal thyroid cells. The biological efficacy of rhTSH was then demonstrated in monkeys, in which it was able to increase serum T_4 and T_3 concentrations and thyroidal radioiodine uptake [5]. In human volunteers, a single dose of 0.1 mg rhTSH was a potent stimulator of thyroid function [6], and single doses higher than 0.1–0.3 mg do not seem to further enhance thyroid hormone or Tg secretion. The serum Tg response to rhTSH occurred later than the serum T_3 and T_4 response, with a peak serum level at day 2. Finally, a single intramuscular (IM) dose of 0.9 mg increases thyroid uptake by approximately 100% [7].

Pharmacokinetic studies showed that the mean peak serum TSH level was achieved within 4–6 hours after each injection. Following the intramuscular injection of 0.9 mg, the mean peak serum level was 116 ± 38 mU/L; serum half-life was 22.3 ± 8.5 hours and serum TSH remained above 30 mU/L for approximately 2 days. The extent of TSH stimulation depends on both the serum TSH level since rhTSH administration and the duration of elevated serum TSH levels and is best expressed by the area under the curve.

The product was approved for human use, upon completion of two phase III pivotal studies on thyroid cancer patients [8,9] with the name of Thyrogen (Genzyme Therapeutics, Cambridge, USA). The cost of the rhTSH test (2 vials) is over 1000 euros. This price may appear to be very high, but it should be considered as relatively modest when weighed against the benefits for the patient (see below). Moreover, knowing that rhTSH is available, patients strongly request treatment with this modality to avoid prolonged episodes of hypothyroidism.

Diagnostic Use of rhTSH

Early Clinical Trials

The availability of large quantities of rhTSH prompted clinical trials in patients with papillary and follicular thyroid cancer to investigate its safety and efficacy in promoting radioiodine uptake and Tg secretion.

Efficacy

A first study (phase I/II), completed in 1994 in 19 patients after a recent thyroidectomy for differentiated thyroid cancer (DTC), demonstrated the safety and the efficacy of rhTSH in promoting ^{131}I uptake [10]. Based on previous dose-finding studies the dose of rhTSH was fixed at 0.9 mg for 2 consecutive days.

The encouraging results of this limited study were confirmed in a larger multicenter phase III study conducted between 1992 and 1995 in the USA in 127 patients [8]. Using a single daily injection of 0.9 mg of rhTSH for 2 consecutive days, the ^{131}I whole-body scan was equal to that obtained after thyroid hormone withdrawal in 86% of the patients and inferior in the remaining patients. This study had some methodological limitations, including the use of non-uniform ^{131}I doses (74–148 MBq, 2–4 mCi), different scanning times and techniques, and the inclusion of only a few patients with metastatic disease. Furthermore, serum Tg testing was not a study endpoint.

To overcome these limitations, a second multicenter phase III trial, including US and European centers, was designed [9]. The study included the comparison of two arms receiving different regimens of rhTSH given at a fixed dose of 0.9 mg (once daily injection for 2 consecutive days versus 3 injections, 3 days apart), a fixed tracer dose of radioiodine (148 MBq, 4 mCi) and the analysis of serum Tg as a marker of disease. Serum Tg testing and ^{131}I-WBS obtained after rhTSH and after thyroid hormone withdrawal were compared: [131]I -WBS were similar in more than 90% of the patients, and serum Tg responses were comparable between the two methods. Among patients with persistent or recurrent disease, 80% had concordant scans, 4% had superior rhTSH scans, and 16% had superior withdrawal scans. Serum Tg was detectable (≥ 2 ng/mL) in only 80% of these patients during L-T$_4$ therapy and was detectable in 100% following both rhTSH and withdrawal. The peak serum Tg was usually observed 2–3 days after the last injection of rhTSH. The shorter duration of stimulation with rhTSH is likely to have an impact on Tg levels and radioiodine uptake. In fact, the serum Tg level attained following rhTSH stimulation was usually lower than following withdrawal, but Tg was still detectable in all patients with persistent or recurrent disease investigated; this underlines why a sensitive IRMA method should be used and why all detectable serum Tg levels should be taken into account, even low levels. Furthermore, radioiodine uptake was also lower with rhTSH, and this was attributed both to a shorter duration of stimulation and to decreased bioavailability of radioiodine after rhTSH (euthyroid status) than following withdrawal (hypothyroid status). In fact, hypothyroidism decreases the renal clearance of iodine and increases its body retention, thus increasing its bioavailability for thyroid cells but also the body radiation dose. This underscores the need for a diagnostic dose of ^{131}I of 4 mCi and not less and for scanning 2 days after the dose using standardized procedures.

In conclusion, the combination of serum Tg and of ^{131}I-WBS was more informative than ^{131}I-WBS alone and even more important, rhTSH-stimulated Tg detected all patients with persistent or recurrent disease.

Tolerance

rhTSH avoids the consequences of prolonged withdrawal, including:

1. The usual signs or symptoms of hypothyroidism, and its consequences for organ function in particular on the brain, heart, liver, and kidney; it avoids the worsening of any associated disease, and also the hazards of any drug therapy induced by a decreased renal or hepatic function; finally, modification of physiology induced by hypothyroidism is avoided and thus any

vital function is conserved and any associated impairment be avoided.

2. Moderate to severe impairment of the ability to work and difficulties in operating a motor vehicle; these consequences are usually underscored by the patients themselves, and are significant because these patients are typically young or middle aged. The number of days of work missed by the patient was reduced by about 14 days when rhTSH was used instead of withdrawal.

3. As a consequence, quality of life was maintained and was much better during rhTSH than during hypothyroidism. Patient preference for rhTSH over withdrawal is universal. Side effects were minimal, being observed in less than 10% of patients, and consisted mainly of mild and transient nausea and headache, and no patient developed detectable anti-rhTSH antibodies.

Protocol

According to the results of these trials, the optimal protocol for using rhTSH in thyroid cancer patients is as follows:

- The dose is fixed at a once daily intramuscular injection of 0.9 mg of rhTSH for 2 consecutive days.
- A ^{131}I dose of at least 148 MBq (4 mCi) is administered on the day following the second injection of rhTSH.
- A whole-body scan is performed 48 h after radioiodine administration, with standardized procedures.
- Serum Tg determination is performed 3 days after the second injection of rhTSH. Indeed, sera containing interferences from antithyroglobulin antibody should be excluded from the analysis, and a sensitive IRMA method should be used to measure serum Tg.
- Serum TSH may also be measured, but only to ensure that rhTSH has been injected. If TSH is measured, it should be measured 1 or 3 days after the second rhTSH injection.
- During this procedure, thyroxine treatment is maintained. Urinary iodine excre-

tion was slightly increased as compared with hypothyroidism, in relation to the iodine content of L-thyroxine, but was always far below 200 μg, and this increase probably did not affect the iodine uptake after a strong stimulation with rhTSH.

Altogether, these clinical trials have clearly shown that rhTSH is an effective and safe alternative to thyroid hormone withdrawal in the postsurgical diagnostic follow-up of patients with papillary and follicular thyroid cancer. The cost of injections is well balanced with the advantages of its use. These studies confirmed the rationale for the use of rhTSH in clinical practice and showed its potential benefit and possible limitations, paving the way for a large series of subsequent clinical studies.

Additional Clinical Studies

Robbins et al. [11] in a retrospective analysis of 289 thyroid cancer patients undergoing routine follow-up testing, including 139 patients with metastatic disease, compared results in patients who were prepared by thyroid hormone withdrawal and patients who received rhTSH. No significant difference in the diagnostic accuracy of ^{131}I-WBS and/or Tg was found, confirming that preparation with either rhTSH or thyroid hormone withdrawal is diagnostically equivalent.

Several authors explored the possibility that rhTSH-stimulated Tg levels may represent the only necessary test to differentiate patients with persistent disease from disease-free patients.

Pacini et al. [12] reported a prospective study in 72 consecutive patients with undetectable (<1 ng/mL) basal serum Tg. They performed an rhTSH-stimulated serum Tg and then withdrew thyroid hormone therapy for ^{131}I-WBS and serum Tg determination. This study showed that rhTSH-stimulated Tg permitted the distinction of disease-free patients (rhTSH/Tg <1 ng/mL) who all had normal ^{131}I-WBS from patients with disease (detectable rhTSH-stimulated Tg) who needed further diagnostic or therapeutic procedures. There was a strong concordance between Tg obtained following rhTSH and withdrawal. However, in 12% of cases, serum Tg was detectable after thyroid hormone withdrawal and undetectable after rhTSH stimulation, but this was always associated with either a negative WBS or faint uptake in the thyroid bed.

Mazzaferri and Kloos [13] retrospectively studied 107 thyroid cancer patients who underwent rhTSH-stimulated testing 10 months to 35 years after initial thyroidectomy and ^{131}I ablation. About 50% of these patients were at high risk of tumor recurrence and five had distant metastases during the course of the follow-up period. Eleven patients (10%), all of whom had rhTSH-stimulated serum Tg levels >2 ng/mL, were found to have persistent disease (4 in lungs, 5 in lymph nodes, 2 in other sites). In no cases did an rhTSH-stimulated ^{131}I-WBS indicate the location of the tumor. A serum Tg <2 ng/mL was found in 87 patients, none of whom had a positive ^{131}I-WBS. In this study an rhTSH-stimulated serum Tg (with a cutoff level of 2 ng/mL) had a sensitivity of 100% and a negative predictive value of 100%. Finally, nine patients had serum Tg above 2 ng/mL and no other evidence of disease. The authors concluded that tumor amenable to early therapy may be found when rhTSH-stimulated serum Tg rises above 2 ng/mL, without performing a diagnostic WBS.

Haugen et al. [14] retrospectively compared the sensitivity of the rhTSH-stimulated Tg test alone in detecting metastatic disease with that of rhTSH-stimulated WBS with or without the Tg test. Of the 83 patients (previously treated with thyroidectomy and ablation), 10 patients had a positive ^{131}I-WBS. Using a cutoff of 2 ng/mL, 25 patients were Tg positive, and using a cutoff of 5 ng/mL, 13 patients were Tg positive. Nine patients combined a positive Tg (cutoff 5 ng/mL) with a negative WBS. After further evaluation, six of these patients appeared to have metastatic disease. The authors concluded that rhTSH-stimulated Tg has a higher sensitivity than rhTSH-stimulated WBS in detecting clinically relevant disease.

Torlontano et al. [15] performed an rhTSH-stimulated Tg determination, a ^{131}I-WBS and a neck ultrasound examination in 99 patients with no uptake outside the thyroid bed on the prior postablative WBS. The study was performed within a year after initial treatment, and its results can be readily applied to clinical practice. The diagnostic ^{131}I-WBS was negative in all cases. rhTSH-stimulated Tg was >1 ng/mL in 21 patients. The ultrasound examination identified lymph node metastases in 4/6 patients with a Tg >5 ng/mL, in 2/15 patients with a Tg between 1 and 5 ng/mL, and in 2/78 patients with a Tg <1 ng/mL. This study showed that adding neck ultrasonography to rhTSH-stimulated Tg testing is useful for the first follow-up of low risk patients. Indeed, some lymph node metastases evidenced by neck ultrasonography were only a few millimeters in diameter; however, the clinical relevance of such an early finding has not yet been demonstrated.

The diagnostic value of combining rhTSH-stimulated Tg and neck ultrasound was confirmed in a larger study by Pacini et al. [16]. They studied 340 consecutive DTC patients treated with near-total thyroidectomy and ^{131}I ablation. On L-T$_4$ therapy, 294 patients had undetectable (<1 ng/mL) serum Tg and negative anti-Tg autoantibodies (TgAb), 25 patients had undetectable serum Tg and positive TgAb, and 21 patients had detectable serum Tg and negative TgAb. rhTSH-stimulated Tg alone had a sensitivity of 85% for detecting disease and a negative predictive value (NPV) of 98.2%. By adding the results of neck ultrasound, the sensitivity increased to 96.3% and the NPV to 99.5%. rhTSH-stimulated ^{131}I-WBS had a sensitivity of only 21% and an NPV of 89%. The combination of rhTSH-stimulated Tg and WBS had a sensitivity of 92.7% and an NPV of 99%. The authors concluded that the rhTSH-stimulated Tg test combined with neck ultrasonography has the highest accuracy in detecting persistent disease in the follow-up of papillary and follicular thyroid carcinoma. A detectable serum Tg level on L-thyroxine, or its conversion from undetectable to detectable after rhTSH and/or suspicious findings at ultrasound will allow the identification of patients requiring therapeutic procedures, without the need for a diagnostic ^{131}I-WBS.

Wartofsky [17] supported the idea that testing serum Tg, both on suppression and after rhTSH stimulation, can help determine therapy. In his multicentric study [18], he found that 18% of patients, including 11% with undetectable Tg on L-T$_4$, ultimately had detectable rhTSH-stimulated Tg. Based on the results of this study, this author suggests that patients with a serum Tg <0.5 ng/mL on suppression, and presumably in a low risk category, may be followed up with an rhTSH-stimulated Tg approach in combination with neck ultrasonography. If the rhTSH-stimulated Tg remains <1 ng/mL and the neck ultrasonography is normal, these patients can be evaluated annually with serum Tg determination on L-T$_4$ treatment and with neck ultrasonography. In patients with slightly higher Tg (up to 2 ng/mL), he suggested obtaining an rhTSH-stimulated Tg and ^{131}I-WBS. In patients with higher Tg, he proposed withdrawing L-T$_4$ for ^{131}I treatment, without previous diagnostic scanning. One of the objectives of this study was to analyze the comparability of serum Tg assays performed in a central reference laboratory (with a third generation radioimmunoassay) with those performed in local laboratories (a variety of immunometric and radioimmunoassays). A strong correlation between central and local laboratory values was found for both baseline ($r = 0.85$) and rhTSH-stimulated ($r = 0.95$) Tg values, and the number of false-negative results was not different with any of the methods used.

Robbins et al. [19] reported a retrospective study on 366 thyroid cancer patients tested using rhTSH and results were partly at variance with the conclusion of the above studies. Using a cutoff of 2 ng/mL, rhTSH Tg testing alone failed to detect 13% of patients with metastatic lesions in whom neoplastic foci were already known, and the diagnostic ^{131}I-WBS was informative in nearly half of these cases. In low risk patients, especially when they already had a negative diagnostic ^{131}I-WBS, the sensitivity of rhTSH-stimulated Tg alone was 97%. In this study, false-negative results were found in patients who had already been treated with ^{131}I, and this is in accordance with a previous report [20] on patients who had repeatedly undergone ^{131}I treatments, and in whom small neoplastic foci were found at surgery despite undetectable stimulated serum Tg levels but with persistent ^{131}I uptake in some. In fact, in these patients the problem is not the diagnosis of persistent or recurrent disease but rather the treatment of previously detected neoplastic foci.

Altogether, the information currently available suggests that patients who have undergone ^{131}I remnant ablation may be followed up by measurement of basal and rhTSH-stimulated serum Tg, and this concept was confirmed in two recent consensus reports, one in the USA and one in Europe [21,22]. Imaging with ^{131}I-WBS is indicated only in patients with detectable basal or stimulated Tg levels (above a cutoff value to be determined at each institution), preferably using therapeutic doses of radioiodine. Patients with undetectable rhTSH-stimulated Tg can be followed up annually on L-thyroxine with serum Tg determination and neck ultrasonography. Indeed, in case of doubt or even in routine practice, rhTSH-stimulated Tg may be obtained every 2 to 5 years to ensure complete remission, but more data are needed to validate this practice.

It is noteworthy that the proposal to use TSH-stimulated serum Tg as the only test in the post-surgical follow-up of thyroid cancer patients is not something new and only derived from experience with rhTSH. In addition, several authors have demonstrated the limited diagnostic value of ^{131}I-WBS when patients are tested in the hypothyroid state. The first observation goes back to 1980, when serum Tg levels were found to be elevated in patients with nonfunctioning metastases [23]. More recently two large retrospective studies, one from Villejuif [24] and one from Pisa [25], developed this concept further.

Conclusion

Studies performed on more than 2000 thyroid cancer patients have confirmed the results of the rhTSH pivotal trials. These studies are also in close agreement with data obtained following withdrawal of L-T$_4$ treatment. The results of these studies in total can be summarized as follows:

1. rhTSH can be effectively used during the follow-up of thyroid cancer patients: hypothyroid and euthyroid rhTSH-stimulated serum Tg levels are comparable in detecting persistent or recurrent disease.
2. Serum Tg measured 3 days after the second injection is a highly sensitive tool for detecting persistent or recurrent disease. Any detectable Tg level (≥1 ng/mL) should be taken into account.
3. Serum Tg converts from undetectable during L-thyroxine treatment to detectable following rhTSH in 10–20% of patients who had no other evidence of disease. The rare false-negative Tg measurements found in this situation are due to isolated small lymph node metastases in the neck, which could be detected by ultrasonography.

4. False-negative serum Tg measurements were also reported in a few patients with neoplastic foci who were previously treated with [131]I: in these patients with a small amount of residual disease, serum Tg may remain undetectable but ^{131}I uptake may still be present.
5. A detectable serum Tg following rhTSH at the first evaluation performed within 1 year after thyroid ablation may subsequently decrease or even normalize in the absence of any treatment; thus, it should be evaluated again a few months later. Then, in patients with a persistent detectable serum Tg level, other procedures are warranted to localize neoplastic foci; one possibility is to administer a high dose of ^{131}I after thyroid hormone withdrawal and to perform a WBS 3–7 days later, in patients with a serum Tg level above some arbitrary threshold (perhaps >5–10 ng/mL) or with an increasing Tg level at consecutive determinations.
6. In contrast, diagnostic ^{131}I-WBS is normal in patients with undetectable rhTSH-stimulated Tg and does not add significant information in most patients with detectable serum Tg levels following rhTSH.
7. Neck ultrasonography is the most sensitive tool for detecting small lymph node metastases not visible on ^{131}I-WBS and not even suggested by an increase in serum Tg level. Thus, neck ultrasonography and serum Tg determination performed 3 days after the second rhTSH injection are advised as first-line tests.

Based on these considerations, the diagnostic algorithm of Figure 17.1 may be proposed. It makes ^{131}I-WBS unnecessary for the follow-up of a large majority of patients with no evidence of disease, thereby reducing the risks of exposure to ^{131}I and the cost of the follow-up protocol.

Therapeutic Use of rhTSH

As mentioned above, withdrawal of L-T$_4$ suppressive therapy in preparation for ^{131}I therapy may expose patients with metastases in critical body structures, such as vertebrae or the brain, to severe complications which are mainly neu-

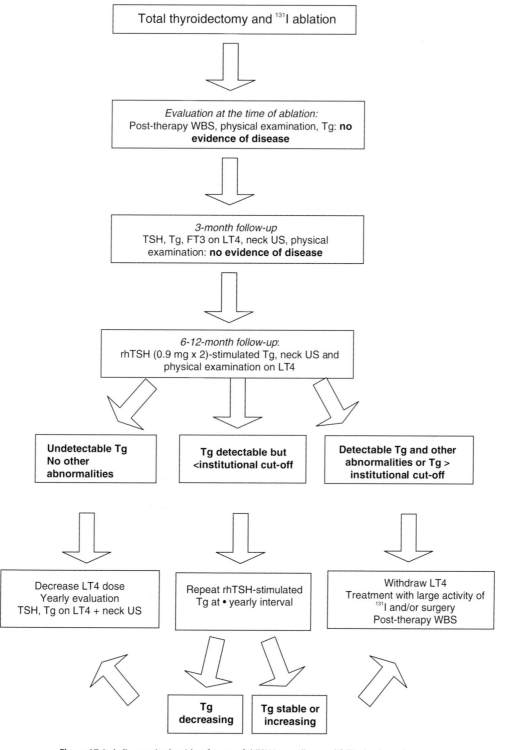

Figure 17.1 A diagnostic algorithm for use of rhTSH in papillary and follicular thyroid cancer.

rological. In addition, a small minority of patients may not be able to elicit a sufficient response of endogenous TSH after thyroid hormone withdrawal, due to older age, long-term suppressive therapy, a concomitant illness, or pituitary insufficiency which prevents adequate uptake of ^{131}I in metastatic foci. Finally, thyroid hormone withdrawal may be contraindicated for medical reasons, such as a coexistent illness. rhTSH is not approved for treatment of patients with ^{131}I uptake in metastatic lesions; however, since 1995, rhTSH has been administered for this purpose to several hundred patients around the world within the framework of a clinical protocol named "compassionate use program."

In publications to date, rhTSH has been applied to stimulate radioiodine treatment in a total of 116 patients from different centers for a total of 155 treatment courses. The large major-ity of these patients were individuals with bulky, widespread, end-stage cancer. The results of the treatment are reported in a detailed and com-prehensive review [26] indicating that rhTSH appeared to promote radioiodine uptake by tumor tissue in nearly all patients and that 66% of 92 patents with adequate follow-up data achieved some clinical benefit. Due to the more rapid renal clearance of ^{131}I in euthyroidism compared to hypothyroidism, a higher ^{131}I dose should theoretically be administered to achieve an equivalent dose to the metastatic lesion, although results from quantitative dosimetric studies are not yet available.

In some patients, swelling and pain due to bone metastases were observed after rhTSH administration. However, the duration of such symptoms was much shorter than was expected when therapy is administered during hypothy-roidism. Caution should be exerted in case of potential neurological complications and corti-costeroids should be used to prevent complica-tions. At this stage, it is not possible to report on the long-term benefits of this treatment modal-ity in comparison with thyroid hormone with-drawal. The general impression is that rhTSH stimulation may become the modality of choice as preparation for radioiodine treatment of metastatic patients provided that additional investigation, particularly in patients with less advanced disease than those included in the "compassionate use program," confirms the pre-liminary observation now available.

Thyroid Remnant Ablation

Another condition for which rhTSH is becom-ing an alternative to prolonged thyroid hormone withdrawal is postsurgical ^{131}I ablation therapy.

Between 2001 and the present, four studies employing rhTSH to promote ^{131}I remnant abla-tion under TSH suppressive therapy have been published. Two studies were performed at Memorial Sloan-Kettering Cancer Center [27,28]. In the first article [27], 10 patients were given rhTSH (0.9 mg IM each day for 2 days) fol-lowed by [131]I (mean dose 110.3 mCi). Follow-up diagnostic scans, obtained 5 to 13 months later, showed no visible uptake in the thyroid bed in any patient. The second study [28] was a retro-spective comparison of 87 patients with differ-entiated thyroid cancer who had undergone thyroid remnant ablation after a regimen of rhTSH ($n = 45$) or L-thyroxine withdrawal ($n = 42$). The mean amounts of radioiodine given for ablation were 110.4 mCi and 128.9 mCi, respec-tively. At follow-up diagnostic scanning done about 11 months after ablation, it was found that 84% of patients prepared using rhTSH and 81% of patients prepared by L-thyroxine withdrawal had complete resolution of visible thyroid bed uptake.

A lower rate of successful ablation for patients prepared with rhTSH compared with patients prepared by withdrawal of thyroid hormone therapy has been reported in a study by Pacini et al. [29] using a fixed dose of 30 mCi [131]I. The authors studied three groups of patients with differentiated thyroid cancer, assigned to a regime of thyroxine withdrawal ($n = 50$), thy-roxine withdrawal plus rhTSH ($n = 42$), and euthyroidism with rhTSH ($n = 70$). Diagnostic scanning then was performed 6 to 10 months later after withdrawal of L-thyroxine. The primary definition of successful ablation was based on no visible uptake of radioiodine in the thyroid bed. The rates of successful ablation in the three groups were 84%, 79%, and 54%, respectively. If successful ablation had been defined as negative scan or undetectable serum Tg (<1 ng/mL while off thyroxine) even with positive uptake on scan, the rates of successful ablation would have been 88.0%, 95.0%, and 74.1% in the thyroxine withdrawal group, the thyroxine withdrawal plus rhTSH group, and the euthyroidism plus rhTSH group, respectively. A possible caveat of this study is that ^{131}I was administered 48 hours after the last injection of rhTSH instead of the usual 24 hours. It remains uncertain whether this delay might partly explain the different outcome of this study compared with the other studies of rhTSH-assisted remnant ablation. Indeed, a higher rate of ablation (81%) has been reported in another study [30] using 30 mCi as a fixed dose in 16 patients with stage I or II papillary or follicular thyroid cancer, in which the therapeutic dose was administered 24 hours after the last rhTSH injection.

More recently, a prospective, randomized clinical trial has been conducted in the USA, Canada, and Europe regarding the ablation of thyroid remnants in patients with well-differentiated thyroid cancer who had recently undergone total or near-total thyroidectomy. After surgery, a total of 63 patients were randomized to receive thyroid ablation with 100 mCi ^{131}I aided by rhTSH while euthyroid ($n = 33$) or by thyroid hormone withdrawal while hypothyroid ($n = 30$). The efficacy of the ablation regimens was assessed 8 months later (± 1 month) using rhTSH-stimulated 4 mCi radioiodine scanning and stimulated serum Tg levels. As a primary endpoint, the definition of successful remnant was a negative neck scan (no visible uptake, or if visible, less than 0.1% uptake in the thyroid bed) 8 ± 1 months following the ablation treatment. Moreover, stimulated serum Tg levels also were used to assess the success of remnant ablation, and a Tg cutoff level of 2 ng/mL was proposed as a widely accepted and appropriate cutoff, although analyses using a cutoff level of 1 ng/mL also were performed. The trial has been completed and the results have been analyzed (manuscript in preparation). The neck scans performed 8 months after ablation showed that 100% of patients with interpretable scans in both treatment groups had successful ablation using the primary endpoint of "no visible uptake, or if visible, <0.1% uptake." Using an rhTSH-stimulated serum Tg level of <2 ng/mL as the criterion, remnant ablation was achieved in 86% of the patients in the hypothyroid group and in 96% of the patients in the euthyroid group (95% CI for difference in ablation rates, euthyroid group minus hypothyroid group, −6.9% to 27.1%, which excluded the clinically relevant difference in the lower bound). If the stimulated

Tg level cutoff of <1 ng/mL is used instead as the criterion for successful ablation, the rates of ablation in the hypothyroid and euthyroid groups were 87% and 83%, respectively, with 95% CI − 24.4% to 16.4%. Therefore, judging by the two objective criteria of quantified thyroid bed uptake or measured serum Tg level, clinically comparable thyroid remnant ablation rates were found in patients with differentiated thyroid cancer when prepared for postoperative radioiodine therapy by L-thyroxine withdrawal or by rhTSH.

There has been concern about whether in the euthyroid condition the iodine content of L-thyroxine medication can alter the uptake of radioiodine compared with patients treated in the hypothyroid state. This issue was addressed in the present study by measuring the urinary iodine excretion at the time of ablation in the two groups of patients. The results have shown that, although the rhTSH-treated group tended to have slightly higher values, the median of urinary iodine (reflecting the total daily intake of iodine) is far below the threshold considered critical for an efficient uptake of radioiodine.

In summary, based on the current experience, the use of rhTSH as an adjunct to radioiodine for the ablation of thyroid remnants is safe and effective and it is predictable that it will become the treatment of choice for thyroid ablation.

References

1. Schlumberger MJ. Papillary and follicular thyroid carcinoma. N Engl J Med 1998; 338:297–306.
2. Dow K, Ferrel B, Anello C. Quality of life changes in patients with thyroid cancer after withdrawal of thyroid hormone therapy. Thyroid 1997; 7:613–619.
3. Schlumberger M, Ricard M, Pacini F. Clinical use of recombinant human TSH in thyroid cancer patients. Eur J Endocrinol 2000; 143:557–563.
4. Mazzaferri EL, Kloos RT. Using recombinant human TSH in the management of well-differentiated thyroid cancer: Current strategies and future directions. Thyroid 2000; 10:767–778.
5. Braverman LE, Pratt BM, Ebner S, Davies TF. Recombinant human thyrotropin stimulates thyroid function and radioactive iodine uptake in rhesus monkey. J Clin Endocrinol Metab 1991; 74:1135–1139.
6. Ramirez L, Braverman L, White B, Emerson C. Recombinant human thyrotropin is a potent stimulator of thyroid function in normal subjects. J Clin Endocrinol Metab 1997; 82:2836–2839.
7. Torres MST, Ramirez L, Simkin PH, Braverman LE, Emerson CH. Effect of various doses of recombinant human thyrotropin on the thyroid radioactive iodine uptake and serum levels of thyroid hormones and thy-

roglobulin in normal subjects. J Clin Endocrinol Metab 2001; 86:1660–1664.

8. Ladenson PW, Braverman LE, Mazzaferri EL, et al. Comparison of administration of recombinant human thyrotropin with withdrawal of thyroid hormone for radioactive iodine scanning in patients with thyroid carcinoma. N Engl J Med 1997; 337:888–895.

9. Haugen BR, Pacini F, Reiners C, et al. A comparison of recombinant human thyrotropin and thyroid hormone withdrawal for the detection of thyroid remnant or cancer. J Clin Endocrinol Metab 1999; 84:3877–3885.

10. Meier CA, Braverman LE, Ebner SA, et al. Diagnostic use of recombinant human thyrotropin in patients with thyroid carcinoma (phase I/II study). J Clin Endocrinol Metab 1994; 78:188–196.

11. Robbins RJ, Tuttle RM, Sharaf RN, et al. Preparation by recombinant human thyrotropin or thyroid hormone withdrawal are comparable for the detection of residual differentiated thyroid carcinoma. J Clin Endocrinol Metab 2001; 86:619–625.

12. Pacini F, Molinaro E, Lippi F, et al. Prediction of disease status by recombinant human TSH-stimulated serum Tg in the postsurgical follow-up of differentiated thyroid carcinoma. J Clin Endocrinol Metab 2001; 86:5686–5690.

13. Mazzaferri EL, Kloos RT. Is diagnostic iodine-131 scanning with recombinant human TSH useful in the follow-up of differentiated thyroid cancer after thyroid ablation?. J Clin Endocrinol Metab 2002; 87:1490–1498.

14. Haugen BR, Ridgway EC, McLaughlin B, McDermott MT. Clinical comparison of whole-body radioiodine scan and serum thyroglobulin after stimulation with recombinant human TSH. Thyroid 2002; 12:37–43.

15. Torlontano M, Crocetti U, D'Aloiso L, et al. Serum thyroglobulin and ^{131}I whole body scan after recombinant human TSH stimulation in the follow-up of low-risk patients with differentiated thyroid carcinoma. The role for neck ultrasonography. Eur J Endocrinol 2003; 148: 18–24.

16. Pacini F, Molinaro E, Castagna MG, et al. rhTSH-stimulated serum thyroglobulin combined with neck ultrasonography has the highest sensitivity in monitoring differentiated thyroid carcinoma. J Clin Endocrinol Metab, 2003; 88:3668–3673.

17. Wartofsky J. Using baseline and recombinant human TSH-stimulated Tg measurements to manage thyroid cancer without diagnostic 131I scanning. J Clin Endocrinol Metab 2002; 87:1486–1489.

18. Wartofsky L. Management of low-risk well-differentiated thyroid cancer based only on thyroglobulin measurement after recombinant human thyrotropin. Thyroid 2002; 12:583–590.

19. Robbins RJ, Larson SM, Sinha N, et al. A retrospective review of the effectiveness of recombinant human TSH as a preparation for radioiodine thyroid remnant ablation. J Nucl Med 2002; 43:1482–1488.

20. Bachelot A, Cailleux AF, Klain M, et al. Relationship between tumor burden and serum thyroglobulin level in patients with papillary and follicular thyroid carcinoma. Thyroid 2002; 12:707–711.

21. Mazzaferri EL, Robbins RJ, Spencer CA, et al. A consensus report of the role of serum thyroglobulin as a monitoring method for low-risk patients with papillary thyroid carcinoma. J Clin Endocrinol Metab 2003; 88:1433–1441.

22. Schlumberger M, Berg G, Cohen O, et al. Follow-up of low-risk patients with differentiated thyroid carcinoma: a European perspective. Eur J Endocrinol 2004; 50:105–112.

23. Pacini F, Pinchera A, Giani C, Baschieri L. Serum thyroglobulin concentrations and 131-I whole body scans in the diagnosis of metastases from differentiated thyroid carcinoma (after thyroidectomy). Clin Endocrinol 1980; 13:107.

24. Cailleux AF, Baudin E, Travagli JP, Ricard M, Schlumberger M. Is diagnostic iodine-131 scanning useful after total thyroid ablation for differentiated thyroid carcinoma? J Clin Endocrinol Metab 2000; 85:175–178.

25. Pacini F, Capezzone M, Elisei R, Ceccarelli C, Taddei D, Pinchera A. Diagnostic 131-iodine whole–body scan may be avoided in thyroid cancer patients who have undetectable stimulated serum Tg levels after initial treatment. J Clin Endocrinol Metab 2002; 87:1499–1501.

26. Luster M, Lippi F, Jarzab B, et al. rhTSH-aided radioiodine ablation and treatment of differentiated thyroid carcinoma: a comprehensive review. Endocr Relat Cancer 2005; 12(1):49–64.

27. Robbins RJ, Tuttle RM, Sonenberg M, Shaha A, et al. Radioioidine ablation of thyroid remnants after preparation with recombinant human thyrotropin. Thyroid 2001; 11:865–869.

28. Robbins RJ, Larson SM, Sinha N, et al. A retrospective review of the effectiveness of recombinant human TSH as a preparation for radioiodine thyroid remnant ablation. J Nucl Med 2002; 43:1482–1488.

29. Pacini F, Molinaro E, Castagna MG, et al. Ablation of thyroid residues with 30 mCi ^{131}I: A comparison in thyroid cancer patients prepared with recombinant human TSH or thyroid hormone withdrawal. J Clin Endocrinol Metab 2002; 87:4063–4068.

30. Barbaro D, Boni G, Meucci G, et al. Radioiodine treatment with 30 mCi after recombinant human thyrotropin stimulation in thyroid cancer: Effectiveness for postsurgical remnants ablation and possible role of iodine content in L-thyroxine in the outcome of ablation. J Clin Endocrinol Metab 2003; 88:4110–4115.

18

Thyroglobulin

Carole A. Spencer and Shireen Fatemi

Serum thyroglobulin (Tg) measurements are a cornerstone for managing patients with differentiated thyroid carcinomas (DTC). The clinical utility of serum Tg testing is predicated on the tissue-specific origin of circulating Tg protein (thyroid follicular cells). However, since the maturation and secretion of a mature Tg molecule is complex, it is not surprising that circulating Tg is heterogeneous, and that as tumors dedifferentiate they can lose their capability to synthesize, iodinate, and secrete conformationally normal Tg protein [1,2]. Consequently, current Tg immunometric assays (IMA), based on monoclonal antibodies with restricted epitope specificity, may only recognize a limited population of Tg isoforms secreted by a neoplasm [3,4]. It follows that specificity differences largely explain the wide method-to-method variability that precludes changing assays when serially monitoring DTC patients. Serum Tg concentrations should be interpreted relative to: (1) the mass of thyroid tissue present (normal remnant and/or tumor); (2) any inflammation of, or injury to, thyroid tissue, such caused by fine-needle aspiration biopsy (FNAB), thyroid surgery, radioactive iodine (RAI) therapy, or thyroiditis; and (3) the thyroid-stimulating hormone (TSH) status of the patient, since the stimulation of TSH receptors by either endogenous or recombinant human TSH (rhTSH), the high human chorionic gonatropin (hCG) of pregnancy, or the thyroid-stimulating immunoglobulins present in Graves' disease, elevate the serum Tg concentration [5–8]. It

follows that when interpreting a serum Tg value, it is important to weigh patient-specific pathology and treatment together with the technical limitations of the method. This chapter will focus on the technical strengths and pitfalls of current Tg methods and the clinical utility of using serum Tg measurement as a tumor-marker for DTC.

Technical Strengths and Pitfalls of Serum Tg Measurement

Over the last decade, IMA methodology has largely replaced radioimmunoassays (RIA) for measuring serum Tg concentrations. IMA methods are favored by laboratories because they can be automated and require a shorter incubation to achieve maximal sensitivity, as compared with RIA [9,10]. Current Tg assays suffer from a number of technical limitations that negatively impact their clinical utility. These include (a) large between-method biases that preclude the use of different methods for serial monitoring of DTC patients; (b) suboptimal between-run precision across the long intervals generally used to monitor DTC patients (~12 months) that can mask clinically important changes; (c) inadequate sensitivity that compromises the early detection of recurrence; and (d) interferences by TgAb and

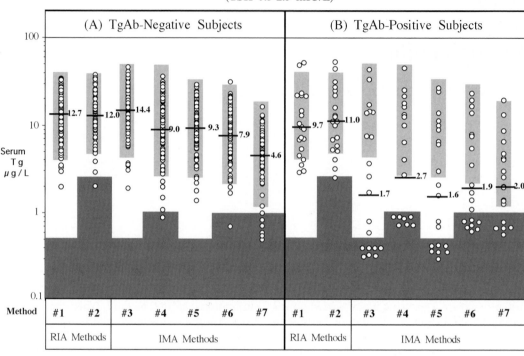

Figure 18.1 Serum Tg concentrations measured in 88 TgAb-negative normal euthyroid volunteers (TSH 0.5–2.5 mlU/L) using different methods. Method #1 = University of Southern California RIA, Los Angeles, CA, USA; method #2 = DSL RIA, Websster, Texas, USA; method #3 = Nichols Advantage ICMA, Nichols Institute Diagnostics ICMA, San Juan Capistrano, CA, USA; method #4 = CIS; method #5 = Access ICMA, Beckman-Coulter, Fullerton, CA, USA; method #6 = Immulite ICMA, Diagnostic Products Corporation, Los Angeles, CA, USA; method #7 = Brahms Kryptor, Berlin, Germany. The shaded area approximates the functional sensitivity. Median values are indicated.

heterophilic antibodies (HAMA) that can lead to the reporting of falsely low or high serum Tg values [7,9,11–13].

Between-Method Biases

Unfortunately, a change in Tg method during the course of monitoring a DTC patient can produce a shift in the serial Tg pattern that can cause clinical confusion. Figure 18.1 shows a representative comparison of Tg measurements made by two RIA and five IMA methods in sera from normal euthyroid subjects with TSH in the 0.5–2.5 mIU/L range, with or without detectable TgAb (Figures 18.1A and 18.1B, respectively). When TgAb was absent, the methods displayed a threefold difference in absolute Tg values

(Figure 18.1A). The new guidelines consider a change in serum Tg during thyroid hormone suppression therapy (THST) in excess of 1.5 μg/L to be clinically significant [10]. Current between-method biases alone could easily produce this magnitude of change, since current biases exceed the within-person variability of serum Tg concentrations (10–15%) [10,14]. Thus, significant assay biases preclude changing methods during long-term monitoring of patients. For example, a change from a Tg method with a positive bias to one with a negative bias has the potential to mask recurrent disease, whereas a change from a method with a negative bias to one with a positive bias would cause concern for recurrence that could potentially lead to unnecessary imaging or RAI treatment. It is now recommended that laboratories consult their physician-users *before* implementing any change in Tg method, and when the bias between the old and proposed new method exceeds 10% the re-baselining of patients is recommended [10]. Practically, the relative bias between methods can be assessed from a comparison between the mean reference range value of the methods in question.

There are a number of reasons for persistent biases between different Tg methods. The biosynthesis of a mature Tg molecule within the follicular cell is a complex vectoral process that is orchestrated by different molecular chaperone proteins [15]. Given the complexity of this, it is not surprising that Tg molecular processing may become unregulated in thyroid tumors, leading to heterogeneity in tumor-derived Tg protein in the circulation. Different Tg assay formulations employ a variety of Tg monoclonal antibody reagents that vary with respect to their specificity for different epitopes on tumor-derived Tg. This can result in the measurement of different Tg isoforms in the specimen and give rise to differences in serum Tg measurements made by assays [4]. Compounding these specificity differences are differences in assay standardization and the use of non-serum calibrator matrices that behave differently from human sera [9].

Between-Run Precision

Current Tg assays have suboptimal between-run precision across the long follow-up interval (6–12 months) typical of monitoring patients with DTC. It is well known that the between-run precision of a biochemical test erodes over time as a consequence of changing reagent lots, instrument calibrations and a myriad of other less well-defined factors. The loss of assay precision over the time between clinical evaluations negatively impacts the ability to detect small clinically significant changes, especially at the extremes of the Tg measurement range. The guidelines suggest that laboratories should archive specimens remaining after serum Tg testing to allow concurrent measurement of the past and current specimens from the patient in the same run, thereby eliminating between-run errors and improving the clinical sensitivity of the test [7,10].

Suboptimal Sensitivity

TSH and Tg assay development share many analogies concerning their quests for improved sensitivity. The clinical utility of TSH measurement has been dramatically enhanced over the last decade by the optimization of IMA methodology, leading to a 100-fold improvement in TSH assay functional sensitivity. Unfortunately, the development of more sensitive Tg assays is still in its infancy. Currently, Tg assay functional sensitivity ranges between 0.3 and 2.5 µg/L (Figure 18.1). As shown in Figure 18.2, a 100-fold improvement in Tg assay functional sensitivity (~0.01 µg/L) would dramatically improve the diagnostic sensitivity of measuring Tg during THST. Specifically, Figure 18.2 shows that there is a striking linear relationship between the serum Tg nadir measured without TSH stimulation in the first postoperative year and long-term (median 8-year) recurrence risk [16]. This suggests that less than 1% of patients with serum Tg below 0.1 µg/L during their first postoperative year would suffer a recurrence [16,17].

As Tg assay sensitivity becomes a marketing issue, there will be increasing commercial pressure for the diagnostic kit manufacturers to make unrealistic claims for the sensitivity of their tests. The guidelines state that the functional sensitivity of a Tg assay should be determined from the lowest Tg value that can be measured with 20% between-run coefficient of variation, using TgAb-negative human sera measured across a 6- to 12-month period and using different lots of reagent [10]. It is critical that Tg method comparisons are made on the basis of functional sensitivity and that descriptive terms such as "ultrasensitive" and "supersensitive" are not used for marketing purposes [10].

Unfortunately, even with Tg assay functional sensitivity determined according to the standardized protocol, the absolute (µg/L) functional sensitivity of different methods cannot be compared because of method biases (Figure 18.1A). The ability to detect small amounts of tumor is related to the degree of discrimination between the assay lower reference limit for normal euthyroid subjects and its functional sensitivity. Currently, there is very little discrimination between the lower reference limit for normal euthyroid subjects and the functional sensitivity limits of current methods, as

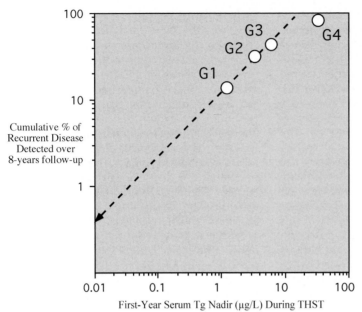

Figure 18.2 The relationship between cumulative percent recurrence in a cohort of 278 papillary thyroid cancer patients followed over a median of 8 years and the median group serum Tg nadir value reported (in the absence of TSH stimulation) during the first year following thyroidectomy. G1 had serum Tg nadirs between 1.0 and 1.9 μg/L; G2 had serum Tg nadirs between 2.0 and 4.9 μg/L; G3 had serum Tg nadirs between 5 and 10 μg/L; G4 had serum Tg nadirs above 10 μg/L [16].

shown in Figure 18.1A. In fact, serum Tg was paradoxically undetectable for some subjects by some methods. A new Tg assay nomenclature system has recently been proposed whereby each "generation" of assay would display an order of magnitude greater discrimination between the lower reference limit and functional sensitivity [13]. Under this proposal, current Tg assays would be defined as "first generation". Ideally, third generation Tg assays, characterized by functional sensitivities in the 0.001 to 0.01 μg/L range would dramatically improve the clinical sensitivity of Tg testing during THST (Figure 18.2) [18,19].

Interferences with Serum Tg Measurements

Thyroglobulin autoantibody (TgAb) and heterophilic antibody (HAMA) interferences with Tg measurements can result in either an under- or overestimation of the serum Tg concentration. Underestimation is the most clinically problematic direction of interference because it has the potential to mask the detection of disease. Although overestimation raises patient and physician concerns for recurrence, imaging

studies can be used to supply reassurance that disease is absent. However, overestimation may lead to the administration of unnecessary empiric radioactive iodine (RAI) treatments, because it is difficult to know if the detection of circulating Tg in a patient with a negative diagnostic RAI scan reflects the insensitivity of RAI imaging or Tg overestimation due to an interference [12,20–22].

TgAb Interference

TgAb interference with serum Tg measurement is undoubtedly the most serious technical problem that currently compromises the use of serum Tg as a tumor marker for patients with DTC. The magnitude of the problem is evident from the high prevalence of TgAb detected in DTC patients (~20%) [10,23,24]. It has been recognized for more than thirty years that endogenous TgAb has the potential to interfere with Tg measurements made by either by IMA or RIA methodology [10,23,25,26]. When TgAb is present, Tg molecules circulate either as free Tg or become complexed with endogenous TgAb. The direction and magnitude of any interference is primarily determined by the characteristics of the assay reagents. Although bi-directional interference is possible with RIA methods, the direction and magnitude of any interference is primarily determined by the affinity and specificity of the endogenous TgAb. Overestimated Tg RIA values would result if the endogenous TgAb sequestered Tg-I^{125} tracer and prevented it from participating in the competitive reaction. Conversely, underestimation would result if the second antibody reagent lacked species specificity and precipitated tracer bound to the endogenous TgAb [25,27]. RIA methods constructed with a combination of high affinity first antibody and species-specific second antibody usually report clinically appropriate total Tg (free Tg plus Tg complexed with TgAb) in the presence of TgAb [13,23,28,29]. The validity of Tg RIA measurement of TgAb-positive sera is supported by the data shown in Figure 18.1 whereby both RIA methods reported that the serum Tg values of TgAb-positive normal euthyroid subjects were essentially indistinguishable from those of TgAb-negative subjects (Figure 18.1B versus 18.1A, respectively). In contrast, each of the five IMA methods reported paradoxically undetectable serum Tg for some of the TgAb-positive normal subjects. Many studies have now established that TgAb interference with Tg IMA measurements is always unidirectional (underestimation) and that paradoxically undetectable Tg IMA values are frequently reported for TgAb-positive DTC patients with documented disease as well as TgAb-positive patients with Graves' thyrotoxicosis [23,24,26,30]. The propensity for TgAb interference is method-dependent and unpredictable since it relates to the characteristics of the endogenous TgAb and the relationship between the free and TgAb-complexed Tg in the circulation [23]. Physicians should be aware that any IMA method has the potential to underestimate the serum Tg concentration even when TgAb levels are very low or below the positive cutoff of the method [23,24,31,32].

When TgAb is present, there is often discordance between the serum Tg reported by an RIA and that reported by an IMA method [23]. In such cases, the RIA value is often detectable whereas the IMA value is typically lower or undetectable (Figure 18.1B). Although an undetectable Tg IMA result would appear appropriate for a thyroidectomized patient, the presence of TgAb in the circulation indicates that the immune system is still sensing the presence of Tg antigen, suggesting that the detectable RIA value is more clinically appropriate [23,29,33]. Given the propensity for IMA methodology to underestimate Tg in the presence of TgAb, the reporting of an undetectable Tg IMA result for a thyroidectomized DTC patient with TgAb has no clinical value. Further, such a report has the potential to mask disease, the risk of which is increased when TgAb is present [23,24,26,34]. This underscores the importance of the guideline (no. 46) that recommends, "laboratories should not report an undetectable serum Tg when TgAb is present if that method produces inappropriately low or undetectable serum Tg for TgAb-positive DTC patients with documented disease" [10]. Currently, most clinical laboratories use IMA methodology to measure serum Tg irrespective of the TgAb status of the patient, and persist in reporting "undetectable" Tg IMA values for sera containing TgAb. This practice persists despite laboratory disclaimers that the result might be unreliable. Some laboratories now limit the use of IMA methodology to TgAb-negative sera and use RIA methodology to measure serum Tg when TgAb is detected [23,35].

Heterophilic Antibody (HAMA) Interferences

In general, the presence of HAMA in the circulation can cause an overestimation of any analyte measured by IMA methodology [11,36]. This is because HAMA can cause a false bridge between the capture and signal monoclonal antibodies employed as IMA reagents, thereby creating a high signal on the solid support that will be read out as a falsely high analyte value. One recent study of an automated Tg IMA method reported that falsely high serum Tg values caused by the presence of HAMA were seen in 2–3% of serum specimens sent for Tg testing [12]. In contrast, RIA methods are not prone to HAMA interference [11].

Tg Testing of TgAb-Negative DTC Patients (Without TSH Stimulation)

As shown in Figure 18.3, serum Tg and TgAb measurements are critical for all phases of managing DTC patients.

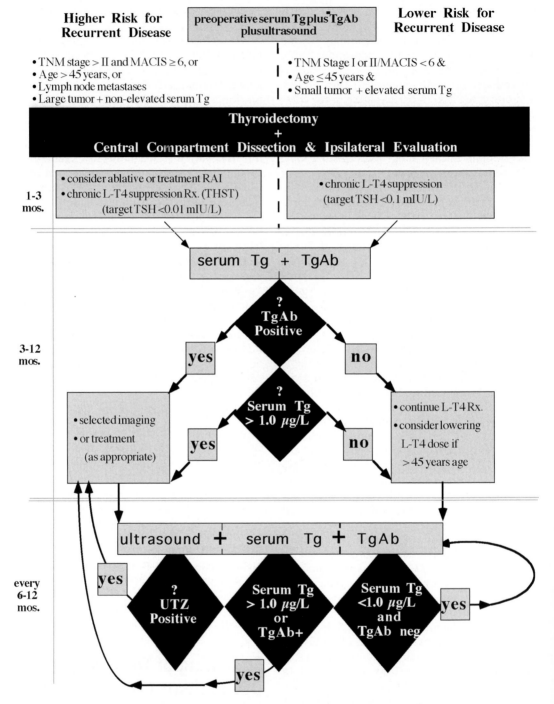

Figure 18.3 Algorithm for risk stratification of patients with DTC. Rx, therapy; UTZ, ultrasound.

Preoperative Serum Tg Measurements

The majority of thyroid tumors, especially follicular and Hürthle cell tumors, are associated with an elevated preoperative serum Tg concentration (relative to the normal reference range) [37–39]. In fact, an elevated serum Tg concentration is a nonspecific risk factor for thyroid malignancy and the degree of preoperative elevation relates to the risk for metastases [38,40,41]. Tumors differ in their ability to synthesize and secrete a conformationally normal Tg protein [1,2,42]. The increased Tg secretion rates and elevated preoperative serum Tg concentrations seen with DTC are likely to result from abnormalities in Tg molecular processing [15,37,38,43]. A preoperative serum Tg measurement provides a gauge of the relationship between tumor mass and Tg secretion and helps with the interpretation of postoperative Tg measurements by authenticating the use of serum Tg as a tumor marker test [38,44]. For example, large tumors that are not associated with an elevated preoperative serum Tg are likely to be poor Tg secretors [38,44]. In such cases, an undetectable postoperative serum Tg report will be less reassuring without evidence that the tumor is capable of secreting Tg protein. In such patients *any* Tg detected in the circulation after thyroidectomy could represent a large mass of residual tumor. It follows that the sensitivity of postoperative Tg measurement will be highest when a small primary tumor is associated with an elevated preoperative serum Tg. Because FNAB increases serum Tg, specimens drawn for the preoperative Tg assessment should be taken either before biopsy and held to await the cytological diagnosis, or deferred for more than 2 weeks after FNAB [45].

Early (<12 months) Postoperative Serum Tg Measurements

Estimates vary, but the half-life of Tg in the circulation approximates 3–4 days [46–48]. Following the postoperative rise in serum Tg secondary to trauma, the dominant influences on postoperative serum Tg concentrations are the mass of thyroid tissue remaining (normal remnant plus any tumor) together with the pre-

vailing TSH status [49]. A number of studies report that 1 month following thyroidectomy when endogenous TSH has become elevated before RAI treatment, an undetectable (<1 µg/L) serum Tg is a good prognostic indicator [8,50–53]. In patients in whom RAI treatment is deferred, thyroid hormone therapy should be initiated immediately after surgery to prevent the rise in TSH. In these patients, postoperative serum Tg concentrations stabilize by 1 to 2 months at a level that reflects the size of the thyroid remnant and the mass of any residual tumor. The tumor's contribution to the postoperative Tg level will relate to its ability to secrete Tg, as judged from the relationship between preoperative Tg and tumor size. There is currently no universally recognized serum Tg cutoff value that distinguishes disease-free patients from those with persistent tumor. A number of factors preclude establishing a universal Tg cutoff value with both good sensitivity as well as specificity for disease [6,54]. These include the technical factors discussed earlier (assay bias and insensitivity) compounded by differences in the amount of remnant tissue left after surgery, differences in the efficiency of tumor-derived Tg secretion and differences in the tumor's sensitivity to TSH. Further, there are differences in the sensitivity of the various modalities used to determine the presence of disease [20,55–59].

The approximate two-gram normal thyroid remnant that is generally left after thyroidectomy is expected to produce a serum Tg concentration approximating 2 µg/L in the absence of TSH stimulation [10,60]. The amount of Tg secreted by the normal remnant depends on the degree of surgery and the effectiveness of any RAI therapy [49,60]. Studies report that the effectiveness of RAI treatment for remnant ablation varies and depends on the dose used and remnant mass [60,61]. Although serum Tg concentrations measured early in the postoperative period have been shown to relate to long-term recurrence risk, patients with a low but detectable (≤3 µg/L) serum Tg early in the postoperative period do not necessarily have persistent disease [7,21,54]. A recent study reports that there is a striking linear relationship between the serum Tg nadir measured in the first postoperative year (without TSH stimulation) and cumulative recurrence (Figure 18.2) [16].

Long-Term Serial Tg Monitoring

A diagnosis of DTC is often made in the third or fourth decade of life. Since recurrences can occur decades after thyroidectomy patients require life-long monitoring for recurrence with clinical examinations, selected imaging, and serial serum Tg and TgAb measurements [62,63]. Historically, a negative diagnostic RAI whole-body scan has been used as the gold standard for the absence of disease [60,64–66]. With the increasing use of imaging modalities such as ultrasound, CT, MRI, and PET, it is now apparent that low dose RAI imaging is less sensitive than Tg testing [20,55,57,59,67–70]. Postoperative serum Tg concentrations reflect the integrated influences of the mass of thyroid tissue remaining (remnant plus any tumor) and the efficiency of the tumor to secrete Tg protein relative to the ambient TSH concentration. Steadily decreasing serum Tg during THST is the hallmark of successful treatment [7,21,54,70]. The pattern of serial Tg measurements made during the TSH-suppressed state is more clinically useful than an isolated Tg value [7,53,71,72]. However, it is critical that the same method is used for serial Tg monitoring because of the biases between assays discussed earlier [10,63]. A progressively decreasing Tg pattern is typical of patients who become disease-free, whereas a persistently detectable or rising Tg pattern is typical of patients with persistent or recurrent disease [7,63,71,72]. The progressive decline in serum Tg seen in RAI-treated patients likely reflects the long-term (2- to 3-year) sterilization effect of RAI, as tumor cells die off as a consequence of radiation damage [7,21,53,54,70,73]. Interestingly, a progressive decline in serum Tg is also often seen in patients who do not receive RAI, presumably reflecting a decrease in thyroid tissue mass secondary to impairment of TSH-dependent mitotic activity [7,54,73].

A rise in serum Tg during serial monitoring is often the first sign of recurrence [7,53,63,72]. However, a rise in serum Tg could reflect either an increase in tumor mass (when TSH is stable) or increased TSH stimulation of a constant mass of thyroid tissue. Many well-differentiated thyroid tumors are exquisitely sensitive to the ambient TSH concentration [7,72]. Before attributing a rise in serum Tg to tumor recurrence, it is important to ensure that the change is not TSH-mediated secondary to noncompliance with L-T_4 therapy, or a switch to a sub-potent generic L-T_4 preparation. Noncompliance cannot necessarily be detected by TSH measurement if patients resume compliance shortly before the clinic visit, since the half-life of TSH in the circulation is much shorter than that of Tg protein (~1 hour versus ~4 days) [46–48,74]. Strategies used to rule out a TSH-mediated rise in serum Tg include counseling the patient about compliance or testing the adequacy of the L-T_4 dose. The latter can be made either by empirically increasing the dose and rechecking serum Tg after 6–8 weeks, or by administering an oral one-milligram loading dose of L-T_4 [75]. A TSH-mediated Tg rise would be suspected if the serum Tg concentration fell 30–50% of basal levels by 8 days following the L-T_4 loading dose [75,76]. A rise in the serum Tg concentration in the face of a stable TSH status likely reflects an increase in tumor mass, since Tg secretion from normal remnant typically does not increase in the absence of a change in TSH [49]. Currently a rise in serum Tg of 1.5 µg/L or >10% is considered clinically significant [10]. Small changes in serum Tg are especially significant when a large tumor has been identified as a poor Tg secretor, as judged from a non-elevated preoperative serum Tg.

Monitoring DTC Patients with TgAb

Tg autoantibodies are more commonly encountered in DTC patients than in the general population (~20% versus ~10%, respectively) [23,24,77]. All sera sent for Tg measurement require adjunctive TgAb testing, because the TgAb status of a patient can change over time from positive to negative and vice versa [10,23,24]. There is now consensus that it is essential to detect TgAb directly by using a sensitive and precise TgAb immunoassay and not an exogenous Tg recovery test [9,10,26,78–80]. Recoveries are not only an unreliable means to detect interfering TgAb but unlike direct TgAb measurement, they cannot be used as a serial quantitative tumor marker [10,23]. In fact, the Guidelines clearly state that, "recovery tests do not reliably detect TgAb and should be discouraged and eliminated" [10]. The propensity for TgAb to interfere with Tg measurements is only weakly related to the TgAb concentration because endogenous Tg antibodies are heterogeneous and their avidity for Tg protein is not necessarily related to the measured TgAb concentration [23,31,32,81]. Failure to detect TgAb in a specimen has serious consequences, since interference leading to the reporting of a false-negative serum Tg result could cause a delay in the detection and treatment of metastatic disease [10,23,26,31,32].

Clinical Utility of Serial TgAb Measurements

A number of studies report that serial TgAb measurements per se can be used as a surrogate tumor marker test for TgAb-positive patients with DTC, since TgAb concentrations respond to changes in circulating Tg antigen [23,24, 33,82,83]. This is evident from the dramatic fall (~50%) in TgAb concentrations during the first 6 months following thyroidectomy or lymph node removal [23,24,84]. In fact, when TgAb-positive patients are rendered athyrotic, serum TgAb concentrations progressively decline and generally become undetectable within the first few postoperative years. In contrast the TgAb in patients with persistent disease characteristically remains detectable, or the serum TgAb concentrations rise over time [23,24,26,31,33,82, 83]. Whereas a rise in serum TgAb is often the first indication of recurrence, a transient rise in TgAb should be expected as a response to increased Tg antigen released by radiolytic destruction of thyroid tissue during the first 1–3 months following RAI treatment [84–87]. In fact, a rise in TgAb following a therapeutic dose of RAI may even be an indicator of the efficacy of RAI treatment of a TgAb-positive patient. Clearly TgAb is heterogeneous, and TgAb methods differ in sensitivity and specificity [23,81]. It is important to recognize that serial TgAb measurements can only be used as a tumor marker when the same manufacturer's method is used, because the absolute TgAb values reported by different methods can differ by as much as 100-fold despite claims that methods are standardized against the MRC 65/93 reference preparation [10,23,88]. It is not uncommon for a patient to be judged TgAb-negative by one manufacturer's method and TgAb-positive by another [23,31,32]. Low concentrations of TgAb that may not be detected by some methods can interfere with Tg measurement [23,31,32]. Failure to detect the presence of

TgAb can lead to the reporting of falsely low or paradoxically undetectable serum Tg IMA values for patients with disease [23,24,26]. TgAb interference with Tg measurements, especially when made by IMA methodology, is likely to remain a problem for the foreseeable future. Fortunately, serial TgAb concentrations can be used as a surrogate tumor marker for monitoring the disease status of TgAb-positive DTC patients.

Tg mRNA Determinations in Peripheral Blood

The reverse transcriptase-polymerase chain reaction (RT-PCR) amplification of tissue-specific mRNAs has been used to detect circulating cancer cells in the peripheral blood of patients with melanoma, prostate and breast malignancies [89]. Detection of Tg mRNA as a marker for DTC was first reported in 1996 [90]. Subsequently, RT-PCR has been used to detect other thyroid-specific mRNAs (TPO, NIS, and TSH-receptor) in peripheral blood or lymph node aspirates of DTC patients [91–94]. Currently, it appears unlikely that Tg mRNA testing will prove useful for facilitating therapeutic decision-making for DTC patients, since studies have reported disparate conclusions regarding the clinical sensitivity and specificity of RT-PCR testing for detecting DTC disease [18,92–101]. It is not clear whether these disparate conclusions reflect the insensitivity of RAI imaging that was used to detect disease in most studies, RT-PCR artifact, primer selection, or illegitimate transcription, the latter being a recognized limitation of RT-PCR methodology [89,94,102]. Even if Tg mRNA testing were proved clinically useful in the future, the expense of this technique compared with that of serum Tg measurement would likely restrict its use to high risk patients or TgAb-positive patients in whom serum Tg measurements were proved to be diagnostically unreliable [93,103].

TSH-Stimulated Tg Testing

TgAb-NegativeDTC Patients

Over the last three decades, many studies have reported that elevated endogenous TSH, or the administration of bovine TSH, increases the serum Tg concentration [104,105]. It is well established that TSH stimulation enhances the sensitivity of using Tg measurements to detect disease [6,8,106,107]. Recently, rhTSH-stimulated Tg testing has become preferred to the practice of withdrawing thyroid hormone to raise endogenous TSH, with its attendant hypothyroid symptoms [108]. There is growing consensus that rhTSH-stimulated Tg testing is superior for detecting recurrent disease compared with diagnostic RAI imaging, even though the serum Tg response to rhTSH administration is only half of the response to the rise in endogenous TSH following thyroid hormone withdrawal [6,20,59,67,68,70,109,110]. There is a linear, approximate 10-fold relationship between the basal (THST) and 72-hour rhTSH-stimulated serum Tg concentrations of both normal control subjects and patients with DTC, as shown in Figure 18.4 [6,72,111,112]. This is in accord with the factors known to influence the degree of TSH-stimulated Tg response, which include: (1) the magnitude and chronicity of the TSH elevation; (2) the mass of remnant thyroid tissue present, and (3) the mass and TSH responsiveness of the tumor [6,72,113]. However, the magnitude of the rhTSH-stimulated response varies considerably among patients (threefold to >20-fold) [6,111,112]. This may relate to differences in body surface area and/or reflect the tumor's intrinsic sensitivity to TSH [6,72,113,114]. Since poorly differentiated tumors display blunted

(less than threefold) increases in serum Tg in response to TSH stimulation, in the future, the magnitude of the rhTSH-stimulated Tg response may prove to be a useful indicator of the tumor's dependence on TSH and thus the efficacy of TSH suppression therapy [72,113]. Because the rhTSH-stimulated Tg response is predictable, rhTSH administration only improves the clinical sensitivity of Tg testing when the basal serum Tg is undetectable during THST. As more sensitive Tg assays become available, the clinical sensitivity of measuring serum Tg during THST will improve (Figure 18.2) and the need for rhTSH stimulation will decline, analogous to the elimination of routine TRH testing after the adoption of more sensitive TSH assays [18,19,115].

When recombinant human TSH was approved for clinical use a 72-hour post rhTSH-stimulated serum Tg value of $\geq 2\,\mu g/L$ was established as the cutoff for a positive response suggestive of disease [6]. Since then, there has been growing recognition that this cutoff level compromises the clinical sensitivity of rhTSH-stimulated Tg testing. Specifically, serum Tg concentrations in the 1–$2\,\mu g/L$ range are close to the lower reference limit for healthy euthyroid subjects with intact thyroid glands, thus making it increasingly difficult to discern between true disease and normal remnant tissue [6,10,20]. It has been recommended that a more conservative rhTSH-stimulated serum Tg cutoff of $\geq 1\,\mu g/L$ should be adopted [69,114].

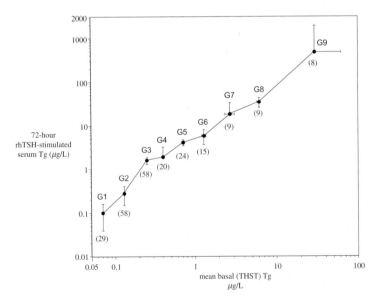

Figure 18.4 Relationship between the mean basal (THST) serum Tg concentration and the mean 72-hour rhTSH-stimulated serum Tg. Tests were grouped according to the basal Tg concentration. G1 had basal Tg between 0.05 and 0.1 µg/L; G2 between 0.2 and 0.3 µg/L; G3 between 0.1 and 0.2 µg/L; G4 between 0.3 and 0.5 µg/L; G5 between 0.5 and 1.0 µg/L; G6 between 1 and 2 µg/L; G7 between 2 and 5 µg/L; G8 between 5 and 10 µg/L; and G9 was >10 µg/L.

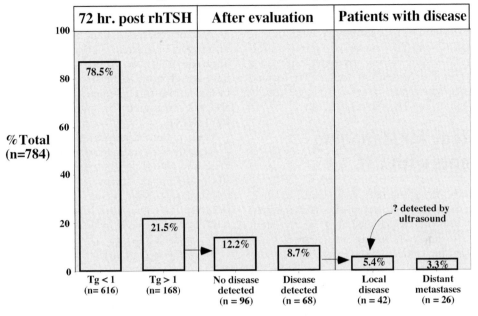

Figure 18.5 Meta-analysis of eight studies [68,110,117,141–144] showing the outcome of rhTSH-stimulated serum Tg testing of 784 patients with undetectable serum Tg during thyroid hormone suppression therapy (THST) [20].

With this lower cutoff, 20% of patients with undetectable (<1 μg/L) serum Tg during THST display detectable serum Tg after rhTSH stimulation [6,20,56]. One important drawback of rhTSH-stimulated serum Tg testing is the high number of patients who have rhTSH-stimulated serum Tg in the 1–10 μg/L range and no evidence of disease [20,57,63,116,117]. In fact, the adoption of the <1 μg/L cutoff is associated with ~15% false-positive responses [20,57,70]. Conversely, ~3% of patients with disease have false-negative rhTSH-stimulated Tg responses because the insensitivity of current Tg assays compromises the clinical sensitivity of Tg testing even when rhTSH stimulation is employed [57,70]. In a recent meta-analysis of 784 patients, ~8% of patients with serum Tg <1 μg/L during THST had disease unmasked by rhTSH-stimulated Tg testing (Figure 18.5) [20]. Most (~5%) of the disease was located in lymph nodes and likely could have been detected by ultrasound, suggesting that few patients would have disease revealed by rhTSH-stimulated Tg testing alone [20,57,63,70]. In fact, it is becoming apparent that rhTSH-stimulated Tg testing

has a low positive predictive value for disease and that the addition of ultrasound to Tg measured during THST dramatically improves the sensitivity and specificity of monitoring patients for recurrent disease [57,63,70,117]. Since only a minority of patients with negative clinical and/or ultrasound examinations have persistent or recurrent disease detected during follow-up, it is not surprising that only a small percentage of patients have disease unmasked by rhTSH-stimulated Tg testing [57,63]. It follows that the high cost and low yield of rhTSH-stimulated serum Tg testing will increasingly raise questions concerning the cost–benefit ratio of using rhTSH stimulation for diagnostic testing as the sensitivity of Tg methodology improves [18,19,118].

TgAb-Positive Patients

Unfortunately, the value of rhTSH stimulation testing is compromised by the presence of TgAb. Specifically, many TgAb-positive patients display blunted or absent TSH-stimulated serum Tg responses, regardless of the class of Tg method used (IMA or RIA) [20]. Currently, the most likely explanation for the paradoxical lack of rhTSH response in the presence of TgAb is that there is enhanced metabolic clearance of Tg complexed with TgAb, as compared with free Tg [119,120]. The rapid removal of TgAb seen following Tg release during thyroidectomy lends support to the contention that newly-formed Tg–TgAb complexes may be more rapidly cleared than free Tg [48,86,119,120].

Strategy for Managing Patients with DTC

As shown in Figure 18.3, risk stratification is the cornerstone of postoperative management of DTC patients. Most recurrent or persistent tumor is detected during the first 5 years following thyroidectomy [62]. Patients are classified as low or high risk for recurrent disease based on a combination of clinical parameters assessed at the time of their initial diagnosis and surgery. Classic prognostic scoring systems, such as TNM and MACIS, combine patient-specific parameters such as age, size of the primary tumor, presence of lymph nodes and distant metastases to predict mortality risk [63,66,121–127]. Most patients with DTC are successfully treated with thyroidectomy followed by chronic thyroid hormone (L-T$_4$) suppression therapy (THST) [60,62]. The use of RAI treatment and the aggressiveness and frequency of follow-up evaluations depends on whether the patient has a high or low risk for recurrent or persistent disease [60,64,65,128–130]. Tumor pathology also influences prognosis, since the prognostic factors for papillary versus follicular thyroid cancers and their variants are distinctively different [60,131,132]. Whereas a preoperative elevation in serum Tg is not an indicator of a neoplasm, an excessively high (>1000 µg/L) preoperative serum Tg value is suspicious for metastatic disease, especially when metastases involve bone [40,85,113]. Further, once a diagnosis of DTC has been made, the relationship between the preoperative Tg level and tumor burden can be used to gauge the significance of postoperative Tg measurements. This is because the sensitivity of postoperative Tg testing for disease will be greatest when patients are diagnosed with small tumors associated with an

elevated preoperative Tg, suggesting that the tumor is an efficient Tg secretor [38,44]. In addition to a preoperative Tg, ultrasound evaluations are now being performed more frequently as part of risk assessment to assess the extent of surgery indicated [133]. This is because approximately two thirds of DTC patients have lymph node metastases, 80% of which are in the central compartment and many of which are not detectable by physical examination [60,133,134].

Thus, patient demographics together with a preoperative Tg measurement, ultrasound, surgical, and pathological findings are used to classify patients as having a low or high risk for disease (~80% versus ~20%, respectively) [63,130]. Patients with a higher risk for recurrent disease have one or more of the following:

- higher prognostic score (TNM > stage II and/or MACIS ≥6);
- age >45 years;
- lymph node metastases;
- large tumor with paradoxically non-elevated serum Tg.

Recent retrospective studies have raised controversy regarding whether RAI treatment influences mortality [129,130]. Radioiodine is usually reserved for patients at higher risk for recurrent or persistent disease, the dose being determined on an individual basis relative to the degree of risk [63,130]. Since the presence of TgAb in the early postoperative period is associated with an increased risk for recurrent disease, RAI treatment may be efficacious for patients with persistent TgAb after the first postoperative year [24,135]. In patients with a lower risk for disease there is a growing consensus that RAI treatment should be deferred [60,129]. Levothyroxine suppression therapy should be initiated immediately in such patients, since serum TSH levels can rise above 30 mIU/L as early as 8 days following thyroidectomy [136]. The degree of TSH suppression targeted for lower risk patients is generally less than that for higher risk patients (<0.1 versus <0.01 mIU/L, respectively) [126,137]. Many studies made in the TSH-stimulated state before RAI therapy have reported that Tg measurements in the early postoperative period are prognostic for disease [8,50,51,70,138]. In view of the relationship between basal and TSH-stimulated Tg shown in Figure 18.4, it follows that any Tg detected above 1 µg/L is suspicious and warrants selective imaging or treatment as appropriate [8,16,50–53].

After the first postoperative year, follow-up evaluations for recurrent disease should be individualized to the risk for recurrence [63,128]. By this time, few patients without TgAb and with a serum Tg below 1 µg/L during THST have a recurrence [16,17,117]. A combination of ultrasound plus serum Tg and TgAb measured during THST (TSH <0.1 mIU/L) is recommended for follow-up surveillance for disease in low risk patients [57,70]. A positive ultrasound and/or a serum Tg above 1 µg/L and/or a rise in TgAb concentration suggests the presence of disease and warrants selected imaging or other treatment as appropriate. Recombinant TSH stimulation is not needed when serum Tg is detectable, because the rhTSH-stimulated Tg response is predictably ~10-fold higher than the basal Tg level (Figure 18.4) [72,117]. Recombinant TSH-stimulated Tg measurements are also generally not helpful in TgAb-positive patients, because the presence of TgAb is associated with an absent or blunted rhTSH-stimulated serum Tg response (see previous section). Patients with a negative baseline ultrasound, no TgAb, and a serum Tg below 1 µg/L are unlikely to have disease unmasked by rhTSH-stimulated diagnostic imaging or Tg testing [16,57,63,70,117,139]. Because thyroid neoplasms grow slowly, long-term monitoring of such patients can be performed relatively infrequently (every 12 months) using serum Tg plus TgAb measured during THST [63,140]. The cost of annual ultrasounds may not be warranted for low risk patients with a negative basal ultrasound and THST serum Tg <1 µg/L [70]. Either a rise in serum Tg or the detection of TgAb in such patients would be an early sign of recurrence that should prompt an individualized more extensive evaluation [19,23,24,84].

Summary

Risk stratification of DTC patients is based on patient demographics, surgical and pathological findings, together with ultrasound and a preoperative Tg measurement. The patient's risk for recurrent or residual disease influences the postoperative treatment and management. Serum Tg and TgAb measurements are critical for each stage of managing both low and high risk patients with DTC. The quality of the Tg and TgAb methods is variable, and will impact the clinical care of DTC patients. Because current Tg or TgAb method is 100% reliable, these biochemical tests should be used in conjunction with clinical examination and ultrasound, together with selected imaging modalities, as dictated by patient-related risk factors. The use of sensitive and specific Tg and TgAb methods for evaluating DTC patients improves the overall cost-effectiveness of management by minimizing costly procedures. However, even when the quality of these biochemical tests is optimal, the results have to be interpreted relative to the patient-specific factors and the physiological factors that control Tg secretion.

References

1. Schneider A, Ikekubo K, Kuma K. Iodine content of serum thyroglobulin in normal individuals and patients with thyroid tumors. J Clin Endocrinol Metab 1983; 57:1251–1256.
2. Druetta L, Croizet K, Bornet H, Rousset B. Analyses of the molecular forms of serum thyroglobulin from patients with Graves' disease, subacute thyroiditis or differentiated thyroid cancer by velocity sedimentation on sucrose gradient and Western blot. Eur J Endocrinol 1999; 139:498–507.
3. Maruyama M, Kato R, Kobayashi S, Kasuga Y. A method to differentiate between thyroglobulin derived from normal thyroid tissue and from thyroid carcinoma based on analysis of reactivity to lectins. Arch Pathol Lab Med 1998; 122:715–720.
4. Schulz R, Bethauser H, Stempka L, Heilig B, Moll A, Hufner M. Evidence for immunological differences between circulating and tissue-derived thyroglobulin in men. Eur J Clin Invest 1989; 19:459–463.
5. Aizawa T, Ishihara M, Koizumi Y, et al. Serum thyroglobulin concentration as an indicator for assessing thyroid stimulation in patients with Graves' disease during antithyroid drug therapy. Am J Med 1990; 89: 175–180.
6. Haugen BR, Pacini F, Reiners C, et al. A comparison of recombinant human thyrotropin and thyroid hormone withdrawal for the detection of thyroid remnant or cancer. J Clin Endocrinol Metab 1999; 84:3877–3885.
7. Spencer CA, Wang CC. Thyroglobulin measurement: Techniques, clinical benefits and pitfalls. Endocrinol Metab Clin North Am 1995; 24:841–863.
8. Lima NCH, Tomimori E, Knobel M, Medeiros-Neto G. Prognostic value of serial serum thyroglobulin determinations after total thyroidectomy for differentiated thyroid cancer. J Endocrinol Invest 2002; 25:110–115.

9. Spencer CA, Takeuchi M, Kazarosyan M. Current status and performance goals for serum thyroglobulin assays. Clin Chem 1996; 42:164–173.

10. Demers LM, Spencer CA. Laboratory medicine practice guidelines: laboratory support for the diagnosis and monitoring of thyroid disease. Thyroid 2003; 13:57–67.

11. Levinson SS. The nature of heterophilic antibodies and their role in immunoassay interference. J Clin Immunoassay 1992; 15:108–115.

12. Preissner CM, O'Kane DJ, Singh RJ, Morris JC, Grebe SKG. Phantoms in the assay tube: heterophile antibody interferences in serum thyroglobulin assays. J Clin Endocrinol Metab 2003; 88:3069–3074.

13. Spencer CA. New insights for using serum thyroglobulin (Tg) measurement for managing patients with differentiated thyroid carcinomas. Thyroid Int 2003; 4:1–14.

14. Feldt-Rasmussen U, Petersen PH, Blaabjerg O, Horder M. Long-term variability in serum thyroglobulin and thyroid related hormones in healthy subjects. Acta Endocrinol (Copenh) 1980; 95:328–334.

15. Arvan P, Kim PS, Kuliawat R, et al. Intracellular protein transport to the thyrocyte plasma membrane: potential implications for thyroid physiology. Thyroid 1997; 7:89–105.

16. Fatemi S, LoPresti J, Guttler R, Singer P, Spencer C. First-year post-thyroidectomy serum thyroglobulin (Tg) concentrations, measured without TSH stimulation, predict long-term recurrence risk in patients with papillary thyroid carcinomas (PTC). J Clin Endocrinol Metab 2005; manuscript in preparation.

17. Schlumberger M, Baudin E. Serum thyroglobulin determination in the follow-up of patients with differentiated thyroid carcinoma. Eur J Endocrinol 1998; 138:249–252.

18. Fugazzola L, Mihalich A, Persani L, et al. Highly sensitive serum thyroglobulin and circulating thyroglobulin mRNA evaluations in the management of patients with differentiated thyroid cancer in apparent remission. J Clin Endocrinol Metab 2002; 87:3201–3208.

19. Zophel K, Wunderlich G, Smith BR. Serum thyroglobulin measurements with a high sensitivity enzyme-linked immunosorbent assay: is there a clinical benefit in patients with differentiated thyroid carcinoma? Thyroid 2003; 13:861–865.

20. Mazzaferri EL, Robbins RJ, Spencer CA, et al. A consensus report of the role of serum thyroglobulin as a monitoring method for low-risk patients with papillary thyroid carcinoma. J Clin Endocrinol Metab 2003; 88:1433–1441.

21. Pacini F, Agate L, Elisei R, et al. Outcome of differentiated thyroid cancer with detectable serum Tg and negative diagnostic ^{131}I whole body scan; Comparison of patients treated with high ^{131}I activities versus untreated patients. J Clin Endocrinol Metab 2001; 86: 4092–4097.

22. Koh JM, Kim ES, Ryu JS, Hong SJ, Kim WB, Shong YK. Effects of therapeutic doses of ^{131}I in thyroid papillary carcinoma patients with elevated thyroglobulin level and negative ^{131}I whole-body scan: comparative study. Clin Endocrinol (Oxf) 2003; 58:421–427.

23. Spencer CA, Takeuchi M, Kazarosyan M, et al. Serum thyroglobulin autoantibodies: prevalence, influence on serum thyroglobulin measurement and prognostic significance in patients with differentiated thyroid carcinoma. J Clin Endocrinol Metab 1998; 83:1121–1127.

24. Chung JK, Park YJ, Kim TY, et al. Clinical significance of elevated level of serum antithyroglobulin antibody in patients with differentiated thyroid cancer after thyroid ablation. Clin Endocrinol (Oxf) 2002; 57:215–221.

25. Schneider AB, Pervos R. Radioimmunoassay of human thyroglobulin: effect of antithyroglobulin autoantibodies. J Clin Endocrinol Metab 1978; 47:126–137.

26. Hjiyiannakis P, Mundy J, Harmer C. Thyroglobulin antibodies in differentiated thyroid cancer. Clin Oncol (R Coll Radiol) 1999; 11:240–244.

27. Feldt-Rasmussen U, Rasmussen AK. Serum thyroglobulin (Tg) in presence of thyroglobulin autoantibodies (TgAb). Clinical and methodological relevance of the interaction between Tg and TgAb in vitro and in vivo. J Endocrinol Invest 1985; 8:571–576.

28. Black EG, Hoffenberg R. Should one measure serum thyroglobulin in the presence of anti-thyroglobulin antibodies? Clin Endocrinol (Oxf) 1983; 19:597–601.

29. Rajashekharrao B, Kumar A, Shah DH, Sharma SM. Interference of antithyroglobulin autoantibodies in serum thyroglobulin estimation by RIA. Indian J Med Res 1988; 88:146–149.

30. Mariotti S, Barbesino G, Caturegli P, et al. Assay of thyroglobulin in serum with thyroglobulin autoantibodies: an unobtainable goal? J Clin Endocrinol Metab 1995; 80:468–472.

31. Larbre H, Schvartz C, Schneider N, et al. Positive antithyroglobulin antibodies in patients with differentiated thyroid carcinoma. What significance? Ann Endocrinol (Paris) 2000; 61(5):422–427.

32. Cubero JM, Rodriquez-Espinosa J, Gelpi C, Estorch M, Corcoy R. Thyroglobulin autoantibody levels below the cut-off for positivity can interfere with thyroglobulin measurement. Thyroid 2003; 13:659–661.

33. Chiovato L, Latrofa F, Braverman LE, et al. Disappearance of humoral thyroid autoimmunity after complete removal of thyroid antigens. Ann Intern Med 2003; 139:346–351.

34. Rubello D, Girelli ME, Casara D, Piccolo M, Perin A, Busnardo B. Usefulness of the combined antithyroglobulin antibodies and thyroglobulin assay in the follow-up of patients with differentiated thyroid cancer. J Endocrinol Invest 1990; 13:737–742.

35. Morris LF, Waxman AD, Braunstein GD. Interlaboratory comparison of thyroglobulin measurements for patients with recurrent or metastatic differentiated thyroid cancer. Clin Chem 2002; 48:1371–1372.

36. Andersen DC, Koch C, Jensen CH, Skjodt K, Brandt J, Teisner B. High prevalence of human anti-bovine IgG antibodies as the major cause of false positive reactions in two-site immunoassays based on monoclonal antibodies. J Immunoassay Immunochem 2004; 25:17–30.

37. Ericsson UB, Tegler L, Lennquist S, Christensen SB, Stahl E, Thorell JI. Serum thyroglobulin in differentiated thyroid carcinoma. Acta Chir Scand 1984; 150:367–375.

38. Sharma AK, Sarda AK, Chattopadhyay TK, Kapur MM. The role of estimation of the ratio of preoperative serum thyroglobulin to the thyroid mass in predicting the behaviour of well differentiated thyroid cancers. J Postgrad Med 1996; 42:39–42.

39. Hocevar M, Auersperg M. Role of serum thyroglobulin in the pre-operative evaluation of follicular thyroid tumours. Eur J Surg Oncol 1998; 24:553–557.

40. Shah DH, Dandekar SR, Jeevanram RK, Kumar A, Sharma SM, Ganatra RD. Serum thyroglobulin in differentiated thyroid carcinoma: histological and metastatic classification. Acta Endocrinol (Copenh) 1981; 98:222–226.

41. Hrafnkelsson J, Tulinius H, Kjeld M, Sigvaldason H, Jonasson JG. Serum thyroglobulin as a risk factor for thyroid carcinoma. Acta Oncol 2000; 39:973–977.

42. Kohno Y, Tarutani O, Sakata S, Nakajima H. Monoclonal antibodies to thyroglobulin elucidate differences in protein structure of thyroglobulin in healthy individuals and those with papillary adenocarcinoma. J Clin Endocrinol Metab 1985; 61:343–350.

43. Tegler L, Ericsson UB, Gillquist J, Lindvall R. Basal and thyrotropin-stimulated secretion rates of thyroglobulin from the human thyroid gland during surgery. Thyroid 1993; 3:213–217.

44. Fatemi S, Nicoloff J, LoPresti J, Guttler R, Spencer C. Clinical utility of a pre-op serum thyroglobulin (Tg) measurement in patients with differentiated papillary thyroid cancer (PTC). American Thyroid Association meeting. Abstract #145, 1999.

45. Bayraktar M, Ergin M, Boyacioglu A, Demir S. A preliminary report of thyroglobulin release after fine needle aspiration biopsy of thyroid nodules. J Int Med Res 1990; 18:253–255.

46. Feldt-Rasmussen U, Petersen PH, Date J, Madsen CM. Serum thyroglobulin in patients undergoing subtotal thyroidectomy for toxic and nontoxic goiter. J Endocrinol Invest 1982; 5:161–164.

47. Izumi M, Kubo I, Taura M, et al. Kinetic study of immunoreactive human thyroglobulin. J Clin Endocrinol Metab 1986; 62:410–412.

48. Hocevar M, Auersperg M, Stanovnik L. The dynamics of serum thyroglobulin elimination from the body after thyroid surgery. Eur J Surg Oncol 1997; 23:208–210.

49. Van Wyngaarden K, McDougall IR. Is serum thyroglobulin a useful marker for thyroid cancer in patients who have not had ablation of residual thyroid tissue? Thyroid 1997; 7:343–346.

50. Ronga G, Filesi M, Ventroni G, Vestri AR, Signore A. Value of the first serum thyroglobulin level after total thyroidectomy for the diagnosis of metastases from differentiated thyroid carcinoma. Eur J Nucl Med 1999; 26:1448–1452.

51. Lin JD, Huang MJ, Hsu BR, et al. Significance of postoperative serum thyroglobulin levels in patients with papillary and follicular thyroid carcinomas. J Surg Oncol 2002; 80:45–51.

52. Roelants V, Nayer PD, Bouckaert A, Beckers C. The predictive value of serum thyroglobulin in the follow-up of differentiated thyroid cancer. The predictive value of serum thyroglobulin in the follow-up of differentiated thyroid cancer. Eur J Nucl Med 1997; 24:722–727.

53. Baudin E, Do Cao C, Cailleux AF, Leboulleux S, Travagli JP, Schlumberger M. Positive predictive value of serum thyroglobulin levels, measured during the first year of follow-up after thyroid hormone withdrawal, in thyroid cancer patients. J Clin Endocrinol Metab 2003; 88:1107–1111.

54. Ozata M, Suzuki S, Miyamoto T, Liu RT, Fierro-Renoy F, DeGroot LJ. Serum thyroglobulin in the follow-up of patients with treated differentiated thyroid cancer. J Clin Endocrinol Metab 1994; 79:98–105.

55. Frilling A, Gorges R, Tecklenborg K, et al. Value of preoperative diagnostic modalities in patients with recurrent thyroid carcinoma. Surgery 2000; 128:1067–1074.

56. Torlontano M, Crocetti U, D'Aloiso L, et al. Serum thyroglobulin and ^{131}I whole body scan after recombinant human TSH stimulation in the follow-up of low-risk patients with differentiated thyroid cancer. Eur J Endocrinol 2003; 148:19–24.

57. Pacini F, Molinaro E, Castagna MG, et al. Recombinant human thyrotropin-stimulated serum thyroglobulin combined with neck ultrasonography has the highest sensitivity in monitoring differentiated thyroid carcinoma. J Clin Endocrinol Metab 2003; 88:3668–3673.

58. Fatourechi V, Hay ID, Mullan BP, et al. Are posttherapy radioiodine scans informative and do they influence subsequent therapy of patients with differentiated thyroid cancer? Thyroid 2000; 10:573–577.

59. Cailleux AF, Baudin E, Travagli JP, Ricard M, Schlumberger M. Is diagnostic iodine-131 scanning useful after total thyroid ablation for differentiated thyroid cancer? J Clin Endocrinol Metab 2000; 85:175–178.

60. Schlumberger MJ. Papillary and Follicular Thyroid Carcinoma. N Engl J Med 1998; 338:297–306.

61. Pacini F, Molinaro E, Castagna MG, et al. Ablation of thyroid residues with 30 mCi [131]I: A comparison in thyroid cancer patients prepared with recombinant human TSH or thyroid hormone withdrawal. J Clin Endocrinol Metab 2002; 87:4063–4068.

62. Mazzaferri EL, Jhiang SM. Long-term impact of initial surgical and medical therapy on papillary and follicular thyroid cancer. Am J Med 1994; 97:418–428.

63. Schlumberger M, Berg G, Cohen O, et al. Follow-up of low-risk patients with differentiated thyroid carcinoma: a European perspective. Eur J Endocrinol 2004; 150:105–112.

64. British Thyroid Association. Guidelines for the management of differentiated thyroid cancer in adults. 2002. http://www.british-thyroid-association.org/guidelines.htm.

65. Singer PA, Cooper DS, Daniels GH, et al. Treatment guidelines for patients with thyroid nodules and well-differentiated thyroid cancer. American Thyroid Association. Arch Intern Med 1996; 156:2165–2172.

66. Sherman SI, Brierley JD, Sperling M, et al. Prospective multicenter study of thyroid carcinoma treatment: initial analysis of staging and outcome. National Thyroid Cancer Treatment Cooperative Study Registry Group. Cancer 1998; 83:1012–1021.

67. Pacini F, Capezzone M, Elisei R, Ceccarelli C, Taddei D, Pinchera A. Diagnostic 131-iodine whole-body scan may be avoided in thyroid cancer patients who have undetectable stimulated serum Tg levels after initial treatment. J Clin Endocrinol Metab 2002; 87:1499–1501.

68. Mazzaferri EL, Kloos RT. Is diagnostic iodine-131 scanning with recombinant human TSH useful in the follow-up of differentiated thyroid cancer after thyroid ablation? J Clin Endocrinol Metab 2002; 87:1490–1498.

69. Wartofsky L. Using baseline and recombinant human TSH-stimulated Tg measurements to manage thyroid

cancer without diagnostic (131)I scanning. J Clin Endocrinol Metab 2002; 87:1486–1489.

70. Torlontano M, Attard M, Crocetti U, et al. Follow-up of low risk patients with papillary thyroid cancer: role of neck ultrasonography in detecting lymph node metastases. J Clin Endocrinol Metab 2004; 89:3402–3407.

71. Black EG, Sheppard MC, Hoffenberg R. Serial serum thyroglobulin measurements in the management of differentiated thyroid carcinoma. Clin Endocrinol 1987; 27:115–120.

72. Spencer CA, LoPresti JS, Fatemi S, Nicoloff JT. Detection of residual and recurrent differentiated thyroid carcinoma by serum thyroglobulin measurement. Thyroid 1999; 9:435–441.

73. Savelli G, Chiti A, Rodari M, et al. Predictive value of thyroglobulin changes for the efficacy of thyroid remnant ablation. Tumori 2001; 87:42–46.

74. Weeke J, Gundersen HJ. Circadian and 30 minute variations in serum TSH and thyroid hormones in normal subjects. Acta Endocrinol 1978; 89:659–672.

75. Spencer CA, LoPresti JS, Nicoloff JT, Dlott R, Schwarzbein D. Multiphasic thyrotropin responses to thyroid hormone administration in man. J Clin Endocrinol Metab 1995; 80:854–859.

76. Gardner DF, Rothman J, Utiger RD. Serum thyroglobulin in normal subjects and patients with hyperthyroidism due to Graves' disease: effects of T3, iodide, ^{131}I and antithyroid drugs. Clin Endocrinol 1979; 11:585–594.

77. Hollowell JG, Staehling NW, Hannon WH, et al. Serum thyrotropin, thyroxine, and thyroid antibodies in the United States population (1988 to 1994): NHANES III. J Clin Endocrinol Metab 2002; 87:489–499.

78. Lindberg B, Svensson J, Ericsson UB, Nilsson P, Svenonius E, Ivarsson SA. Comparison of some different methods for analysis of thyroid autoantibodies: importance of thyroglobulin autoantibodies. Thyroid 2001; 11:265–269.

79. Massart C, Maugendre D. Importance of the detection method for thyroglobulin antibodies for the validity of thyroglobulin measurements in sera from patients with Graves disease. Clin Chem 2002; 48:102–107.

80. Zophel K, Wunderlich G, Liepach U, Koch R, Bredow J, Franke WG. Recovery test or immunoradiometric measurement of anti-thyroglobulin autoantibodies for interpretation of thyroglobulin determination in the follow-up of different thyroid carcinoma. Nuklearmedizin 2001; 40:155–163.

81. Benvenga S, Burek CL, Talor M, Rose NR, Trimarchi F. Heterogeneity of the thyroglobulin epitopes associated with circulating thyroid hormone autoantibodies in Hashimoto's thyroiditis and non-autoimmune thyroid diseases. J Endocrinol Invest 2002; 25:977–982.

82. Pacini F, Mariotti S, Formica N, Elisei R. Thyroid autoantibodies in thyroid cancer: Incidence and relationship with tumor outcome. Acta Endocrinol 1988; 119:373–380.

83. Rubello D, Casara D, Girelli ME, Piccolo M, Busnardo B. Clinical meaning of circulating antithyroglobulin antibodies in differentiated thyroid cancer: a prospective study. J Nucl Med 1992; 33:1478–1480.

84. Fatemi S, Nicoloff J, LoPresti J, Guttler R, Spencer C. Clinical significance of serial serum Tg autoantibody (TgAb) patterns in patients with differentiated thyroid cancers (DTC). 12th International Congress of Thyroidology. Kyoto, 2000.

85. Pacini F, Pinchera A, Giani C, Grasso L, Doveri F, Baschieri L. Serum thyroglobulin in thyroid carcinoma and other disorders. J Endocrinol Invest 1980; 3:283–292.

86. Franke WG, Zophel K, Wunderlich GR, et al. Thyroperoxidase: a tumor marker for post-therapeutic follow-up of differentiated thyroid carcinomas? Results of a time course study. Cancer Detect Prev 2000; 24:524–530.

87. Nakazato N, Yoshida K, Mori K, et al. Antithyroid drugs inhibit radioiodine-induced increases in thyroid autoantibodies in hyperthyroid Graves' disease. Thyroid 1999; 9:775–779.

88. Sapin R, d'Herbomez M, Gasser F, Meyer L, Schlienger JL. Increased sensitivity of a new assay for antithyroglobulin antibody detection in patients with autoimmune thyroid disease. Clin Biochem 2003; 36: 611–616.

89. Ghossein RA, Bhattacharya S. Molecular detection and characterisation of circulating tumour cells and micrometastases in solid tumours. Eur J Cancer 2000; 36:1681–1694.

90. Ditkoff BA, Marvin MR, Yemul S, et al. Detection of circulating thyroid cells in peripheral blood. Surgery 1996; 120:959–965.

91. Arturi F, Russo D, Giuffrida D, et al. Early diagnosis by genetic analysis of differentiated thyroid cancer metastases in small lymph nodes. J Clin Endocrinol Metab 1997; 82:1638–1641.

92. Elisei R, Vivaldi A, Agate L, et al. Low specificity of blood thyroglobulin messenger ribonucleic acid assay prevents its use in the follow-up of differentiated thyroid cancer patients. J Clin Endocrinol Metab 2004; 89:33–39.

93. Chinnappa P, Taguba L, Arciaga R, et al. Detection of TSH-receptor mRNA and thyroglobulin mRNA transcripts in peripheral blood of patients with thyroid disease: sensitive and specific markers for thyroid cancer. J Clin Endocrinol Metab 2004; 89(8):3705–3709.

94. Verburg FA, Lips CJ, Lentjes EG, de Klerk JM. Detection of circulating Tg-mRNA in the follow-up of papillary and follicular thyroid cancer: how useful is it? Br J Cancer 2004; 91:1–5.

95. Ringel MD, Balducci-Silano PL, Anderson JS, et al. Quantitative reverse transcription-polymerase chain reaction of circulating thyroglobulin messenger ribonucleic acid for monitoring patients with thyroid carcinoma. J Clin Endocrinol Metab 1998; 84:4037–4042.

96. Savagner F, Rodien P, Reynier P, Rohmer V, Bigorgne JC, Malthiery Y. Analysis of Tg transcripts by real-time RT-PCR in the blood of thyroid cancer patients. J Clin Endocrinol Metab 2002; 87:635–639.

97. Takano T, Miyauchi A, Yoshida H, Hasegawa Y, Kuma K, Amino N. Quantitative measurement of thyroglobulin mRNA in peripheral blood of patients after total thyroidectomy. Br J Cancer 2001; 85:102–106.

98. Bugalho MJ, Domingues RS, Pinto AC, et al. Detection of thyroglobulin mRNA transcripts in peripheral blood of individuals with and without thyroid glands: evidence for thyroglobulin expression by blood cells. Eur J Endocrinol 2001; 145:409–413.

99. Bellantone R, Lombardi CP, Bossola M, et al. Validity of thyroglobulin mRNA assay in peripheral blood of postoperative thyroid carcinoma patients in predicting tumor recurrence varies according to the histologic

type: results of a prospective study. Cancer 2001; 92: 2273–2279.

100. Bojunga J, Roddiger S, Stanisch M, et al. Molecular detection of thyroglobulin mRNA transcripts in peripheral blood of patients with thyroid disease by RT-PCR. Br J Cancer 2000; 82:1650–1655.

101. Biscolla RP, Cerutti JM, Maciel RM. Detection of recurrent thyroid cancer by sensitive nested reverse transcription-polymerase chain reaction of thyroglobulin and sodium/iodide symporter messenger ribonucleic acid transcripts in peripheral blood. J Clin Endocrinol Metab 2000; 85:3623–3627.

102. Chelly J, Concordet JP, Kaplan JC, Kahn A. Illegitimate transcription: transcription of any gene in any cell type. Proc Natl Acad Sci USA 1989; 86:2617–2621.

103. Spencer CA. Challenges of serum thyroglobulin (Tg) measurement in the presence of Tg autoantibodies (TgAb). J Clin Endocrinol Metab 2004; 89:3702–3704.

104. Belfiore A, Runello F, Sava L, La Rosa G, Vigneri R. Thyroglobulin release after graded endogenous thyrotropin stimulation in man: lack of correlation with thyroid hormone response. J Clin Endocrinol Metab 1984; 59:974–978.

105. Schafgen W, Grebe SF, Schatz H. Dissociation of thyroglobulin and thyroid hormone secretion following endogenous thyrotropin stimulation by oral TRH. Horm Metab Res 1984; 16:615–616.

106. Schneider AB, Line BR, Goldman JM, Robbins J. Sequential serum thyroglobulin determinations, ^{131}I scans, and ^{131}I uptakes after triiodothyronine withdrawal in patients with thyroid cancer. J Clin Endocrinol Metab 1981; 53:1199–1206.

107. Pacini F, Lari R, Mazzeo S, Grasso L, Taddei D, Pinchera A. Diagnostic value of a single serum thyroglobulin determination on and off thyroid suppressive therapy in the follow-up of patients with differentiated thyroid cancer. Clin Endocrinol 1985; 23:405–411.

108. Dow KH, Ferrell BR, Anello C. Quality-of-life changes in patients with thyroid cancer after withdrawal of thyroid hormone therapy. Thyroid 1997; 7:613–619.

109. Schlumberger M, Ricard M, Pacini F. Clinical use of recombinant human TSH in thyroid cancer patients. Eur J Endocrinol 2000; 143:557–563.

110. Pacini F, Molinaro E, Lippi F, et al. Prediction of disease status by recombinant human TSH-stimulated serum Tg in the postsurgical follow-up of differentiated thyroid carcinoma. J Clin Endocrinol Metab 2001; 86: 5686–5690.

111. Torres MS, Ramirez L, Simkin PH, Braverman LE, Emerson CH. Effect of various doses of recombinant human thyrotropin on the thyroid radioactive iodine uptake and serum levels of thyroid hormones and thyroglobulin in normal subjects. J Clin Endocrinol Metab 2001; 86:1660–1664.

112. Nielsen VE, Bonnema SJ, Hegedus L. Effects of 0.9 mg recombinant human thyrotropin on thyroid size and function in normal subjects: a randomized, double-blind, cross-over trial. J Clin Endocrinol Metab 2004; 89:2242–2247.

113. Schlumberger M, Charbord P, Fragu P, Lumbroso J, Parmentier C, Tubiana M. Circulating thyrotropin and thyroid hormones in patients with metastases of differentiated thyroid cancer: relationship to serum thyrotropin levels. J Clin Endocrinol Metab 1980; 51:513–519.

114. Pellegriti G, Scollo C, Regalbuto C, et al. The diagnostic use of the rhTSH/thyroglobulin test in differentiated thyroid cancer patients with persistent disease and low thyroglobulin levels. Clin Endocrinol (Oxf) 2003; 58:556–561.

115. Spencer C, Schwarzbein D, Guttler R, LoPresti J, Nicoloff J. TRH stimulation test responses employing 3rd. and 4th. generation TSH assay technology. J Clin Endocrinol Metab 1993; 76:494–499.

116. Fatemi S, Nicoloff J, LoPresti J, Guttler R, Spencer C. TSH-stimulated serum thyroglobulin in the 1–10 ng/ml range suggests a low long-term recurrence risk for papillary thyroid cancer (PTC). Annual Meeting American Thyroid Association, Washington, DC, November 6–10, 2001: 280 (Abstract).

117. Haugen BR, Ridgway EC, McLaughlin BA, McDermott MT. Clinical comparison of whole-body radioiodine scan and serum thyroglobulin after stimulation with recombinant human thyrotropin. Thyroid 2002; 12: 37–43.

118. Fatemi S, LoPresti JS. A consensus report of the role of serum thyroglobulin as a monitoring method for low-risk patients with papillary thyroid carcinoma. J Clin Endocrinol Metab 2003; 88:4507–4508.

119. Feldt-Rasmussen U, Petersen PH, Date J, Madsen CM. Sequential changes in serum thyroglobulin (Tg) and its autoantibodies (TgAb) following subtotal thyroidectomy of patients with preoperatively detectable TgAb. Clin Endocrinol 1980; 12:29–38.

120. Weigle WO, High GJ. The behaviour of autologous thyroglobulin in the circulation of rabbits immunized with either heterologous or altered homologous thyroglobulin. J Immunol 1967; 98:1105–1114.

121. Hay ID, Bergstralh EJ, Goellner JR, Ebersold JR, Grant CS. Predicting outcome in papillary thyroid carcinoma: development of a reliable prognostic scoring system in a cohort of 1779 patients surgically treated at one institution during 1940 through 1989. Surgery 1993; 114:1050–1057.

122. Hay ID, Taylor WF, McConahey WM. A prognostic score for predicting outcome in papillary thyroid carcinoma. Endocrinology 1986; 119:1–15.

123. Hay ID. Papillary thyroid carcinoma. Endocrinol Metab Clin North Am 1990; 19:545–576.

124. TNM American Joint Committee on Cancer. Manual for staging of cancer, 4th edn. Philadelphia: JB Lippincott, 1992: 53.

125. Hay ID GC, van Heerden JA, Goellner JR, Ebersold JR. Papillary thyroid microcarcinoma: a study of 535 cases observed in a 50-year period. Surgery 1992; 112:1139–1147.

126. Cooper DS, Specker B, Ho M, et al. Thyrotropin suppression and disease progression in patients with differentiated thyroid cancer: results from the National Thyroid Cancer Treatment Cooperative Registry. Thyroid 1998; 8(9):737–744.

127. Eichhorn W, Tabler H, Lippold R, Lochmann M, Schreckenberger M, Bartenstein P. Prognostic factors determining long-term survival in well-differentiated thyroid cancer: an analysis of four hundred eighty-four patients undergoing therapy and aftercare at the same institution. Thyroid 2003; 13:949–958.

128. Conrad MF, Pandurangi KK, Parikshak M, Castillo ED, Talpos GB. Postoperative surveillance of differentiated thyroid carcinoma: a selective approach. Am Surg 2003; 69:244–250.

129. Wartofsky L, Sherman SI, Gopal J, Schlumberger M, Hay ID. The use of radioactive iodine in patients with papillary and follicular thyroid cancer. J Clin Endocrinol Metab 1998; 83:4195–4203.

130. Kim S, Wei JP, Braveman JM, Brams DM. Predicting outcome and directing therapy for papillary thyroid carcinoma. Arch Surg 2004; 139:390–394.

131. Marchesi M, Biffoni M, Biancari F, Berni A, Campana FP. Predictors of outcome for patients with differentiated and aggressive thyroid carcinoma. Eur J Surg Suppl 2003; 588:46–50.

132. Passler C, Scheuba C, Prager G, et al. Prognostic factors of papillary and follicular thyroid cancer: differences in an iodine-replete endemic goiter region. Endocr Relat Cancer 2004; 11:131–139.

133. Kouvaraki MA, Shapiro SE, Fornage BD, et al. Role of preoperative ultrasonography in the surgical management of patients with thyroid cancer. Surgery 2003; 134:946–954.

134. Grebe SK, Hay ID. Thyroid cancer nodal metastases: biologic significance and therapeutic considerations. Surg Oncol Clin N Am 1996; 5:43–63.

135. Fatemi S, Guttler R, LoPresti J, et al. TgAb-negative differentiated thyroid cancer (DTC) patients with lymphocytic thyroiditis detected at thyroidectomy have a lower risk of recurrence during long-term follow-up. American Thyroid Association meeting Abstract #36. 2003.

136. Serhal DI, Nasrallah MP, Arafah BM. Rapid rise in serum thyrotropin concentrations after thyroidectomy or withdrawal of suppressive thyroxine therapy in preparation for radioactive iodine administration to patients with differentiated thyroid cancer. J Clin Endocrinol Metab 2004; 89:3285–3289.

137. Pujol P, Daures JP, Nsakala N, Baldet L, Bringer J, Jaffiol C. Degree of thyrotropin suppression as a prognostic determinant in differentiated thyroid cancer. J Clin Endocrinol Metab 1996; 81:4318–4323.

138. Toubeau M, Touzery C, Arveux P, et al. Predictive value for disease progression of serum thyroglobulin levels measured in the postoperative period and after (131)I ablation therapy in patients with differentiated thyroid cancer. J Nucl Med 2004; 45:988–994.

139. Frasoldati A, Pesenti M, Gallo M, Caroggio A, Salvo D, Valcavi R. Diagnosis of neck recurrences in patients with differentiated thyroid cancer. Cancer 2003; 97: 90–96.

140. Ito Y, Uruno T, Nakano K, et al. An observation trial without surgical treatment in patients with papillary microcarcinoma of the thyroid. Thyroid 2003; 13:381–387.

141. David A, Blotta A, Bondanelli M, et al. Serum thyroglobulin concentrations and (131)I whole-body scan results in patients with differentiated thyroid carcinoma after administration of recombinant human thyroid-stimulating hormone. J Nucl Med 2001; 42: 1470–1475.

142. Giovanni V, Arianna LG, Antonio C, et al. The use of recombinant human TSH in the follow-up of differentiated thyroid cancer: experience from a large patient cohort in a single centre. Clin Endocrinol (Oxf) 2002; 56:247–252.

143. Robbins RJ, Chon JT, Fleisher M, Larson SM, Tuttle RM. Is the serum thyroglobulin response to recombinant human thyrotropin sufficient, by itself, to monitor for residual thyroid carcinoma? J Clin Endocrinol Metab 2002; 87:3242–3247.

144. Wartofsky L. Management of low-risk well-differentiated thyroid cancer based only on thyroglobulin measurement after recombinant human thyrotropin. Thyroid 2002; 12:583–590.

19

Follow-up of Patients with Differentiated Thyroid Carcinoma

Martin J. Schlumberger, Sophie M. Leboulleux, and Furio Pacini

Introduction

Differentiated (papillary and follicular) thyroid carcinoma (DTC) generally is characterized by an indolent course with low morbidity and mortality and is among the most curable cancers [1]. In most cases, initial treatment for DTC is total thyroidectomy, with lymph node dissection in case of papillary thyroid carcinoma. In case of persistent disease or when the TNM (tumor, node, metastasis) or any other scoring system predicts a high risk of recurrence, the surgery may be followed by administration of a large activity of 131-iodine (^{131}I) to ablate remnant tissue and any residual disease. Patients then are placed on levothyroxine (L-T_4) treatment to decrease serum thyroid-stimulating hormone (TSH), while avoiding L-T_4 overdosage.

Because DTC may recur at any time for years after initial treatment, and L-T_4 therapy is life-long, long-term follow-up is necessary. Since the estimated European population of DTC patients and survivors is 200 000 [2], any follow-up protocol will affect the safety and quality of life of a large population and exert an important impact on health economics.

In recent years, the spectrum of patients with DTC has changed. In part due to incidental findings on neck ultrasonography (US) for non-thyroid indications, a larger number of thyroid tumors, mainly papillary, are being discovered at an earlier stage, accounting for the increased incidence of the disease [2–4]. Also, the quality

of initial surgery has improved, as well as the sensitivity of the methods used for detecting persistent disease. As a result, the risk of recurrence in patients with no obvious disease after initial treatment is much lower than previously reported, and is probably less than 5%. In these patients, follow-up should be guided by a protocol with a high negative predictive value, to exclude from unnecessary investigations those with a nonsignificant risk of recurrence. It should also be sensitive enough to identify the few individuals who have a previously unrecognized risk of recurrence and therefore merit a closer follow-up. Indeed, patients with distant metastases or persistent disease after incomplete thyroid surgery should be treated and followed up according to specific protocols, and will not be considered in this review.

The follow-up protocol of patients with no clinically obvious residual disease after initial treatment includes three important elements addressing recent findings (Figure 19.1) [5,6]. First, up to now the same protocol is applied to all DTC patients who have been treated postoperatively with radioiodine. Second, the protocol uses recombinant human thyroid-stimulating hormone (rhTSH) as the "gold standard" to obtain TSH stimulation for diagnostic follow-up. Third, the protocol virtually obviates diagnostic total-body scan (dxTBS) and highlights the importance of neck US in the follow-up.

This review details the follow-up protocol that can be applied to the majority of

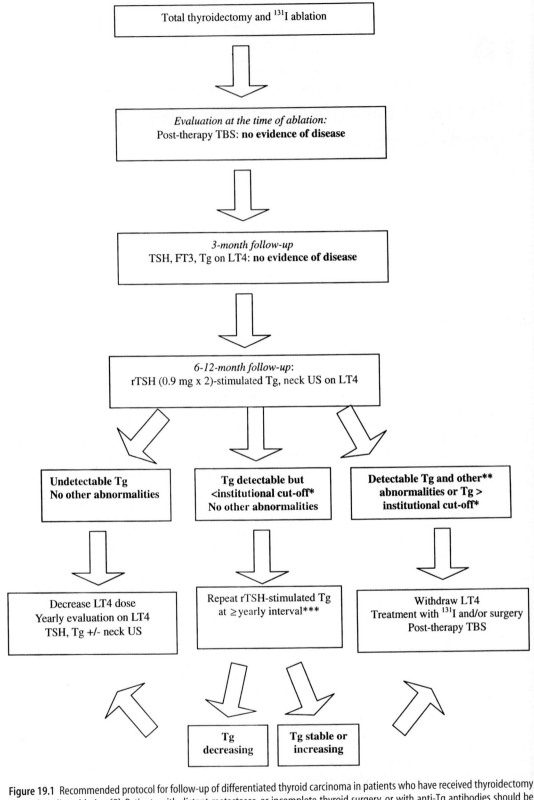

Figure 19.1 Recommended protocol for follow-up of differentiated thyroid carcinoma in patients who have received thyroidectomy and radioiodine ablation [5]. Patients with distant metastases, or incomplete thyroid surgery, or with anti-Tg antibodies should be followed up according to other specific protocols. FT$_3$, free triiodothyronine; L-T$_4$, L-thyroxine, rhTSH, recombinant human thyroid-stimulating hormone; Tg, serum thyroglobulin measurement; TSH, thyroid-stimulating hormone; US, ultrasonography; TBS, total-body scan. *In each institution, the Tg threshold should be determined after rhTSH stimulation for each assay method. **Any suspicious finding on neck US warrants FNA with cytological evaluation and measurement of Tg concentration in the aspirate. ***This interval depends on exact Tg level and on the clinical context.

DTC patients and then describes particular conditions.

Objectives and Stages of Follow-up

After initial treatment, the follow-up of patients with DTC has two objectives: (1) to discover at the earliest possible time persistent or recurrent disease, allowing for treatment that may extend survival [1,7], and (2) to ensure that the patient receives the lowest effective L-T$_4$ dose, that is one that provides no more TSH suppression than necessary [8,9].

Monitoring patients with DTC comprises four stages: (1) evaluation at the time of radioiodine ablation of thyroid remnants; (2) ~3-month follow-up while the patient is on L-T$_4$ treatment; (3) 6- to 12-month follow-up, after TSH stimulation; and (4) subsequent follow-up.

The follow-up strategy is mainly based on serum thyroglobulin (Tg) measurement, which should always employ an immunometric assay with a functional sensitivity of <1 ng/mL. To aid in the interpretation of Tg results and identify the ~20% of cases with anti-Tg antibodies (TgAb) [10], Tg testing should be accompanied by a TgAb assay, or by recovery testing. In cases of interference with Tg measurements by TgAb, which are evidenced by the recovery test in about 1% of patients and may lead to falsely low or even undetectable values, patients should be monitored according to a modified protocol (see below). Of note, a detectable serum Tg in the presence of TgAb is generally observed in patients with persistent or recurrent disease. Also of note, in the absence of disease, TgAb will progressively decrease and disappear within the first 2 years of follow-up [10,11].

Early Follow-up

Evaluation at the Time of Radioiodine Ablation of Thyroid Remnants

Evaluation at the time of ablation consists of "posttherapy" TBS 3–7 days after administration of the ablative activity of [131]I. TBS is performed using a large field-of-view gamma camera with thick crystals and high-energy collimators. Whole-body images are taken with spot images of the neck and any other suspicious area [9]. An accurate anatomical view of any neck uptake will differentiate whether the uptake is present in normal thyroid remnants or lymph node metastases. Indeed, high uptake in thyroid remnants will obliterate visualization of lower uptake in neck lymph nodes. This emphasizes the paramount importance of performing a total thyroidectomy with the aim of achieving an uptake in thyroid remnants lower than 1–2% of the administered activity. The risk of artifacts should be minimized by having the patient drink lemon juice and large amounts of liquid, chew gum, and shower and change clothes before scanning. Iodine contamination should be avoided by the patient's following a low iodine diet for a few weeks before radioiodine treatment, and is ruled out by testing of urinary iodine concentration. A diagnostic TBS or even a measurement of neck uptake is usually not performed before ^{131}I treatment in patients in whom an experienced surgeon has performed a total thyroidectomy; in these patients, it does not afford any benefit but may decrease the subsequent uptake of the ablation dose. However, when a limited thyroid surgery has been performed, it may be preferable to measure neck uptake before treatment because patients with a thyroid uptake >5–15% should be considered for additional surgery.

Serum Tg is measured on the day when the ablative activity of ^{131}I is administered. A low or undetectable serum Tg at that time generally announces a favorable outcome. Elevated values have questionable prognostic significance and may be related to persistent disease or to lingering leakage from postsurgical thyroid residues. Neck US performed at this time may be useful in detecting previously undiagnosed lymph node metastases, although images may be uninformative due to the recency of surgery.

Evaluation at 3 Months

The ~3-month follow-up consists of serum TSH, free triiodothyronine (FT$_3$) and Tg determinations [12] while the patient is on L-T$_4$ treatment. TSH testing is not conducted until ~3 months after ablation because elevated TSH levels may persist until that point and may lead to overtreatment with L-T$_4$. At this stage of follow-up, a TSH concentration around 0.1 µU/mL, with normal FT_3 levels, denotes an appropriate dose of $L-T_4$.

The results of the postablation and ~3-month follow-ups should be used to distinguish two groups of patients: those (1) with evidence of disease, who should be referred for treatment, and (2) without evidence of disease, if they have complete tumor resection according to the surgeon's report, no uptake outside the thyroid bed on postablative ^{131}I TBS, undetectable serum Tg level (<1 ng/mL) during $L-T_4$ treatment, and no abnormality on neck US. Also, patients whose evidence of disease comprises only detectable but low Tg at the time of ablation and/or at any subsequent follow-up should undergo the same follow-up protocol.

Six- to 12-Month Follow-up

For patients without evidence of disease at the 3-month follow-up, the 6- to 12-month follow-up should consist of Tg testing after rhTSH stimulation and of neck US. rhTSH should be administered in two consecutive daily intramuscular injections of 0.9 mg and blood should be drawn for Tg measurement 3 days after the second injection.

The rationale for use of TSH stimulation is the well-documented appreciable percentage of patients with persistent or recurrent disease having false-negative Tg measurements during $L-T_4$ treatment. When the functional sensitivity of the method used for measuring Tg is 1 ng/mL, serum Tg is undetectable during $L-T_4$ treatment in more than 20% of patients with lymph node metastases, and about 5% of patients with distant metastases but normal plain radiographs [1]. TSH stimulation increases the sensitivity of serum Tg measurement and it appears that there is no detectable serum Tg value below which the presence of persistent or recurrent disease can be excluded; in parallel, TSH stimulation decreases the specificity of serum Tg measurement, the negative predictive value then being only 50%. On the other hand, the use of a highly sensitive assay provides a higher sensitivity for detecting persistent or recurrent disease, but a much lower specificity, and it does not improve the quality of follow-up (manuscript in preparation).

It should be noted that only a small minority of patients with no clinically obvious disease will have persistent or recurrent disease at follow-up examination; therefore, the number of patients for whom any testing following TSH stimulation will permit the discovery of disease is low. In our view, TSH stimulation with serum Tg determination combined with neck US still is warranted because it will both obviate other tests and provide reassurance for the majority of patients and in the others will indicate further testing and/or treatment.

The rationale for using rhTSH instead of $L-T_4$ withdrawal for TSH stimulation is threefold. First, the sensitivity of rhTSH-stimulated serum Tg measurement has been amply demonstrated [13–23]. Second, rhTSH stimulation avoids the discomfort and quality-of-life impairment and decreases the safety risks associated with the hypothyroidism that is secondary to $L-T_4$ withdrawal [15,24]. Third, use of rhTSH stimulation largely avoids the negative economic and professional consequences of that hypothyroidism.

The rationale for avoiding dxTBS in the 6- to 12-month follow-up of patients with no evidence of disease up to that time is fourfold. First, total ablation defined as the absence of uptake or a low but not measurable uptake in the thyroid bed at a subsequent dxTBS is achieved in almost all patients with small thyroid remnants [25]. Second, in patients with low uptake (<1–2%) in thyroid remnants, the TBS performed some days after the ablation dose is more sensitive for detecting uptake outside the thyroid bed than a TBS performed some months later with a lower activity of [131]I [1,9,23,25]. Third, recent studies totaling more than 2500 consecutive patients given $L-T_4$ withdrawal [25–27], rhTSH [13,14,16–20,22], or a combination of these methods [15,23] have shown that no patient who was Tg-negative, defined as having a value below the limits of detectability, was TBS-positive, defined as having uptake outside the thyroid bed. A single study [21] shows a small percentage of Tg-negative, TBS-positive patients. However, this study appears to include some patients who received further therapy after initial treatment and presumably had evidence of disease at the postablation or 6–12-month follow-up: not the population in which our protocol suggests avoidance of dxTBS. It must be stressed that the number of metastatic patients so far reported following rhTSH stimulation is limited, and that false-negative serum Tg may be recognized only some years or decades later. Four, obviation of dxTBS prevents possible impairment of uptake of any necessary therapeutic activity of radioiodine due to stunning from a diagnostic activity [28,29].

The rationale for using neck US in patients with no evidence of disease before the 6- to 12-month follow-up is the efficacy of neck US in detecting neck recurrences, documented by four recent large studies [13,20,27,30]. In these studies, the sensitivity of the combination of serum Tg obtained following TSH stimulation and of neck US for detecting lymph node metastases ranged from 97% to 100%. In comparison, the sensitivity of either neck palpation or TBS is much lower.

In patients with papillary thyroid carcinoma, neck lymph nodes are the most frequent site of recurrence, and almost the only site in patients with undetectable Tg during L-T$_4$ treatment [1,9,14,20,27,30]. Neck US should employ a probe containing a linear transducer of at least 7.5 megahertz, and results should be reported on a diagram. Lymph nodes are suspicious when they are hypoechogenic, lack an echogenic central line, have a round shape, and/or have a hypervascularized appearance on color Doppler. Microcalcifications or a cystic component are highly suspicious. It is essential that neck US be performed by an operator with day-to-day experience in evaluating patients with thyroid cancer, not just thyroid disease in general. Likewise, US-guided fine-needle aspiration (FNA) should be performed by an operator experienced in that procedure.

Neck US can detect lymph node metastases as small as 2–3 mm in diameter. In these patients, the above characteristics cannot be reliably assessed and serum Tg may remain undetectable even following TSH stimulation. Indeed, it is estimated [31,32] that 1 g of neoplastic tissue will increase serum Tg obtained during L-T$_4$ treatment by about 0.5–1 ng/mL, and that TSH stimulation will increase serum Tg values about 10-fold over baseline levels. Thus, all suspicious lesions that are accessible to puncture should be subjected to FNA with cytological evaluation. Measurement of Tg concentration in the aspirate is an easy procedure that should be routinely performed because it increases the reliability of FNA [33,34]. Tg

reverse transcription polymerase chain reaction may serve as an alternative to such measurement [35].

In conclusion, the use of neck US permits the detection of small lymph node metastases. The benefits of their early discovery is far from being demonstrated, while the routine use of neck US may lead to the discovery of benign lymph nodes in a large number of patients and thus to unnecessary FNA being carried out in many patients.

Subsequent Follow-up and Management

In almost 85% of patients with favorable prognostic indicators, rhTSH-stimulated Tg was undetectable and findings on neck US were normal at the 6- to 12-month follow-up. In these patients, the risk of subsequent recurrence is less than 0.5% [20,25,27]. These patients can be reassured and the dose of L-T$_4$ may be safely decreased to obtain a normal TSH concentration (0.5–2.5 µU/mL). These patients are followed yearly with TSH and Tg and eventually neck US. Tg testing may be conducted during L-T$_4$ therapy without rhTSH stimulation; whether such stimulation, for instance after an interval of 5 years, is justified by providing added benefits needs to be ascertained.

In patients with detectable rhTSH-stimulated Tg concentrations at the 6- to 12-month follow-up, subsequent management depends on the Tg levels and the presence or absence of abnormalities on neck US and any other evaluation methods that may have been performed. Detectable serum Tg may be produced for some months after initial treatment by irradiated cancer cells that eventually will disappear, or by neoplastic foci that will progress. The slope between the 6- to 12-month and subsequent Tg values obtained following rhTSH can differentiate between these two sources of detectable Tg.

Therefore, patients with a Tg concentration that is detectable but at a low level (below an institutional cutoff determined following rhTSH stimulation for each particular assay employed) and no other abnormalities should be followed with rhTSH-stimulated Tg measurement one year or more later depending on the Tg level and the clinical context. Serum Tg will decrease in about two thirds of these patients and subsequent monitoring should be conducted in the same manner as in patients without any evidence of disease up to the 6- to 12-month follow-up. In individuals who show a stable or increasing Tg concentration between the 6- to 12-month follow-up and the subsequent testing point, persistent or recurrent disease should be carefully sought [36,37].

Patients who at the 6- to 12-month follow-up have detectable rhTSH-stimulated Tg levels above the institutional cutoff also should receive such management, starting with the administration of a large activity of ^{131}I. If the posttherapy TBS does not show any uptake, other imaging modalities may be employed: spiral computed tomography of the neck and chest, bone scintigraphy, and [^{18}F] fluorodeoxyglucose positron emission tomography (FDG-PET). FDG-PET may be more sensitive when performed following rhTSH stimulation [38,39]. Its main role is to provide a reliable investigation of the mediastinum.

Particular Conditions

Patients with Evidence of Disease

Persistent disease is more frequently found in patients with extensive disease in the neck, including those with large thyroid tumor, tumor extension beyond the thyroid capsule, or with extensive lymph node metastases. Similarly, recurrent disease occurs more frequently in these patients, the recurrence rate after the 6- to 12-month follow-up being around 10%. Of note, most patients who will experience a recurrence during the subsequent follow-up can be individualized at the 6- to 12-month follow-up because they already have a detectable serum Tg.

Patients with evidence of disease are treated according to the location of the disease.

Patients with Large Thyroid Remnants

In patients with large thyroid remnants who are treated with radioiodine, immediate postablation TBS may be poorly sensitive for detecting uptake outside the thyroid bed; also, the ablation rate is lower than in patients with small thyroid remnants. Detectable serum Tg may be related to persistent thyroid remnants. For these reasons, a dxTBS at 6 to 12 months may be indicated. Whenever rhTSH is used to provide TSH elevation for dxTBS, an activity of at least 148 MBq (4 mCi) of ^{131}I should be administered one day after the last injection of rhTSH. This underlines that performing a total thyroidectomy in all DTC patients will improve the quality and ease of the follow-up.

Patients with Anti-Tg Antibodies

In such cases, follow-up cannot rely on serum Tg determination and should comprise neck US and ^{131}I TBS. The persistence of anti-Tg antibodies for more than 2 years after initial treatment is suspicious of persistent disease [10,11].

Patients Who Did Not Receive ^{131}I Ablation Therapy

By definition, the risk of recurrence according to initial prognostic indicators and completeness of surgery is low in these patients. Follow-up is based on serum Tg determination during L-T$_4$ treatment, which should be undetectable, and on neck US. In the presence of any abnormality, an ablative activity of ^{131}I may be administered some months or even years after surgery, with a TBS performed some days later.

Conclusion

The monitoring of patients with DTC is entering an era of still greater safety, simplicity, convenience, and cost savings with the recent documentation of (1) the lack of sensitivity of dxTBS in identifying individuals suspicious for disease among patients without evidence of DTC up to the 6- to 12-month follow-up who also are receiving TSH-stimulated Tg testing; (2) the efficacy of rhTSH stimulation and its safety and preservation of patients' work productivity relative to L-T$_4$ withdrawal and concomitant hypothyroidism; and (3) the superior efficacy of neck US in detecting neck recurrences.

References

1. Schlumberger MJ. Medical progress: papillary and follicular thyroid carcinoma. N Engl J Med 1998; 338:297–306.
2. Parkin DM, Whelan SL, Ferlay J, Raymond L, Young J. Cancer incidence in five continents, Vol. VII. Lyon: IARC Scientific Publications No 143, 1997.
3. Colonna M, Grosclaude P, Remontet L, et al. Incidence of thyroid cancer in adults recorded by French Cancer registries (1978–1997). Eur J Cancer 2002; 38:1762–1768.
4. Leenhardt L, Bernier MO, Boin-Pineau MH, et al. Advances in diagnostic practices affect thyroid cancer incidence in France. Eur J Endocrinol 2004; 50:133–139.
5. Schlumberger M, Berg G, Cohen O, et al. Follow-up of low-risk patients with differentiated thyroid carcinoma: a European perspective. Eur J Endocrinol 2004; 50:105–112.
6. Mazzaferri EL, Robbins RJ, Spencer CA, et al. A consensus report of the role of serum thyroglobulin as a monitoring method for low-risk patients with papillary thyroid carcinoma. J Clin Endocrinol Metab 2003; 88: 1433–1441.
7. Schlumberger MJ, Challeton C, De Vathaire F, et al. Radioactive iodine treatment and external radiotherapy for lung and bone metastases from thyroid carcinoma. J Nucl Med 1996; 37:598–605.
8. Biondi B, Palmieri EA, Lombardi G, Fazio S. Effects of subclinical thyroid dysfunction on the heart. Ann Intern Med 2002; 137:909–914.
9. Schlumberger MJ, Pacini F. Thyroid tumors, 2nd edn. Paris: Editions Nucleon, 2003.
10. Spencer CA, Takeuchi M, Kazarosyan M, et al. Serum thyroglobulin antibodies: prevalence, influence on serum thyroglobulin measurements, and prognostic significance in patients with differentiated thyroid carcinoma. J Clin Endocrinol Metab 1998; 83:1121–1127.
11. Chiovato L, Latrofa F, Braverman LE, et al. Disappearance of humoral thyroid autoimmunity after complete removal of thyroid antigens. Ann Intern Med 2003; 139: 346–351.
12. Bartalena L, Martino E, Pacchiarotti A, et al. Factors affecting suppression of endogenous thyrotropin secretion by thyroxine treatment: retrospective analysis in athyreotic and goitrous patients J Clin Endocrinol Metab 1987; 64:849–855.
13. Torlontano M, Crocetti U, D'Aloiso L, et al. Serum thyroglobulin and ^{131}I whole body scan after recombinant human TSH stimulation in the follow-up of low-risk patients with differentiated thyroid cancer. The role for neck ultrasonography. Eur J Endocrinol 2003; 148:18–24.
14. David A, Blotta A, Bondanelli M, et al. Serum thyroglobulin concentrations and ^{131}I whole-body scan results in patients with differentiated thyroid carcinoma after administration of recombinant human thyroid-stimulating hormone. J Nucl Med 2001; 42:1470–1475.
15. Haugen BR, Pacini F, Reiners C, et al. A comparison of recombinant human thyrotropin and thyroid hormone withdrawal for the detection of thyroid remnant or cancer. J Clin Endocrinol Metab 1999; 84:3877–3885.
16. Haugen BR, Ridgway EC, McLaughlin B, McDermott MT. Clinical comparison of whole-body radioiodine scan and serum thyroglobulin after stimulation with recombinant human TSH. Thyroid 2002; 12:37–43.
17. Ladenson PW, Braverman LE, Mazzaferri EL, et al. Comparison of administration of recombinant human thyrotropin with withdrawal of thyroid hormone for radioactive iodine scanning in patients with thyroid carcinoma. N Engl J Med 1997; 337:888–896.
18. Mazzaferri EL, Kloos RT. Is diagnostic iodine-131 scanning with recombinant human TSH useful in the follow-up of differentiated thyroid cancer after thyroid ablation? J Clin Endocrinol Metab 2002; 87:1490–1498.
19. Meier CA, Braverman LE, Ebner SA, et al. Diagnostic use of recombinant human thyrotropin in patients with thyroid carcinoma (Phase I/II Study). J Clin Endocrinol Metab 1994; 78:188–196.
20. Pacini F, Molinaro E, Castagna MG, et al. rhTSH-stimulated serum thyroglobulin combined with neck ultrasonography has the highest sensitivity in monitoring differentiated thyroid carcinoma. J Clin Endocrinol Metab 2003; 88:3668–3673.
21. Robbins RJ, Chon JT, Fleisher M, Larson SM, Tuttle RM. Is the serum thyroglobulin response to recombinant human thyrotropin sufficient, by itself, to monitor for residual thyroid carcinoma? J Clin Endocrinol Metab 2002; 87:3242–3247.
22. Wartofsky L. Management of low risk well-differentiated thyroid cancer based only upon thyroglobulin measurement after recombinant human thyrotropin. Thyroid 2002; 12:583–590.
23. Pacini F, Molinaro E, Lippi F, et al. Prediction of disease status by recombinant human TSH stimulated serum Tg in the postsurgical follow-up of differentiated thyroid carcinoma. J Clin Endocrinol Metab 2001; 86:5686–5690.
24. Dow KH, Ferrell BR, Anello C. Quality-of-life changes in patients with thyroid cancer after withdrawal of thyroid hormone therapy. Thyroid 1997; 7:613–619.
25. Cailleux AF, Baudin E, Travagli JP, Ricard M, Schlumberger M. Is diagnostic iodine-131 scanning useful after total thyroid ablation for differentiated thyroid cancer? J Clin Endocrinol Metab 2000; 85:175–178.
26. Pacini F, Capezzone M, Elisei R, Ceccarelli C, Taddei D, Pinchera A. Diagnostic 131-iodine whole-body scan may be avoided in thyroid cancer patients who have undetectable stimulated serum Tg levels after initial treatment. J Clin Endocrinol Metab 2002; 87:1499–1501.
27. Torlontano M, Attard M, Crocetti U, et al. Follow-up of low risk patients with papillary thyroid cancer: role of neck ultrasonography in detecting lymph node metastases. J Clin Endocrinol Metab 2004; 89:3402–3407.
28. Park HM, Perkins OW, Edmondson JW, Schnute RB, Manatunga A. Influence of diagnostic radioiodines on the uptake of ablative dose of iodine-131. Thyroid 1994; 4:49–54.
29. Postgard P, Jimmelman J, Lindencrona U, et al. Stunning of iodine transport by (131)I irradiation in cultured thyroid epithelial cells. J Nucl Med 2002; 43:828–834.
30. Frasoldati A, Presenti M, Gallo M, Caroggio A, Salvo D, Valcavi R. Diagnosis of neck recurrences in patients with differentiated thyroid carcinoma. Cancer 2003; 97: 90–96.

31. Bachelot A, Cailleux AF, Klain M, et al. Relationship between tumor burden and serum thyroglobulin level in patients with papillary and follicular thyroid carcinoma. Thyroid 2002; 12:707–711.
32. Demers LM, Spencer CA. 7–13–2002 Laboratory support for the diagnosis and monitoring of thyroid disease. http://www.nacb.org/lmpg/thyroid/LMPH.stm.
33. Pacini F, Fugazzola L, Lippi F, et al. Detection of thyroglobulin in fine needle aspirates of nonthyroidal neck masses: a clue to the diagnosis of metastatic differentiated thyroid cancer. J Clin Endocrinol Metab 1992; 74: 1401–1404.
34. Frasoldati A, Toschi E, Zini M, et al. Role of thyroglobulin measurement in fine-needle aspiration biopsies of cervical lymph nodes in patients with differentiated thyroid cancer. Thyroid 1999; 9:105–111.
35. Arturi F, Russo D, Giuffrida D, et al. Early diagnosis by genetic analysis of differentiated thyroid cancer metastases in small lymph nodes. J Clin Endocrinol Metab 1997; 82:1638–1641.
36. Baudin E, Do Cao C, Cailleux AF, Leboulleux S, Travagli JP, Schlumberger M. Positive predictive value of serum thyroglobulin levels, measured during the first year of follow-up after thyroid hormone withdrawal in thyroid cancer patients. J Clin Endocrinol Metab 2003; 88:1107–1111.
37. Pacini F, Agate L, Elisei R, et al. Outcome of differentiated thyroid cancer with detectable serum Tg and negative diagnostic ^{131}I whole body scan: comparison of patients treated with high ^{131}I activities versus untreated patients. J Clin Endocrinol Metab 2001; 86:4092–4097.
38. Petrich T, Börner AR, Otto D, Hofmann M, Knapp WH. Influence of rhTSH on [^{18}F]fluorodeoxyglucose uptake by differentiated thyroid carcinoma. Eur J Nucl Med Mol Imaging 2002; 29:641–647.
39. Chin BB, Patel P, Cohade C, Ewertz M, Wahl R, Ladenson P. Recombinant human thyrotropin stimulation of fluoro-D-glucose positron emission tomography uptake in well-differentiated thyroid carcinoma. J Clin Endocrinol Metab 2004; 89:91–95.

20

Management of Differentiated Thyroid Carcinoma Patients with Negative Whole-Body Radioiodine Scans and Elevated Serum Thyroglobulin Levels

Ernest L. Mazzaferri

Abbreviations

CT	Computed tomography scans
DTC	Differentiated thyroid carcinoma
DxWBS	Diagnostic whole body ^{131}I scan
[18]FDG-PET	[18]Fluorodeoxyglucose positron emission tomography
HAB	Heterophile antibody
IMA	Immunometric assay
rhTSH	Recombinant human TSH
RIA	Radioimmunoassay
RxWBS	Posttherapy whole body ^{131}I scan
Tg	Thyroglobulin
TgAb	Antithyroglobulin antibody
THST	Thyroid hormone suppression of TSH
THW	Thyroid hormone withdrawal
TSH	Thyrotropin

Introduction

For patients with differentiated thyroid carcinoma (DTC), the main goal of follow-up is to identify tumor at the earliest stage possible while simultaneously distinguishing those who are free of disease. Although a thin diagnostic line separates the two groups, it is important to differentiate them because therapy has the greatest potential to extend survival in the first group while the second group should be reassured and spared from unnecessary treatment, especially thyroid hormone suppression of TSH with its potential for producing adverse cardiac events and loss of bone mineral density. Tumor is identified in its earliest stages when the TSH-stimulated serum thyroglobulin (Tg) concentration rises above 2μg/L, whereas in the absence of tumor, the Tg remains undetectable, even during TSH stimulation.

Classification of Tumor Status after Initial Therapy

Patients are classified as being free of disease after total or near-total thyroidectomy and ^{131}I remnant ablation when *all* of the following criteria are fulfilled:

- Complete resection of identifiable tumor.
- No uptake outside the thyroid bed on the posttherapy whole body ^{131}I scan.
- Negative neck ultrasound examination.
- Undetectable serum Tg levels (<1μg/L) during both:
  thyroid hormone suppression of TSH and TSH stimulation.

TSH stimulation of Tg can be achieved either by administering recombinant human TSH (rhTSH, Thyrogen, Figure 20.1) or by withdrawing thyroid hormone (THW) long enough, usually 2 to 3 weeks, to raise TSH levels above 30 mIU/L [1,2]. This is necessary because meas-

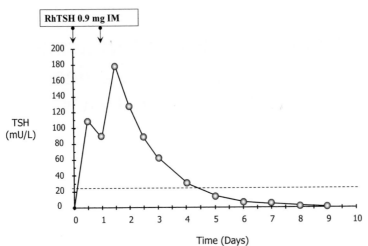

Figure 20.1 Serum rhTSH levels achieved after intramuscular (IM) injection of rhTSH (recombinant human TSH, Thyrogen). (Data reproduced with permission of the Genzyme Corporation, Boston, MA, USA.)

uring serum Tg concentrations during thyroid hormone suppression of TSH (THST) frequently fails to identify persistent tumor or identifies it late in its course when it is at a more advanced stage [3–6]. Likewise, performing diagnostic whole-body scans (DxWBS), whether after THW or with rhTSH administration, often fails to identify persistent tumor. On the other hand, posttreatment whole-body ^{131}I scans (RxWBS) and neck ultrasonography are powerful tools with which tumor may be identified at an early stage [3–6].

The Problem of Delayed Identification of Tumor

In older studies that used less sensitive follow-up techniques, tumor was often first identified 10 or more years after initial therapy, often at an advanced stage that was unresponsive to therapy (Figure 20.2) [7]. Delayed treatment, whether caused by failure to recognize malignancy in a thyroid nodule [8], or by withholding contralateral lobectomy (completion thyroidectomy) until long after hemithyroidectomy has been done [9], or by failing to promptly identify persistent tumor after initial therapy [7], all increase the likelihood that tumor will be found at a more advanced stage, thus increasing cancer mortality rates [10]. In our studies, for example, 15% of regional

relapses and 25% of distant metastases were first noted more than 10 years and in some cases as long as 35 years after initial treatment.

Newer diagnostic paradigms that rely heavily upon measuring TSH-stimulated serum Tg levels now identify persistent tumor within 3 to 18 months of initial therapy, sometimes at such an early stage that the tumor site is only visible with sensitive neck ultrasound studies or on RxWBS or ^{18}FDG-PET imaging (Figure 20.3 and Chapter 1) [1,2,5,11]. Albeit is considerably more sensitive than older follow-up paradigms, this new approach has caused a troubling new problem: identifying the source of a high serum Tg level when the DxWBS studies are negative. An even more difficult problem arises when the post-^{131}I ablation RxWBS study is negative, which is currently the most common reason patients are referred to our clinic. Although controversy swirls around the treatment of such patients [12–15], contemporary studies give considerable insight into their management.

Clinical Evaluation

Serum Tg Levels

High Serum Tg Concentrations and Tumor Mass

After total or near-total thyroidectomy and ^{131}I remnant ablation when the TSH level is stable

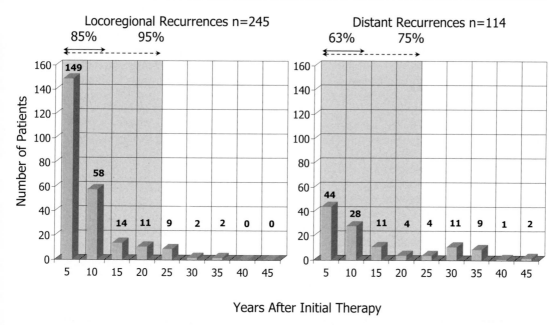

Figure 20.2 Recurrence rates of differentiated thyroid cancer over time. (Drawn from the data of Mazzaferri and Kloos [14].)

during THST, any alteration in the serum Tg level usually reflects a change in tumor mass [16,17]. Still, an undetectable basal (THST) Tg level, using current commercial assays, is not a reliable criterion to exclude tumor in patients who have been treated with total thyroidectomy and [131]I [17]. This requires TSH stimulation. The magnitude of rise in serum Tg levels in response to TSH stimulation, whether by THW or rhTSH, gives a good estimate of tumor mass, providing the cells are capable of secreting Tg [16,17]. Patients with higher serum Tg levels generally have more extensive disease and require more aggressive treatment than those with minimally elevated serum Tg levels [1,2,5,6,17]. In a recent study of 169 patients with metastatic disease, Robbins et al. [18] found that the basal Tg level directly correlated with the number of metastatic lesions, and that it was highest in patients with follicular and lowest in those with papillary thyroid carcinoma. Moreover, the basal Tg level was highest in those with bone metastases and lowest in patients with cervical metastases. The increase in serum Tg after rhTSH was highest in papillary thyroid carcinoma and lowest in Hürthle cell carcinoma, but was not influenced by tumor volume or by the site of metastatic lesions.

Accurate measurement and interpretation of serum Tg levels (see Chapter 18) is a prerequisite for distinguishing patients who are free of disease from those with persistent tumor, especially when its presence is signaled only by an elevated serum Tg level [1,2,5,6]. Several things spuriously lower or elevate serum Tg concentrations, which must be taken into account in the evaluation of patients with a high serum Tg level and a negative DxWBS.

Misleadingly Low Serum Tg Measurements

Following thyroidectomy and ^{131}I ablation, the serum Tg level should be undetectable (<1 µg/L) during THW and after rhTSH stimulation [1,2,16], but both tests may be falsely low in patients with persistent tumor when anti-Tg antibodies (TgAb) are present in the serum specimen in which Tg is measured [16]. This is an important problem because TgAbs are present in 25% of patients with DTC [19]. Still, among patients who are free of disease, the TgAb levels progressively decrease and disappear within a median of 3 years (2 to 4 years) after complete thyroid ablation, thus serving as a surrogate tumor marker [20]. Although Tg recovery assays are commonly used to circumvent this problem, some question the accuracy of this methodology [16].

Serum Tg levels also may be erroneously undetectable, even after TSH stimulation, in patients with lymph node metastases [17,21], particularly when Tg is measured by recovery Tg assays [5,11,21,22]. Although circulating Tg mRNA is a potentially more sensitive marker of thyroid tissue or persistent tumor than is the serum Tg concentration, especially in serum specimens with circulating TgAb, it has not yet gained widespread clinical use [23,24]. Negative thyroid ultrasonography and RxWBS remain the best indicators that a patient is free of tumor when TgAbs are present. Perhaps the most dangerously misleading situation occurs when tumor becomes more undifferentiated and fails to secrete Tg, even in response to TSH stimulation, and also fails to concentrate ^{131}I on RxWBS.

Misleadingly High Serum Tg Measurements

This is also of importance, especially considering the trend of treating high serum Tg levels with ^{131}I when the DxWBS is negative. Heterophile antibodies (HAB), which are human anti-animal (often anti-mouse) antibodies, may interfere with Tg measurements made by immunometric assays (IMA). Unlike the situation with TgAb, interference caused by HAB tends to artifactually raise serum Tg levels. A recent study [25] of one commonly used automated IMA system found that 3% of 1106 specimens with a serum Tg >1 μg/L fell an average of 57%, going to levels <1 μg/L and in some cases to <0.1 μg/L after the serum had been incubated in HAB-blocking tubes. The artifactually elevated serum Tg levels ranged from 1 to 15 600 μg/L, averaging 123.3 μg/L with a median of 14 μg/L. Most of these specimens were Tg-negative. HAB interference thus can lead to artifactually high serum Tg levels that are well within the range being empirically treated with [131]I. It is likely that other commercial Tg IMA tests have a similar problem. Unless a Tg assay is confirmed to be free of HAB interference, this problem should be suspected if the Tg results do not fit the clinical picture or fail to rise with TSH stimulation or to fall with THST.

Even without assay artifacts, a high Tg may not necessarily reflect the presence of tumor. It occurs, for example, with a large thyroid remnant [16]. Tg levels are also high for 4–6 weeks immediately after thyroidectomy [16], and may rise again after diagnostic ^{131}I scanning, falling spontaneously after about 2 weeks [26], and may remain high for months after ^{131}I remnant ablation or tumor treatment [11].

Measuring Serum Tg Levels over Time

Persistently high post-^{131}I ablation serum Tg levels sometimes decline spontaneously over several years to undetectable levels without further treatment [11,27]. The pattern of serial serum Tg measurements, made while the patient has a stable TSH, is thus more useful than an isolated Tg value[11], providing the Tg measurements are made in the same laboratory using the same assay method [16].

Serum Tg Concentrations During TSH Suppression and after TSH Stimulation

TSH-stimulated serum Tg concentrations, which typically rise >10-fold above basal (THST) levels [16], increase about twofold higher in response to THW than they do with rhTSH [16]. Although the exact Tg cutoff level varies with the assay being used, a TSH-stimulated serum Tg level >2 μg/L [1,28] after rhTSH administration or during endogenous TSH elevation (THW) is suspicious of tumor in a patient who has undergone total thyroidectomy and thyroid remnant ablation [1,5,11]. This is a much more sensitive test than measuring Tg levels during THST. Without TSH stimulation, ~20% of patients with lymph node metastases and 5% of those with distant metastases are missed by a Tg <1 μg/L during THST [2]. Examined from another perspective, 20% of 784 patients who had no clinical evidence of tumor, and baseline serum Tg levels <1 μg/L during THST, developed a serum Tg >2 μg/L 72 hours after rhTSH administration [1]. Of the group with an rhTSH-stimulated Tg >2 μg/L, 36% had metastases, over one third of which were in distant sites [1]. An rhTSH-stimulated Tg >2 mg/mL identified 91% of those with metastases, whereas DxWBS after either rhTSH or THW identified only 19% [1]. It is important to note that these studies employed a variety of commercial Tg assays. Using a TSH-stimulated

Tg cutoff of 2 μg/L, either after THW or 72 hours after rhTSH, along with neck ultrasonography, is sufficiently sensitive to be used alone in the follow-up of patients with DTC, providing there is no uptake outside the thyroid bed on the post ^{131}I-remnant ablation RxWBS [1,2,5,11]. A serum Tg above a cutoff of 2 μg/L should be considered high enough to warrant further study or more frequent surveillance, but the exact Tg cutoff should be determined for each institution and can be related to the above data by considering the normal reference range of the Tg assay being used. Chapter 18 provides information about new sensitive Tg assays, which may replace TSH-Tg stimulation. However, before this becomes widely used, careful studies will be necessary to identify the optimal Tg cutoffs using these new sensitive Tg assays, which must be gauged against the gold standard, which currently is Tg-stimulated serum Tg measurement.

Imaging Studies

Diagnostic Whole-Body [131]I Scans

This is generally performed 48 to 72 hours after 185 MBq (5 mCi) of [131]I. The technique used for performing the DxWBS may be the cause of a negative imaging study. Smaller amounts of ^{131}I for DxWBS often fail to show thyroid bed or tumor uptake, while larger amounts may have a sufficiently harmful effect to interfere with subsequent uptake of therapeutic doses of ^{131}I on RxWBS [29]. Referred to as "thyroid stunning," this effect is not always seen [29] but occurs with as little as 111 MBq (3 mCi) of ^{131}I and becomes increasingly greater with larger amounts of ^{131}I, but it is not produced by [123]I [30]. Perhaps of most importance, the DxWBS is usually unnecessary, even before the first postoperative ^{131}I treatment in low risk patients who are clinically free of tumor after surgery [1,2].

Posttreatment Whole-Body [131]I Scans

An RxWBS should always be done to document the site and extent of ^{131}I uptake. Up to 25% of RxWBS studies show tumor not detected by the DxWBS, regardless of the amount of ^{131}I used for

the latter [14,15]. The RxWBS is most likely to yield important new information in young patients with high serum Tg concentrations and negative DxWBS, especially if they have been previously treated with [131]I [31]. Older patients with bulky disease visualized on X-rays or CT, and those without ^{131}I uptake on previous RxWBS, rarely show uptake on subsequent RxWBS [31]. A recent study of 106 patients with DTC found that the RxWBS after the first ^{131}I ablation changed the disease stage in 8.3% of the patients and the therapeutic approach in another 15%, and provided clinically relevant information for 26% of the patients who had undergone a previous ablation [32].

Neck Ultrasonography (US)

Study of the central and lateral cervical compartments by neck US often detects small malignant lymph nodes and other neck tumors in patients with an elevated serum Tg level. Size alone is not a good criterion for malignancy. A 1 cm cutoff for differentiating benign from malignant lymph nodes fails to identify the majority of malignant lymph nodes, which are more reliably recognized by their shape and other characteristics [33]. Benign lymph nodes tend to be elongated (oval to fusiform) with a Solbiati index (SI = ratio of largest to smallest diameter) >2 [34] and often show a string-like hyperechoic central structure (hilar sign) with a central hilar pattern of blood flow on power Doppler [33]. Malignant lymph nodes have a rounded or oval appearance with an SI ≤2 in over 80% of cases and do not have a hilar sign [33]. Perhaps the best indicators of malignancy in a lymph node are its heterogeneous echo pattern or irregular hyperechoic small intranodal structures and the presence of irregular diffuse intranodal blood flow on power Doppler study [33].

Neck US combined with TSH-stimulated serum Tg levels has the highest diagnostic accuracy for detecting persistent neck tumors. A study of 294 patients [35] comparing rhTSH-stimulated serum Tg levels, DxWBS, and US found that US and rhTSH-stimulated serum Tg used together had the highest sensitivity (96%) and negative predictive values (99.5%). Others report similarly good results with US, even in children [22,36]. In one study [5], neck US identified lymph node metastases in 67% of the patients with rhTSH-Tg levels >5 μg/L, in 13% with a Tg from 1 to <5 μg/L, and in only 3% with a Tg <1 μg/L.

[18]Fluorodeoxyglucose Positron Emission Tomography (FDG-PET)

An elevated serum Tg level with a negative RxWBS is a major indication for FDG-PET scanning [37–40]. It usually performs better than ^{99m}Tc sestamibi scintigraphy and DxWBS and often identifies tumor that is amenable to surgery [41,42]. Depending upon the serum Tg level, its sensitivity for detecting metastases in one study was 11%, 50%, and 93% of patients with Tg levels, respectively, of <10, 10–20, and >100 μg/L. Sensitivity is enhanced by raising serum TSH levels either by THW [38] or by rhTSH administration [43]. Unlike tumors that concentrate ^{131}I, RxWBS-negative metastases that demonstrate FDG uptake tend to be poorly differentiated and to display rapid growth, making FDG-PET scanning of value in providing prognostic information. In one study [44], for example, the 3-year survival probability was 96% and 18% for patients with FDG-PET volumes, respectively, of ≤125 mL and >125 mL. No cancer deaths occurred in 66 FDG-negative

patients, including 10 with distant metastases who were alive and well at the end of the follow-up period, whereas almost 70% of 59 FDG-PET-positive patients died during the same period. This test often changes the clinical management of patients with elevated serum Tg levels and negative RxWBS. In one study [40], FDG-PET was positive in 70% of 27 patients, 14 of whom had tumor in cervical lymph nodes, 2 in mediastinal lymph nodes, 3 in lung, and 2 in bone, which resulted in surgical intervention in 17 of the patients, 82% of whom achieved a disease-free status.

Testing Sequence

The testing sequence varies among clinicians (see Chapter 19), but the one we use is shown in Figure 20.3. In a patient with no uptake outside the thyroid bed on the RxWBS after ^{131}I remnant ablation who is clinically free of disease, the first step is to perform a serum Tg measurement during TSHT. If the serum Tg is undetectable, neck ultrasonography is done and 0.9 mg of rhTSH is administered intramuscularly for 2 consecutive days; 72 hours after the last rhTSH injection a serum Tg is measured. This can be done with THW, but the TSH levels are less con-

Testing Sequence after Negative [131]I DxWBS and High Tg

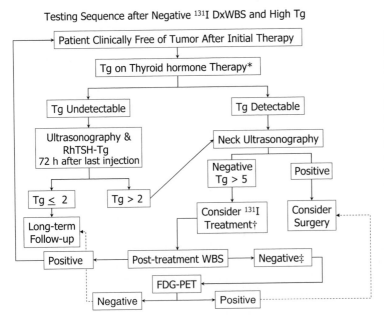

Figure 20.3 Sequence of tests during follow-up after total thyroidectomy and thyroid ^{131}I remnant ablation when Tg is elevated and RxWBS is negative. Tg is thyroglobulin, rhTSH is recombinant human TSH-α administered at a dosage of 0.9 mg on 2 consecutive days with serum Tg measurement 72 hours after the last injection. * This may occur at any time during follow-up, but is more likely to be encountered immediately after initial therapy. † Urine iodine should be <100 μg/g creatinine, TSH should be >30 mIU/L following thyroid hormone withdrawal, lithium pretreatment should be considered. If the patient cannot become hypothyroid or the TSH will not rise in response to THW, rhTSH can be used to stimulate ^{131}I uptake. ‡ The differential diagnosis of this condition is detailed in the text.

sistent during withdrawal [45], making the Tg cutoff levels used for making therapeutic decisions more variable unless the TSH is >30 mIU/L [28]. If the serum Tg is less than 2 µg/L, the patient simply is followed at 6- to 12-month intervals with serum Tg measurements during THST. If on the other hand, the serum Tg rises above 2 µg/L after rhTSH stimulation and the neck ultrasonography is negative, ^{131}I therapy should be considered, particularly if the Tg rises above 5 µg/L after rhTSH. The exact Tg level to consider ^{131}I treatment is a matter of debate, but in general the higher the Tg level is at the time of treatment, the more likely ^{131}I uptake will be seen on the RxWBS [14]. The levels we use to consider further study is a serum Tg level >2 µg/L after rhTSH and a level >5 µg/L after THW. If there is no uptake on the RxWBS, then an [18]FDG-PET scan should be done.

Treatment

We consider empiric ^{131}I treatment of some patients with negative whole-body ^{131}I scans if the serum Tg rises >5 µg/L after rhTSH administration or >10 µg/L after THW. Yet before empiric ^{131}I therapy is administered, the causes of a high serum Tg level and a negative whole-body ^{131}I scan must be considered, to avoid unnecessary treatment in some patients and missing an important therapeutic opportunity in others.

The Differential Diagnosis of High Tg and Negative Whole-Body Scans

High Tg and Negative DxWBS

When the serum THST-Tg is detectable (>1 µg/L) or Tg rises above a cutoff of 2 µg/L during rhTSH stimulation and the DxWBS is negative, there are at least six situations that must be differentiated [46]:

- TSH is too low to maximally stimulate ^{131}I uptake (usually a problem only with THW).
- Iodine contamination, usually from radiographic contrast material or drugs.
- Metastases too small to see on the DxWBS.

- Heterophile antibody interference with Tg assays [25].
- Insufficient ^{131}I activity administered for DxWBS.
- Tumor dedifferentiation with reduced/absent sodium-iodine symporter function.

High Tg and Negative RxWBS

This is a more serious situation than a negative DxWBS. When the serum Tg is elevated and the RxWBS fails to show ^{131}I uptake after 3700 MBq (100 mCi) has been administered, the usual presumption is that the tumor does not concentrate [131]I. Yet before this hypothesis can be accepted, one must be absolutely certain that there were no technical problems in the preparation of the patient and administration of the isotope and that "stunning" did not occur during a recent preceding DxWBS [29]. Indeed, the differential diagnosis for a negative RxWBS is the same as summarized above for a negative DxWBS. In our experience these technical problems are common, particularly when physicians are unfamiliar with the usual routines in preparing patients for ^{131}I treatment.

Insufficient TSH Stimulation of [131]I Uptake

After thyroidectomy, ^{131}I uptake by thyroid remnants and metastases is increased by high serum TSH levels. To maximize the therapeutic effect of ^{131}I, one must closely adhere to a protocol that ensures serum TSH reaches levels of at least 30 mIU/L. This may be done by administering oral T_3 (liothyronine, Cytomel) alone for 4 weeks then withdrawing it for 2 weeks, after which the patient is hypothyroid and the serum TSH usually is about 70 mIU/L, but it ranges from just over 30 to nearly 300 mIU/L, depending upon the size of the thyroid remnant [47]. T_3 may be withdrawn for 4 weeks, which raises the TSH even further, but careful studies [47] show that this does not improve ^{131}I uptake by remnants or tumors more than that achieved with 2 weeks' withdrawal of T_3. Another way to do this is to simply withdraw thyroid hormone therapy and to measure serum TSH levels several times a week. One recent study [45] found that serum TSH concentrations reached more than 30 mU/L 8 to 26 days (14.2 ± 4.8 days) after thyroidectomy and 9 to 29 (18.1 ± 4.1) days after THW. This level was achieved in 95% of patients, and only minimal symptoms of hypothyroidism were noted.

High serum TSH levels can also be achieved by administering 0.9 mg of rhTSH on 2 successive days, after which serum rhTSH levels peak to ~180 mIU/L and rapidly return to baseline concentrations within about 5 days (Figure 20.1). This has been used both for diagnostic [28] and for therapeutic [48–50] purposes. The latter is an off-label use of the drug, but rhTSH is associated with greater compliance [51] and with improved patient comfort as compared with THW [52]. The half-life of ^{131}I in thyroid remnants and metastases, however, may be substantially shorter after rhTSH stimulation than it is after THW [53]. Then again some [54] find prolongation of ^{131}I in the thyroid remnant and decreased radiation to the blood when patients are given rhTSH for preparation compared with being hypothyroid. All the patients in the latter study received diagnostic ^{131}I in the same order: first while euthyroid, followed by hypothyroidism, and it is possible that thyroid remnant "stunning" seen on RxWBS accounted for these observations [54]. Lithium pretreatment, however, improves ^{131}I retention both in thyroid remnants and in metastases [55] (see Chapter 1).

Lithium Augmentation of [131]I Therapy

Studies [55] from the US National Institutes of Health show that lithium is a useful adjuvant for ^{131}I therapy of thyroid cancer, augmenting both accumulation and retention of ^{131}I in tumor and thyroid remnants (see Chapter 1). A comparison of ^{131}I retention during lithium treatment with that during a control period showed a mean increase in the biological half-life (cell retention) of 50% in tumors and 90% in remnants. This increase was proportionally greater in lesions with poor ^{131}I retention. When the control biological half-life was less than 3 days, lithium therapy prolonged the effective half-life (a combination of biological turnover and isotope decay; see Figure 1.9 in Chapter 1) in metastases by more than 50%. More ^{131}I accumulated within metastases or the thyroid remnant during lithium therapy, probably as a consequence of its dampening effect on iodine release. The increase in accumulated ^{131}I and the lengthening of the effective half-life combined to increase the estimated ^{131}I radiation dose in

metastases nearly threefold. As a result of these studies, we regularly use lithium (10 mg/kg) for one week prior to ^{131}I therapy in patients with a negative RxWBS if there is any question about the quality of the original study. Doing this requires measuring blood lithium levels on a daily basis, which should be maintained within the usual therapeutic limits. The drug is excreted by the kidney and should be used with caution in patients with renal impairment, heart failure or those taking a number of drugs that interfere with lithium excretion. The physician should be familiar with the pharmacology and contraindications to the drug.

Iodine Contamination

Before ^{131}I treatment is administered, the total body iodine pool should be low and urine iodine levels should be less than 100 μg/g of creatinine. This requires at least 2 full weeks of a low iodine diet [56] and absolute avoidance of iodine-containing medicines or iodinated radiographic contrast materials that may expand the iodine pool for 3 months or longer, depending upon the contrast material and the patient's age and renal function. The time to excrete the iodine load increases with the number of studies with radiographic contrast material that the patient has undergone. We always obtain urine iodine levels before treating patients who have received radiographic contrast agents in the past 6 months because even small amounts of iodine can interfere with ^{131}I uptake by thyroid remnants or metastases. A recent study [57] found that 1110 MBq (30 mCi) of ^{131}I failed to ablate the thyroid remnant in almost half the euthyroid patients prepared with rhTSH, whereas a similar study [49] using the same preparation and ^{131}I activity achieved about an 80% rate of total ablation by simply by withholding thyroxine (50 μg of iodine/tablet) for 3 days before and 1 day after ^{131}I administration, which lowered urine iodine levels to ~38 μg/L.

Low Diagnostic [131]I Activity as a Cause of a Negative DxWBS

The amount of ^{131}I administered to perform a DxWBS may be too small to visualize a thyroid remnant or metastases. This is especially true when small amounts of [131]I (<111 MBq (3 mCi)) are administered. This can be improved by using larger ^{131}I activities, but doing this increases the risk of thyroid stunning proportionally [58].

Metastases Too Small to See on RxWBS

If the patient's iodine pool has not been expanded with iodine, a high serum Tg concentration and negative RxWBS is commonly due to small lymph node metastases that can be seen only on ultrasonography. However, lung metastases are usually marked by higher baseline and TSH-stimulated Tg levels than those occurring with lymph node metastases, and usually can be visualized on the DxWBS early in their course. Tg levels due to tumor, regardless of its location, continue to rise over time. If the RxWBS is negative, an [18]FDG-PET should be performed, and if it is negative, watchful waiting with the serum Tg levels generally clarifies the patient's tumor status.

Heterophile Antibody Interference

This should be suspected when the elevated serum Tg levels do not change with THST or THW. The Tg should be remeasured in another laboratory, preferably one that runs specific tests to eliminate HAB interference [25].

Tumor Dedifferentiation with Impaired Sodium-Iodine Symporter Function

This is characterized by failure of tumor to concentrate ^{131}I after the patient has been carefully prepared for treatment, including high TSH levels, lithium pretreatment, and low urine iodine excretion. If the RxWBS is negative, no further ^{131}I is administered, especially when the [18]FDG-PET scan reveals tumor (Figure 20.4) [59]. A few patients with tumor that does not concentrate ^{131}I may benefit from 13-*cis*-retinoic acid therapy, which has the potential to redifferentiate thyroid cancer cells in vitro. Given orally for at least 2 months to 12 patients with DTC that could not be otherwise treated, retinoic acid induced ^{131}I uptake in two and a faint response in three patients [60]. Subsequent studies, however, have shown less of an effect [61].

Choice of Therapy

Surgery Versus [131]I Versus External Beam Radiotherapy (EBRT) Therapy Versus No Therapy

Patients with high serum Tg levels should be treated with surgery, whenever possible (Figure 20.3). Patients should not be treated with ^{131}I if they have any of the following five conditions: (1) HAB Tg interference; (2) after adequate preparation, there is no ^{131}I uptake on RxWBS; (3) there is no fall in Tg within a year after ^{131}I therapy; (4) there is intense uptake of [18]FDG-PET by metastases; or (5) anatomical imaging such as ultrasonography reveals tumor deposits amenable to surgery. EBRT should be considered in patients over 45 years who have locally invasive (pT4 tumors), unresectable regional

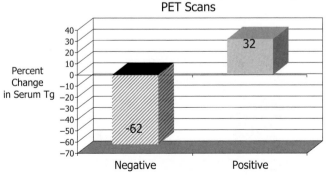

PET Results and Therapeutic Response to [131]I Among Patients with Distant metastases and positive or negative FDG-PET Scans

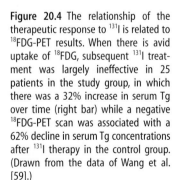

Figure 20.4 The relationship of the therapeutic response to ^{131}I is related to [18]FDG-PET results. When there is avid uptake of [18]FDG, subsequent ^{131}I treatment was largely ineffective in 25 patients in the study group, in which there was a 32% increase in serum Tg over time (right bar) while a negative [18]FDG-PET scan was associated with a 62% decline in serum Tg concentrations after ^{131}I therapy in the control group. (Drawn from the data of Wang et al. [59].)

tumor that does not concentrate [131]I (Figure 20.3).

Efficacy of [131]I Therapy

When the DxWBS and neck ultrasonography are both negative, patients are often empirically treated with ^{131}I, both to locate and to treat persistent tumor [4]. Whether this benefits patients has sparked much controversy [12–15], mainly because there are few studies with long-term follow-up of such treatment, there are no randomized prospective trials of this treatment, and there are considerable differences in patient cohorts and endpoints among studies of empiric ^{131}I treatment. Still, there is one consistent observation: serum Tg levels decline when ^{131}I uptake is seen on the RxWBS after 3700 to 5550 MBq (100 to 150 mCi) of ^{131}I, particularly in patients with lung metastases (Figures 20.5 and 20.6) [27,62]. Empiric ^{131}I treatment must be considered with caution, however, in the light of studies that show a slow fall in high serum Tg levels months to years after ^{131}I ablation without further treatment [11,27]. Long-term follow-up of our cohort of patients [6] undergoing follow-up studies showed that about half the patients whose rhTSH-stimulated Tg increased above the detectable range but remained ≤2 μg/L had a spontaneous fall in serum Tg to undetectable levels over 3 to 5 years, whereas this occurred in only 5% of patients with an rhTSH-stimulated serum Tg >2 μg/L.

Follow-up is too short in most studies to know if empirically treating high serum Tg levels when the DxWBS is negative enhances

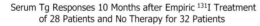

Serum Tg Responses in 17 Patients with DTC Empirically Treated with [131]I

Figure 20.5 Serum Tg levels after ^{131}I treatment of thyroid cancer in 17 patients with elevated serum Tg levels and negative DxWBS scans. Evaluations were performed within 1 year of a positive RxWBS and/or Tg measurement greater than 5 μg/L, and 1 to 2 years after a negative RxWBS or Tg measurement of 5 μg/L or less. The amount of ^{131}I administered at each evaluation ranged from none in some patients to 3700 to 11 100 MBq (100 to 300 mCi) in others. (Drawn from the data of Pineda et al. [62].)

survival, but several studies suggest that this occurs. The survival benefit from ^{131}I therapy appears to be inversely related to tumor mass. Schlumberger [63], for example, reported complete remission and 10-year survival rates, respectively, of 96% and 100% in 19 patients with tumor found only on a positive RxWBS,

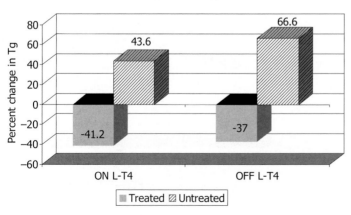

Figure 20.6 Mean change in serum Tg levels 10 months after empiric ^{131}I therapy of 28 patients with high serum Tg concentrations and negative DxWBS studies compared with 32 control patients who did not undergo ^{131}I therapy for elevated serum Tg concentrations and negative DxWBS. The differences between the two groups are statistically significant ($P < 0.001$). (Drawn from the data of Koh et al. [68].)

compared with 83% and 91% among 55 patients with metastases seen on both the DxWBS and RxWBS, and 53% and 63% among 64 patients with micronodules seen on chest X-ray, and with 14% and 11% among 77 patients with macronodules seen on chest X-ray.

In another study [64], 56 patients with DTC were treated with 5550 MBq (150 mCi) of ^{131}I because of an elevated serum Tg level after THW and a negative 370 MBq [131]I (10 mCi) DxWBS. After empiric ^{131}I therapy, half had ^{131}I uptake on the RxWBS and half did not. After a median of 4.2 years (0.5 to 13.5 years) and treatment with a median cumulative ^{131}I activity of 150 mCi (range 50–650), 64% of the 28 patients with positive RxWBS achieved complete remission defined as a negative RxWBS and a serum Tg <1.5 µg/L on THST, compared with only 36% of the 28 patients with a negative RxWBS. None of those with a positive RxWBS died of thyroid cancer, whereas 9 without ^{131}I uptake died of cancer, producing a 5-year survival rate of 100% in the former and 76% in the latter (P < 0.001). However, it may be that patients who had no uptake of ^{131}I on the RxWBS had less well-differentiated tumor, which in itself might explain the differences in survival benefit from empiric ^{131}I therapy.

In another study of 23 patients treated with ^{131}I for diffuse pulmonary metastases detected only by ^{131}I imaging, 87% had no lung uptake on subsequent scans [65]. After ^{131}I therapy, serum Tg became undetectable and lung CT scans showed disappearance of the micronodules in almost half the patients, while lung biopsy showed no evidence of disease in two.

Others also report a substantial fall in serum Tg levels after ^{131}I treatment with little or no progression of disease compared with a rise in serum Tg over time and progression of disease in patients who have been treated [62]. Others report a reduction of metastatic disease in most patients whose lung metastases concentrate ^{131}I, but find that a complete remission is uncommon [66,67]. Still, a partial response with reduction of metastatic disease is usually possible and patients generally have a good quality of life with no further disease progression.

In another study [68], in which 28 patients with high serum Tg levels and negative DxWBS studies were treated with ^{131}I and 32 were not treated, the decreases in serum Tg during THST and THW in the treated group were 41.2% and 37.0%, respectively, levels that were significantly higher (P < 0.001) than those in the untreated group, which were 43.6% and 66.6%, respectively (Figure 20.6). The serum Tg levels were undetectable (<1 µg/L) in four cases, both on and off thyroid hormone 15 to 22 months after the administration of ^{131}I, and these negative serum Tg levels persisted for 24 to 70 months; however, this was not observed in any of the untreated group. The RxWBS studies revealed pathologic uptake in 12 of 28 cases (43%). Most of the patients in the treated group (89%) had stable disease or experienced a partial remission, while only 11% had progression of their disease, whereas the comparable figures in the untreated group were, respectively, 53% and 47% (Figure 20.7).

Eleven studies of empiric ^{131}I therapy are summarized in Table 20.1 [13,14,27,62,64,68–73]. In

Location of Uptake

▨ No Pathologic Uptake

▨ Multiple Lung Uptake

▨ Loco-regional recurrence

Effects of Therapy

▨ Progressive Disease

▨ Stable Disease

▨ Partial Remission

Figure 20.7 Location of tumor and disease progression in the same group of patients whose data are shown in Figure 20.6. The panel on the left shows the location of ^{131}I uptake in the treated group and the panel on the right shows the effect of therapy in the two groups. (Drawn from the data of Koh et al. [68].)

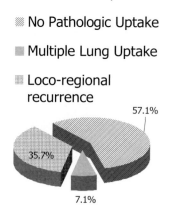

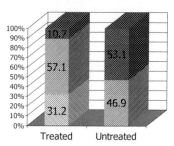

Table 20.1 Studies of empiric ^{131}I therapy

Authors	Total in study	Number of patients		Follow-Up duration	Results
		Negative DxWBS and empirically treated	Positive RxWBS after empiric treatment		
Pachucki and Burmeister [69]	21	7 (33%)	4 (57%)	1.5–34 months	No data
Mazzaferri and Kloos [14]	10	10 (100%)	8 (80%)	2–4 years	3 no uptake on RxWBS and Tg-off <5 µg/L
Ronga et al. [70]	61	11 (18%)	8 (73%)	Not given	No follow-up data in pos. RxWBS group. One of 3 patients with neg. RxWBS had progressive disease within 5 months
De Keizer et al. [71]	22	16 (73%)	11 (69%)	1 year	Decrease in Tg-off in 9 patients with RxWBS pos. and in 3 with RxWBS neg. Tg-off 8–608 µg/L
Pacini et al. [72]	17	17 (100%)	16 (94%)	12 patients; 30 months to 5 years	At last follow-up decrease in serum Tg (-off) in 7 and an increase in 1 patient
Pineda et al. [62]	17	17 (100%)	16 (94%)	6 months to 5 years	Decrease in Tg-off in 81% after 1st empiric treatment and in 5 patients after 3rd empiric ^{131}I treatment. 50% of patients had Tg-on <5 µg/L. RxWBS neg. in 50%; Tg-off never <5 µg/L
Fatourechi et al. [13]	24	24 (100%)	6 (25%)	6–33 months	Tg-on increased after ^{131}I in 75% of patients; 5 died, 4 with negative RxWBS, 1 with partial neg. RxWBS (no uptake in bone metastases)
Schaap et al. [73]	39	39 (100%)	22 (60%)	Up to 15 months	Tg-on after RxWBS pos. decreased and increased in RxWBS-neg. group ($P = 0.006$.)
Pacini et al. [27]	70	42 (60%)	30 (71%)	Mean 6.7 years ± 3.8 years	Decrease in Tg-off in 19 patients with RxWBS pos. Complete remission in 33% of patients with RxWBS pos., in 17% with RxWBS neg., and in 68% of untreated group
Van Tol et al. [64]	56	56 (100%)	28 (50%)	Mean 4.5 ± 2.9 years	No change in Tg-off before and after empiric ^{131}I therapy in both groups. Complete remission in 64% of patients with RxWBS pos., and in 36% with RxWBS neg. 5-year cancer survival 100% in RxWBS-pos. and 76% in RxWBS-neg. group
Koh et al. [68]	60	28 (47%)	12 (43%)	23.8 ± 19.6 months	Tg-on and Tg-off decreased, respectively 41% and 37% in treated group versus a Tg rise of 44% and 67%, respectively in untreated group
Total	397	267 (67%)	161 (60%)	23.8 ± 19.6 months	Tg-on and Tg-off decreased, respectively 41% and 37% in treated group versus a Tg rise of 44% and 67%, respectively in untreated group

Updated and modified from van Tol et al. [64]. DxWBS, diagnostic ^{131}I whole-body scan; RxWBS, posttreatment whole-body scan; Tg-on, serum Tg measured during thyroid hormone therapy; Tg-off, Tg measured off thyroid hormone or under rhTSH stimulation; pos., positive; neg., negative.

these studies, 60% of 161 patients had ^{131}I uptake on the RxWBS. The best responses occur in children and young adults with diffuse pulmonary metastases not seen on any imaging studies except on the RxWBS [15,74]. This is not uncommon. We found uptake in the lung only on the RxWBS study in 13% of 89 consecutive paired DxWBS and RxWBS studies performed in 79 patients (15% of the patients) with serum THW-Tg levels that were almost always above 15 μg/L [14]. Two to 4 years later, three of them (25%), all under 45 years, had no uptake on RxWBS and serum Tg levels <5 μg/L during THW.

Summary

The situation of a high serum Tg concentration and a negative DxWBS is common in patients with DTC and requires a careful search for tumor while excluding factitial causes for an elevated serum Tg or a negative RxWBS. Empiric ^{131}I therapy should be considered only after certain criteria are fulfilled, such as negative neck ultrasonography, and should be done only after impeccable patient preparation. There are certain situations in which empiric therapy usually should not be given. This includes tumors that previously have failed to concentrate ^{131}I even after the patient has been carefully prepared for the treatment. No prospective randomized studies have been done to substantiate the long-term effect of treatment of these patients, but studies now show that serum Tg levels consistently decline after uptake is seen on the RxWBS after empiric ^{131}I therapy, and that tumor may regress to the point that mortality rates are improved in some patients.

References

1. Mazzaferri EL, Robbins RJ, Spencer CA, et al. A consensus report of the role of serum thyroglobulin as a monitoring method for low-risk patients with papillary thyroid carcinoma. J Clin Endocrinol Metab 2003; 88(4): 1433–1441.
2. Schlumberger M, Berg G, Cohen O, et al. Follow-up of low-risk patients with differentiated thyroid carcinoma: a European perspective. Eur J Endocrinol 2004; 150(2): 105–112.
3. Pacini F, Capezzone M, Elisei R, Ceccarelli C, Taddei D, Pinchera A. Diagnostic 131-iodine whole-body scan

4. Cailleux AF, Baudin E, Travagli JP, Ricard M, Schlumberger M. Is diagnostic iodine-131 scanning useful after total thyroid ablation for differentiated thyroid cancer? J Clin Endocrinol Metab 2000; 85(1):175–178.
5. Torlontano M, Crocetti U, D'Aloiso L, Bonfitto N, Di Giorgio A, Modoni S et al. Serum thyroglobulin and ^{131}I whole body scan after recombinant human TSH stimulation in the follow-up of low-risk patients with differentiated thyroid cancer. Eur J Endocrinol 2003; 148(1): 19–24.
6. Mazzaferri EL, Kloos RT. Is Diagnostic iodine-131 scanning with recombinant human TSH (rhTSH) useful in the follow-up of differentiated thyroid cancer after thyroid ablation? J Clin Endocrinol Metab 2002; 87: 1490–1498.
7. Mazzaferri EL, Kloos RT. Using recombinant human TSH in the management of well-differentiated thyroid cancer: current strategies and future directions. Thyroid 2000; 10(9):767–778.
8. Yeh MW, Demircan O, Ituarte P, Clark OH. False-negative fine-needle aspiration cytology results delay treatment and adversely affect outcome in patients with thyroid carcinoma. Thyroid 2004; 14(3):207–215.
9. Scheumann GFW, Seeliger H, Musholt TJ, et al. Completion thyroidectomy in 131 patients with differentiated thyroid carcinoma. Eur J Surg 1996; 162:677–684.
10. Mazzaferri EL. Thyroid cancer. In: Bar RS (ed.) Early Diagnosis and treatment of endocrine disorders. Totowa, NJ: Humana Press, 2003: 1–36.
11. Baudin E, Cao CD, Cailleux AF, Leboulleux S, Travagli JP, Schlumberger M. Positive predictive value of serum thyroglobulin levels, measured during the first year of follow-up after thyroid hormone withdrawal, in thyroid cancer patients. J Clin Endocrinol Metab 2003; 88(3): 1107–1111.
12. McDougall IR. [131]I treatment of ^{131}I negative whole body scan, and positive thyroglobulin in differentiated thyroid carcinoma: what is being treated? Thyroid 1997; 7(4):669–672.
13. Fatourechi V, Hay ID, Javedan H, Wiseman GA, Mullan BP, Gorman CA. Lack of impact of radioiodine therapy in Tg-positive, diagnostic whole-body scan-negative patients with follicular cell-derived thyroid cancer. J Clin Endocrinol Metab 2002; 87(4):1521–1526.
14. Mazzaferri EL, Kloos RT. Current approaches to primary therapy for papillary and follicular thyroid cancer. J Clin Endocrinol Metab 2001; 86(4):1447–1463.
15. Schlumberger M, Mancusi F, Baudin E, Pacini F. 131-I Therapy for elevated thyroglobulin levels. Thyroid 1997; 7:273–276.
16. Baloch Z, Carayon P, Conte-Devolx B, et al. Laboratory medicine practice guidelines. Laboratory support for the diagnosis and monitoring of thyroid disease. Thyroid 2003; 13(1):3–126.
17. Bachelot A, Cailleux AF, Klain M, et al. Relationship between tumor burden and serum thyroglobulin level in patients with papillary and follicular thyroid carcinoma. Thyroid 2002; 12(8):707–711.
18. Robbins RJ, Srivastava S, Shaha A, et al. Factors influencing the basal and recombinant human thy-

The situation of a high serum Tg concentration and a negative DxWBS is common in patients with DTC and requires a careful search for tumor while excluding factitial causes for an elevated serum Tg or a negative RxWBS. Empiric ^{131}I therapy may be avoided in thyroid cancer patients who have undetectable stimulated serum Tg levels after initial treatment. J Clin Endocrinol Metab 2002; 87(4):1499–1501.

rotropin-stimulated serum thyroglobulin in patients with metastatic thyroid carcinoma. J Clin Endocrinol Metab 2004; 89(12):6010–6016.

19. Spencer CA, Wang CC. Thyroglobulin measurement – techniques, clinical benefits, and pitfalls. Endocrinol Metab Clin North Am 1995; 24:841–863.

20. Chiovato L, Latrofa F, Braverman LE, et al. Disappearance of humoral thyroid autoimmunity after complete removal of thyroid antigens. Ann Intern Med 2003; 139(5 Pt 1):346–351.

21. Robbins RJ, Chon JT, Fleisher M, Larson S, Tuttle RM. Is the serum thyroglobulin response to recombinant human TSH sufficient, by itself, to monitor for residual thyroid carcinoma? J Clin Endocrinol Metab 2002; 87:3242–3247.

22. Frasoldati A, Pesenti M, Gallo M, Caroggio A, Salvo D, Valcavi R. Diagnosis of neck recurrences in patients with differentiated thyroid carcinoma. Cancer 2003; 97(1):90–96.

23. Ringel MD. Molecular detection of thyroid cancer: differentiating "signal" and "noise" in clinical assays. J Clin Endocrinol Metab 2004; 89(1):29–32.

24. Elisei R, Vivaldi A, Agate L, et al. Low specificity of blood thyroglobulin messenger ribonucleic acid assay prevents its use in the follow-up of differentiated thyroid cancer patients. J Clin Endocrinol Metab 2004; 89(1):33–39.

25. Preissner CM, O'Kane DJ, Singh RJ, Morris JC, Grebe SK. Phantoms in the assay tube: heterophile antibody interferences in serum thyroglobulin assays. J Clin Endocrinol Metab 2003; 88(7):3069–3074.

26. Muratet JP, Giraud P, Daver A, Minier JF, Gamelin E, Larra F. Predicting the efficacy of first iodine-131 treatment in differentiated thyroid carcinoma. J Nucl Med 1997; 38:1362–1368.

27. Pacini F, Agate L, Elisei R, et al. Outcome of differentiated thyroid cancer with detectable serum Tg and negative diagnostic 131-I whole body scan: comparison of patients treated with high 131-I activities versus untreated patients. J Clin Endocrinol Metab 2001; 86(9): 4092–4097.

28. Haugen BR, Pacini F, Reiners C, et al. A comparison of recombinant human thyrotropin and thyroid hormone withdrawal for the detection of thyroid remnant or cancer. J Clin Endocrinol Metab 1999; 84:3877–3885.

29. Morris LF, Waxman AD, Braunstein GD. Thyroid stunning. Thyroid 2003; 13(4):333–340.

30. Anderson GS, Fish S, Nakhoda K, Zhuang H, Alavi A, Mandel SJ. Comparison of I-123 and I-131 for whole-body imaging after stimulation by recombinant human thyrotropin: a preliminary report. Clin Nucl Med 2003; 28(2):93–96.

31. Sherman SI, Tielens ET, Sostre S, Wharam MD, Jr, Ladenson PW. Clinical utility of posttreatment radioiodine scans in the management of patients with thyroid carcinoma. J Clin Endocrinol Metab 1994; 78:629–634.

32. Souza Rosario PW, Barroso AL, Rezende LL, et al. Post I-131 therapy scanning in patients with thyroid carcinoma metastases: an unnecessary cost or a relevant contribution? Clin Nucl Med 2004; 29(12):795–798.

33. Gorges R, Eising EG, Fotescu D, et al. Diagnostic value of high-resolution B-mode and power-mode sonography in the follow-up of thyroid cancer. Eur J Ultrasound 2003; 16(3):191–206.

34. Solbiati L, Osti V, Cova L, Tonolini M. Ultrasound of thyroid, parathyroid glands and neck lymph nodes. Eur Radiol 2001; 11(12):2411–2424.

35. Pacini F, Molinaro E, Castagna MG, et al. Recombinant human thyrotropin-stimulated serum thyroglobulin combined with neck ultrasonography has the highest sensitivity in monitoring differentiated thyroid carcinoma. J Clin Endocrinol Metab 2003; 88(8):3668–3673.

36. Antonelli A, Miccoli P, Fallahi P, et al. Role of neck ultrasonography in the follow-up of children operated on for thyroid papillary cancer. Thyroid 2003; 13(5):479–484.

37. Wang W, Macapinlac H, Larson SM, et al. [18F]-2-fluoro-2-deoxy-D-glucose positron emission tomography localizes residual thyroid cancer in patients with negative diagnostic (131)I whole body scans and elevated serum thyroglobulin levels. J Clin Endocrinol Metab 1999; 84(7):2291–2302.

38. Lind P, Kresnik E, Kumnig G, et al. 18F-FDG-PET in the follow-up of thyroid cancer. Acta Med Austriaca 2003; 30(1):17–21.

39. Lowe VJ, Mullan BP, Hay ID, McIver B, Kasperbauer JL. 18F-FDG PET of patients with Hurthle cell carcinoma. J Nucl Med 2003; 44(9):1402–1406.

40. Helal BO, Merlet P, Toubert ME, et al. Clinical impact of (18)F-FDG PET in thyroid carcinoma patients with elevated thyroglobulin levels and negative (131)I scanning results after therapy. J Nucl Med 2001; 42(10):1464–1469.

41. Kresnik E, Mikosch P, Gallowitsch HJ, et al. Evaluation of head and neck cancer with 18F-FDG PET: a comparison with conventional methods. Eur J Nucl Med 2001; 28(7):816–821.

42. Grunwald F, Menzel C, Bender H, et al. Comparison of [18]FDG-PET with [131]iodine and ^{99m}Tc-sestamibi scintigraphy in differentiated thyroid cancer. Thyroid 1997; 7(3):327–335.

43. Chin BB, Patel P, Cohade C, Ewertz M, Wahl R, Ladenson P. Recombinant human thyrotropin stimulation of fluoro-d-glucose positron emission tomography uptake in well-differentiated thyroid carcinoma. J Clin Endocrinol Metab 2004; 89(1):91–95.

44. Wang W, Larson SM, Fazzari M, et al. Prognostic value of [18F]fluorodeoxyglucose positron emission tomographic scanning in patients with thyroid cancer. J Clin Endocrinol Metab 2000; 85(3):1107–1113.

45. Serhal DI, Nasrallah MP, Arafah BM. Rapid rise in serum thyrotropin concentrations after thyroidectomy or withdrawal of suppressive thyroxine therapy in preparation for radioactive iodine administration to patients with differentiated thyroid cancer. J Clin Endocrinol Metab 2004; 89(7):3285–3289.

46. Mazzaferri EL. Treating high thyroglobulins with radioiodine. A magic bullet or a shot in the dark? J Clin Endocrinol Metab 1995; 80:1485–1487.

47. Goldman JM, Line BR, Aamodt RL, Robbins J. Influence of triiodothyronine withdrawal time on 131-I uptake postthyroidectomy for thyroid cancer. J Clin Endocrinol Metab 1980; 50:734–739.

48. Jarzab B, Handkiewicz-Junak D, Roskosz J, et al. Recombinant human TSH-aided radioiodine treatment of advanced differentiated thyroid carcinoma: a single-centre study of 54 patients. Eur J Nucl Med Mol Imaging 2003; 30(8):1077–1086.

49. Barbaro D, Boni G, Meucci G, et al. Radioiodine treatment with 30 mCi after recombinant human thy-

rotropin stimulation in thyroid cancer: effectiveness for postsurgical remnants ablation and possible role of iodine content in L-thyroxine in the outcome of ablation. J Clin Endocrinol Metab 2003; 88(9):4110–4115.

50. Robbins RJ, Larson SM, Sinha N, et al. A retrospective review of the effectiveness of recombinant human TSH as a preparation for radioiodine thyroid remnant ablation. J Nucl Med 2002; 43(11):1482–1488.

51. Cohen O, Dabhi S, Karasik A, Zila ZS. Compliance with follow-up and the informative value of diagnostic whole-body scan in patients with differentiated thyroid carcinoma given recombinant human TSH. Eur J Endocrinol 2004; 150(3):285–290.

52. Berg G, Lindstedt G, Suurkula M, Jansson S. Radioiodine ablation and therapy in differentiated thyroid cancer under stimulation with recombinant human thyroid-stimulating hormone. J Endocrinol Invest 2002; 25(1):44–52.

53. Menzel C, Kranert WT, Dobert N, et al. rhTSH stimulation before radioiodine therapy in thyroid cancer reduces the effective half-life of (131)I. J Nucl Med 2003; 44(7):1065–1068.

54. Luster M, Sherman SI, Skarulis MC, et al. Comparison of radioiodine biokinetics following the administration of recombinant human thyroid stimulating hormone and after thyroid hormone withdrawal in thyroid carcinoma. Eur J Nucl Med Mol Imaging 2003; 30(10):1371–1377.

55. Koong SS, Reynolds JC, Movius EG, et al. Lithium as a potential adjunvant to ^{131}I therapy of metastatic, well differentiated thyroid carcinoma. J Clin Endocrinol Metab 1999; 84:912–916.

56. Park JT, Hennessey JV. Two-week low iodine diet is necessary for adequate outpatient preparation for radioiodine rhTSH scanning in patients taking levothyroxine. Thyroid 2004; 14(1):57–63.

57. Pacini F, Molinaro E, Castagna MG, et al. Ablation of thyroid residues with 30 mCi (131)I: a comparison in thyroid cancer patients prepared with recombinant human TSH or thyroid hormone withdrawal. J Clin Endocrinol Metab 2002; 87(9):4063–4068.

58. Morris LF, Waxman AD, Braunstein GD. The nonimpact of thyroid stunning: remnant ablation rates in (131)I-scanned and nonscanned individuals. J Clin Endocrinol Metab 2001; 86(8):3507–3511.

59. Wang W, Larson SM, Tuttle RM, et al. Resistance of [18F]-fluorodeoxyglucose-avid metastatic thyroid cancer lesions to treatment with high-dose radioactive iodine. Thyroid 2001; 11(12):1169–1175.

60. Grünwald F, Menzel C, Bender H, et al. Redifferentiation therapy-induced radioiodine uptake in thyroid cancer. J Nucl Med 1998; 39:1903–1906.

61. Gruning T, Tiepolt C, Zophel K, Bredow J, Kropp J, Franke WG. Retinoic acid for redifferentiation of thyroid cancer – does it hold its promise? Eur J Endocrinol 2003; 148(4):395–402.

62. Pineda JD, Lee T, Ain K, Reynolds J, Robbins J. Iodine-131 therapy for thyroid cancer patients with elevated thyroglobulin and negative diagnostic scan. J Clin Endocrinol Metab 1995; 80:1488–1492.

63. Schlumberger MJ. Diagnostic follow-up of well-differentiated thyroid carcinoma: Historical perspective and current status. J Endocrinol Invest 1999; 22(Suppl to No. 11):3–7.

64. Van Tol KM, Jager PL, De Vries EG, et al. Outcome in patients with differentiated thyroid cancer with negative diagnostic whole-body scanning and detectable stimulated thyroglobulin. Eur J Endocrinol 2003; 148(6):589–596.

65. Schlumberger M, Arcangioli O, Piekarski JD, Tubiana M, Parmentier C. Detection and treatment of lung metastases of differentiated thyroid carcinoma in patients with normal chest X-rays. J Nucl Med 1988; 29:1790–1794.

66. Sisson JC, Giordano TJ, Jamadar DA, et al. 131-I treatment of micronodular pulmonary metastases from papillary thyroid carcinoma. Cancer 1996; 78:2184–2192.

67. Samuel AM, Rajashekharrao B, Shah DH. Pulmonary metastases in children and adolescents with well-differentiated thyroid cancer. J Nucl Med 1998; 39:1531–1536.

68. Koh JM, Kim ES, Ryu JS, Hong SJ, Kim WB, Shong YK. Effects of therapeutic doses of ^{131}I in thyroid papillary carcinoma patients with elevated thyroglobulin level and negative ^{131}I whole-body scan: comparative study. Clin Endocrinol (Oxf) 2003; 58(4):421–427.

69. Pachucki J, Burmeister LA. Evaluation and treatment of persistent thyroglobulinemia in patients with well-differentiated thyroid cancer. Eur J Endocrinol 1997; 137:254–261.

70. Ronga G, Fiorentino A, Paserio E, Signore A, et al. Can iodine-131 whole-body scan be replaced by thyroglobulin measurement in the post-surgical follow-up of differentiated thyroid carcinoma? J Nucl Med 1990; 31:1766–1771.

71. de Keizer B, Koppeschaar HP, Zelissen PM, et al. Efficacy of high therapeutic doses of iodine-131 in patients with differentiated thyroid cancer and detectable serum thyroglobulin. Eur J Nucl Med 2001; 28(2):198–202.

72. Pacini F, Lippi F, Formica N, Elisei R, Anelli S, Ceccarelli C. Therapeutic doses of iodine-131 reveal undiagnosed metastases in thyroid cancer patients with detectable serum thyroglobulin levels. J Nucl Med 1987; 28:1888–1891.

73. Schaap J, Eustatia-Rutten CF, Stokkel M, et al. Does radioiodine therapy have disadvantageous effects in non-iodine accumulating differentiated thyroid carcinoma? Clin Endocrinol (Oxf) 2002; 57(1):117–124.

74. Casara D, Rubello D, Saladini G, et al. Different features of pulmonary metastases in differentiated thyroid cancer: Natural history and multivariate statistical analysis of prognostic variables. J Nucl Med 1993; 34:1626–1631.

Section VI

Medullary Thyroid Carcinoma

21

Medullary Thyroid Cancer: Diagnosis and Management

Aldo Pinchera and Rossella Elisei

Introduction

Medullary thyroid carcinoma is a well-differentiated thyroid tumor maintaining the biochemical and pathological features of the parafollicular or calcitonin-producing C cells from which it derives [1,2]. Its origin makes it a separate entity from the other differentiated thyroid carcinomas.

The overall frequency of medullary thyroid carcinoma is not well established, while its prevalence is 5–10% in all thyroid malignancies, 0.4–1.4% in all thyroid nodules, and less than 1% in the thyroids of subjects submitted to autopsy. Contrary to papillary and follicular carcinomas, no difference in distribution between females and males is observed. The clinical appearance is mainly in the fourth and fifth decades, but a wide range of age at onset is present [3–6].

No significant environmental factors or ethnic differences associated with the development of medullary thyroid carcinoma have been identified, although associations with prior thyroid diseases and other disorders such as hypertension, allergies, and gallbladder disease have been reported in a pooled analysis of epidemiological studies [7].

The pathogenetic mechanism has been recognized in the activation of the *RET* proto-oncogene [8–10]. According to the somatic or germline localization of the activated *RET* oncogene, two different forms are recognized: the sporadic form, which accounts for about 75% of cases, and the hereditary or familial form, which accounts for the remaining 25%. Only the hereditary form affects children and, generally, the most aggressive is the multiple endocrine neoplasia type 2B (MEN2B) syndrome in the clinically affected child [11–13].

The biological behavior of medullary thyroid carcinoma is much less favorable when compared with that of the other well-differentiated thyroid carcinomas even though it is not as unfavorable as that of anaplastic carcinoma [14] (Figure 21.1). A 10-year survival of about 50% of medullary thyroid carcinoma patients is reported in several series. Both the cure and survival of these patients are positively affected by an early diagnosis [15,16].

Clinical Presentation

Sporadic Form

The most common clinical presentation of sporadic medullary thyroid carcinoma is a thyroid nodule, either single or belonging to a series of nodules configuring the clinical picture of a multinodular goiter. With the exception of the simultaneous presence of diarrhea and/or flushing syndrome, which is however rare and usually related to an advanced metastatic disease, patients do not generally have any specific symptom. The association of thyroid nodular disease with a lump in the neck may

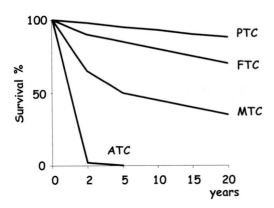

Figure 21.1 Survival rate of patients affected by different histotypes of thyroid carcinoma. MTC patients have a 10-year survival rate of about 50%, which is lower than that of patients with papillary and follicular thyroid carcinoma but higher than that of patients with anaplastic thyroid carcinoma.

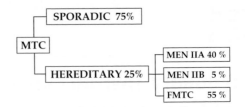

Figure 21.2 Classification and relative prevalence of different forms of medullary thyroid carcinoma according to *RET* genetic screening and clinical manifestations.

lead the clinician to suspect a thyroid malignancy but not specifically a medullary thyroid carcinoma.

Hereditary Forms

In about 25% of cases the medullary thyroid carcinoma is one of the components of the multiple endocrine neoplasia type 2 syndrome, which is an autosomal dominant inherited syndrome with a variable degree of expressivity and an age-related penetrance. As shown in Table 21.1, three different hereditary syndromes can be classified according to the involved organs: (a) multiple endocrine neoplasia type 2A (MEN2A), a syndrome consisting of medullary thyroid carcinoma, pheochromocytoma, and parathyroid neoplasia [17]; (b) MEN2B, a syndrome consisting of medullary thyroid carcinoma, pheochromocytoma, mucosal neuromas, and ganglioneuromatosis [18]; (c) familial medullary thyroid carcinoma (FMTC), which is characterized by the presence of an inheritable medullary thyroid carcinoma with no apparent association with other endocrine neoplasia [19]. After the introduction of *RET* genetic screening, the relative prevalence of the FMTC syndrome has been found to be much higher (from 10% to 50% of all MEN syndromes) (Figure 21.2). The increased number of FMTC cases is mainly due to the high number of apparently sporadic medullary thyroid carcinomas demonstrated to be familial cases by the *RET* mutation analysis [20,21].

The clinical appearance of medullary thyroid carcinoma in MEN syndromes is that of a thyroid nodular disease, similar to that of the sporadic form with the exception that it is usually bilateral, multicentric, and almost invariably associated with C-cell hyperplasia [22–24]. The clinical course of the medullary thyroid carcinoma varies considerably in the three syndromes. It is very aggressive and almost invariably unfavorable in MEN2B, with affected patients rarely surviving after adolescence. It is most indolent in the majority of patients with the FMTC form and shows variable degrees of aggressiveness in patients with MEN2A. Different types of *RET* gene mutations account for different biological behavior [25–28] and separate therapeutic protocols have been defined for the treatment of medullary thyroid carcinoma occurring in the three different syndromes [29].

Table 21.1 Prevalence of different endocrine neoplasia and other clinical manifestations in MEN2 syndromes

	Clinical manifestation	Prevalence (%)
MEN2A	Medullary thyroid carcinoma	100
	Pheochromocytoma	50
	Parathyroid adenomas	10–30
	Cutaneous lichen amyloidosis	<10
MEN2B	Medullary thyroid carcinoma	100
	Mucosal neuromas (tongue, subconjunctivas)	100
	Ganglioneuromatosis	100
	Marfanoid habitus	65
	Pheochromocytoma	45
FMTC	Medullary thyroid carcinoma	100

Between 10% and 30% of patients with MEN2A develop hyperparathyroidism during the third to fourth decades of life. The clinical findings are superimposable on those of the sporadic form of hyperparathyroidism and very often no specific symptoms are present. At variance with the sporadic form, multiple parathyroid hyperplasia or adenomatosis is most commonly found [17,30]. Hyperparathyroidism has only occasionally been reported in patients with MEN2B [18].

About 50% of MEN2A and 40–45% of MEN2B patients develop pheochromocytoma, which shares the same characteristics in both syndromes. Contrary to the sporadic form of pheochromocytoma, the adrenal tumors of MEN syndromes are usually bilateral and multicentric. However, the two adrenal glands are rarely simultaneously involved and a mean period of 10 years usually elapses between the development of the tumor in the two glands.

The MEN2B syndrome is characterized by the association with mucosal neuromas, which are mainly located on the distal tongue and subconjunctival areas, and ganglioneuromatosis affecting the gastrointestinal tract. MEN2B patients may be easily recognized on physical examination by the typical marfanoid habitus characterized by thin and inappropriately long extremities and pectus excavatum [18,31–33]. Thick lips and eyelids are frequently observed in the presence of mucosal neuromas, and are usually clearly evident when eyes and mouth are explored (Figure 21.3). Gastrointestinal disorders due to the intestinal neuromas throughout the intestinal tract, including obstructive symptoms, cramping and diarrhea, are frequently observed in early childhood.

An association with cutaneous lichen amyloidosis (CLA), a characteristically a pigmented and itchy skin lesion specifically localized in the interscapular region of the back (Figure 21.4),

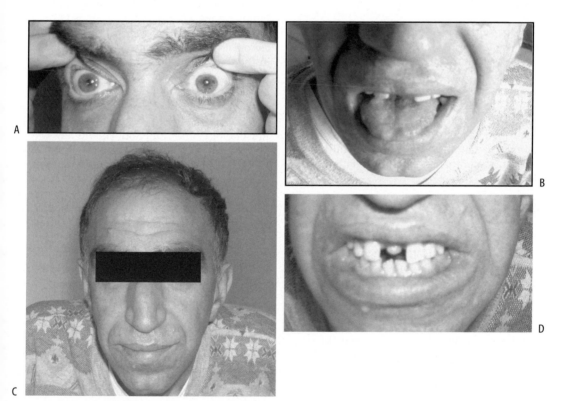

A

B

C

D

Figure 21.3 Clinical features of MEN2B syndrome. **A** Characteristic mucosal neurinomas of subconjunctivas are apparent. **B** Characteristic mucosal neurinomas of the distal part of the tongue are apparent. **C** Characteristic thick lips and marfanoid habitus. **D** Thick lips and mucosal neurinomas.

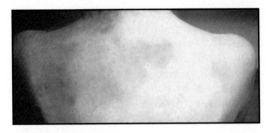

Figure 21.4 Cutaneous lichen amyloidosis (CLA) in a patient affected by MEN2A. The figure shows the characteristic location in the interscapular regions.

has been reported in less than 10% of MEN2A families [34,35]. The development of CLA may precede the development of the medullary thyroid carcinoma: thus, when present it is almost invariably diagnostic of MEN2A and may be considered a predictor of the syndrome.

Diagnosis

Thyroid ultrasonography, ultrasound-guided fine-needle aspiration cytology, and measurement of serum calcitonin levels (basal and after injection of calcitonin-stimulating reagents, e.g. pentagastrin) represent the most sensitive diagnostic tools for medullary thyroid carcinoma. *RET* genetic analysis should always be performed when the diagnosis of medullary thyroid carcinoma has been established to verify the sporadic or hereditary nature of the thyroid malignancy.

Sporadic Form

Physical examination of the neck does not offer any significant diagnostic elements. A palpable single or multi nodular goiter is usually present. A classical workup for thyroid nodular disease is then performed. Thyroid ultrasonography usually shows a hypoechoic nodule, sometimes with microcalcifications; ^{131}I and/or ^{99}Tc thyroid scintiscan reveals a cold nodule and the diagnosis is made by fine-needle aspiration cytology and/or by elevated serum calcitonin levels. Several studies have demonstrated that routine measurement of serum calcitonin is the most accurate diagnostic tool for the detection of medullary thyroid carcinoma in patients with thyroid nodules [36–42]. Subjects with elevated

basal serum calcitonin should be submitted to a pentagastrin stimulation test (0.5 µg/kg intravenously) to distinguish calcitonin secreted by a medullary thyroid carcinoma: a significant increase in serum calcitonin is observed in patients with medullary thyroid carcinoma [43,44] but not in those with elevated basal serum calcitonin deriving from other sources (Table 21.2) or those due to artifacts [45–47]. Although the routine measurement of serum calcitonin in all subjects with thyroid nodules is still controversial [48,49], evidence has been provided that this approach allows an early diagnosis and treatment, thus significantly improving the outcome of this potentially lethal disease [50].

Taking into account the relevance of completeness of the first surgical treatment [51], the suspicion or clinical diagnosis of medullary thyroid carcinoma requires an accurate examination of the neck to plan the best surgical treatment for the patient. A neck ultrasound should be performed in order to identify suspicious lymph nodes with metastatic lesions to be submitted to a fine-needle aspiration for cytological examination or measurement of calcitonin in the washout of the needle used.

Since at least 5–7% of apparently sporadic medullary thyroid carcinoma are found to be hereditary cases [20,21], a preoperative evaluation of both the adrenal and parathyroid morphology and function should always be performed. The familial history should also be carefully reconsidered with particular regard to the occurrence of pheochromocytoma and hyperparathyroidism in other family members.

Measurement of the serum carcinoembryonic antigen (CEA) is also indicated in the preoperative phase because elevated levels are strongly suggestive of advanced disease. Cases with advanced local disease demonstrated by neck ultrasound and associated with elevated

Table 21.2 Hypercalcitoninemia in conditions other than MTC

"Small cell" lung carcinoma
Various neuroendocrine tumors
Chronic renal failure
Pernicious anemia
Zollinger's syndrome
Lymphocytic thyroiditis
Follicular and papillary thyroid microcarcinoma

serum CEA levels should be studied by computerized tomography (CT) to better evaluate the relationship of the disease with the large veins, trachea, and esophagus and plan the most appropriate surgical treatment [52–54].

Hereditary Forms

The hereditary nature of the tumor may be suspected on the basis of a positive family history (other members already affected), or the association with other endocrine neoplasia (pheochromocytoma and/or parathyroid adenomas) or other disorders (neuromas, marfanoid features, CLA). The evaluation of thyroid nodule in the hereditary form is performed in the same way as that recommended for sporadic cases, while the hereditary forms require mandatory simultaneous examination of adrenal and parathyroid glands.

With the exception of a few examples [55,56], the development and the diagnosis of pheochromocytoma usually follows the development and the diagnosis of medullary thyroid carcinoma. Symptoms of pheochromocytoma are not specific and may be confused with those caused by anxiety. Hypertension is very rare, especially at the beginning of the disease. An elevated value of the daily urinary excretion of epinephrine is observed as the first alteration of catecholamine production. Norepinephrine usually increases only later in the course of the disease; thus the earliest biochemical abnormality is an elevated ratio of epinephrine to norepinephrine [57,58]. It has recently been demonstrated that the measurement of plasma metanephrines, the o-methylated metabolites of catecholamines, offer great advantages for an early diagnosis of pheochromocytoma over standard measurements of plasmatic catecholamines. Tests for plasma metanephrines are more specific and sensitive than those for catecholamines: while normal plasma concentrations of metanephrines exclude the diagnosis of pheochromocytoma, normal plasma concentrations of catecholamines do not [59,60]. Once the biochemical suspicion of a pheochromocytoma has arisen, an abdomen ultrasound with or without computerized tomography (CT) and/or magnetic resonance imaging (MRI) may be useful for the localization of the adrenal mass [61,62]. If there is no demonstrable adrenal mass by CT or MRI scanning, ^{131}I metaiodoben-

zylguanidine, a catecholamine analogue actively concentrated by chromaffin tissue, can be used to investigate the presence of an extra-adrenal tumor [63].

Parathyroid glands may also be involved in MEN2A. Both adenomas and hyperplasia may be associated with an increase of the parathyroid hormone secretion, resulting in hypercalcemia and hypercalciuria in more advanced cases [64]. The earliest serum abnormality detected is a moderately elevated level of serum parathyroid hormone with normal–high levels of calcemia. In doubtful cases, a calcium infusion test that is unable to suppress the parathyroid hormone secretion will be helpful for the diagnosis [65].

RET genetic analysis is fundamental for the early discovery of gene carriers who have to be submitted to a clinical evaluation as soon as the mutation has been revealed in their constitutive DNA. Thyroid ultrasound and a serum calcitonin measurement should be performed in gene carriers. If both of them are negative a pentagastrin stimulation test is usually required. Therapeutic strategies and follow-up protocols will be adjusted according to the guidelines for the diagnosis and treatment of the multiple endocrine neoplasia as reported below [29].

Follow-up and Diagnosis of Persistent Disease

After the initial therapy has been performed, serum basal and pentagastrin-stimulated calcitonin should be measured to verify the completeness of the treatment. The first control after surgery should be done 3 months after the surgical treatment, including physical examination, neck ultrasound and measurement of serum free triiodothyronine (FT$_3$), free thyroxine (FT$_4$), thyroid-stimulating hormone (TSH), calcitonin, and CEA. Measurement of FT$_3$, FT$_4$, and TSH are requested for monitoring the levothyroxine (L-T$_4$) replacement therapy. Serum calcitonin and CEA measurement and neck ultrasound are necessary for follow-up of the medullary thyroid disease. Due to the prolonged half-lives, if performed too early, measurement of serum calcitonin may be misleading, especially if a high serum concentration was present preoperatively [66] (Figure 21.5). If basal calcitonin is undetectable, a pentagastrin

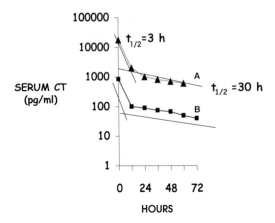

Figure 21.5 Disappearance rate of serum calcitonin (CT) after total thyroidectomy in two patients affected by MTC (A and B): two different half-lives of 3 and 30 hours respectively have been observed in both patients. (Modified from Fugazzola et al. [66].)

stimulation test is recommended. Patients with a negative pentagastrin stimulation test should be reevaluated one year later. A large series of patients with prolonged follow-up has shown that 3.3% of patients with one postoperative negative pentagastrin tests subsequently become positive [67]. Two negative pentagastrin tests on two follow-up evaluations strongly suggest that the patient is disease-free. Thus, basal serum calcitonin measurement on an annual basis is recommended, while the pentagastrin stimulation test may be performed at longer intervals (e.g. every 5 years). In patients with undetectable levels of serum calcitonin, measurement of CEA is not necessary.

Frequently basal and/or pentagastrin-stimulated serum calcitonin is persistently elevated after initial surgery. Because serum calcitonin is a very sensitive and specific tumor marker, the finding of detectable serum levels of basal or stimulated calcitonin is an indication of persistent disease. In patients with persistent disease, serum CEA concentration should be monitored because both high and increasing levels are strongly suggestive of a progressive disease [68,69]. In the majority of cases, the challenge is to find the source of production of calcitonin and CEA. An accurate neck ultrasound is the first localization technique to be performed due to the high frequency of local recurrence and cervical node metastases. A total body CT scan and bone scintigraphy are also suggested in the workup of a patient with detectable values of serum calcitonin. Other imaging techniques such as Octreoscan, ^{123}I-MIBG, and positron emission tomography (PET) may be useful although at present they do not appear to be particularly sensitive, especially in the presence of micrometastases [70–73]. The most accurate technique for the localization of occult metastases is probably the measurement of serum calcitonin after selective venous sampling catheterization: the presence of a gradient in the neck, in the mediastinum or in the suprahepatic veins suggests the presence of metastatic disease in the area where the higher levels of serum calcitonin have been found. It should be taken into account that this method is rather invasive and does not significantly improve the rate of cure [74–76].

About 50% of patients not cured at surgery have no evidence of metastatic disease when studied with the traditional imaging techniques (CT, MRI, PET). In this condition of "biochemical disease," characterized by the persistence of detectable levels of basal and/or pentagastrin-stimulated serum calcitonin but without evidence of metastatic lesions, the most widely accepted therapeutic strategy is that of "wait and see." A detectable serum calcitonin level is in fact compatible with long-term survival, during which calcitonin may remain stable with time or slowly increase. These patients are periodically monitored at intervals of 6 months to 1 year (Figure 21.6).

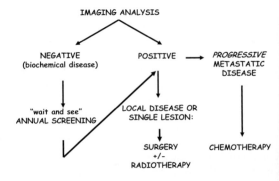

Figure 21.6 Flow chart for the management of patients with detectable serum levels of calcitonin after total thyroidectomy.

Diagnostic Tools

Fine-Needle Aspiration Cytology (FNAC)

Fine-needle aspiration is performed according to the standard procedure. In a typical cytological smear of a medullary thyroid carcinoma, cells are usually isolated, with shape varying from oval to round, large polygonal or spindled. Cytoplasm may be abundant or scanty and usually contains acidophilic granulation visible with specific stains (May–Grünwald–Giemsa). Nuclei, of which there are two or even more, are preferentially round and eccentrically localized (Figure 21.7). Amyloid is frequently detectable as clumps of amorphous material, and revealed by Congo red staining [77,78]. Immunocytochemistry for calcitonin and/or chromogranin should be performed if a diagnostic uncertainty is present [79,80]. Although the cytological pattern of medullary thyroid carcinoma is generally typical, there are several series that show a high percentage of failure in making a presurgical diagnosis [81,36–38]. Among other explanations, negative results might be due to the fact that medullary thyroid carcinoma could be present in one nodule not submitted to FNAC, especially when multinodular goiter is the clinical diagnosis. In this condition, serum calcitonin measurement is more reliable, since it is elevated even in the presence of microfoci of medullary thyroid carcinoma [36,39].

Serum Basal and Stimulated Calcitonin

Calcitonin is the most specific and sensitive medullary thyroid tumor marker, both before and after thyroidectomy [2,82,83]. It is a small polypeptide hormone of 32 amino acids normally produced almost exclusively by C cells. The gene encoding for calcitonin is located on chromosome 11p and yields two distinct messenger RNAs (mRNA) by alternative splicing: calcitonin and calcitonin gene-related peptide (CGRP) [84,85]. Calcitonin mRNA is found almost exclusively in the thyroid and CGRP mRNA in the nervous system. However, aberrant expression of CGRP may be observed in medullary thyroid carcinoma [86–88].

Release and secretion of calcitonin is mainly regulated by extracellular calcium concentration [89]. Other substances, such as pentagastrin, β-adrenergic agonists, growth hormone-releasing hormone and other gastrointestinal peptides [90–92], can stimulate calcitonin release from C cells.

The physiological role of calcitonin is still not well defined. It binds specifically to the osteoclasts and inhibits bone resorption in this site [93]. Experimental data obtained from mice

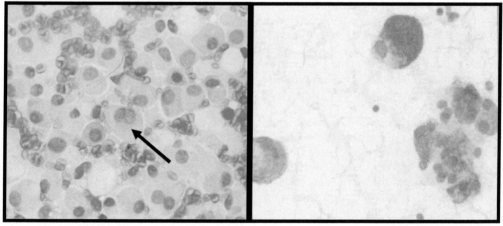

A   *B*

Figure 21.7 Cytological appearance of MTC. **A** Cells with abundant cytoplasm are visible; arrow indicates one cell with two nuclei, eccentrically localized (Papanicolaou staining, ×500). **B** Positive cytoplasmic staining for calcitonin confirms the suspicion of medullary carcinoma (immunocytochemistry for calcitonin, ×630). (Kindly provided by Dr G. Di Coscio, Department of Pathology, University of Pisa, Italy.)

homozygous null for the calcitonin gene have demonstrated a significant increase in bone formation at 1 and 3 months of age [94]. However, in normal adult human subjects even quite large doses of calcitonin have little effect on serum calcium levels. It is only in subjects with an increased bone turnover that calcitonin treatment acutely inhibits bone resorption and lowers the serum calcium [95]. Recently, evidence has been reported suggesting that the actions of calcitonin may not be limited to bone. Calcitonin receptors have also been identified in the central nervous system, testes, skeletal muscle, lymphocytes, and the placenta [96].

Ten years after the recognition of medullary thyroid carcinoma as a distinct histological type of thyroid carcinoma [1], high levels of calcitonin were demonstrated to be present both in the tumoral tissue and serum of patients with medullary thyroid carcinoma [2]. Elevated basal levels of serum calcitonin are diagnostic of medullary thyroid carcinoma. However, there are several other conditions, both physiological and pathological, in which basal levels of serum calcitonin may be found to be elevated and a differential diagnosis may be indicated [45,97–101]. Since the release of calcitonin in these diseases does not appear to be regulated by the same factors that stimulate calcitonin release in the C cells, differential diagnosis can be performed by either the calcium (2 mg/kg) or pentagastrin (0.5 mg/kg intravenously) rapid stimulation test [102]. While in patients with medullary thyroid carcinoma and elevated basal levels of calcitonin, the pentagastrin stimulation determines a 5–10-fold increase in serum levels of calcitonin, in other diseases the calcitonin increase is limited or absent. In patients with an endocrine tumor of another origin, an increase may be observed but is not usually greater than twofold [43,102].

Routine measurement of serum calcitonin in nodular thyroid diseases allows the preoperative diagnosis of unsuspected sporadic medullary thyroid carcinoma [36–42]. Calcitonin screening determines the early diagnosis of medullary thyroid carcinoma, usually when the tumor is still at stage I, thus favoring successful surgical treatment. A comparison of the outcome of two groups of patients, one diagnosed by serum calcitonin screening and the other by cytology or histology, has demon-

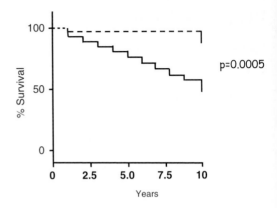

Figure 21.8 Significant difference in survival rate between patients with MTC diagnosed by serum calcitonin screening (dashed line) and those with MTC diagnosed at surgery and/or by preoperative cytology (solid line). (Modified from Elisei at al. [50].)

strated a significantly better prognosis in the first group [50] (Figure 21.8).

It is worth noting that calcitonin precursors (pre- and pro-calcitonin) and post-translational deriving peptides (katacalcin and N-terminal peptide) are also present in the blood and may interfere in the measurement of serum calcitonin. Artifactual recognition of larger calcitonin precursors is commonly observed with one-site radioimmunoassay. This problem seems to be overcome by the most recent generation of calcitonin two-site immunoradiometric assays (IRMA) that are able to specifically recognize the mature molecule of calcitonin [103]. Artifacts may be also determined by the presence of heterophilic antibodies in the blood of patients, which can interfere with the assay, thus producing false-positive results [47]. The absence of a significant increase in the serum calcitonin levels after pentagastrin or calcium stimulation test strongly suggests the artifactual nature of these false-positive values.

As an additional tool for the diagnosis of medullary thyroid carcinoma, calcitonin measurement in the washout of the needle used for the puncture of a suspected thyroid nodule may be useful. This approach is of particular diagnostic utility to ascertain the nature of neck lymph nodes, especially before thyroidectomy, to plan the surgical approach or the most appropriate therapeutic strategies.

Other Secretory Products

Although calcitonin is the most reliable tumor marker due to its high sensitivity and specificity, there are some other proteins that may be released by the malignant transformed C cell.

Serum CEA is usually elevated when the disease is diffuse and distant metastases are present [68,69]. Unlike calcitonin, CEA does not show any response to the pentagastrin stimulus. It is most useful in monitoring the progression of the disease since its level increases when the disease becomes rapidly progressive.

Serum chromogranin may also be elevated in patients with medullary thyroid carcinoma. It is not specific since elevated values have been reported in patients with neither clinical nor biochemical evidence of a primary medullary thyroid carcinoma [104].

As in many other neuroendocrine tumors, somatostatin, gastrin-releasing peptide, vasoactive intestinal peptide, neuron-specific enolase, and other neuroendocrine substances may be produced abnormally but none of these peptides are useful for diagnosis [105–107].

Some of the products of medullary thyroid carcinoma may result in significant clinical manifestations: not just CGRP, but also vasoactive intestinal peptide, serotonin and prostag-landins, may all contribute to the flushing and diarrhea syndrome [108,109].

Histology

Normal C Cells

The parafollicular C cells represent about 1% of all thyroid cells and are located at the basal layer of the follicle (Figure 21.9). At variance with thyroid follicular cells, which derive from endoderm, C cells originate from the neural crest and migrate to the final location along with the ultimobranchial body, during embryonic development [110,111]. Although C cells have several features that differentiate them from follicular epithelium, there is evidence to suggest the possible origin of the follicular and parafollicular C cells from a common ancestral cell. Critical neurotrophic growth factors, including glial-derived neurotrophic factor (GDNF), which is a natural ligand of RET receptor, as well as nerve growth factor (NGF) and other neurotrophins, seem to play a central role in promoting the differentiation of cells deriving from the neural crest [112].

There are specific features that make the C cell a separate entity from a follicular cell: (a) the peculiar distribution in the thyroid gland,

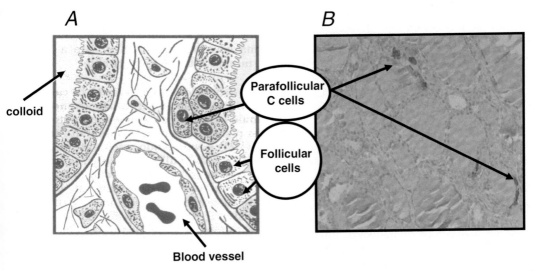

Figure 21.9 Schematic representation (**A**) and immunohistochemistry for calcitonin showing normal parafollicular C cells in normal thyroid tissue (**B**, ×100): the parafollicular C cells are located at the basal layer of the follicle.

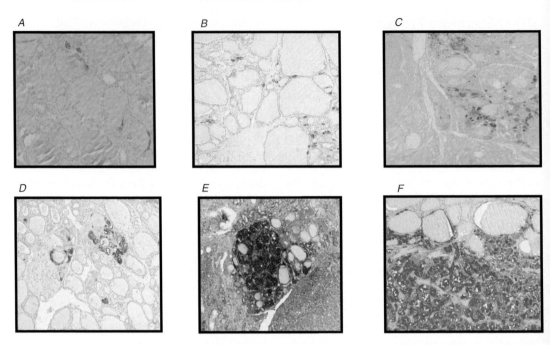

Figure 21.10 Different stages in the development of hereditary MTC. **A** Normal parafollicular C cells; **B** slight C-cell hyperplasia (CCH); **C** diffuse CCH; **D** focal CCH; **E** nodular CCH; **F** MTC. Immunohistochemistry for calcitonin (Ventana Medical System antibody, 1:100; ×100). (Kindly provided by Professor F. Basolo, Department of Pathology, University of Pisa, Italy.)

which is prevalent at the junction of the upper third and the lower two thirds and along the central vertical axis of each thyroid lobe; (b) the growth and functional independence from TSH, as well as the inability to take up iodine; and (c) the production and secretion of calcitonin, a biogenic amine, which is almost exclusively produced by both normal and malignant C cells.

C-Cell Hyperplasia

The definition of C-cell hyperplasia has changed over the years, especially after the introduction of *RET* genetic screening and the histological examination of apparently normal thyroid glands of mutated gene carriers that usually show an increased number of C cells. Studies of both human normal thyroid and thyroids affected by lymphocytic thyroiditis have demonstrated that one can see up to 50 C cells per 1 and 3 low power fields respectively, without correlation with any pathological status [98,113]. According to these findings, this is at present the most widely accepted definition of

C-cell hyperplasia, even though this criterion may be not respected in the presence of cytologically evident atypia [114].

According to the number and the distribution of C cells either a diffuse, focal, or nodular C-cell hyperplasia can be distinguished (Figure 21.10). It is likely that they represent progressive stages through which the normal C cell is transformed into a tumoral cell. While there is general agreement in considering C-cell hyperplasia the preneoplastic lesion of the hereditary form of medullary thyroid carcinoma, little is known about the relationship between C-cell hyperplasia and the sporadic form. Nevertheless, about 30% of sporadic medullary thyroid carcinoma is associated with C-cell hyperplasia [115].

Several authors would like to distinguish two types of C-cell hyperplasia: primary or neoplastic C-cell hyperplasia, which is related to the hereditary form of medullary thyroid carcinoma, and secondary or non-neoplastic C-cell hyperplasia, which may be observed in other thyroid diseases (thyroiditis and follicular or papillary microcarcinoma) and in about 20% of normal subjects [116,117]. However, the pathological definition and clinical significance of secondary C-cell hyperplasia remains unclear.

Medullary Thyroid Carcinoma

Under macroscopic examination, medullary thyroid carcinoma shows a hard and firm consistency and is either chalky white or red in color on cross-section. Histologically, medullary thyroid carcinoma is pleomorphic with spindle-shaped or rounded cells characteristically organized in a nested pattern. Mitoses are not very frequent, nuclei are usually uniform, and the eosinophilic cytoplasm is characterized by the presence of secretory granules. Deposits of amyloid substance are frequently (60–80%) observed between tumoral cells [118].

Sometimes there is difficulty distinguishing medullary thyroid carcinoma from anaplastic carcinoma, Hürthle cell carcinoma or insular carcinoma, especially if pseudopapillary elements or giants cells are present. Positive immunohistochemistry for calcitonin is diagnostic of medullary thyroid carcinoma. Immunohistochemistry for chromogranin A and carcinoembryonic antigen may also be useful [115] (Figure 21.11).

Histopathological description of medullary thyroid carcinoma must include the number and the distribution of tumoral foci as well as the simultaneous presence of C-cell hyperplasia. This information is of practical usefulness because bilaterality, multicentricity, and C-cell hyperplasia are considered the histological hallmarks of the hereditary forms [22].

A mixed form of medullary thyroid carcinoma is also described [119]. It is characterized by the simultaneous presence of parafollicular and follicular cell features, with positive immunohistochemistry for both calcitonin and thyroglobulin. In this regard, it is worth noting that the association of medullary and papillary thyroid carcinoma in the same thyroid gland seems to be quite frequent [120,121]. Molecular studies have shown that genes theoretically specific for the parafollicular C cells (i.e. normal RET gene) are expressed in papillary thyroid carcinoma and that genes theoretically specific for follicular cells (e.g. thyroglobulin, TSH receptor, thyroid transcription factor 1) are expressed in medullary thyroid carcinoma [122–124]. Despite all these observations, it is still controversial whether the mixed medullary thyroid carcinoma is a real separate histological entity, originating from an ancestral stem cell able to differentiate as both follicular and parafollicular cell, or the consequence of the collision of two distinct tumors, medullary and papillary, originating in the same thyroid gland.

RET Genetic Analysis

RET mutation analysis represents one of the most useful genetic screening tests in clinical practice. The mutation is inherited as an autosomal dominant trait: since the penetrance of RET mutations is near 100%, all gene heterozygous carriers will develop medullary thyroid

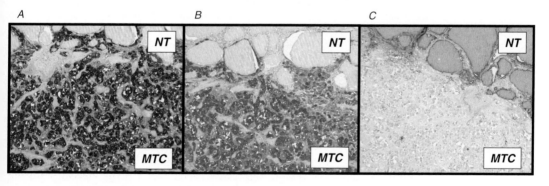

Figure 21.11 Medullary thyroid carcinoma (MTC) and normal adjacent thyroid tissue (NT). **A** Immunohistochemistry for calcitonin. **B** Immunohistochemistry for chromogranin. **C** Immunohistochemistry for thyroglobulin. Both calcitonin and chromogranin, but not thyroglobulin, are positive in MTC. A positive immunostaining for thyroglobulin is present in NT (×100, Ventana Medical System antibodies). (Kindly provided by Professor F. Basolo, Department of Pathology, University of Pisa, Italy.)

carcinoma, which is lethal in almost 50% of cases if not adequately treated. The genotype–phenotype correlation has been well demonstrated by the analysis of 477 MEN2 families studied by the International RET Consortium: no evidence of false-positive *RET* mutation was described and all patients who underwent thyroidectomy on the basis of the genetic screening were found to have medullary thyroid cancer [27]. Recently, a new mutation at codon 883 in exon 15 has been reported to result in the development of medullary thyroid carcinoma only in the homozygous condition [125].

Screening for *RET* gene mutations allows the early discovery of gene carriers, who can be treated with precocious and even prophylactic thyroidectomy, which may provide a definitive cure of this potentially lethal thyroid disease [126].

RET Gene

The *RET* proto-oncogene is a 21 exon gene that lies on chromosome 10q11-2 and encodes for a tyrosine kinase transmembrane receptor. The receptor is composed of an extracellular domain (EC), with a distal cadherin-like region and a juxta-membrane cystine-rich region, a transmembrane domain and an intracellular domain with tryosine kinase activity (TK) (Figure 21.12). *RET* is expressed in a variety of neuronal cell lineages including thyroid C cells and adrenal medulla. Recently data indicate that

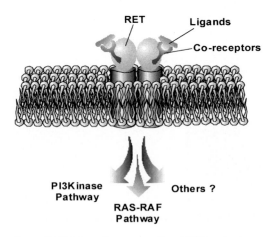

Figure 21.12 Schematic representation of RET tyrosine kinase receptor. The interaction with the ligand and corresponding co-receptor induces the dimerization and phosphorylation of the receptor, resulting in the activation of the intracellular signaling pathway.

RET gene expression may also occur in follicular thyroid cells [122]. In physiological conditions, the activation of RET protein is secondary to its dimerization due to the interaction with one of its ligands. Four different ligands have so far been recognized: GDNF, neurturin (NTN), persepin (PNS), and artemin (ART). The interaction is mediated by a ligand specific co-receptor (e.g. the GFRα-1 is the co-receptor for the GDNF). The dimerization of RET protein induces autophosphorylation of the TK domain and the activation of downstream signaling pathways [127].

In 1987 genetic linkage analysis localized MEN2 to the centromeric region of chromosome 10 [128,129]. In 1993 two independent groups reported that activating germline point mutations of the *RET* proto-oncogene are causative events in MEN2A and in FMTC [8,9] (Figure 21.13). One year later, MEN2B was also associated with germline *RET* proto-oncogene mutations [130]. Since then, a large number of publications have addressed the relationship between *RET* mutations and the clinical phenotype of MEN2 patients and the clinical implication of screening MEN2 family members for *RET* gene mutations.

About 98% of MEN2A cases are associated with *RET* mutations in the cystine-rich extracellular domain, in particular in codons 609, 611, 618, 620, and 634 of exons 10 and 11. Mutations at codon 634 of exon 11 (mainly TGC to CGC) are the most common, accounting for 85% of MEN2A cases [27–29,131]. Interestingly, mutation of cystine 634 significantly correlates with the presence of pheochromocytoma and parathyroid adenomas (Table 21.3).

A specific mutation in exon 16, at codon 918 (ATG to ACG) is almost invariably associated with MEN2B. The substitution of methionine with threonine causes alterations in the substrate recognition pocket of the catalytic probe determining the activation of the intra-signaling pathways. Other rare mutations of the intracellular domain have been reported in codon 883 of exon 15 [132]. A double *RET* mutation at codon 804 and 904 has also been described [133]. The Met918Thr mutation is associated with a very aggressive MTC that usually develops during childhood, often only a few years after birth.

In FMTC, the mutations are widely distributed among the five cystine codons 609, 611, 618, 620, and 634 but also in other non-cystine codons, such as codon 804 in exon 14, 891 in

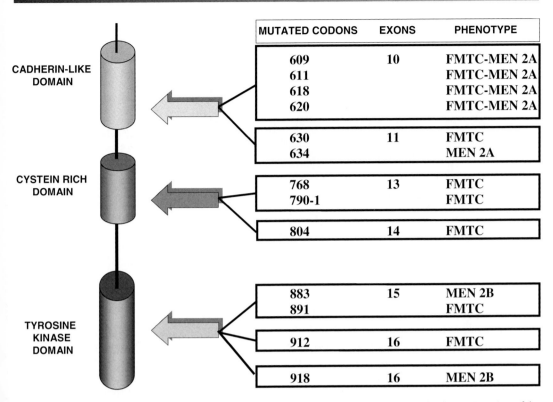

MUTATED CODONS	EXONS	PHENOTYPE
609	10	FMTC-MEN 2A
611		FMTC-MEN 2A
618		FMTC-MEN 2A
620		FMTC-MEN 2A
630	11	FMTC
634		MEN 2A
768	13	FMTC
790-1		FMTC
804	14	FMTC
883	15	MEN 2B
891		FMTC
912	16	FMTC
918	16	MEN 2B

CADHERIN-LIKE DOMAIN

CYSTEIN RICH DOMAIN

TYROSINE KINASE DOMAIN

Figure 21.13 Schematic representation of *RET* gene with the location of all known mutated codons in the three main regions of the gene and the relationship with the MEN syndromes.

exon 15 and others (Figure 21.14). A different biological behavior, characterized by a lower aggressiveness and an older mean age at diagnosis, has been described for FMTC associated with mutations in non cystine codons with respect to both MEN2A and FMTC with mutations in cystine codons [28].

In about 4–10% of MEN2A or FMTC patients and in about 95% of those with MEN2B, the germline *RET* mutation is a "de novo" mutation,

Table 21.3 Correlation between phenotype and *RET* gene mutations

	Most frequently involved codons[a]							
	609	611	618	620	634	768	804	918
MEN2A								
MEN2A (1) (MTC + pheochromocytoma + hyperparathyroidism)			6%	2%	92%			
MEN2A (2) (MTC + pheochromocytoma)		3%	4%	13%	80%			
MEN2A (3) (MTC + hyperparathyroidism)	8%	15%	8%		69%			
MEN2B								97%
FMTC	7%	3%	33%	17%	30%		3%	
Sporadic FMTC								95%

[a] As a percentage of patients with somatic *RET* gene mutations.
[b] Somatic mutations detectable in about 40% of sporadic MTC.

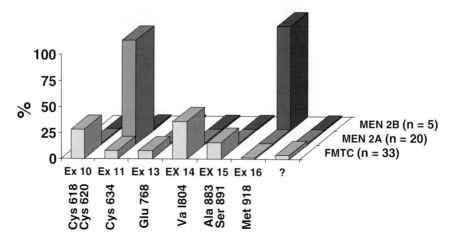

Figure 21.14 Different MEN2 syndromes and corresponding germline *RET* mutations in an Italian series of MEN2 kindreds (*n* = 58). (Series of the Department of Endocrinology, University of Pisa, Italy.)

as demonstrated by the negative finding of the *RET* genetic analysis in the patients' parents. In these cases the mutation is usually located in the allele inherited from the patient's father [134].

Somatic *RET* mutations are found in about 40% of sporadic cases of MTC mainly consisting of a Met918Thr mutation in exon 16, which is the same mutation also occurring in MEN2B (Figure 21.15). Other *RET* somatic mutations and also some small deletions have been reported in other codons [135]. Several studies indicate that MTC patients with somatic *RET* mutations have a poorer prognosis than those with no evidence of *RET* mutation [136].

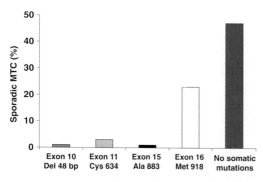

Figure 21.15 Somatic *RET* gene mutations in an Italian series of 77 sporadic MTC. About 50% of cases do not harbor any known *RET* mutation. The most frequent somatic mutation is the Met918Thr substitution at exon 16. (Series of the Department of Endocrinology, University of Pisa, Italy.)

Several *RET* gene polymorphisms have been found both in MTC affected patients and in normal subjects. It is still controversial whether some of these polymorphisms have a higher prevalence in MTC with respect to normal individuals and if they play any role in the development of MTC [137–139].

Screening for *RET* Gene Mutations in MEN2 Family Members

The recognition of the role of RET mutation in MEN2 provided a reliable method to screen family members of an affected proband carrying a germline mutation. From a practical point of view, once the germline *RET* mutation of the index case has been recognized, blood is taken from all first degree family members. Informed consent and adequate genetic counseling are requested. This allows the identification of "gene carriers" at the time they are still clinically unaffected or at an early stage of the disease. It also has the advantage of excluding "non gene carriers" from further testing for the rest of their life. Although the presence of a germline *RET* mutation is diagnostic of MEN2 syndrome, gene carriers must be submitted to further clinical and biochemical evaluations to ascertain the actual development of the MTC and its extension, if already present. The involvement of other endocrine organs must also be assessed [29,140].

Screening for *RET* Gene Mutations in Apparently Sporadic Cases

All patients with MTC, independently from their apparent sporadic origin, should be submitted to genetic screening of the *RET* gene by analyzing their constitutional DNA derived from blood and, whenever possible, also from tumoral tissue. It is well known that from 5% to 10% of apparently sporadic MTC cases are found to harbor a germline *RET* mutation being "de novo" or misdiagnosed familial cases. This finding is of great relevance for the early discovery of the other gene carriers in the family who are unaware of their condition.

In sporadic MTC cases, *RET* gene analysis should be in any case performed also in the tumoral tissue, collected at surgery and kept at −80°C or in the paraffin-embedded tumoral tissue. There are at least three main reasons to justify this procedure: (a) the discovery of a somatic mutation, which usually occurs in 45% of cases, strongly supports the sporadic nature of the tumor; (b) the prognostic value of the presence/absence of the somatic mutation; (c) the future possibility for *RET* mutated patients to be treated with drugs specifically aimed at inhibiting the altered *RET* gene.

Therapy

Initial Treatment

An early diagnosis and complete surgical treatment are the bases for a definitive cure of patients affected by medullary thyroid carcinoma (Figure 21.16). The minimal standard procedure is total (or near-total) thyroidectomy with central neck lymph node dissection, in both sporadic and familial forms. The need for total thyroidectomy is supported by the multicentricity and bilaterality of the medullary thyroid carcinoma that occurs in about 100% of the hereditary form and 30% of sporadic form [22]. Furthermore, C-cell hyperplasia, which is considered a preneoplastic lesion, is almost invariably associated with the hereditary form of medullary thyroid carcinoma and, to a lesser extent, with the sporadic form [24]. An additional reason in favor of total thyroidectomy is the fact that, as mentioned above, 5–7% of apparently sporadic cases are in fact hereditary

forms, which almost invariably have bilateral disease [20,21].

Central node dissection, from the hyoid bone to the innominate veins, is mandatory during the initial operation. This node compartment is in fact the primary lymphatic drainage of the thyroid and 50–60% of medullary thyroid carcinomas show node metastases in this area at the time of presentation [51,141]. The removal of the central compartment also has a prophylactic significance and must be performed independently of the size of the primary tumor and the presurgical evidence of lymph node involvement. This surgical approach is also suggested in *RET* gene carriers without clinical evidence of the disease, which can be completely cured by surgical treatment. It is still controversial as to whether the central node dissection has to be performed in child gene carriers without clinical and biochemical (undetectable levels of basal and stimulated calcitonin) evidence of disease [142–144].

Whenever a presurgical clinical diagnosis of node metastases is achieved, the surgical dissection of the corresponding lateral node compartment should be included. It is still debated whether a modified radical neck dissection with removal of nodes in the ipsilateral or bilateral compartment should be performed in any case. Since unilateral or bilateral cervical nodal metastases occur in up to 90% of patients with medullary thyroid carcinoma, especially when

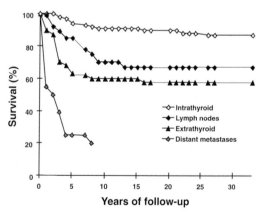

Figure 21.16 Different survival rates of patients affected by MTC according to the tumor extension at the time of the diagnosis: The best prognosis is observed in patients with MTC at stage I. (Modified from Gharib et al. [15].)

the primary tumor is palpable [39,55], several authors strongly suggest an "en bloc" dissection of both central and bilateral neck compartments together with the thyroid gland [145]. This is of great clinical significance because the adequacy of the initial surgical treatment is a prerequisite for the effective cure of the MTC, thus the choice of the most appropriate initial procedure is fundamental. In this regard it is worth considering that radical neck dissection may result in significant morbidity and has not been clearly shown to improve the prognosis of the disease, which in fact is dependent on several other factors such as the local extent of the disease at the time of diagnosis, the presence or absence of other endocrine neoplasia, and, the presence of cervical lymph node metastases. Patients who are cured by the initial treatment are usually those with a lower stage of disease, with no involvement of lateral nodes in the neck. Several reports indicate that when lateral node metastases are present at diagnosis, achievement of a definitive cure with the initial treatment is uncommon regardless of the extent of the surgical procedure [67,146,147].

C cells are not able to actively concentrate radioiodine and, as consequence, ^{131}I radioactive ablation is not useful in medullary thyroid carcinoma. There are only a few anecdotal reports indicating a beneficial effect of ^{131}I treatment of the postsurgical remnant presumably due to death of C cells adjacent to follicular cells as consequence of a bystander effect [148,149].

In patients with a locally aggressive disease not completely removed by the primary resection, surgical treatment should be followed by external-beam radiotherapy as adjuvant treatment. Although bulky medullary thyroid carcinoma deposits are consistently resistant to external radiotherapy, there is evidence of a potential benefit from radiotherapy in terms of a lower risk (from two- to fourfold) of local recurrence in patients with residual disease [150,151]. This procedure should be reserved for patients who have undergone complete central compartment and lateral neck dissection and postponed to a second surgical treatment in those who have been approached with a less aggressive primary resection. Radiation therapy after thyroidectomy and node dissection is not generally recommended on a prophylactic basis but it is worth mentioning that there is some evidence that external beam radiation in patients with residual malignant disease after

surgery may increase the 5-year survival rate from 60% to 95% [152].

Hormone replacement therapy with L-thyroxine (L-T$_4$) should be started immediately after thyroidectomy. Unlike papillary and follicular thyroid tumors, medullary carcinoma is not dependent on TSH for both growth and function, thus there is no need to treat patients with L-T$_4$ suppressive therapy: the daily dose should be tailored by measuring serum FT$_3$, FT$_4$, and TSH aiming to keep their values within the normal range. Unilateral or bilateral adrenalectomy must be performed before total thyroidectomy, when a pheochromocytoma has been documented, because of the risk of a life-threatening hypertensive crisis during the induction of anesthesia for the neck surgical treatment. Preoperative screening for pheochromocytoma should be conducted in all patients with a diagnosis of medullary thyroid carcinoma since the patient may be an index case of a familial form, presented as apparently sporadic. Although pheochromocytoma is usually bilateral, a 10-year interval is the mean period between the first and the contralateral adrenal mass appearance. Different approaches to the management of adrenal medullary disease are suggested when only one adrenal gland is involved at the time of the diagnosis. Bilateral adrenalectomy in principle eliminates the need for a second intervention later in the patient's life, but implies the risk associated with the corticosteroid deficiency. Since a laparoscopic surgical approach has been introduced [153], the preferred strategy is to remove only the affected adrenal gland and periodically monitor the morphology and function of the other adrenal gland. Whatever the final decision, all patients to be submitted to adrenalectomy should be treated preoperatively with pharmacological α- and β-adrenergic antagonists [154,155].

Grossly enlarged parathyroid glands should be resected during the first operation for patients with hereditary forms of medullary thyroid carcinoma and documented clinical hyperparathyroidism. An intraoperative serum parathyroid hormone measurement is recommended to ensure the precise and total removal of the affected gland(s). This procedure is of practical importance especially when the macroscopic appearance of the removed parathyroid is not indicative of the presence of adenoma, suggesting the presence of multiple adenomatosis or diffuse hyperplasia [156]. In some centers normal or hyperplastic parathyroid glands of patients with hereditary forms are always removed, even in the presence of normal serum parathyroid hormone levels. They are appropriately marked, for making their localization easier whenever it might be necessary, and totally or partially implanted in a muscle [157]. It is worth noting that an aggressive management of normal parathyroid glands is associated with a higher incidence of hypoparathyroidism. In this regard, a greater concern is represented by young *RET* gene carriers who, if rendered hypoparathyroid, would be exposed to the need for calcium and vitamin D supplementation for the rest of their lives.

Gene Carrier Treatment

Once a gene carrier has been diagnosed by genetic analysis, the therapeutic strategy should be defined according to the guidelines for the diagnosis and treatment of multiple endocrine neoplasia [29], which take into account the different biological behavior of the medullary thyroid carcinoma in the three forms of multiple endocrine neoplasia. In MEN2B total thyroidectomy should be performed as soon as possible, even under 2 years of age if the diagnosis is available. In MEN2A, total thyroidectomy should be performed at 10 years of age or less if the pentagastrin stimulation test for calcitonin is positive. In FMTC, yearly based follow-up should be performed with a pentagastrin stimulation test and thyroid surgical treatment is indicated at the first positive test.

Parathyroid and adrenal gland morphology and function must be assessed and an adequate treatment should be performed if needed. If no abnormalities of these glands are found at the time of diagnosis, their morphology and function should be monitored annually because both hyperparathyroidism and pheochromocytoma may show up later in life.

Further Treatments

When patients are not cured by the primary surgical treatment, other therapeutic procedures are indicated according to the localization and the number of lesions. In planning a therapeutic strategy it should be taken into account that most distant metastases found during follow-up are small at the time of their recognition and that their growth is usually very slow. These lesions are compatible with a long period of good quality of life. In these cases, an aggressive therapeutic approach may not be indicated, unless an evident rapidly progressive disease is demonstrated.

Local Recurrence and Regional Lymph Node Metastases

In the first years following surgical treatment the regional lymph nodes of the neck and mediastinum are most frequently responsible for persistent disease. A second surgical treatment with a curative intent is recommended only for minimal residual disease. To this purpose an extensive modified neck dissection involving microdissection of all node-bearing compartments from the clavicle to the skull is recommended [158]. Unfortunately, less than 30% of patients affected by MTC with extrathyroidal invasion can be cured by a second surgical treatment [159,160]. Capsular invasion and more than 10 lymph node metastases [145] in the primary surgical specimens are significant predictors of poor response to reoperation. In the clinical management of patients with MTC the identification of those who might benefit from this treatment is of great practical importance to avoid false expectation.

If a reasonable prospect of a definitive cure is not foreseen, a second surgical treatment should only be performed for symptomatic lesions or when their growth may cause significant morbidity as may happen for lymph nodes of the mediastinum adjacent to the great vessels, tracheoesophageal groove, carotid sheath, and brachial plexus. A second operation with palliative intent may be strongly indicated in patients with compressive symptoms who can benefit from a surgical debulking. Local external radiotherapy may be indicated in these advanced situations.

Distant Metastases

Surgical treatment of distant metastases is not indicated, except for those lesions whose growth may compromise some vital functions. Surgical debulking of vertebral metastases that could impair spinal cord function is an example of a non-curative but appropriate procedure.

Chemotherapy for advanced, metastatic medullary thyroid carcinoma has shown limited response rates in several small-scale trials published to date [161]. Thus, chemotherapy should only be used in patients with a diffuse and well-documented progressive disease. In these cases the reduction in the growth rate and the stabilization of the disease represent a satisfactory result. A high dose of doxorubicin (75 mg/m^2 every 3–4 weeks) is the most effective chemotherapeutic agent with a response rate of 15–20% in terms of stabilization of the disease. The same response rate is obtained when doxorubicin is used alone or in combination with other drugs such as 5-fluorouracil, dacarbazine, streptozocin, cyclophosphamide, and vincristine [162,163]. Since major toxic effects are frequently observed and the response is only partial and short-lived, chemotherapy should not be used in patients with stable or slowly progressive disease.

Medullary thyroid carcinoma is a neuroendocrine tumor and 30–50% of cases express somatostatin receptors as ascertained by Octreoscan [70]. Over the years, different types of octreotide, from the native to the long-acting analogues, have been explored as potential therapeutic agents. In the majority of cases, a significant reduction in serum calcitonin has been demonstrated [164]. Unfortunately, no evidence of a parallel reduction in the number and/or the size of tumor lesions has been shown. Inconstant and transient effects in reducing symptoms such as flushing and diarrhea are not sufficient to recommend the administration of somatostatin analogues in metastatic medullary thyroid cancer patients. No improvement in the therapeutic effect has been observed when the somatostatin analogues have been combined with α-interferon [164]. Recently, specific somatostatin receptors have been identified both in cell lines deriving from human medullary thyroid carcinoma and in tissue surgical specimens of medullary thyroid carcinoma [165–167]. The possibility of using analogues that specifically recognize these receptors is currently under evaluation.

Treatment with several radioactive elements has been widely explored. There is no clinical evidence to encourage treatment with ^{131}I, which has been demonstrated to be ineffective in large series of patients with metastatic medullary thyroid carcinoma [148,149]. A more promising use of radioactive iodine has been shown when iodine is linked to metaiodobenzylguanidine [168,169]. However, only a small proportion of patients (30%) have a positive result and the treatment is relatively ineffective. Other radioimmunotherapeutic agents have been explored and, in particular, the bi-specific antibodies directed against the carcinoembryonic antigen (CEA), which is expressed on the surface of the majority of metastatic medullary thyroid cells, but unfortunately no significant benefits have been found in treated patients [170]. Preliminary data have been reported on the use of somatostatin analogues labeled with yttrium-90 or other radionuclides, in patients with metastatic medullary thyroid carcinoma showing octreotide uptake at Octreoscan [169,171]. Further studies are needed to establish the therapeutic effectiveness of this procedure.

As reported above, external beam radiotherapy is indicated in medullary thyroid carcinoma when local aggressive unresectable disease is present. Although the radiosensitivity of medullary thyroid carcinoma is moderate and no survival benefit has been so far demonstrated, available data suggest that improved local control of the disease with a longer interval between treatment and the recurrence of regional or local disease may be obtained by external postsurgical radiotherapy compared with those not treated [151,152]. When bone metastases are present, external beam radiation is indicated to prevent pathological fractures and for palliation of symptoms. Brain metastases also may be treated with external radiotherapy and a rapid and reliable response may be obtained. Other therapeutic strategies are indicated for lung and liver metastases. Radiation therapy of lung metastases carries risk of radiation fibrosis and respiratory dysfunction. Chemotherapy is better indicated if progression of pulmonary disease is observed. Liver metastases may be amenable to surgical resection, especially if preceded by transarterial chemoembolization. This procedure has been demonstrated to be of particular benefit when liver metastases are smaller than 3 cm and the liver involvement is less than 30% [172].

Discomfortable Syndrome

Particular care should be taken to reduce severe symptoms such as diarrhea, flushes, and pain. Diarrhea is of particular discomfort for patients, deeply disturbing their quality of life and resulting in severe loss of weight. Symptomatic therapy should be performed using loperamide. Histamine receptor inhibitors may be employed to control the flushing syndrome. Analgesic drugs, as appropriate, should be used to give some pain relief to patients with very advanced metastatic disease.

Future Therapeutic Strategies

At present, the treatment of advanced and metastatic medullary thyroid carcinoma is unsatisfactory. Novel alternative therapeutic approaches are under investigation and several experimental studies are already ongoing [173]. Tissue-specific cancer gene therapy has been evaluated for several years. Adenovirus-mediated tumor-specific combined gene therapy using the herpes simplex virus thymidine/ganciclovir system and murine interleukin-12 seems very promising. An effective growth suppression of tumor has been observed in rat models affected by medullary thyroid carcinoma and treated with this system [174]. Other interesting approaches are based on immunotherapy, for example stimulation of immune response and vaccination with tumor lysate [175,176].

Inhibitors of tyrosine kinase receptors are currently under investigation for their potential role as therapeutic agents in human cancers related to a structural alteration of these receptors [177]. As a general mechanism, they compete with adenosine triphosphate, thus hampering autophosphorylation and signal transduction downstream from the targeted kinase receptor. At present, two drugs have been shown to produce beneficial effects: STI571 (imatinib or Gleevec), which has been documented to inhibit BCR-ABL in chronic myeloid leukemia and c-KIT and PDGFR in gastrointestinal stromal tumors, and ZD1839 (gefitinib or Iressa), which has been documented to inhibit EGFR in non-small cell lung carcinoma [178,179]. A further very promising agent is ZD6474, which has been demonstrated to have an inhibiting activity on the growth of cell lines harboring RET gene activating alterations and on the formation of tumors after injection of these cells into nude mice [180–182]. ZD6474 also exerts an inhibiting effect on the vascular endothelial growth factor receptor (VEGFR), resulting in antiangiogenic activity. At present, a phase I trial has been completed with no significant adverse events. Clinical trials of phase II and III are required to establish the therapeutic potential of this and other compounds in RET-positive cancer patients.

References

1. Hazard JB, Hawk WA, Crile G Jr. Medullary (solid) carcinoma of the thyroid; a clinicopathologic entity. J Clin Endocrinol Metab 1959; 19:152–161.
2. Melvin KE, Tashjian AH Jr. The syndrome of excessive thyrocalcitonin produced by medullary carcinoma of the thyroid. Proc Natl Acad Sci USA 1968; 59:1216–1222.
3. Bergholm U, Adami HO, Telenius-Berg M, Johansson H, Wilander E. Incidence of sporadic and familial medullary thyroid carcinoma in Sweden 1959 through 1981. A nationwide study in 126 patients. Swedish MCT Study Group. Acta Oncol 1990; 29:9–15.
4. Christensen SB, Ljungberg O, Tibblin S. A clinical epidemiologic study of thyroid carcinoma in Malmo, Sweden. Curr Probl Cancer 1984; 8:1–49.
5. Bondeson L, Ljungberg O. Occult thyroid carcinoma at autopsy in Malmo, Sweden. Cancer 1981; 47:319–323.
6. Bhattacharyya N. A population-based analysis of survival factors in differentiated and medullary thyroid carcinoma. Otolaryngol Head Neck Surg 2003; 128:115–123.
7. Negri E, Ron E, Franceschi S, et al. Risk factors for medullary thyroid carcinoma: a pooled analysis. Cancer Causes Control 2002; 13:365–372.
8. Mulligan LM, Kwok JBJ, Healey CS, et al. Germline mutations of the RET proto-oncogene in multiple endocrine neoplasia type 2A (MEN 2A). Nature 1993; 363:458–460.
9. Donis-Keller H, Shenshen D, Chi D, et al. Mutations in the RET proto-oncogene are associated with MEN 2A and FMTC. Hum Mol Genet 1993; 2:851–856.
10. Mulligan MN, Marsh DJ, Robinson BG, et al. Genotype-phenotype correlation in multiple endocrine neoplasia type 2: report of the international RET mutation consortium. J Intern Med 1995; 238:343–346.
11. Machens A, Niccoli-Sire P, Hoegel J, et al.; European Multiple Endocrine Neoplasia (EUROMEN) Study Group. Early malignant progression of hereditary medullary thyroid cancer. N Engl J Med 2003; 349:1517–1525.
12. Niccoli-Sire P, Murat A, Baudin E, et al. Early or prophylactic thyroidectomy in MEN 2/FMTC gene carriers: results in 71 thyroidectomized patients. The French Calcitonin Tumours Study Group (GETC). Eur J Endocrinol 1999; 141:468–474.
13. Sanso GE, Domene HM, Garcia R, et al. Very early detection of RET proto-oncogene mutation is crucial for preventive thyroidectomy in multiple endocrine neoplasia type 2 children: presence of C-cell malignant disease in asymptomatic carriers Cancer. 2002; 94:323–330.

14. Christensen SB, Ljungberg O. Mortality from thyroid carcinoma in Malmo, Sweden 1960–1977. A clinical and pathologic study of 38 fatal cases. Cancer 1984; 54: 1629–1634.

15. Gharib H, McConahey WM, Tiegs RD, et al. Medullary thyroid carcinoma: clinicopathologic features and long-term follow-up of 65 patients treated during 1946 through 1970. Mayo Clin Proc 1992; 67:934–940.

16. Kebebew E, Ituarte PH, Siperstein AE, Duh QY, Clark OH. Medullary thyroid carcinoma: clinical characteristics, treatment, prognostic factors, and a comparison of staging systems. Cancer 2000; 88:1139–1148.

17. Keiser HR, Beaven MA, Doppman J, et al. Sipple's syndrome: medullary thyroid carcinoma, pheochromocytoma, and hyperparathyroidism. Ann Intern Med 1973; 78:561–579.

18. Cunliffe WJ, Hudgson P, Fulthorpe JJ, et al. A calcitonin-secreting medullary thyroid carcinoma associated with mucosal neuromas, marfanoid features, myopathy and pigmentation. Am J Med 1970; 48:120–126.

19. Farndon JR, Leight GS, Dilley WG, et al. Familial medullary thyroid carcinoma without associated endocrinopathies: a distinct clinical entity. Br J Surg 1986; 73:278–281.

20. Eng C, Mulligan LM, Smith DP, et al. Low frequency of germline mutations in the RET proto-oncogene in patients with apparently sporadic medullary thyroid carcinoma. Clin Endocrinol (Oxf). 1995; 43:123–127.

21. Wiench M, Wygoda Z, Gubala E, et al. Estimation of risk of inherited medullary thyroid carcinoma in apparent sporadic patients. J Clin Oncol 2001; 19:1374–1380.

22. Block MA, Jackson CE, Greenawald KA, et al. Clinical characteristics distinguishing hereditary from sporadic medullary thyroid carcinoma. Arch Surg 1980; 115:142–148.

23. Baylin SB, Gann DS, Hsu SH. Clonal origin of inherited medullary thyroid carcinoma and pheochromocytoma. Science 1976; 193:321–323.

24. Wolfe HJ, DeLellis RA. Familial medullary thyroid carcinoma and C-cell hyperplasia. Baillières Clin Endocrinol Metab 1981; 10:351–365.

25. Cirafici AM, Salvatore G, De Vita G, et al. Only the substitution of methionine 918 with a threonine and not with other residues activates RET transforming potential. Endocrinology 1997; 138:1450–1455.

26. Carlomagno F, Salvatore G, Cirafici AM, et al. The different RET-activating capability of mutations of cysteine 620 or cysteine 634 correlates with the multiple endocrine neoplasia type 2 disease phenotype. Cancer Res 1997; 57:391–395.

27. Eng C, Clayton D, Schuffenecker I, et al. The relationship between specific RET proto-oncogene mutations and disease phenotype in multiple endocrine neoplasia type 2. International RET mutation consortium analysis. JAMA 1996; 276:1575–1579.

28. Niccoli-Sire P, Murat A, Rohmer V, et al.; French Calcitonin Tumors Group (GETC). Familial medullary thyroid carcinoma with noncysteine ret mutations: phenotype-genotype relationship in a large series of patients. J Clin Endocrinol Metab 2001; 86:3746–53.

29. Brandi ML, Gagel RF, Angeli A, et al. Guidelines for diagnosis and therapy of MEN type 1 and type 2. J Clin Endocrinol Metab 2001; 86:5658–5671.

30. Carney JA, Roth SI, Heath H III, Sizemore GW, Hayles AB. The parathyroid glands in multiple endocrine neoplasia type 2b. Am J Pathol 1980; 99:387–398.

31. Williams ED, Pollok DJ. Multiple mucosal neuromata with endocrine tumours: a syndrome allied to Von Recklinghausen's disease. J Pathol Bacteriol 1966; 91: 71–80.

32. Carney JA, Sizemore GW, Hayles AV. C-cell disease of the thyroid gland in multiple endocrine neoplasia type 2b. Cancer 1979; 44:2173–2183.

33. Rashid M, Khairi MR, Dexter RN, Burzynski NJ, Johnston CC Jr. Mucosal neuroma, pheochromocytoma and medullary thyroid carcinoma: multiple endocrine neoplasia type 3. Medicine (Baltimore) 1975; 54:89–112.

34. Gagel RF, Levy ML, Donovan DT, Alford BR, Wheeler T, Tschen JA. The association of multiple endocrine neoplasia, type 2a and cutaneous lichen amyloidosis. Ann Intern Med 1990; 112:551–552.

35. Ceccherini I, Romei C, Barone V, et al. Identification of the Cys634→Tyr mutation of the RET proto-oncogene in a pedigree with multiple endocrine neoplasia type 2A and localized cutaneous lichen amyloidosis. J Endocrinol Invest 1994; 17:201–204.

36. Pacini F, Fontanelli M, Fugazzola L, et al. Routine measurement of serum calcitonin in nodular thyroid diseases allows the preoperative diagnosis of unsuspected sporadic medullary thyroid carcinoma. Clin Endocrinol Metab 1994; 78:826–829.

37. Rieu M, Lame MC, Richard A, et al. Prevalence of sporadic medullary thyroid carcinoma: the importance of routine measurement of serum calcitonin in the diagnostic evaluation of thyroid nodules. Clin Endocrinol (Oxf) 1995; 42:453–460.

38. Niccoli P, Wion-Barbot N, Caron P, et al. Interest of routine measurement of serum calcitonin: study in a large series of thyroidectomized patients. The French Medullary Study Group. J Clin Endocrinol Metab 1997; 82:338–341.

39. Vierhapper H, Raber W, Bieglmayer C, Kaserer K, Weinhausl A, Niederle B. Routine measurement of plasma calcitonin in nodular thyroid diseases. J Clin Endocrinol Metab 1997; 82:1589–1593.

40. Kaserer K, Scheuba C, Neuhold N, et al. C-cell hyperplasia and medullary thyroid carcinoma in patients routinely screened for serum calcitonin. Am J Surg Pathol 1998; 22:722–728.

41. Ozgen AG, Hamulu F, Bayraktar F, et al. Evaluation of routine basal serum calcitonin measurement for early diagnosis of medullary thyroid carcinoma in seven hundred seventy-three patients with nodular goiter. Thyroid 1999; 9:579–582.

42. Hahm JR, Lee MS, Min YK, et al. Routine measurement of serum calcitonin is useful for early detection of medullary thyroid carcinoma in patients with nodular thyroid diseases. Thyroid 2001; 11:73–80.

43. Karanikas G, Moameni A, Poetzi C, et al. Frequency and relevance of elevated calcitonin levels in patients with neoplastic and nonneoplastic thyroid disease and in healthy subjects. J Clin Endocrinol Metab 2004; 89:515–519.

44. Barbot N, Calmettes C, Schuffenecker I, et al. Pentagastrin stimulation test and early diagnosis of medullary thyroid carcinoma using an immunoradiometric assay of calcitonin: comparison with genetic

screening in hereditary medullary thyroid carcinoma. J Clin Endocrinol Metab 1994; 78:114–120.

45. Samaan NA, Castillo S, Schultz PN, Khalil KG, Johnston DA. Serum calcitonin after pentagastrin stimulation in patients with bronchogenic and breast cancer compared to that in patients with medullary thyroid carcinoma. J Clin Endocrinol Metab 1980; 51:237–241.

46. Ichimura T, Kondo S, Okushiba S, Morikawa T, Katoh H. A calcitonin and vasoactive intestinal peptide-producing pancreatic endocrine tumor associated with the WDHA syndrome. Int J Gastrointest Cancer 2003; 33:99–102.

47. Tommasi M, Brocchi A, Cappellini A, Raspanti S, Mannelli M. False serum calcitonin high levels using a non-competitive two-site IRMA. Endocrinol Invest 2001; 24:356–360.

48. Hodak SP, Barman KD. The calcitonin conundrum – is it time for routine measurement of serum calcitonin in patients with thyroid nodules? J Clin Endocrinol Metab 2004; 89:511–514.

49. Deftos LJ. Should serum calcitonin be routinely measured in patients with thyroid nodules – will the law answer before endocrinologists do? J Clin Endocrinol Metab 2004; 89:4768–4769.

50. Elisei R, Bottici V, Luchetti F, et al. Impact of routine measurement of serum calcitonin on the diagnosis and outcome of medullary thyroid cancer: experience in 10,864 patients with nodular thyroid disorders. J Clin Endocrinol Metab 2004; 89:163–168.

51. Ukkat J, Gimm O, Brauckhoff M, Bilkenroth U, Dralle H. Single center experience in primary surgery for medullary thyroid carcinoma. World J Surg 2004; 28:1271–1274.

52. DeLellis RA, Rule AH, Spiler I, et al. Calcitonin and carcinoembryonic antigen as tumor markers in medullary thyroid carcinoma. Am J Clin Pathol 1978; 70:587–594.

53. Kodama T. Identification of carcinoembryonic antigen in the C-cell of the normal thyroid. Cancer 1980; 45:98.

54. Jackson CE, Norum RA, Talpos GB, Feldkamp CS, Tashjian AH Jr. Clinical value of calcitonin and carcinoembryonic antigen doubling times in medullary thyroid carcinoma. Henry Ford Hosp Med J 1987; 35:120–121.

55. Jadoul M, Leo JR, Berends HH, et al. Pheochromocytoma-induced hypertensive encephalopathy revealing MEN IIa syndrome in a 13-year-old boy. Horm Metab Res 1989; 21(Suppl):46–49.

56. Lips KJ, Van der Sluys Veer J, Struyvenberg A, et al. Bilateral occurrence of pheochromocytoma in patients with the multiple endocrine neoplasia syndrome type 2A (Sipple's syndrome). Am J Med 1981; 70:1051–1060.

57. Hamilton BP, Landsberg L, Levine RJ. Measurement of urinary epinephrine in screening for pheochromocytoma in multiple endocrine neoplasia type II. Am J Med 1978; 65:1027–1032.

58. Miyauchi A, Masuo K, Ogihara T, et al. Urinary epinephrine and norepinephrine excretion in patients with medullary thyroid carcinoma and their relatives. Nippon Naibunpi Gakkai Zasshi 1982; 58:1505–1516.

59. Lenders JW, Keiser HR, Goldstein DS, et al. Plasma metanephrines in the diagnosis of pheochromocytoma. Ann Intern Med 1995; 123:101–109.

60. Weise M, Merke DP, Pacak K, Walther MM, Eisenhofer G. Utility of plasma free metanephrines for detecting childhood pheochromocytoma. J Clin Endocrinol Metab 2002; 87:1955–1960.

61. DeLellis RA, Wolfe HJ, Gagel RF, et al. Adrenal medullary hyperplasia. A morphometric analysis in patients with familial medullary thyroid carcinoma. Am J Pathol 1976; 83:177–196.

62. Carney JA, Sizemore GW, Tyce GM. Bilateral adrenal medullary hyperplasia in multiple endocrine neoplasia, type 2: the precursor of bilateral pheochromocytoma. Mayo Clin Proc 1975; 50:3–10.

63. Sisson JC, Shapiro B, Beierwaltes WH. Scintigraphy with I-131 MIBG as an aid to the treatment of pheochromocytoma in patients with the multiple endocrine neoplasia type 2 syndromes. Henry Ford Hosp Med J 1984; 32:254–261.

64. Silverberg SJ, Shane E, Jacobs TP, Siris E, Bilezikian JP. A 10-year prospective study of primary hyperparathyroidism with or without parathyroid surgery. N Engl J Med 1999; 341:1249–1255.

65. Heath H III, Sizemore GW, Carney JA. Preoperative diagnosis of occult parathyroid hyperplasia by calcium infusion in patients with multiple endocrine neoplasia type 2a. J Clin Endocrinol Metab 1976; 43:428–435.

66. Fugazzola L, Pinchera A, Luchetti F, et al. Disappearance rate of serum calcitonin after total thyroidectomy for medullary thyroid carcinoma. Int J Biol Markers 1994; 9:21–24.

67. Franc S, Niccoli-Sire P, Cohen R, et al.; French Medullary Study Group (GETC). Complete surgical lymph node resection does not prevent authentic recurrences of medullary thyroid carcinoma. Clin Endocrinol (Oxf). 2001; 55:403–409.

68. Busnardo B, Girelli ME, Simioni N, Nacamulli D, Busetto E. Nonparallel patterns of calcitonin and carcinoembryonic antigen levels in the follow-up of medullary thyroid carcinoma. Cancer 1984; 53:278–285.

69. Rougier P, Calmettes C, Laplanche A, et al. The values of calcitonin and carcinoembryonic antigen in the treatment and management of nonfamilial medullary thyroid carcinoma. Cancer 1983; 51:855–862.

70. Baudin E, Lumbroso J, Schlumberger M, et al. Comparison of octreotide scintigraphy and conventional imaging in medullary thyroid carcinoma. J Nucl Med 1996; 37:912–916.

71. Szakall S Jr, Esik O, Bajzik G, et al. 18F-FDG PET detection of lymph node metastases in medullary thyroid carcinoma. J Nucl Med 2002; 43:66–71.

72. Arslan N, Ilgan S, Yuksel D, et al. Comparison of In-111 octreotide and Tc-99m (V) DMSA scintigraphy in the detection of medullary thyroid tumor foci in patients with elevated levels of tumor markers after surgery. Clin Nucl Med 2001; 26:683–688.

73. Gotthardt M, Battmann A, Hoffken H, et al. 18F-FDG PET, somatostatin receptor scintigraphy, and CT in metastatic medullary thyroid carcinoma: a clinical study and an analysis of the literature. Nucl Med Commun 2004; 25:439–443.

74. Abdelmoumene N, Schlumberger M, Gardet P, et al. Selective venous sampling catheterisation for localisation of persisting medullary thyroid carcinoma. Br J Cancer 1994; 69:1141–1144.

75. Frank-Raue K, Raue F, Buhr HJ, Baldauf G, Lorenz D, Ziegler R. Localization of occult persisting medullary thyroid carcinoma before microsurgical reoperation: high sensitivity of selective venous catheterization. Thyroid 1992; 2:113–117.

76. Ben Mrad MD, Gardet P, Roche A, et al. Value of venous catheterization and calcitonin studies in the treatment and management of clinically inapparent medullary thyroid carcinoma. Cancer 1989; 63:133–138.

77. Soderstrom N, Telenius-Berg M, Akerman M. Diagnosis of medullary carcinoma of the thyroid by fine needle aspiration biopsy. Acta Med Scand 1975; 197:71–76.

78. Mendonca ME, Ramos S, Soares J. Medullary carcinoma of thyroid: a re-evaluation of the cytological criteria of diagnosis. Cytopathology 1991; 2:93–102.

79. Takeichi N, Ito H, Okamoto H, Matsuyama T, Tahara E, Dohi K. The significance of immunochemically staining calcitonin and CEA in fine-needle aspiration biopsy materials from medullary carcinoma of the thyroid. Jpn J Surg 1989; 19:674–678.

80. Papaparaskeva K, Nagel H, Droese M. Cytologic diagnosis of medullary carcinoma of the thyroid gland. Diagn Cytopathol 2000; 22:351–358.

81. Forrest CH, Frost FA, de Boer WB, Spagnolo DV, Whitaker D, Sterrett BF. Medullary carcinoma of the thyroid: accuracy of diagnosis of fine-needle aspiration cytology. Cancer 1998; 84:295–302.

82. Tashjian AH Jr, Melvin EW. Medullary carcinoma of the thyroid gland. Studies of thyrocalcitonin in plasma and tumor extracts. N Engl J Med 1968; 279:279–283.

83. Dube WJ, Bell GO, Aliapoulios MA. Thyrocalcitonin activity in metastatic medullary thyroid carcinoma. Further evidence for its parafollicular cell origin. Arch Intern Med 1969; 123:423–427.

84. Przepiorka D, Baylin SB, McBride OW, Testa JR, de Bustros A, Nelkin BD. The human calcitonin gene is located on the short arm of chromosome 11. Biochem Biophys Res Commun 1984; 120:493–499.

85. Hoppener JW, Steenbergh PH, Zandberg J, et al. The second human calcitonin/CGRP gene is located on chromosome 11. Hum Genet 1985; 70:259–263.

86. Zaidi M, Breimer LH, MacIntyre I. Biology of peptides from the calcitonin genes. Q J Exp Physiol 1987; 72:371–408.

87. Pacini F, Fugazzola L, Basolo F, Elisei R, Pinchera A. Expression of calcitonin gene-related peptide in medullary thyroid cancer. J Endocrinol Invest 1992; 15:539–542.

88. Schifter S, Williams ED, Craig RK, Hansen HH. Calcitonin gene-related peptide and calcitonin in medullary thyroid carcinoma. Clin Endocrinol (Oxf) 1986; 25:703–710.

89. Cooper CW, Deftos LJ, Potts JT Jr. Direct measurement of in vivo secretion of pig thyrocalcitonin by radioimmunoassay. Endocrinology 1971; 88:747–754.

90. Emmertsen KK, Nielsen HE, Mosekilde L, Hansen HH. Pentagastrin, calcium and whisky stimulated serum calcitonin in medullary carcinoma of the thyroid. Acta Radiol Oncol 1980; 19:85–89.

91. Vitale G, Ciccarelli A, Caraglia M, et al. Comparison of two provocative tests for calcitonin in medullary thyroid carcinoma: omeprazole vs pentagastrin. Clin Chem 2002; 48:1505–1510.

92. Oishi S, Yamauchi J, Fujimoto Y, Hamasaki S, Umeda T, Sato T. Calcitonin release from medullary thyroid carcinoma by thyrotropin-releasing hormone: comparison with calcium injection. Acta Endocrinol (Copenh) 1992; 126:325–328.

93. Lin HY, Harris TL, Flannery MS, et al. Expression cloning of an adenylate cyclase-coupled calcitonin receptor. Science 1991; 254:1022–1024.

94. Hoff AO, Catala-Lehnen P, Thomas PM, et al. Increased bone mass is an unexpected phenotype associated with deletion of the calcitonin gene. Clin Invest 2002; 110:1849–1857.

95. Deftos LJ, First BP. Calcitonin as a drug. Ann Intern Med 1981; 95:192–197.

96. Purdue BW, Tilakaratne N, Sexton PM. Molecular pharmacology of the calcitonin receptor. Receptors Channels 2002; 8:243–255.

97. Niccoli P, Conte-Devolx B, Lejeune PJ, et al. Hypercalcitoninemia in conditions other than medullary cancers of the thyroid, Ann Endocrinol (Paris) 1996; 57:15–21.

98. Guyetant S, Wion-Barbot N, Rousselet MC, Franc B, Bigorgne JC, Saint-Andre JP. C-cell hyperplasia associated with chronic lymphocytic thyroiditis: a retrospective quantitative study of 112 cases. Hum Pathol 1994; 25:514–521.

99. Albores-Saavedra J, Monforte H, Nadji M, Morales AR. C-cell hyperplasia in thyroid tissue adjacent to follicular cell tumors. Hum Pathol 1988; 19:795–799.

100. Tsolakis AV, Portela-Gomes GM, Stridsberg M, et al. Malignant gastric ghrelinoma with hyperghrelinemia. J Clin Endocrinol Metab 2004; 89:3739–3744.

101. Mullerpatan PM, Joshi SR, Shah RC, et al. Calcitonin-secreting tumor of the pancreas. Dig Surg 2004; 21:321–324.

102. Demers LM, Spencer CA. Laboratory medicine practice guidelines: Calcitonin (Ct) and RET proto-oncogene measurement. Thyroid 2003; 13:68–74.

103. Engelbach M, Gorges R, Forst T, Pfutzner A, et al. Improved diagnostic methods in the follow-up of medullary thyroid carcinoma by highly specific calcitonin measurements. J Clin Endocrinol Metab 2000; 85:1890–1894.

104. Baudin E, Bidart JM, Bachelot A, et al. Impact of chromogranin A measurement in the work-up of neuroendocrine tumors. Ann Oncol 2001; Suppl 2:S79–S82.

105. Barakat MT, Meeran K, Bloom SR. Neuroendocrine tumours. Endocr Relat Cancer 2004; 11:1–18.

106. Pacini F, Elisei R, Anelli S, Gasperini L, Schipani E, Pinchera A. Circulating neuron-specific enolase in medullary thyroid cancer. Int J Biol Markers 1986; 1:85–88.

107. Pacini F, Basolo F, Elisei R, Fugazzola L, Cola A, Pinchera A. Medullary thyroid cancer. An immunohistochemical and humoral study using six separate antigens. Am J Clin Pathol 1991; 95:300–308.

108. Wyon Y, Frisk J, Lundeberg T, Theodorsson E, Hammar M. Postmenopausal women with vasomotor symptoms have increased urinary excretion of calcitonin gene-related peptide. Maturitas 1998; 30:289–294.

109. Jaffe BM. Prostaglandins and serotonin: nonpeptide diarrheogenic hormones. World J Surg 1979; 3:565–578.

110. Le Douarin N, Le Lievre C. Demonstration of neural origin of calcitonin cells of ultimobranchial body of

chick embryo. C R Acad Sci Hebd Seances Acad Sci D 1970; 270:2857–2860.

111. Wolfe HJ, Voelkel EF, Tashjian AH Jr. Distribution of calcitonin-containing cells in the normal adult human thyroid gland: a correlation of morphology with peptide content. J Clin Endocrinol Metab 1974; 38:688–694.

112. Robertson K, Mason I. The GDNF-RET signalling partnership. Trends Genet 1997; 13:1–3.

113. de Lellis RA, Wolfe HJ. The pathobiology of the human calcitonin (C)-cell: a review. Pathol Annu 1981; 16(Pt2): 25–52.

114. LiVolsi VA. C cell hyperplasia/neoplasia. J Clin Endocrinol Metab 1997; 82:39–41.

115. Rosai J, Carcangiu ML, De Lellis RA. Tumors of the thyroid gland. In: Atlas of tumor pathology, 3rd series. Washington, DC: Armed Forces Institute of Pathology, 1992.

116. Perry A, Molberg K, Albores-Saavedra J. Physiologic versus neoplastic C-cell hyperplasia of the thyroid: separation of distinct histologic and biologic entities. Cancer 1996; 77:750–756.

117. Komminoth P, Roth J, Saremaslani P, Matias-Guiu X, Wolfe HJ, Heitz PU. Polysialic acid of the neural cell adhesion molecule in the human thyroid: a marker for medullary thyroid carcinoma and primary C-cell hyperplasia. An immunohistochemical study on 79 thyroid lesions. Am J Surg Pathol 1994; 18:399–411.

118. Sletten K, Westermark P, Natvig JB. Characterization of amyloid fibril proteins from medullary carcinoma of the thyroid. J Exp Med 1976; 143:993.

119. Matias-Guiu X. Mixed medullary and follicular carcinoma of the thyroid. On the search for its histogenesis. Am J Pathol 1999; 155:1413–1418.

120. Biscolla RP, Ugolini C, Sculli M, et al. Medullary and papillary tumors are frequently associated in the same thyroid gland without evidence of reciprocal influence in their biologic behavior. Thyroid 2004; 14:946–952.

121. Vantyghem MC, Pigny P, Leteurtre E, et al. Thyroid carcinomas involving follicular and parafollicular C cells: seventeen cases with characterization of RET oncogenic activation. Thyroid 2004; 14:842–847.

122. Fluge O, Haugen DR, Akslen LA, et al. Expression and alternative splicing of c-ret RNA in papillary thyroid carcinomas. Oncogene 2001; 20:885–892.

123. Elisei R, Pinchera A, Romei C, et al. Expression of thyrotropin receptor (TSH-R), thyroglobulin, thyroperoxidase, and calcitonin messenger ribonucleic acids in thyroid carcinomas: evidence of TSH-R gene transcript in medullary histotype. J Clin Endocrinol Metab 1994; 78:867–871.

124. Katoh R, Miyagi E, Nakamura N, et al. Expression of thyroid transcription factor-1 (TTF-1) in human C cells and medullary thyroid carcinomas. Hum Pathol 2000; 31:386–393.

125. Elisei R, Cosci B, Romei C, et al. Identification of a novel point mutation in the RET gene (Ala883Thr), which is associated with medullary thyroid carcinoma phenotype only in homozygous condition. J Clin Endocrinol Metab 2004; 89:5823–5827.

126. Pacini F, Romei C, Miccoli P, et al. Early treatment of hereditary medullary thyroid carcinoma after attribution of multiple endocrine neoplasia type 2 gene carrier status by screening for ret gene mutations. Surgery 1995; 118:1031–1035.

127. Santoro M, Melillo RM, Carlomagno F, Vecchio G, Fusco A. Minireview: RET: normal and abnormal functions. Endocrinology 2004; 145:5448–5451.

128. Mathew CG, Chin KS, Easton DF, et al. A linked genetic marker for multiple endocrine neoplasia type 2A on chromosome 10. Nature 1987; 328:527–528.

129. Simpson NE, Kidd KK, Goodfellow PJ, et al. Assignment of multiple endocrine neoplasia type 2A to chromosome 10 by linkage. Nature 1987; 328:528–530.

130. Eng C, Smith DP, Mulligan LM, et al. Point mutation within the tyrosine kinase domain of the RET proto-oncogene in multiple endocrine neoplasia type 2B and related sporadic tumours. Hum Mol Genet 1994; 3:237–241.

131. Machens A, Gimm O, Hinze R, Hoppner W, Boehm BO, Dralle H. Genotype-phenotype correlations in hereditary medullary thyroid carcinoma: oncological features and biochemical properties. J Clin Endocrinol Metab 2001; 86:1104–1109.

132. Gimm O, Marsh DJ, Andrew SD, et al. Germline dinucleotide mutation in codon 883 of the RET proto-oncogene in multiple endocrine neoplasia type 2B without codon 918 mutation. J Clin Endocrinol Metab 1997; 82:3902–3904.

133. Menko FH, van der Luijt RB, de Valk IA, et al. Atypical MEN type 2B associated with two germline RET mutations on the same allele not involving codon 918. J Clin Endocrinol Metab 2002; 87:393–397.

134. Schuffenecker I, Ginet N, Goldgar D, et al. Prevalence and parental origin of de novo RET mutations in multiple endocrine neoplasia type 2A and familial medullary thyroid carcinoma. Le Groupe d'Etude des Tumeurs a Calcitonine. Am J Hum Genet 1997; 60: 233–237.

135. Romei C, Elisei R, Pinchera A, et al. Somatic mutations of the ret protooncogene in sporadic medullary thyroid carcinoma are not restricted to exon 16 and are associated with tumor recurrence. J Clin Endocrinol Metab 1996; 81:1619–1622.

136. Zedenius J, Larsson C, Bergholm U, et al. Mutations of codon 918 in the RET proto-oncogene correlate to poor prognosis in sporadic medullary thyroid carcinomas. J Clin Endocrinol Metab 1995; 80:3088–3090.

137. Elisei R, Cosci B, Romei C, et al. RET exon 11 (G691S) polymorphism is significantly more frequent in sporadic medullary thyroid carcinoma than in the general population. J Clin Endocrinol Metab 2004; 89:3579–3584.

138. Gimm O, Neuberg DS, Marsh DJ, et al. Over-representation of a germline RET sequence variant in patients with sporadic medullary thyroid carcinoma and somatic RET codon 918 mutation. Oncogene 1999; 18:1369–1373.

139. Ruiz A, Antinolo G, Fernandez RM, Eng C, Marcos I, Borrego S. Germline sequence variant S836S in the RET proto-oncogene is associated with low level predisposition to sporadic medullary thyroid carcinoma in the Spanish population. Clin Endocrinol (Oxf) 2001; 55:399–402.

140. Jimenez C, Gagel RF. Genetic testing in endocrinology: lessons learned from experience with multiple endocrine neoplasia type 2 (MEN2). Growth Horm IGF Res 2004; 14 Suppl A:S150–S157.

141. Moley JF, DeBenedetti MK. Patterns of nodal metastases in palpable medullary thyroid carcinoma: rec-

ommendations for extent of node dissection. Ann Surg 1999; 229:880–887; discussion 887–888.

142. Fleming JB, Lee JE, Bouvet M, et al. Surgical strategy for the treatment of medullary thyroid carcinoma. Ann Surg 1999; 230:697–707.

143. Machens A, Holzhausen HJ, Thanh PN, Dralle H. Malignant progression from C-cell hyperplasia to medullary thyroid carcinoma in 167 carriers of RET germline mutations. Surgery 2003; 134:425–431.

144. Dralle H, Gimm O, Simon D, et al. Prophylactic thyroidectomy in 75 children and adolescents with hereditary medullary thyroid carcinoma: German and Austrian experience. World J Surg 1998; 22:744–50; discussion 750–751.

145. Scollo C, Baudin E, Travagli JP, et al. Rationale for central and bilateral lymph node dissection in sporadic and hereditary medullary thyroid cancer. J Clin Endocrinol Metab 2003; 88:2070–2075.

146. Dralle H, Damm I, Scheumann GF, Kotzerke J, Kupsch E. Frequency and significance of cervicomediastinal lymph node metastases in medullary thyroid carcinoma: results of a compartment-oriented microdissection method. Henry Ford Hosp Med J 1992; 40:264–267.

147. Gimm O, Ukkat J, Dralle H. Determinative factors of biochemical cure after primary and reoperative surgery for sporadic medullary thyroid carcinoma. World J Surg. 1998; 22:562–567; discussion 567–568.

148. Nieuwenhuijzen Kruseman AC, Bussemaker JK, Frolich M. Radioiodine in the treatment of hereditary medullary carcinoma of the thyroid. J Clin Endocrinol Metab 1984; 59:491–494.

149. Nusynowitz ML, Pollard E, Benedetto AR, Lecklitner ML, Ware RW. Treatment of medullary carcinoma of the thyroid with I-131. J Nucl Med 1982; 23:143–146.

150. Brierley J, Tsang R, Simpson WJ, Gospodarowicz M, Sutcliffe S, Panzarella T. Medullary thyroid cancer: analyses of survival and prognostic factors and the role of radiation therapy in local control. Thyroid 1996; 6:305–310.

151. Fersht N, Vini L, A'Hern R, Harmer C. The role of radiotherapy in the management of elevated calcitonin after surgery for medullary thyroid cancer. Thyroid 2001; 11:1161–1168.

152. Fife KM, Bower M, Harmer CL. Medullary thyroid cancer: the role of radiotherapy in local control. Eur J Surg Oncol 1996; 22:588–591.

153. Assalia A, Gagner M. Laparoscopic adrenalectomy. Br J Surg 2004; 91:1259–1274.

154. Kocak S, Aydintug S, Canakci N. Alpha blockade in preoperative preparation of patients with pheochromocytomas. Int Surg 2002; 87:191–194.

155. Cubeddu LX, Zarate NA, Rosales CB, Zschaeck DW. Prazosin and propranolol in preoperative management of pheochromocytoma. Clin Pharmacol Ther 1982; 32:156–160.

156. Sokoll LJ. Measurement of parathyroid hormone and application of parathyroid hormone in intraoperative monitoring. Clin Lab Med 2004; 24:199–216.

157. Niederle B, Roka R, Brennan MF. The transplantation of parathyroid tissue in man: development, indications, technique, and results. Endocr Rev 1982; 3:245–79.

158. Moley JF, Wells SA, Dilley WG, Tisell LE. Reoperation for recurrent or persistent medullary thyroid cancer. Surgery 1993; 114:1090–1095; discussion 1095–1096.

159. Jackson CE, Talpos GB, Kambouris A, Yott JB, Tashjian AH Jr, Block MA. The clinical course after definitive operation for medullary thyroid carcinoma. Surgery 1983; 94:995–1001.

160. Tisell LE, Hansson G, Jansson S, Salander H. Reoperation in the treatment of asymptomatic metastasizing medullary thyroid carcinoma. Surgery 1986; 99:60–66.

161. Orlandi F, Caraci P, Mussa A, Saggiorato E, Pancani G, Angeli A. Treatment of medullary thyroid carcinoma: an update. Endocr Relat Cancer 2001; 8:135–147.

162. Schlumberger M, Abdelmoumene N, Delisle MJ, Couette JE. Treatment of advanced medullary thyroid cancer with an alternating combination of 5 FU-streptozocin and 5 FU-dacarbazine. The Groupe d'Etude des Tumeurs a Calcitonine (GETC). Br J Cancer 1995; 71: 363–365.

163. Nocera M, Baudin E, Pellegriti G, Cailleux AF, Mechelany-Corone C, Schlumberger M. Treatment of advanced medullary thyroid cancer with an alternating combination of doxorubicin-streptozocin and 5 FU-dacarbazine. Groupe d'Etude des Tumeurs Ã Calcitonine (GETC). Br J Cancer. 2000; 83:715–718.

164. Lupoli GA, Fonderico F, Fittipaldi MR, et al. The role of somatostatin analogs in the management of medullary thyroid carcinoma. J Endocrinol Invest 2003; 26(8 Suppl): 72–74.

165. Zatelli MC, Tagliati F, Taylor JE, Piccin D, Culler MD, degli Uberti EC. Somatostatin, but not somatostatin receptor subtypes 2 and 5 selective agonists, inhibits calcitonin secretion and gene expression in the human medullary thyroid carcinoma cell line, TT. Horm Metab Res 2002; 34:229–233.

166. Zatelli MC, Tagliati F, Piccin D, et al. Somatostatin receptor subtype 1-selective activation reduces cell growth and calcitonin secretion in a human medullary thyroid carcinoma cell line. Biochem Biophys Res Commun 2002; 297:828–834.

167. Papotti M, Kumar U, Volante M, Pecchioni C, Patel YC. Immunohistochemical detection of somatostatin receptor types 1–5 in medullary carcinoma of the thyroid. Clin Endocrinol (Oxf) 2001; 54:641–649.

168. Mukherjee JJ, Kaltsas GA, Islam N, et al. Treatment of metastatic carcinoid tumours, phaeochromocytoma, paraganglioma and medullary carcinoma of the thyroid with (131)I-meta-iodobenzylguanidine [(131)I-mIBG]. Clin Endocrinol (Oxf) 2001; 55:47–60.

169. Kaltsas G, Rockall A, Papadogias D, Reznek R, Grossman AB. Recent advances in radiological and radionuclide imaging and therapy of neuroendocrine tumours. Eur J Endocrinol 2004; 151:15–27.

170. Kraeber-Bodere F, Faivre-Chauvet A, Ferrer L, et al. Pharmacokinetics and dosimetry studies for optimization of anti-carcinoembryonic antigen x anti-hapten bispecific antibody-mediated pretargeting of iodine-131-labeled hapten in a phase I radioimmunotherapy trial. Clin Cancer Res 2003; 9:3973S–3981S.

171. Bodei L, Handkiewicz-Junak D, Grana C, et al. Receptor radionuclide therapy with 90Y-DOTATOC in patients with medullary thyroid carcinomas. Cancer Biother Radiopharm 2004; 19:65–71.

172. Roche A, Girish BV, de Baere T, et al. Trans-catheter arterial chemoembolization as first-line treatment for hepatic metastases from endocrine tumors. Eur Radiol 2003; 13:136–140.

173. Drosten M, Putzer BM. Gene therapeutic approaches for medullary thyroid carcinoma treatment. J Mol Med 2003; 81:411–419.

174. DeGroot LJ, Zhang R. Viral mediated gene therapy for the management of metastatic thyroid carcinoma. Curr Drug Targets Immune Endocr Metabol Disord 2004; 4: 235–244.

175. Stift A, Sachet M, Yagubian R, et al. Dendritic cell vaccination in medullary thyroid carcinoma. Clin Cancer Res 2004; 10:2944–2953.

176. Maio M, Coral S, Sigalotti L, et al. Analysis of cancer/testis antigens in sporadic medullary thyroid carcinoma: expression and humoral response to NY-ESO-1. J Clin Endocrinol Metab 2003; 88:748–754.

177. Gschwind A, Fischer OM, Ullrich A. The discovery of receptor tyrosine kinases: targets for cancer therapy. Nat Rev Cancer 2004; 4:361–370.

178. Mughal TI, Goldman JM. Chronic myeloid leukemia: current status and controversies. Oncology (Huntingt) 2004; 18:837–844.

179. Tanovic A, Alfaro V. Gefitinib: current status in the treatment of non-small cell lung cancer. Drugs Today (Barc) 2004; 40:809–827.

180. Bates D. ZD-6474. AstraZeneca Curr Opin Investig Drugs 2003; 4:1468–1472.

181. Ciardiello F, Caputo R, Damiano V, et al. Antitumor effects of ZD6474, a small molecule vascular endothelial growth factor receptor tyrosine kinase inhibitor, with additional activity against epidermal growth factor receptor tyrosine kinase. Clin Cancer Res 2003; 9:1546–1556.

182. Carlomagno F, Vitagliano D, Guida T, et al. ZD6474, an orally available inhibitor of KDR tyrosine kinase activity, efficiently blocks oncogenic RET kinases. Cancer Res 2002; 62:7284–7290.

22

Nonmedullary Thyroid Cancer and the Role of the Geneticist

Sanjay Popat and Richard S. Houlston

Genetics of Nonmedullary Thyroid Cancer

Introduction

The overall incidence of thyroid cancer in the UK is around 0.7 per 100 000 in males and 1.9 per 100 000 in females (http://www.cancerresearchuk.org/aboutcancer/statistics/). The most common form of thyroid cancer is nonmedullary thyroid cancer (NMTC). This accounts for ~90% of all cases and originates in the follicular cells, which synthesize and secrete thyroxine. NMTC has two major subtypes, follicular (FTC) and papillary (PTC). These two biologically distinct groups of tumors arise from the normal follicular cell, and multiple stages in transformation can be identified in both, culminating rarely in the highly aggressive anaplastic carcinoma [1].

A familial predisposition to medullary thyroid carcinoma (MTC) is recognized in about 25% of all cases, and is due to activating mutations in the *RET* oncogene [2]. Understanding the molecular genetics of MTC as well as multiple endocrine neoplasia syndromes (MEN) 2A and 2B has revolutionized the clinical approach to these patients, both in terms of managing their familial risks, and in terms of screening for related cancers.

Until recently, NMTC had not been considered to have a familial basis. However, there is now increasing evidence that a proportion of cases can be attributed to an underlying inherited susceptibility. Although most NMTCs are sporadic, familial NMTC, and familial PTC in particular, is well recognized. Familial NMTC and can be arbitrarily dichotomized into cancer predisposition syndrome-associated and non-syndromic variants. Whilst disease-causing alleles have been identified for a proportion of such syndromic familial PTCs, no such alleles have been unequivocally identified for the majority of cases of familial PTC or indeed familial NMTC, and remain a focus on ongoing research.

The molecular genetics and management of patients with MTC have been covered elsewhere in this book. In this chapter, we concentrate on the molecular genetics underlying the inherited predisposition to NMTC. We then go on to review the role of the clinical geneticist with respect to cancer families, and give special reference to NMTC families.

Evidence for a Genetic Predisposition to Nonmedullary Thyroid Cancer

A number of epidemiological studies have investigated the risk of malignancy associated with a family history of thyroid cancer (Table 22.1). Ron et al. [3] performed a small case-control study of 159 cases and 285 controls, and demonstrated an odds ratio (OR) of 5 for a

Table 22.1 Familial risks of thyroid and other cancers in epidemiological studies

Author	First site	Second site	Relative risk (95% CI)
Stoffer et al. [4]	Thyroid	Thyroid	4.7 (2.0–9.3)
Ron et al. [3]	Thyroid	Thyroid	5.2 (0.2–544)
Goldgar et al. [6]	Thyroid	Thyroid	8.6 (4.7–13.8)
Pal et al. [5]	Thyroid	Thyroid	10.3 (2.2–47.6)
Hemminki et al. [7]	Thyroid (PTC or FTC)	Thyroid (PTC or FTC) in sons	7.8 (3.9–13.2)
Hemminki et al. [7]	Thyroid (PTC or FTC)	Thyroid (PTC or FTC) in daughters	2.8 (1.5–4.5)
Hemminki et al. [7]	Thyroid (anaplastic)	Thyroid (anaplastic) in sons	239 (86.2–469)
Hemminki et al. [7]	Thyroid (anaplastic)	Thyroid (anaplastic) in daughters	168 (66.4–315)
Hemminki et al. [8]	Thyroid (PTC)	Thyroid (PTC)	4.2 (1.9–8.1)
Pal et al. [5]	Thyroid	Breast	1.7 (1.0–3.0)
Pal et al. [5]	Thyroid	Hormone-related cancers[a]	1.8 (1.2–2.7)
Ron et al. [3]	Breast	Thyroid	1.2 (0.6–2.6)
Peto et al. [10]	Breast	Thyroid	1.7 (0.7–3.4)
Goldgar et al. [6]	Thyroid	Soft tissue	2.9 (0.9–4.0)
	Thyroid	Lymphocytic leukemia	2.7 (1.1–5.5)
	Thyroid	Prostate	1.4 (1.1–1.9)
	Thyroid	Breast	1.7 (1.3–2.2)
Goldgar et al. [6]	Breast	Thyroid	1.7 (1.3–2.2)
	Larynx	Thyroid	3.0 (0.8–7.9)
	Lymphocytic leukemia	Thyroid	2.4 (0.9–6.5)
	Soft tissue	Thyroid	2.8 (0.9–6.5)
Hemminki et al. [7]	Breast	Thyroid	1.1 (0.9–1.3)

CI, confidence interval; FTC, follicular thyroid cancer; PTC, papillary thyroid cancer.
[a] Defined by the authors as breast, ovarian, endometrial, or prostate cancers.

family history of NMTC. Similarly, a systematic analysis of families of 222 consecutive PTC patients by Stoffer et al. [4] demonstrated that up to 6% of patients reported a first-degree relative with cancer, with a fivefold increased risk in first-degree relatives.

In a hospital-based case-control study, Pal et al. [5] identified 339 unselected patients with NMTC and 319 unaffected ethnically matched controls. Family histories of cancer were obtained from cases, controls, and 3292 first-degree relatives. At least one first-degree relative with thyroid cancer was observed in 17 of the cases (5.0%) and two of the controls (0.6%), resulting in a relative risk of 10.3. In these 17 familial cases, none of the pedigrees were consistent with known familial cancer syndromes.

In order to overcome the potential biases encountered in studies of familial risk (e.g. criteria for selection of probands, method of determining cancer frequency in relatives), two large, population-based analyses have been performed. In the first, Goldgar et al. [6] used the Utah Population Database resource to systematically study familial clustering among 399 786 first-degree relatives of index cancer patients. This analysis demonstrated a ninefold increase

in risk of thyroid cancer, the highest of a number of cancers studied in this cohort.

The second population-based analysis was performed by Hemminki et al. [7], who analyzed the Swedish cancer registry, a database of cases based on compulsory notification estimated to be at near 100% completeness. Relative risks were calculated from the data, which included 2435 thyroid cancers among offspring. Seventy-eight families were identified in which both a parent and offspring had thyroid cancer. The relative risks for papillary and follicular cancers combined were 7.8 and 2.8, for male and female cancers, respectively, giving a sex ratio of 2.8. Restricting analysis to families in which parents and offspring developed the same type of thyroid cancer, the relative risks for all PTCs and FTCs combined were 7.8 and 2.8, for sons and daughters, respectively. Whilst the relative risks for concordant anaplastic cancers were reported as 239 and 168, for sons and daughters, respectively, compared to parents, this may have been biased, since medullary cancers were likely to have been reported as anaplastic in the dataset pre-1985. Intriguingly, this study also demonstrated that the risk of NMTC in relatives of MTC cases is similarly elevated to that observed in relatives of NMTC cases, suggesting that part of the familial risk of all thyroid cancers has a common etiology.

Hemminki et al. [8] have further reported from this population registry, and assessed the relative risks for a number of common cancers occurring both in parents or offspring. Analysis of all thyroid cancers demonstrated a risk of 7.5, and in PTCs in which the same disease occurred in offspring and parent the relative risk was 4.2.

Whilst these analyses have clearly demonstrated an increased familial risk for thyroid cancer, some have also assessed the association between thyroid cancer and other types of cancer (Table 22.1). In the study by Pal et al. [5], an increased relative risk (RR) of breast cancer and an increased risk of hormone-related cancers, defined by the authors as breast, ovarian, endometrial, or prostate cancers, was observed (RR = 1.7 and 1.8, respectively). No other significant associations were detected. Further support of an association between breast and thyroid malignancies has come from the smaller case-control and cohort studies of Ron et al. [9] and Peto et al. [10].

The two population-based analyses have also assessed these relationships. Goldgar et al [6] identified a relationship between thyroid cancer and cancers at other sites, principally with breast cancer. The risk of breast cancer in relatives of thyroid cancer patients in this study was increased twofold. However, this association was not observed in the Swedish dataset [7], where the relative risk of all types of thyroid cancer in offspring of mothers with breast cancer was 1.1 (0.9–1.3).

Although the association between thyroid and other cancers, such as breast cancer in particular, remains equivocal, a true association might reflect the pleiotropic effects of an inherited predisposition, with a susceptibility allele accounting for cancer at several sites. A good example of this phenomenon is Li–Fraumeni syndrome, in which *TP53* germline mutations cause soft tissue sarcomas, leukemia, and brain and breast cancers [11].

Cancer Predisposition Syndrome-Associated Nonmedullary Thyroid Cancer

A number of families have been reported which show clustering of PTC and other NMTCs. Review of these reports suggests that NMTCs can be arbitrarily divided into two groups: a syndromic variant, in which NMTC is associated with other cancers in the context of a cancer predisposition syndrome, and a non-syndromic variant, in which NMTC is independent of an accompanying disorder. We first focus on syndromes associated with NMTC.

Familial Adenomatous Polyposis: Role of APC

Familial adenomatous polyposis (FAP) is an autosomal dominantly inherited disease, affecting around 1 in 8000 of the population. It is characterized by the presence of florid polyposis of the colorectum, and the inevitable development of colorectal cancer if left untreated. The disease was first described with clear dominant inheritance by Lockhart-Mummery in 1925 [12]. The clinical diagnosis of FAP depends on detection of hundreds to thousands of adenomatous polyps in the colon and rectum of affected individuals. Polyps usually appear by adolescence or the third decade of life and if untreated, colorectal cancer usually develops by the early forties. Annual colonoscopy is therefore indicated from adolescence, followed by prophylactic colectomy or proctocolectomy to eliminate the risk of colorectal cancer [13]. FAP is caused by germline mutations in the adenomatous polyposis coli (*APC*) gene, which maps to chromosome 5q21 [14–16].

Although principally associated with colorectal cancers, a number of extracolonic malignancies associated with FAP are recognized. Gardner's syndrome refers to the association of colonic polyps with epidermoid skin cysts and benign mandibular or long bone osteoid tumors [17], whilst Turcot's syndrome refers to the association of colonic polyps with cerebellar medulloblastoma [18,19]. Desmoids (benign fibromatosis) are also seen in FAP patients and are a significant cause of morbidity and mortality [20]. They usually arise in the abdominal wall or bowel mesentery, and commonly recur after surgical resection. Other malignancies associated with the FAP phenotype include hepatoblastoma [21,22] and PTC.

An association between FAP and thyroid cancer was first described by Crail in 1949 [23], and since then over 50 other cases have been reported (Table 22.2). The great majority (over 90%) of cases reported have been PTCs, usually detected within 10 years of a diagnosis of FAP. Although thyroid cancer has a female

Table 22.2 Reported associations of familial adenomatous polyposis coli (FAP) and thyroid cancer

Authors	Sex	Age Thyroid cancer	Age FAP	Thyroid cancer histology
Crail [23]	M	24	24	Papillary
Ogata et al. [90]	M	31	–	Adenocarcinoma
Raynham and Louw [91]	F	20	20	?[a]
Smith [92]	M	29	39	Papillary[a]
		–	–	?
		–	–	?
Camiel et al. [93]	F	19	28	Papillary
	F	20	29	Papillary[a]
Smith and Kern [94]	F	–	–	?
	F	–	–	?
	–	–	–	?
	–	–	–	?
Mathias and Smith [95]	F	<30	–	Papillary
Keshgegian and Enterline [96]	F	21	14	Papillary[a]
Takahashi et al. [97]	M	58	–	Papillary
Ida et al. [98]	M	26	–	?
	F	26	–	?
Ushio et al. [99]	M	27	–	?
Harada et al. [100]	F	22	–	Papillary
Okamura et al. [101]	F	29	–	Papillary
Hamilton et al. [102]	F	18	17	Papillary
Miura et al. [103]	F	27	–	?
Lee and MacKinnon [104]	F	23	32	Papillary[a]
Delamarre et al. [105]	F	21	27	Follicular
Thompson et al. [106]	F	34	22	Papillary[a]
Schneider et al. [107]	F	37	33	Papillary
Masuyama et al. [108]	F	26	–	Papillary
Plail et al. [24]	F	22	21	Papillary[a]
	F	26	19	Papillary[a]
	F	34	31	Papillary
	F	23	27	Papillary[a]
	F	20	20	?[a]
	F	16	28	?
	F	34	17	?
Piffer [109]	F	26	24	Follicular[a]
	F	28	–	Papillary
	F	55	–	?
Delamarre et al. [110]	F	29	16	Papillary[a]
	F	19	17	Papillary[a]
Bulow et al. [25]	F	19	17	Papillary
	F	–	–	Papillary
	F	40	26	Papillary
van Erpecum et al. [111]	F	34	31	Papillary
Herrera et al. [112]	F	27	23	Papillary
	F	–	–	Papillary
Ono et al. [113]	F	50	50	Follicular
Bell and Mazzaferri [114]	F	24	24	Papillary
Giardiello et al. [26]	M	29	–	
	F	27	–	
	F	27	–	3 Papillary
	F	29	–	2 Papillary and follicular
	F	18	–	

[a] Multifocal.

preponderance in the general population (F/M ratio 2:1), this is more so the case in FAP-associated cancers (F/M ratio 5.8:1).

Three systematic studies have investigated the risks of thyroid cancer in FAP. In a retrospective review of 316 FAP patients on the St Mark's Hospital registry, Plail et al. [24] reported four women with PTC, and estimated a relative risk of PTC in females under 35 years of age to be 160 (95% confidence interval (CI): 44–410). A subsequent retrospective analysis of 245 patients on the Danish polyposis register [25] demonstrated two thyroid cancer cases, both in women, giving a relative risk of 100 (95% CI: 12–361). A more conservative estimate of risk of thyroid cancer was, however, demonstrated in a study of 197 FAP patients registered at Johns Hopkins Hospital [26]. Five patients with FAP developed thyroid cancer, and the relative risk, irrespective of sex or age, was around 8 (95% CI: 2.5–17.7).

Although the differences in the relative risks calculated in the above studies might be ascribed to a variety of factors including differing analytical methods, and age stratification effects in the study populations, it is likely that there results represent a true increased risk of thyroid cancer in FAP patients. Whilst the relative risk of NMTC is elevated in FAP, the overall absolute risk of developing the disease is only around 2% [27].

This association between NMTC and FAP undoubtedly implicates *APC* inactivation in sporadic thyroid carcinogenesis. However, the precise mechanism for APC inactivation remains uncertain. Although, *APC* is expressed in normal as well as malignant human thyroid tissue [28,29], loss of the *APC* wild-type allele and tumor-specific *APC* mutations were not found in a small series of PTCs associated with FAP [30], raising the possibility that epigenetic phenomena, or a dominant negative effect of the single abnormal *APC* allele may be the mechanism of pathogenesis in thyroid follicular cells. In sporadic NMTC, a failure to demonstrate mutations in *APC* in over 100 cases at a variety of stages of differentiation implies that *APC* mutations are an infrequent event in thyroid tumorigenesis [31–34]. Thus, whilst *APC* inactivation undoubtedly contributes to the development of a distinctive form of thyroid cancer seen in FAP, it is unlikely to be important in the development of thyroid cancer outside FAP.

Cowden Syndrome: Role of PTEN

Papillary or follicular thyroid carcinoma is also recognized as a manifestation of the dominantly inherited disorder Cowden syndrome [35,36]. Cowden syndrome is a complex disorder of malignant and benign (hamartomatous) lesions affecting derivatives of all three germ layers [37], affecting around 1 in 200 000 of the population [38]. It is characterized by multiple hamartomas, macrocephaly, trichilemmomas, as well as a high risk of both benign and malignant cancers of the thyroid, breast, uterus, and skin.

When defined by strict operational diagnostic criteria, around 80% of Cowden syndrome is thought to be due to pathogenic mutations in *PTEN*, a tumor suppressor that maps to chromosome 10q23 [39]. A wide spectrum of phenotypes are observed, with considerable overlap with that of Bannayan–Riley–Ruvalcaba syndrome (characterized by macrocephaly, lipomatosis, hemangiomatosis, and pigmented glans penis macules).

The lifetime risk for breast cancer in Cowden syndrome is around 40% [37,40], and the risk for thyroid cancer is around 10% [36,37]. These thyroid cancers are typically follicular, but occasionally papillary. Benign thyroid abnormalities such as adenomatous goiter and hyper- or hypothyroidism are common, and a variety of benign tumors of muscular and neuronal origin have been described. Because Cowden syndrome is rare, the overall contribution of the disorder to the total burden of thyroid cancer is small.

Thyroid Cancer with Other Syndromic Associations

Thyroid cancer has been anecdotally reported in association with a number of other cancer-predisposing syndromes including ataxia telangiectasia (AT) [41], Peutz–Jeghers syndrome [42], and hereditary non-polyposis colorectal cancer (HNPCC). Systematic studies have, however, failed to show that PTC forms part of the spectrum of HNPCC [43,44]. Similarly, a systematic study of Peutz–Jeghers patients did not show an increased risk of thyroid cancer [45]. In a study of 110 AT families reported by Swift et al. [46], a 2.7-fold increase in risk of thyroid cancer was seen in AT heterozygotes, albeit nonsignificantly (95% CI 0.7–6.8). Other studies, however, have failed to established an increased risk of thyroid cancer in AT [47,48].

Non-Syndromic Familial Nonmedullary Thyroid Cancer

In addition to an association with readily identifiable cancer predisposition syndromes such as FAP, a number of families with non-syndromic clustering of thyroid cancers (primarily PTCs) have been described (Table 22.3).

Although on first inspection it might be thought that familial clustering is secondary to ascertainment bias, this is statistically highly unlikely. For example, a nuclear family with two offspring with NMTC (e.g. the family reported by Lote et al. [49]) would be expected to occur by chance alone less than once every 100 years. Furthermore, analysis of the familial cases has shown a marked excess of bilateral and multiple primary or multicentric cancer, compatible with an inherited predisposition. In addition, nodal involvement and distant spread are frequent at the time of presentation, suggesting an aggressive phenotype. There is also evidence of sex limitation, with a preponderance of female cases, and a number of the published pedigrees are consistent with vertical transmission of thyroid cancer.

NMTC in Association with Benign Thyroid Disease: Role of MNG1

There is evidence that some forms of NMTC may be caused by a predisposition to developing multinodular goiter (MNG) or other forms of benign thyroid disease. A high incidence of benign thyroid disease was documented in a number of families segregating NMTC [4]. This is supported by systematic studies of risks of thyroid disease in cancer in relatives of patients with NMTC. The risk of benign thyroid disease is increased three- to fourfold in relatives of patients with thyroid disease or NMTC [50,51]. Furthermore, the risk of NMTC is elevated up to fivefold in individuals with a history of benign thyroid disease [3,52]. Based on a survey of 159 patients, Ron et al. [3] estimated that about 20% of thyroid cancers are attributable to a prior history of benign thyroid disease. Taken

together, these observations suggest the existence of relatively common disease-causing alleles conferring a high risk of benign thyroid disease (usually nonfunctioning adenomatous goiter), but a moderate risk of invasive disease. Although the underlying basis of this remains unclear, this hypothesis is concordant with the observation that chronic iodine-deficient diets can lead to thyroid cancer through stages of follicular hyperplasia, hypertrophy, nodule, and adenoma formation [53]. It is also possible that the inherited predisposition to MNG may also mediate, in part, the association between thyroid and breast cancer, since nontoxic goiter is twice as common in women with breast cancer [54].

Based on the possibility of a common MNG and NMTC disease-predisposition, a genome-wide linkage based study of a large Canadian family segregating 18 cases of nontoxic NMG and two cases of PTC led to the identification of a locus on chromosome 14q, termed MNG1 [55]. One possible candidate gene for this locus is the thyroid-stimulating hormone receptor gene (TSHR) on chromosome 14q. This gene is somatically mutated in a proportion of hyperfunctioning thyroid follicular adenomas [56]. Whilst TSHR is within 20 Mb of MNG1, no mutations in the gene were detected in affected family members, and the recombinants between the disease and TSHR confirmed that TSHR is not MNG1 [55]. Although MNG1 appears to cause some forms of NMTC, linkage analysis in 37 small NMTC families has shown that it does not make a major contribution to the overall burden of familial NMTC [55].

PTC in Association with Papillary Renal Tumors: Role of fPTC/PRN

Malchoff et al. [57] have reported a large three-generation kindred segregating PTC in which two members had papillary renal tumors (PRN) in addition. One of these affected individuals had multifocal papillary renal adenomas [57]. In order to investigate the underlying genetic predisposition to this syndrome further, Malchoff et al. [58] performed a genome-wide linkage analysis of this family. Significant linkage to chromosome 1q21 was observed, which they termed fPTC/PRN. The deleterious allele at this locus, however, remains to be identified. Three candidate genes map to the linked chromosome

Table 22.3 Reported familial occurrence of nonmedullary thyroid cancers

Author	Proband					Relative				
	No.	M:F	Tumor type	Nodal metastasis	Radiation exposure	No.	M:F	Tumor type	Nodal metastasis	Radiation exposure
Robinson and Orr [115]	1	0:1	P	+	−	2	0:2	P	+	−
Elman [116]a	1	0:1	P	?	−	1	0:1	F	?	−
Lacour et al. [117]	1	0:1	P	+	+	1	1:0	P	+	−
Nemec et al. [118]	1	1:0	P/F	+	−	1	0:1	F	?	−
Palestro et al. [119]	1	1:0	P	?	?	1	1:0	P	?	?
Fisher and Edmonds [120]	1	1:0	P	+	+	1	1:0	P	−	+
Lote et al. [49]b	2	0:2	2P	?	−	10	3:7	9P,1?	?	−
Phade et al. [121]	1	1:0	P	?	−	2	0:2	2P	?	−
Lamberg et al. [122]	2	0:2	2M	−	?	2	1:1	2P	?	−
Flannigan et al. [123]	1	1:0	1P	+	−	1	1:0	P	+	−
Christensen et al. [50]	3	0:3	2P,P/M	?	−	3	1:2	3P	+	−
Suzuki and Watanabe [124]	1	0:1	P	+	−	2	0:2	2P	+	−
Stoffer et al. [4]	7	1:6	7P	?	?	14	4:8:2?	14P	?	?
Ozaki et al. [125]	10	1:9	10P	5+,4−,1?	−	11	1:10	7P,1?,2A,F	8+,3?	5−,6?
Austoni [126]	1	0:1	P	−	?	2	0:2	P	−	?
Dzwonkowski et al. [127]	1	1:0	P	?	?	1	0:1	P	+	?
Fischer et al. [128]	1	1:0	P	+	+	1	0:1	P	?	?
Samaan [129]	3	0:3	3P	?	?	3	0:3	3P	?	?
Szanto et al. [130]	1	0:1	P	−	?	1	0:1	P	−	?
Ron et al. [9]	4	?	?	?	?	4	2:2	?	?	?
Grossman et al.[131]	14	6:8	12P,P/F,H	8+,6−	3+,11−	16	3:2:11?	?	?	2−,2+
Takami et al. [132]	34	?	?	?	?	72a	17:55a	64P,6F,A2	61	?

A, anaplastic; P, papillary; F, follicular; M, medullary; +, present; −, absent; ?, unknown.
a Associated with familial nerve deafness and goiter; one sister with genital hypoplasia the other with endometrial carcinoma.
b Age range of cases 17–67; mean 37.6 years.

1q21 region: *NRAS*, *PRCC*, and *NTRK1*. Mutations in the exonic regions of *NRAS* or *PRCC* have not been detected [59] and *NTRK1* is unlikely to be implicated since it is expressed neither in normal thyroid tissue nor in normal thyroid tissue of patients with the familial PTC/PRN syndrome. Further work is still required to identify disease-causing alleles in the linked region.

NMTC in Association with Cell Oxyphilia: Role of *TCO*

A subset of thyroid cancers are characterized by cell oxyphilia. Oxyphilic cells are found in a minority of either benign or malignant thyroid tumors, and are characterized by a large volume of granular eosinophilic cytoplasm, and a large number of mitochondria. Oxyphilic thyroid malignancies are frequently associated with autoimmune thyroiditis. A large multigenerational family segregating six cases of MNG and three of PTC from a non-endemic-goiter area of western France [60] was used for a genome-wide linkage search [61]. Five of the cases had histology available and in four, oxyphilia was noted. Significant linkage to chromosome 19p13.2 was detected, and the locus termed *TCO* (*t*hyroid tumors with *c*ell *o*xyphilia). The pathogenic allele at this locus remains to be identified, but candidate genes include *ICAM1*.

This and other previously described predisposition loci have been comprehensively assessed by Bevan et al. [62]. They assessed 22 families segregating NMTC, all of which had a clinical diagnosis of FAP and Cowden syndrome excluded. Four established (*MNG1*, *TCO*, *fPTC*, *PTEN*) and two putative predisposition loci (*TSHR* and *TRKA*) were assessed by linkage-based methods. The latter two loci were chosen on the basis of their role in the pathogenesis of nonmalignant thyroid disease a priori [63,64]. None of the families showed significant linkage to *MNG1* or *fPTC*. One of the families did, however, show linkage to chromosome 19p13.2, providing independent confirmation of *TCO* as an NMTC predisposition locus. By contrast to the previous thyroid cancers linked to *TCO* [61], the cancers in the family reported by Bevan et al. [62] were papillary, with no suggestion of oxyphilia.

Familial PTC Alone: the Chromosome 2q21 Locus

Despite identification of the NMTC predisposition loci *TCO* [61], *MNG1* [55], *fPTC/PRN* [58] described above, the majority of familial PTC kindreds are not linked to these loci [65,66], highlighting the marked genetic heterogeneity of NMTC. McKay et al. [67] investigated this further by performing a genome-wide linkage analysis on a large Tasmanian family segregating PTC, with no cell oxyphilia, or renal malignancy. Significant linkage to chromosome 2q21 was detected, which was subsequently verified by analysis of 80 pedigrees, all again with no cell oxyphilia, or renal malignancy.

Evidence for a predisposition locus on chromosome 2q21 has been supported by loss of heterozygosity and cytogenetic studies, suggesting the existence of one or more tumor suppressor genes in this region [68,69]. Again, the causative allele at the chromosome 2q21 locus remains to be identified. Candidate genes include *ACVR2*, which has been implicated in thyroid growth, *RAB6/RALB*, members of the Ras-like family, and *LRP-DIT*. The *Pax8* gene has been implicated in NMTC carcinogenesis [70], but can be excluded from a role in carcinogenesis in the dataset assessed by McKay et al. [67], since it maps to a location centromeric to the linked region.

Familial NMTC with No Specific Clinical Association: Role of *TG*

The NMTC loci chromosome 2q21, *fPTC/PRN*, *TCO*, and *NMG1* have all been identified through analysis of single large families. Other families segregating NMTC have not shown linkage to these loci [62,65], and it is very unlikely that sequence changes at these loci will account for the majority of the familial risk. Part of the residual familial risk could be due to high penetrance mutations in as yet undefined genes. Alternatively, a polygenic mechanism could account for at least part of the familial risk. Alleles conferring relative risks of ~2.0 will rarely cause multiple-case families and are difficult or impossible to identify through linkage-based methods [71]. The search for low penetrance alleles has therefore centered on association studies based on comparing the frequency of polymorphic sequence variants in cases to controls. Variants (alleles) observed in greater frequency in cases compared to controls may be either causally related to disease risk or in linkage disequilibrium with a nearby disease-causing sequence variant [72].

Matakidou et al. [73] have published the first allelic association study of NMTC. Three hundred and four UK and Canadian NMTC cases, the great majority of which had PTC, and 400 controls were assessed at two polymorphisms in *TSHR* (P52T, and D727E) and at one sequence variant (Q2511R) in the thyroglobulin gene (*TG*). These genes were chosen on the basis of the observed linkage between *TSHR* mutations and thyroid cancer [74], and the association between level of circulating thyroglobulin and NMTC development [75]. Although no evidence of an increased risk of NMTC associated with the *TSHR* variants was detected, the *TG* Q2511R polymorphism was associated with an increased risk of 1.6 and 2.0 for hetero- and homozygotes, respectively. If confirmed by independent datasets, given that the allele frequency of the *TG* 2511 "R" allele is ~50% in Caucasians, this variant may underlie NMTC risk in around one third of all NMTC cases.

Table 22.4 Scope of clinical cancer genetics

1. Assessment of hereditary risk of cancer and options to reduce risk:
   - Identification of hereditary syndromes or patterns of inheritance predisposing to cancer
   - Assessment of risk of recurrence, additional related cancer, additional unrelated cancer to affected individuals and unrelated cancers to unaffected family members
   - Options for genetic testing, pretest counseling, posttest counseling
   - Options for screening and prevention
   - Recommendations for risk-reducing behavior
2. Genetic counseling for cancer survivors, or for their families, regarding reproductive risks:
   - Post-chemotherapy risks for sterility and teratogenicity
   - Options for prenatal diagnosis to determine genotype in known germline mutation carriers
3. Interpretation of genetic tests for the diagnosis of malignancy:
   - The ordering of appropriate genetic tests, at most suitable time point
   - Interpretation of test results
4. Interpretation of genetic tests with prognostic utility for cancer patients:
   - Selection of therapeutic approaches based on prognostic markers

The Role of the Clinical Geneticist

Scope of Cancer Genetics Clinics

Until recently, the activities in clinical cancer genetics have traditionally been confined to the management of familial cancer syndromes. With the realization that a significant proportion of most common cancers are due to an inherited predisposition, cancer genetics clinics have been established.

These clinics have a wide remit and have evolved depending on the sub-specialties of their staff. The scope of clinical cancer genetics is overviewed in Table 22.4. Although assessment of hereditary risk of cancer and options to reduce risk for unaffected relatives of probands as well as genetic counseling for patients with cancer or their families remains the mainstay of work, other areas that are increasingly becoming important are counseling regarding reproductive risks, interpretation of genetic tests for the diagnosis of malignancy, and the develop-

ment of genetic tests with prognostic utility for cancer patients.

The current provision of genetics services in the UK is based on a regional organization, with 25 local providers of clinical genetics services across the UK. The ideal cancer genetics clinic is staffed by personnel not only familiar with genetics, but also with a background in oncology, supported by counselors and psychologists. These clinics are therefore most likely to be established at joint clinics serving a geographical locality, and are likely to be staffed by clinicians in secondary or primary care, as well as other healthcare professionals.

The activities in cancer genetics cover a range of activities including the keeping of accurate personal and family records according to local and national guidelines, linking familial data via family registers, training of other healthcare professionals in guidelines for appropriate referral, the providing of a resource for research and development, as well as genetic testing and interpretation of these results. Data management is therefore crucial to the smooth running of these clinics, not only for research and audit purposes, but also for service activities such as confirming diagnoses from medical records and death certificates. In addition, liaison with a diagnostics laboratory (usually within a regional genetics service) is vital in ensuring storage, retrieval, and testing of blood and tumor samples.

Referral to Cancer Genetics Clinics

There is currently considerable variability in the threshold for referring patients to such clinics, and this is dependent not only on local policy, but on the experience of local clinicians managing patients with cancer. Since completion of sequencing the human genome, the profile of clinical genetics and cancer genetics per se has never been higher, both in terms of media interest (http://www.bbc.co.uk/genes/) and the political agenda [76]. Increasingly patients, as well as their clinicians, are recognizing that cancers may be attributable to an inherited predisposition. Due to numbers of individuals with the common cancers, it will be impossible for all patients subjectively perceived to be at risk to be seen in the secondary care setting; nor do all these individuals require such specialized services. A key role for primary care clinicians is in identifying those most in need of secondary care services. In the absence of computer-based criteria, catering for every possible familial cancer pattern, this in turn depends on high quality referral guidelines issued by the service provider.

Genetic Counseling

Genetic counseling is a term used to describe the interview that occurs when an individual attends a genetics clinic. Counseling is one of the most important features of a genetics consultation, and is based on a nondirective model, aiming to offer choices to patients. Currently, much of the initial consultation relates to the diagnosis and management of the disease, and exploration of the individual's family history. However, as preventative options become available, with the possibility of novel intervention strategies, the dynamics of this approach will undoubtedly change, and a more proscriptive approach may become evident.

Genetic counselors are degree-level healthcare professionals with training in both the psychosocial and medical aspects of inherited diseases. In most clinics this role is undertaken by both clinicians and specialist nurses, alike. Although the premise of the model for genetic counseling was primarily developed in the prenatal and pediatric setting, since this is the basis of most clinical genetics, it is equally applicable to risk counseling for adult-onset disorders. Even though the instigation of counseling may be driven by the requirement to obtain informed consent, the basic elements of the counseling process are still relevant even if the individual concerned chooses not to undergo DNA testing.

A number of definitions of genetic counseling exist, but perhaps one of the most popular is "a communication process which deals with the human problems associated with the occurrence, or risk of occurrence, of a genetic disorder in a family ... involving an attempt to help the individual or family (1) comprehend the medical facts ... and the available management; (2) appreciate the way heredity contributes to the disorder ... ; (3) understand the options for dealing with the risk of recurrence; (4) choose the course of action which seems appropriate ... ; and (5) make the best possible adjustment to the disorder" [77]. Cancer genetic counseling per se has a strong emphasis on communication, risk assessment, guidance, and support. The basic areas covered in a typical genetic counseling session are: contracting, baseline risk perception, pedigree construction, pedigree documentation, medical history, physical examination, genetic risk assessment, strategies to prevent cancer or early detection, pretest counseling, response to questions and support together with follow-up plans.

Contracting

The term "contracting" has been taken from the concept of the therapeutic contract in psychotherapy and refers to the process of interaction and alliance between the genetic counselor (e.g. doctor or nurse specialist) and the referred individual (i.e. the probands: individual affected with disease or healthy relative of affected individual). In this process the counselor elicits the proband's perceptions of the reason for the clinic attendance, and their notion of what information they intend to glean from the clinic visit. While many are referred without even a basic premise of the reason for clinic attendance, other individuals will have already have done much in the way of background reading, and have a preconceived agenda. These perceptions are then reconciled with what can actually be accomplished during the clinic visit, with an explanation of what the session will entail, and a reinforcement of the goal of working together to reach decisions.

The Family History

The establishment of the individual's family history is central in coming to a conclusion as to the risk of disease. It is therefore essential to establish a pedigree that is as accurate as possible. Since many patients will often not have clinical details of relatives that they have lost contact with, many centers routinely send a "family history questionnaire" to patients when they send the clinic appointment. Patients are then asked to return this questionnaire prior to the first consultation. This questionnaire allows individuals to document demographic details and diagnoses of first- and second-degree relatives, as well as any other relatives with a diagnosis of cancer within the extended family, prior to the initial clinic visit, thereby maximizing the information gleaned at this consultation. Family information can then be assembled into a traditional pedigree during the consultation and updated as necessary. Sending out such a questionnaire prior to the clinic appointment has a number of advantages. Not only might it save around 20 minutes of consultation time, there by increasing throughput, but it also allows probands to discuss and confirm clinical details of distant relatives with other members of the family, thereby allowing other individuals at risk of disease to think about their personal and familial risks, and their relationship to the proband's risk.

Pedigree Construction

Although traditionally regarded as a rather minor part of the new patient medical history, the accurate documentation of a proband's family history is essential to assessing risk. The family structure, including all relevant known relatives, alive and dead, should be represented

as a pedigree. The symbols commonly used to construct pedigrees are shown in Figure 22.1, and an example of the documentation of relationships between family members is represented in Figure 22.2.

Several computer-based software packages exist for the drawing of pedigrees, and the type of software used by the clinic will depend on needs. Packages available range from those that will simply draw pedigrees (PedDraw, San Antonio, TX) to those that can deal with genetic marker data and include integrated relational databases (Progeny, South Bend, IN).

Medical History and Examination

The proband should first be identified as being either an affected or unaffected individual. The past medical history should be as complete as possible, giving specific reference to known preoplastic lesions such as benign thyroid disease, goiter, adenomatous bowel polyps, and dysplastic nevi. Specific associated clinical features of cancer syndromes should be sought in either the probands, or in the cancers of the relatives. Such features might include, for example, a history of multinodular goiter, colonic polyps, epidermoid cysts, in a family segregating FAP-associated NMTC, or trichilemmomas and macrocephaly suggestive of Cowden syndrome. A personal or familial history of developmental delay might further indicate Cowden syndrome, as might a history of hamartomatous polyps or breast fibroadenomas, or uterine leiomyomas. Alternatively, a history of supernumerary or impacted teeth might indicate an underlying diagnosis of FAP, as might a history of duodenal or gastric polyps. A history of polypectomy should be investigated further by requesting histological reports, in order to assess presence of adenomatous lesions. It is, however, more likely than not, given the rarity of FAP and Cowden syndrome, that for the majority of probands presenting with an increased risk of the common cancers a previous medical history will be unremarkable.

A history of exposure to environmental risk factors should be sought. In individuals previously treated for cancer, previous treatments should be documented in order to be able to accurately assess secondary cancer risk. Previous and current levels of tobacco smoking and alcohol consumption should be clearly documented. Individuals should be questioned on symptoms indicative of cancer or underlying congenital abnormalities.

The ethnic background of all probands should also be sought, given the increased probability of deleterious alleles in individuals from particular backgrounds. For example, the I1307K allele of APC is primarily restricted to individuals of Jewish ancestry [78]. Similarly a history of consanguinity, which may be commonplace in some cultures [79], and associated with a higher than expected risk of disease, should be sought.

The type and scope of a physical examination when conducted within a genetic counseling session will entirely depend on the background of the counselor. Examination should be performed to detect an underlying malignancy or

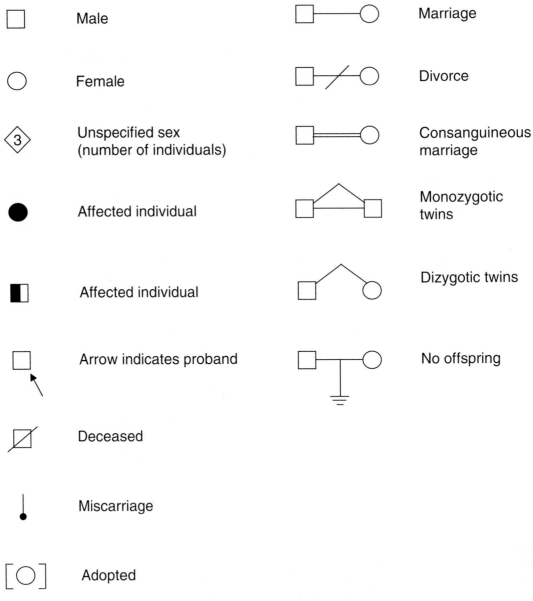

Male	Marriage
Female	Divorce
Unspecified sex (number of individuals)	Consanguineous marriage
Affected individual	Monozygotic twins
Affected individual	Dizygotic twins
Arrow indicates proband	No offspring
Deceased	
Miscarriage	
Adopted	

Figure 22.1 Symbols used for pedigree construction.

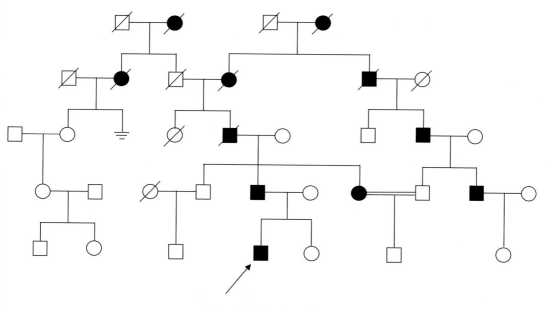

Figure 22.2 Sample pedigree.

clinical features that might suggest an inherited predisposition syndrome. For example, the skin should be fully examined in order to exclude Cowden syndrome (verrucous skin lesions of the face and limbs, lipomas, hemangiomas, and cobblestone-like hyperkeratotic papules of the gingiva and buccal mucosa) and FAP (sebaceous or epidermoid cysts). Macrocephaly (>97th percentile) should be excluded. The body should be examined for presence of desmoids, particularly the abdomen, and also for osteomas, particularly at the mandible. Primary as well as associated malignant neoplasia should be excluded. Thus, examination of the thyroid gland should be performed in order to exclude primary malignant disease, but also benign disease (e.g. multinodular goiter). Breast examination (for malignant disease and giant breast fibroadenomas in the case of Cowden syndrome) is therefore warranted. Retinal examination (for retinal gliomas in the case of Cowden syndrome, and congenital hypertrophy of the retinal pigment epithelium in the case of FAP) should also be performed.

Genetic Risk Assessment

After ascertaining the proband's perception on their personal risk, it is important to give some objective estimate of risk, based on the family history. There are considerable epidemiological data available to give a quantitative risk estimate, based on the pedigree analysis. The advantage of such data is that they are applicable to the majority of individuals referred to the clinic and have either a negligible or modestly increased risk of cancer over the general population. Some estimates of risk can be derived from models that have been validated from follow-up datasets [80–82]. More precise risk estimates may be derived after genetic testing.

Predictive Gene Testing

The decision to undertake genetic testing should not be undertaken lightly, and never without fully informed consent. Pretest counseling is required in order to deliver all the possible options to the proband, and to prepare them for the possible consequences of a test, both medical and psychological, and possibly economic. Integral to this is education about what the genetic tests themselves can deliver, and the possibility of type II error (false negative).

The consenting process should first begin with provisions for patient autonomy (the right of the individual to act freely, with adequate information). Here, information on the specific test being performed should be given, together with implications of a positive and negative result. The possibility that the test result may be inconclusive should also be highlighted. Options for the determination of genetic risk from epidemiological data, without gene testing, should be highlighted, as well as the risks of passing any mutations on to children. Second, options for medical surveillance either following or in place of testing should be discussed, as well as specific measures to reduce risk if identified as a mutation carrier.

A number of issues pertaining to non-maleficence (doing no harm) should be discussed. These include the technical accuracy of the test, and the time-scale expected for a result. The possibility of psychological distress should also be addressed, as well as the risks of discrimination, either from insurance provider or from employer. Public perception of this problem is high, and probably overly fearful [83], with a current UK moratorium on the use of genetic test results by the UK Insurance industry [84].

Finally, issues governing the notification of family members on the basis of the test result should be discussed, as well as the risks that nonpaternity may be discovered, and how this information will (or will not) be disclosed.

Risk Reduction Strategies

Physicians involved in the management of individuals at increased risk of malignancy are uniquely placed to be able to direct risk reduction strategies. These would include either a screening program in order to either prevent disease, or pick it up at an early stage, or more active measures, such as prophylactic surgery. The level of involvement that the physician wishes to maintain will vary and depend on the level of primary care responsibilities they are willing to assume. In many cases, the physician is best placed in the role of screening facilitator and coordinator.

Many probands attending clinic may be only at the population risk of cancer, and no specific risk reduction strategies would be appropriate. For others, either at moderate or high risk of future malignancy, strategies to reduce risk will depend on the underling diagnosis. However, in all cases, individuals who continue to smoke tobacco should be vehemently counseled

against this. Strategies to reduce alcohol intake should also be explored, in those in whom this is a risk factor.

For most probands, issues pertaining to risk reduction will involve cancer screening and referral to appropriate specialists or units. The role of such screening strategies should be discussed fully with patients, especially those for which no unequivocally proven benefit has been demonstrated [85]. Alternatively, these patients may be ideal candidates to recruit into studies of chemoprevention with either well-established or novel agents, and entry into such studies should be discussed.

In a minority of probands, prophylactic surgery may be considered. This strategy has been shown to be highly successful in the case of thyroidectomy [86]. However, the timing of such surgery will need to be discussed [87], as well as the risks of recurrent disease despite surgery. The opinion of a psychologist in such situations may be invaluable [88].

Clinical Management of NMTC Families

Despite the identification of a familial component to NMTCs, the recognition that some NMTCs are occasionally seen in association with rare cancer predisposition syndromes coupled with major advances in mapping predisposition loci in large NMTC-segregating families, there has been little progress in unequivocally identifying the disease-causing alleles accounting for familial NMTC outside that seen in rare cancer predisposition syndromes such as Cowden syndrome. The paucity of unequivocally identified disease-causing alleles has hampered the clinical management of familial NMTC, compared to medullary thyroid cancer, and means that germline gene testing in affected individuals in familial or early onset NMTC is limited to those in which there is a high likelihood of an underlying cancer predisposition syndrome.

Individuals with Cowden and other such syndromes should receive genetic counseling. Guidelines for diagnosis, counseling, and screening for associated disease with these syndromes are discussed elsewhere [36,89]. Families of probands should also be screened for NMTC, given their increased risk.

In patients with PTC, a family history should be extracted with special reference to family members with either NMTC or PRN. Presence of either of these should suggest a familial PTC syndrome. If such a familial PTC syndrome is identified, the first-degree relatives should be screened for underlying thyroid disease. The optimum screening method has yet to be identified. Although indicated in families with MEN2A and MEN2B, the value of prophylactic thyroidectomy has not been proven and should not routinely be recommended, not only since PTC is generally more indolent than medullary thyroid cancer, but also since no germline mutations can be unequivocally associated with affection status. There has yet to be formal consensus on the most effective screening program for PTC in high risk families. First-degree relatives of affected familial PTC kindred members should be assessed with a yearly physical examination of the thyroid gland, probably starting at the age of 20 years. The role of ultrasound monitoring of the thyroid gland may also be of use due to its greater sensitivity and ability to identify unrelated and clinically unimportant abnormalities. The role of ultrasound in screening for PRN is limited, as an increased incidence of PRN is not observed in most familial PTC kindreds. Moreover, in those kindreds segregating PTC and PRN, the frequency of PRN is far lower than that of PTC.

Finally, any size of families segregating NMTC, from affected sibling pairs upwards, should be accrued whenever possible, after host institution ethical review board approval, for gene mapping studies. If participating in such studies, and when disease-causing alleles have not been unequivocally identified, results should not influence clinical management of participating families, due to the statistical probabilities concerned and the lack of an identified mutant allele.

Summary and Conclusions

A familial component to NMTC is now well recognized. A number of families segregating NMTC outside that seen in cancer predisposition syndromes have been reported and genome-wide linkage analyses have mapped at least four predisposition loci (chromosome 2q21, fPTC/PRN, TCO, NMG1). However, the disease-causing alleles at these loci have yet to be identified. These loci are unlikely to account for the majority of the familial risk observed in relatives of NMTC cases and are unlikely to account for the majority of cases of NMTC observed. There is therefore marked genetic heterogeneity underlying the predisposition to NMTC.

A significant component of NMTC may, however, be mediated through a number of disease-causing alleles, each conferring modest risks. Association based methods have identified a polymorphic variant of TG as conferring such modestly increased risks of NMTC. Although alleles of this type confer only modest risks, due to their high frequency in the general population, they may, in fact, account for the majority of NMTC cases.

The lack of unequivocally identified disease-causing alleles has hampered the clinical management of familial NMTC. Identification of a familial component to NMTC cases, by taking a careful family history and cross-referencing cases with local cancer registries in the public domain, is clearly important. Affected individuals should be assessed by taking a good personal and family history, and by careful clinical examination, together with review of associated pathology reports for any evidence that their NMTC forms part of a cancer predisposition syndrome such as Cowden syndrome. Family members of individuals at risk should be offered thyroid screening, although the best program for this remains unclear.

References

1. Wynford-Thomas D. In vitro models of thyroid cancer. Cancer Surv 1993; 16:115–134.
2. Mulligan LM, Eng C, Healey CS, et al. Specific mutations of the RET proto-oncogene are related to disease phenotype in MEN 2A and FMTC. Nat Genet 1994; 6(1):70–74.
3. Ron E, Kleinerman RA, Boice JD, Jr, LiVolsi VA, Flannery JT, Fraumeni JF, Jr. A population-based case-control study of thyroid cancer. J Natl Cancer Inst 1987; 79(1):1–12.
4. Stoffer SS, Van Dyke DL, Bach JV, Szpunar W, Weiss L. Familial papillary carcinoma of the thyroid. Am J Med Genet 1986; 25(4):775–782.
5. Pal T, Vogl FD, Chappuis PO, et al. Increased risk for nonmedullary thyroid cancer in the first degree relatives of prevalent cases of nonmedullary thyroid cancer: a hospital-based study. J Clin Endocrinol Metab 2001; 86(11):5307–5312.

6. Goldgar DE, Easton DF, Cannon-Albright LA, Skolnick MH. Systematic population-based assessment of cancer risk in first-degree relatives of cancer probands. J Natl Cancer Inst 1994; 86(21):1600–1608.

7. Hemminki K, Dong C. Familial relationships in thyroid cancer by histo-pathological type. Int J Cancer 2000; 85(2):201–205.

8. Hemminki K, Li X. Familial risk of cancer by site and histopathology. Int J Cancer 2003; 103(1):105–109.

9. Ron E, Kleinerman RA, LiVolsi VA, Fraumeni JF, Jr. Familial nonmedullary thyroid cancer. Oncology 1991; 48(4):309–311.

10. Peto J, Easton DF, Matthews FE, Ford D, Swerdlow AJ. Cancer mortality in relatives of women with breast cancer: the OPCS Study. Office of Population Censuses and Surveys. Int J Cancer 1996; 65(3):275–283.

11. Malkin D, Li FP, Strong LC, et al. Germ line p53 mutations in a familial syndrome of breast cancer, sarcomas, and other neoplasms. Science 1990; 250(4985): 1233–1238.

12. Lockhart-Mummery A. Cancer and heredity. Lancet 1925; i:427–429.

13. Popat S, Houlston RS. Inherited susceptibility to colorectal cancer. In: Cunningham D, Topham C, Miles A (eds) The effective management of colorectal cancer. London: Aesculapius Medical Press, 2003: 3–20.

14. Bodmer WF, Bailey CJ, Bodmer J, et al. Localization of the gene for familial adenomatous polyposis on chromosome 5. Nature 1987; 328(6131):614–616.

15. Groden J, Thliveris A, Samowitz W, et al. Identification and characterization of the familial adenomatous polyposis coli gene. Cell 1991; 66(3):589–600.

16. Kinzler KW, Nilbert MC, Su LK, et al. Identification of FAP locus genes from chromosome 5q21. Science 1991; 253(5020):661–665.

17. Gardner EJ. Follow-up study of a family group exhibiting dominant inheritance for a syndrome including intestinal polyps, osteomas, fibromas and epidermal cysts. Am J Hum Genet 1962; 14:376–390.

18. Hamilton SR, Liu B, Parsons RE, et al. The molecular basis of Turcot's syndrome. N Engl J Med 1995; 332(13): 839–847.

19. Paraf F, Jothy S, Van Meir EG. Brain tumor-polyposis syndrome: two genetic diseases? J Clin Oncol 1997; 15(7):2744–2758.

20. Lotfi AM, Dozois RR, Gordon H, et al. Mesenteric fibromatosis complicating familial adenomatous polyposis: predisposing factors and results of treatment. Int J Colorectal Dis 1989; 4(1):30–36.

21. Garber JE, Li FP, Kingston JE, et al. Hepatoblastoma and familial adenomatous polyposis. J Natl Cancer Inst 1988; 80(20):1626–1628.

22. Giardiello FM, Offerhaus GJ, Krush AJ, et al. Risk of hepatoblastoma in familial adenomatous polyposis. J Pediatr 1991; 119(5):766–768.

23. Crail HW. Multiple primary malignancy arising in the rectum, brain and thyroid. Report of cases. UN Navy Med Bull 1949; 49:123–128.

24. Plail RO, Bussey HJ, Glazer G, Thomson JP. Adenomatous polyposis: an association with carcinoma of the thyroid. Br J Surg 1987; 74(5):377–380.

25. Bulow S, Holm NV, Mellemgaard A. Papillary thyroid carcinoma in Danish patients with familial adenomatous polyposis. Int J Colorectal Dis 1988; 3(1):29–31.

26. Giardiello FM, Offerhaus GJ, Lee DH, et al. Increased risk of thyroid and pancreatic carcinoma in familial adenomatous polyposis. Gut 1993; 34(10):1394–1396.

27. Houlston RS, Stratton MR. Genetics of non-medullary thyroid cancer. QJM 1995; 88(10):685–693.

28. Zeki K, Tang S-H, Gonsky R, Fagin JA. Mutations of the adenomatous polyposis coli gene in sporadic thyroid neoplasms. 65th Meeting of the American Thyroid Association 3 (Suppl), T111. 1993.

29. Horii A, Nakatsuru S, Ichii S, Nagase H, Nakamura Y. Multiple forms of the APC gene transcripts and their tissue-specific expression. Hum Mol Genet 1993; 2(3): 283–287.

30. Cetta F, Curia MC, Montalto G, et al. Thyroid carcinoma usually occurs in patients with familial adenomatous polyposis in the absence of biallelic inactivation of the adenomatous polyposis coli gene. J Clin Endocrinol Metab 2001; 86(1):427–432.

31. Curtis L, Wyllie AH, Shaw JJ, et al. Evidence against involvement of APC mutation in papillary thyroid carcinoma. Eur J Cancer 1994; 30A(7):984–987.

32. Colletta G, Sciacchitano S, Palmirotta R, et al. Analysis of adenomatous polyposis coli gene in thyroid tumours. Br J Cancer 1994; 70(6):1085–1088.

33. Varesco L, Gismondi I, De Benedetti L, Bafico A, Ferara GB. Germline and somatic mutations of adenomatous polyposis coli (APC) gene. First Italian congress on molecular oncology, abstract book, 121. 1993.

34. Zeki K, Spambalg D, Sharifi N, Gonsky R, Fagin JA. Mutations of the adenomatous polyposis coli gene in sporadic thyroid neoplasms. J Clin Endocrinol Metab 1994; 79(5):1317–1321.

35. Chen YM, Ott DJ, Wu WC, Gelfand DW. Cowden's disease: a case report and literature review. Gastrointest Radiol 1987; 12(4):325–329.

36. Pilarski R, Eng C. Will the real Cowden syndrome please stand up (again)? Expanding mutational and clinical spectra of the PTEN hamartoma tumour syndrome. J Med Genet 2004; 41(5):323–326.

37. Starink TM, van der Veen JP, Arwert F, et al. The Cowden syndrome: a clinical and genetic study in 21 patients. Clin Genet 1986; 29(3):222–233.

38. Nelen MR, van Staveren WC, Peeters EA, et al. Germline mutations in the PTEN/MMAC1 gene in patients with Cowden disease. Hum Mol Genet 1997; 6(8):1383–1387.

39. Nelen MR, Padberg GW, Peeters EA, et al. Localization of the gene for Cowden disease to chromosome 10q22–23. Nat Genet 1996; 13(1):114–116.

40. Brownstein MH, Wolf M, Bikowski JB. Cowden's disease: a cutaneous marker of breast cancer. Cancer 1978; 41(6):2393–2398.

41. Ohta S, Katsura T, Shimada M, Shima A, Chishiro H, Matsubara H. Ataxia-telangiectasia with papillary carcinoma of the thyroid. Am J Pediatr Hematol Oncol 1986; 8(3):255–257.

42. Reed MW, Harris SC, Quayle AR, Talbot CH. The association between thyroid neoplasia and intestinal polyps. Ann R Coll Surg Engl 1990; 72(6):357–359.

43. Mecklin JP, Jarvinen HJ. Tumor spectrum in cancer family syndrome (hereditary nonpolyposis colorectal cancer). Cancer 1991; 68(5):1109–1112.

44. Watson P, Lynch HT. Extracolonic cancer in hereditary nonpolyposis colorectal cancer. Cancer 1993; 71(3): 677–685.

45. Giardiello FM, Welsh SB, Hamilton SR, et al. Increased risk of cancer in the Peutz–Jeghers syndrome. N Engl J Med 1987; 316(24):1511–1514.
46. Swift M, Reitnauer PJ, Morrell D, Chase CL. Breast and other cancers in families with ataxia-telangiectasia. N Engl J Med 1987; 316(21):1289–1294.
47. Borresen AL, Andersen TI, Tretli S, Heiberg A, Moller P. Breast cancer and other cancers in Norwegian families with ataxia-telangiectasia. Genes Chromosomes Cancer 1990; 2(4):339–340.
48. Pippard EC, Hall AJ, Barker DJ, Bridges BA. Cancer in homozygotes and heterozygotes of ataxia-telangiectasia and xeroderma pigmentosum in Britain. Cancer Res 1988; 48(10):2929–2932.
49. Lote K, Andersen K, Nordal E, Brennhovd IO. Familial occurrence of papillary thyroid carcinoma. Cancer 1980; 46(5):1291–1297.
50. Christensen SB, Ljungberg O, Tibblin S. A clinical epidemiologic study of thyroid carcinoma in Malmo, Sweden. Curr Probl Cancer 1984; 8(14):1–49.
51. Levi F, Franceschi S, La Vecchia C, et al. Previous thyroid disease and risk of thyroid cancer in Switzerland. Eur J Cancer 1991; 27(1):85–88.
52. Preston-Martin S, Bernstein L, Pike MC, Maldonado AA, Henderson BE. Thyroid cancer among young women related to prior thyroid disease and pregnancy history. Br J Cancer 1987; 55(2):191–195.
53. Williams ED, Doniach I, Bjarnason O, Michie W. Thyroid cancer in an iodide rich area: a histopathological study. Cancer 1977; 39(1):215–222.
54. Shering SG, Zbar AP, Moriarty M, McDermott EW, O'Higgins NJ, Smyth PP. Thyroid disorders and breast cancer. Eur J Cancer Prev 1996; 5(6):504–506.
55. Bignell GR, Canzian F, Shayeghi M, et al. Familial nontoxic multinodular thyroid goiter locus maps to chromosome 14q but does not account for familial nonmedullary thyroid cancer. Am J Hum Genet 1997; 61(5):1123–1130.
56. Parma J, Duprez L, Van Sande J, et al. Somatic mutations in the thyrotropin receptor gene cause hyperfunctioning thyroid adenomas. Nature 1993; 365(6447):649–651.
57. Malchoff CD, Sarfarazi M, Tendler B, Forouhar F, Whalen G, Malchoff DM. Familial papillary thyroid carcinoma is genetically distinct from familial adenomatous polyposis coli. Thyroid 1999; 9(3):247–252.
58. Malchoff CD, Sarfarazi M, Tendler B, et al. Papillary thyroid carcinoma associated with papillary renal neoplasia: genetic linkage analysis of a distinct heritable tumor syndrome. J Clin Endocrinol Metab 2000; 85(5):1758–1764.
59. Malchoff DM, Joshi V, Tendler B, Whalen B, Whalen G, Malchoff CD. The syndrome of familial papillary thyroid carcinoma with papillary renal neoplasia: evaluation of linked candidate genes. Program of the 82nd Annual Meeting of the Endocrine Society, Toronto, Ontario, 574. 2000.
60. Kraimps JL, Bouin-Pineau MH, Amati P, et al. Familial papillary carcinoma of the thyroid. Surgery 1997; 121(6):715–718.
61. Canzian F, Amati P, Harach HR, et al. A gene predisposing to familial thyroid tumors with cell oxyphilia maps to chromosome 19p13.2. Am J Hum Genet 1998; 63(6):1743–1748.

62. Bevan S, Pal T, Greenberg CR, et al. A comprehensive analysis of MNG1, TCO1, fPTC, PTEN, TSHR, and TRKA in familial nonmedullary thyroid cancer: confirmation of linkage to TCO1. J Clin Endocrinol Metab 2001; 86(8):3701–3704.
63. Pierotti MA, Vigneri P, Bongarzone I. Rearrangements of RET and NTRK1 tyrosine kinase receptors in papillary thyroid carcinomas. Recent Results Cancer Res 1998; 154:237–247.
64. Duprez L, Parma J, Van Sande J, et al. Germline mutations in the thyrotropin receptor gene cause nonautoimmune autosomal dominant hyperthyroidism. Nat Genet 1994; 7(3):396–401.
65. Lesueur F, Stark M, Tocco T, et al. Genetic heterogeneity in familial nonmedullary thyroid carcinoma: exclusion of linkage to RET, MNG1, and TCO in 56 families. NMTC Consortium. J Clin Endocrinol Metab 1999; 84(6):2157–2162.
66. McKay JD, Williamson J, Lesueur F, et al. At least three genes account for familial papillary thyroid carcinoma: TCO and MNG1 excluded as susceptibility loci from a large Tasmanian family. Eur J Endocrinol 1999; 141(2):122–125.
67. McKay JD, Lesueur F, Jonard L, et al. Localization of a susceptibility gene for familial nonmedullary thyroid carcinoma to chromosome 2q21. Am J Hum Genet 2001; 69(2):440–446.
68. Sozzi G, Miozzo M, Cariani TC, et al. A t(2;3) (q12–13;p24–25) in follicular thyroid adenomas. Cancer Genet Cytogenet 1992; 64(1):38–41.
69. Zedenius J, Wallin G, Svensson A, et al. Allelotyping of follicular thyroid tumors. Hum Genet 1995; 96(1):27–32.
70. Kroll TG, Sarraf P, Pecciarini L, et al. PAX8-PPARgamma1 fusion oncogene in human thyroid carcinoma. Science 2000; 289(5483):1357–1360.
71. Risch N, Merikangas K. The future of genetic studies of complex human diseases. Science 1996; 273(5281):1516–1517.
72. Cardon LR, Bell JI. Association study designs for complex diseases. Nat Rev Genet 2001; 2(2):91–99.
73. Matakidou A, Hamel N, Popat S, et al. Risk of nonmedullary thyroid cancer influenced by polymorphic variation in the thyroglobulin gene. Carcinogenesis 2004; 25(3):369–373.
74. Ohno M, Endo T, Ohta K, Gunji K, Onaya T. Point mutations in the thyrotropin receptor in human thyroid tumors. Thyroid 1995; 5(2):97–100.
75. Hrafnkelsson J, Tulinius H, Kjeld M, Sigvaldason H, Jonasson JG. Serum thyroglobulin as a risk factor for thyroid carcinoma. Acta Oncol 2000; 39(8):973–977.
76. Our inheritance, our future – realising the potential of genetics in the NHS. Cm5791. 2003.
77. Anonymous. Genetic counseling. Am J Hum Genet 1975; 27(2):240–242.
78. Niell BL, Long JC, Rennert G, Gruber SB. Genetic anthropology of the colorectal cancer-susceptibility allele APC I1307K: evidence of genetic drift within the Ashkenazim. Am J Hum Genet 2003; 73(6):1250–1260.
79. Corry PC. Intellectual disability and cerebral palsy in a UK community. Community Genet 2002; 5(3):201–204.
80. Gail MH, Brinton LA, Byar DP, et al. Projecting individualized probabilities of developing breast cancer for

white females who are being examined annually. J Natl Cancer Inst 1989; 81(24):1879–1886.

81. Claus EB, Risch N, Thompson WD. Autosomal dominant inheritance of early-onset breast cancer. Implications for risk prediction. Cancer 1994; 73(3):643–651.

82. Colditz GA, Willett WC, Hunter DJ, et al. Family history, age, and risk of breast cancer. Prospective data from the Nurses' Health Study. JAMA 1993; 270(3):338–343.

83. Hodgson SV, Popat S. Polymorphic sequence variants in medicine: a challenge and an opportunity. Clin Med 2003; 3(3):260–264.

84. Wilkie T. Genetics and insurance in Britain: why more than just the Atlantic divides the English-speaking nations. Nat Genet 1998; 20(2):119–121.

85. Collins WP, Bourne TH, Campbell S. Screening strategies for ovarian cancer. Curr Opin Obstet Gynecol 1998; 10(1):33–39.

86. Kebebew E, Clark OH. Medullary thyroid cancer. Curr Treat Options Oncol 2000; 1(4):359–367.

87. Machens A, Niccoli-Sire P, Hoegel J, et al. Early malignant progression of hereditary medullary thyroid cancer. N Engl J Med 2003; 349(16):1517–1525.

88. Bleiker EM, Hahn DE, Aaronson NK. Psychosocial issues in cancer genetics – current status and future directions. Acta Oncol 2003; 42(4):276–286.

89. Anonymous. NCCN colorectal cancer screening practice guidelines. National Comprehensive Cancer Network. Oncology (Huntingt) 1999; 13(5A):152–179.

90. Ogata H, Ohtsuka K, Tanaka K. A case of rectal cancer which presented an interesting metastasis. Natl Def Med J 1964; 11(137):138.

91. Raynham WH, Louw JH. Familial polyposis of the colon. S Afr Med J 1966; 40(35):857–865.

92. Smith WG. Familial multiple polyposis: research tool for investigating the etiology of carcinoma of the colon? Dis Colon Rectum 1968; 11(1):17–31.

93. Camiel MR, Mule JE, Alexander LL, Benninghoff DL. Association of thyroid carcinoma with Gardner's syndrome in siblings. N Engl J Med 1968; 278(19):1056–1058.

94. Smith WG, Kern BB. The nature of the mutation in familial multiple polyposis: papillary carcinoma of the thyroid, brain tumors, and familial multiple polyposis. Dis Colon Rectum 1973; 16(4):264–271.

95. Mathias JR, Smith WG. Mesenteric fibromatosis associated with familial polyposis. Am J Dig Dis 1977; 22(8):741–744.

96. Keshgegian AA, Enterline HT. Gardner's syndrome with duodenal adenomas, gastric adenomyoma and thyroid papillary – follicular adenocarcinoma. Dis Colon Rectum 1978; 21(4):255–260.

97. Takahasi S, Okuno Y, Nakamura A, et al. Gardner's syndrome in association with thyroid carcinoma. Rinsho Geka (J Clin Surg) 1976; 31:795–800.

98. Ida M, Yao Y, Ohgushi H, et al. Gastric lesions in familial adenomatosis of the colon; on their characteristics and follow-up studies. I To Cho (Stom Intest) 1977; 12:1365–1374.

99. Ushio K, Abe S, Mitsushima T, et al. Gastric and duodenal lesions associated with familial polyposis. I To Cho (Stom Intest) 1977; 12:1547–1557.

100. Harada M, Murakami T, Shishido Y, et al. Two cases of unusual extracolonic phenotypes accompanying familial polyposis of the colon – one with papillary carcinoma of the thyroid and the other with mesenteric fibromatosis. Nippon Shokakibyo Gakkai Zasshi 1977; 74(11):1567–1574.

101. Okamura S, Kusugami K, Kurokawa S, Miwa M, Oka Y, Hattori T. A case of familial polyposis coli with interesting findings. Saishin Igaku 1979; 34:2697–2700.

102. Hamilton SR, Bussey HJ, Mendelsohn G, et al. Ileal adenomas after colectomy in nine patients with adenomatous polyposis coli/Gardner's syndrome. Gastroenterology 1979; 77(6):1252–1257.

103. Miura K, Yamaguchi A, Kawase K, et al. A case of adenomatous coli associated with carcinoma of the colon, ovary and thyroid gland and nodular hyperplasia of the adrenal cortex. Nippon Shokakibyo Gakkai Zasshi 1980; 13:328–332.

104. Lee FI, MacKinnon MD. Papillary thyroid carcinoma associated with polyposis coli. A case of Gardner's syndrome. Am J Gastroenterol 1981; 76(2):138–140.

105. Delamarre J, Duppas JL, Capron JP, et al. Polypose rectocolique familiale, syndrome et Gardner et cancer thyroidien: estude de deux cas. Gastroenterol Clin Biol 1982; 10:659–662.

106. Thompson JS, Harned RK, Anderson JC, Hodgson PE. Papillary carcinoma of the thyroid and familial polyposis coli. Dis Colon Rectum 1983; 26(9):583–585.

107. Schneider NR, Cubilla AL, Chaganti RS. Association of endocrine neoplasia with multiple polyposis of the colon. Cancer 1983; 51(6):1171–1175.

108. Masuyama K, Kawahara M, Mori T, et al. An atypical case of familial adenomatous polyposis with multiple thyroid cancers and colonic cancers. Nippon Shokakai Byou Gakiai Zasshi (Jpn J Gastroenterol Surg) 1986; 19:1316.

109. Piffer S. Gardner's syndrome and thyroid cancer – a case report and review of the literature. Acta Oncol 1988; 27(4):413–415.

110. Delamarre J, Capron JP, Armand A, Dupas JL, Deschepper B, Davion T. Thyroid carcinoma in two sisters with familial polyposis of the colon. Case reports and review of the literature. J Clin Gastroenterol 1988; 10(6):659–662.

111. van Erpecum KJ, Berge Henegouwen GP, Meinders AE, Bronkhorst FB, Eggink WF, Jonkers M. Papillary thyroid carcinoma and characteristic pigmented ocular fundus lesions in a patient with Gardner's syndrome. Neth J Med 1988; 32(3–4):136–142.

112. Herrera L, Carrel A, Rao U, Castillo N, Petrelli N. Familial adenomatous polyposis in association with thyroiditis. Report of two cases. Dis Colon Rectum 1989; 32(10):893–896.

113. Ono C, Iwama T, Mishima Y. A case of familial adenomatous polyposis complicated by thyroid carcinoma, carcinoma of the ampulla of Vater and adrenocortical adenoma. Jpn J Surg 1991; 21(2):234–240.

114. Bell B, Mazzaferri EL. Familial adenomatous polyposis (Gardner's syndrome) and thyroid carcinoma. A case report and review of the literature. Dig Dis Sci 1993; 381:185–190.

115. Robinson DW, Orr TG. Carcinoma of the thyroid and other diseases of the thyroid in identical twins. AMA Arch Surg 1955; 70(6):923–928.

116. Elman DS. Familial association of nerve deafness with nodular goiter and thyroid carcinoma. N Engl J Med 1958; 259(5):219–223.

117. Lacour J, Vignalou J, Perez R, Gerard-Marchant R. Papillary epithelioma of the thyroid gland. Apropos of 2 familial cases. Nouv Presse Med 1973; 2(34):2249–2252.

118. Nemec J, Soumar J, Zamrazil V, Pohunkova D, Motlik K, Mirejovsky P. Familial occurrence of differentiated (non-medullary) thyroid cancer. Oncology 1975; 32 (3–4):151–157.

119. Palestro G, Navone R, Coda R, Mussa A, Abeatici S. Aspetti dell'immunita cellulare in due casi di carcinoma tiroideo nella stessa famiglia. Tumori 1975; 61(4):333–337.

120. Fisher C, Edmonds CJ. Papillary carcinoma of the thyroid in two brothers after chest fluoroscopy in childhood. BMJ 1980; 281(6255):1600–1601.

121. Phade VR, Lawrence WR, Max MH. Familial papillary carcinoma of the thyroid. Arch Surg 1981; 116(6):836–837.

122. Lamberg BA, Reissel P, Stenman S, et al. Concurrent medullary and papillary thyroid carcinoma in the same thyroid lobe and in siblings. Acta Med Scand 1981; 209(5):421–424.

123. Flannigan GM, Clifford RP, Winslet M, Lawrence DA, Fiddian RV. Simultaneous presentation of papillary carcinoma of thyroid in a father and son. Br J Surg 1983; 70(3):181–182.

124. Suzuki S, Watanabe I. Familial occurrence of papillary thyroid carcinoma. Gan No Rinsho 1985; 31(4):414–419.

125. Ozaki O, Ito K, Kobayashi K, Suzuki A, Manabe Y, Hosoda Y. Familial occurrence of differentiated, nonmedullary thyroid carcinoma. World J Surg 1988; 12(4): 565–571.

126. Austoni M. Thyroid papillary carcinoma in identical twins. Lancet 1988; i(8594):1115.

127. Dzwonkowski P, O'Leary J, Farid NR. Thyroid papillary carcinoma in HLA identical sibs. Lancet 1988; ii(8617):971.

128. Fischer DK, Groves MD, Thomas SJ, Jr, Johnson PC, Jr. Papillary carcinoma of the thyroid: additional evidence in support of a familial component. Cancer Invest 1989; 7(4):323–325.

129. Samaan NA. Papillary carcinoma of the thyroid: hereditary or radiation-induced? Cancer Invest 1989; 7(4): 399–400.

130. Szanto J, Gundy C, Toth K, Kasler M. Coincidental papillary carcinoma of the thyroid in two sisters. Oncology 1990; 47(1):92–94.

131. Grossman RF, Tu SH, Duh QY, Siperstein AE, Novosolov F, Clark OH. Familial nonmedullary thyroid cancer. An emerging entity that warrants aggressive treatment. Arch Surg 1995; 130(8):892–897.

132. Takami H, Ozaki O, Ito K. Familial nonmedullary thyroid cancer: an emerging entity that warrants aggressive treatment. Arch Surg 1996; 131(6): 676.

Section VII

Thyroid Cancer in Children

23

Thyroid Cancer in Childhood

Nicholas J. Sarlis and Wellington Hung

Abbreviations

ATC	Anaplastic thyroid carcinoma
CCH	C-cell hyperplasia
CNS	Central nervous system
CXR	Chest X-ray
EBRT	External beam radiation therapy
EGF	Epidermal growth factor
ERK	Extracellular signal-regulated kinase
FAP	Familial adenomatous polyposis
FGF	Fibroblast growth factor
FMTC	Familial medullary thyroid cancer
FNAB	Fine-needle aspiration biopsy
FTC	Follicular thyroid carcinoma
GH	Growth hormone
IGF-1	Insulin-like growth factor-1
JNK	c-Jun N-terminal kinase
L-T$_3$	L-triiodothyronine; liothyronine
L-T$_4$	Levothyroxine
MAPK	Mitogen-activated protein kinase
MEN	Multiple endocrine neoplasia
MRI	Magnetic resonance imaging
MTC	Medullary thyroid carcinoma
NED	No evidence of disease (status)
PI3K	Phosphatidylinositol 3-kinase
PPARγ	Peroxisome proliferator-activated receptor-γ
PTC	Papillary thyroid carcinoma
RAI	Radioactive iodine; radioiodine
rhTSH	Recombinant human TSH
RTK	Receptor tyrosine kinase
T$_3$	Triiodothyronine
T$_4$	Thyroxine
TC	Thyroid cancer
Tg	Thyroglobulin
TH	Thyroid hormone
THST	Thyroid hormone suppression therapy
T/NTT	Total/near-total thyroidectomy
TSH	Thyrotropin
U/S	Ultrasonography
VEGF	Vascular endothelial growth factor
WBS	Whole-body scan (or scanning)
WDTC	Well-differentiated thyroid carcinoma

Introduction

Thyroid carcinoma (TC) in the pediatric age group is rare, constituting only 1.3% of all newly diagnosed pediatric malignancies in the United States between 1973 and 1987, as determined from the Surveillance, Epidemiology, and End Results Program data collected by the National Cancer Institute of the National Institutes of Health [1]. Two thirds of TCs occur in girls, with a peak incidence between 7 and 12 years of age [2]. In general, TCs in children and adolescents have a better prognosis than other malignancies in children or even same-stage TCs of the same histological type in adults. Most pediatric studies designate papillary and follicular thyroid carcinomas (PTCs and FTCs, respectively) as well-differentiated thyroid carcinomas (WDTCs), and this convention will be followed in this chapter. The other two major histopathological types of TCs are medullary and anaplastic TCs (MTCs and ATCs, respectively).

Epidemiology and Molecular Pathogenesis

Well-Differentiated Thyroid Carcinoma

The epidemiology of WDTC is not well understood, and the relative proportion of PTC versus FTC varies geographically, perhaps as a function of the iodine content of the diet [3]. Iodine deficiency alters the pathology of TC in adults by increasing the relative prevalence of FTCs and ATCs, whereas the percentage of PTCs is higher in iodine-sufficient areas [4]; it is likely that similar effects of iodine sufficiency may affect the relative incidence of various TC types in pediatric populations.

One cause of TC is the external beam radiotherapy widely used from 1920 to 1960 in children for treating benign conditions of the head, neck, and upper chest, such as tinea capitis, acne, tonsillar hypertrophy, and thymic enlargement. In 1949, Quimby and Werner [5] suggested a relationship between neck irradiation and the development of TC later in life. The thyroid gland in childhood is highly sensitive to radiation. After 1950, the use of radiotherapy for benign conditions gradually diminished. Currently, certain diagnostic techniques, especially fluoroscopy, can also involve radiation exposure in the range implicated in the pathogenesis of thyroid tumors [6]. Moreover, medically indicated radiation therapy for the treatment of assorted malignancies, especially acute lymphocytic leukemia and Hodgkin's disease, continues to be administered. Scattered radiation from the primary fields of therapy, which transverses thyroid tissue, results in sublethal thyroid irradiation in such patients.

Exposure to γ-radiation and higher-energy β-emitters, such as radioiodines (RAIs), in atomic fallout is also associated with the development of TC [7]. The accident at the nuclear power plant in Chernobyl, Ukraine, on 26 April 1986, released into the atmosphere approximately 1800 PBq (49 MCi) of ^{131}I, 2500 PBq (68 MCi) of ^{133}I, and 1000 PBq (27 MCi) of ^{132}Te, which decays rapidly to ^{132}I [8,9]. Of note, released iodine isotopes had much shorter half-lives than ^{131}I, but are believed to be more carcinogenic. As early as 4 years after the accident, the incidence of PTC in pediatric patients in the most contaminated region, the province of Gomel, Belarus, increased dramatically [10,11]. These findings provide evidence that this marked increase in the incidence of TC was a direct consequence of exposure to fallout heavily enriched by radioactive iodine compounds [12]. The short latency period of 4 years for the development of TC in this cohort of patients is in contrast to 18+ years of latency observed in PTCs associated with other types of radiation exposure [13].

Cytogenetic studies of PTCs and FTCs from pediatric patients exposed to radiation in Belarus were performed to study the pathogenetic mechanisms of carcinogenic induction by ionizing radiation. Proto-oncogenes encode protein products that promote cell growth. When proto-oncogenes undergo activating mutations, they become oncogenes and contribute to uncontrolled proliferation and growth. The RET proto-oncogene (human chromosome locus on 10q11.2) encodes a transmembrane receptor with a tyrosine kinase domain (RTK) [14]. The protein product, RET, is a member of a large class of RTKs that function as signal transduction molecules to regulate cellular function and proliferation [15]. Native transmembrane RET is not expressed (or possibly expressed in extremely minute amounts) in normal follicular thyrocytes. On the other hand, in some PTCs, chromosomal rearrangements result in the illegitimate fusion of the tyrosine kinase domain of RET with 5′-located regulatory parts of other ubiquitously expressed genes, such as ELE1, leading to constitutive activation of the resultant fusion genes, called RET/PTCs [16]. The products of these genes, the RET/PTC oncoproteins, exist in the intracellular compartment of the thyrocyte and strongly activate downstream signaling systems dependent on RET activation, including the Ras/extracellular signal-regulated kinase (ERK), phosphatidylinositol 3-kinase (PI3K)/Akt, p38 mitogen-activated protein kinase (MAPK), and c-Jun N-terminal kinase (JNK) pathways [17]. Three main RET/PTC rearrangements (i.e., RET/PTC1, RET/PTC2, and RET/PTC3) lead to the production of the corresponding oncoproteins and have been identified in thyroid epithelial tumors. Of note, additional, rarer subtypes of RET/PTC exist (RET/PTC4–RET/PTC8), but are not well studied.

In children in Belarus who developed PTC after the Chernobyl accident, RET/PTC rearrangements were detected in 60–80% of tumors [18]. This RET/PTC1 rearrangement is correlated with radiation-induced carcinogenesis; however, it is also observed in 3–35% of spontaneous (non-radiation-induced) PTCs [19,20]. Interestingly, although only RET/PTC1 rearrangements were observed in adults, both RET/PTC1 and RET/PTC3 rearrangements were seen in children of the Chernobyl cohort, with the latter being slightly predominant [18]. Some investigators have suggested that the RET/PTC3 rearrangement is preferentially formed after exposure to high radiation and is related to a more aggressive pattern of PTC growth [21]. Point gene mutations of the oncogenes RAS and GSP (GNAS) were very rarely found in PTCs that developed after the Chernobyl accident, thereby differing in that aspect from sporadic cases of PTC [22,23]. Additionally, a loss of expression of or mutations in the p53 tumor suppressor gene was also rare in pediatric PTCs among the Chernobyl cohort [23]. Another cytogenetic change observed in Belarussian children with TC was rearrangement of the gene NTRK1 (also known as TrkA, coding for another RTK; locus on 1q22) in some of the PTCs [20,24]. Subsequently, Santoro et al. [25] concluded that activation of RTK genes played the predominant role in thyroid carcinogenesis in these children.

Activating point mutations of the RAS genes (locus on 11p15.5-p15.1) are frequently found not only in thyroid follicular adenomas, but also in FTCs, a finding suggesting that RAS mutations may be an early event in thyroid tumorigenesis, yielding a morphological phenotype consistent with follicular formations [26,27]. FTCs can also develop through another distinct and virtually nonoverlapping molecular pathway involving another fusion protein, the product of the Pax8-peroxisome proliferator-activated receptor (PPARγ) oncogene. The latter is formed though a t(2;3)(q13;p25) translocation involving the in-frame juxtaposition of the PAX8 gene, which encodes a paired domain transcription factor, with the PPARγ gene [28,29]. The downstream signaling pathways that operate after the formation of an active Pax8-PPARγ oncoprotein are not known at present but may involve interactions with Wnt, cyclooxygenase-2, and assorted apoptosis-regulating systems [30]. Notably, FTCs are quite rare in children and adolescents, constituting only about 5% of TCs [31].

Thyroid growth is induced by other stimuli, including – among others – thyrotropin (TSH), epidermal growth factor (EGF), fibroblast growth factor (FGF), vascular endothelial growth factor (VEGF), insulin-like growth factor-1 (IGF-1), prostaglandins, and growth hormone (GH) [32], which are thought to have a growth-promoting effect in benign thyroid disease. It is not clear to date that these stimuli have an effect on the development of WDTC, with the notable exception of TSH, which is believed to be a bona fide growth stimulator for most WDTCs [32].

Survival rates for children with many pediatric malignancies have improved, but the radiotherapy and chemotherapy used to treat these children have been implicated in the development of secondary TCs in some patients [33,34]. Genetic factors have also been implicated in TC development, with several reports of a thyroid growth advantage occurring in familial syndromes (with mutations of the corresponding responsible genes shown in parentheses), such as McCune–Albright syndrome (postzygotic mutations of GNAS; locus on 20q13.2-q13.3); Pendred syndrome (SLC26A4 or PDS; locus on 7q22–31.1); Peutz–Jeghers syndrome (LKB1 or STK11; locus on 19p13.3); Cowden syndrome (PTEN; locus on 10q23.3); Carney complex (PRKAR1A, locus on 17q22–24); and familial adenomatoid polyposis coli (FAP), including its subtype, Gardner syndrome (APC; locus on 5q21) [32,35]. Furthermore, Pal et al. [36] have suggested that there may be additional, yet unknown, familial factors that predispose children to TC.

Medullary Thyroid Carcinoma

MTC originates in calcitonin-producing cells (C cells) of the thyroid. C cells are of neuroectodermal origin and do not accumulate iodine. There exist both familial and sporadic variants of MTC. Patients with MTC or its precursor condition, C-cell hyperplasia (CCH), have elevated basal plasma calcitonin levels and exaggerated responses of calcitonin to various stimuli. Multiple endocrine neoplasia type 2 (MEN2) is an autosomal dominant syndrome caused by germline mutations of the *RET* proto-oncogene and characterized by high penetrance for MTC [15]. The MEN2A variant is characterized by the presence of MTC, pheochromocytoma, and hyperparathyroidism [37]. On the other hand, the MEN2B variant is characterized by MTC, pheochromocytoma, mucosal ganglioneuromas, and a marfanoid habitus [38]. MEN2B is the more aggressive of the two variants [39]. In the third variant, familial MTC (FMTC), MTC occurs without other endocrine neoplasms [40].

Specific codon mutations within the *RET* gene are present in each of the above forms of MTC, correlate with the phenotypic expression of each familial MTC variant, and partially determine the aggressiveness of the resultant malignancies [39]. The *RET* mutations are believed to be the initiating event responsible for the development of neoplasia in MTC developing in the context of MEN2 syndromes [41]. Additionally, *RET* mutations are found in as many as 40% of sporadic MTCs [42]. This also means that other, yet unknown, genes are responsible for the development of the remaining 60% of sporadic MTCs. Of note, the overwhelming majority of MTCs that occur in childhood are due to either de novo or inherited mutations of the *RET* oncogene and, hence, occur in the context of a familial syndrome [43].

Anaplastic Thyroid Carcinoma

ATCs probably represent the terminal stage in the dedifferentiation process of WDTCs [44]. The cause of this dedifferentiation is not known.

RAS oncogene activation is a rather frequent event in ATCs, but it also occurs in WDTCs [27] as an early event in thyroid tumorigenesis [26]. The *p53* gene (locus on 17p13.1) is a tumor suppressor gene and is the most commonly affected gene in human cancers [45]. The *p53* gene product, the TP53 protein, plays an essential role in cell cycle regulation, specifically in the transition from G0 to G1. Inactivating point mutations of *p53* are frequently present in anaplastic TC but not in differentiated TC, suggesting that *p53* mutations play an important role in the pro-gression from the differentiated to undifferentiated/anaplastic phenotype [45]. ATC is thought to be exceedingly rare in the pediatric age group [46], although a very limited number of cases end up being referred to and managed in tertiary comprehensive cancer centers in the United States, as has been our experience.

Histopathology and Elements of Biological Behavior

Papillary Thyroid Carcinoma

PTC usually is unencapsulated, well differentiated, and sharply circumscribed from the surrounding thyroid parenchyma. PTCs bear almost pathognomonic cytomorphological changes, including nuclear grooves, folds, and invaginations, in addition to central nuclear clearing [47]. The cancer may be multicentric. PTC foci have a moderately dense fibrous stroma and tend to invade the space between follicles. Psammoma bodies are a cardinal feature of PTC [47]. The tumors may spread to normal surrounding thyroid parenchyma and regional lymph nodes. However, they are capable of distant dissemination as well. PTCs characteristically grow slowly [48].

Follicular Thyroid Carcinoma

FTCs are characterized by well-developed follicles and an absence of well-defined papillae. They are usually encapsulated and show a marked tendency toward vascular invasion [47]. These malignancies typically spread hematogenously to lung and bone, and more rarely to the central nervous system (CNS) and elsewhere [48].

Medullary Thyroid Carcinoma

MTCs vary in size from those that are barely visible grossly to those that replace the entire thyroid gland. Most MTCs (both sporadic and familial) are unencapsulated and show a solid pattern of growth. They exhibit a wide spectrum of histological patterns that mimic other types of thyroid malignancies. The presence of amyloid and positive immunohistochemical reactions for markers of neuroendocrine differentiation are diagnostic. CCH is usually present either adjacent to the carcinoma or at a distance from it. MTCs occurring in the context of familial syndromes characteristically involve both lobes [47]. MTCs initially metastasize to lymph nodes of the neck and mediastinum. The tumor may replace an entire lobe and extend into perithyroidal soft tissues. Distant dissemination can occur to the lung, bone, liver, and CNS or rarely to more atypical locations [48].

Anaplastic Thyroid Carcinoma

ATCs are usually large and widely invasive. Three major distinct microscopic morphological patterns exist: (1) squamoid, (2) spindle cell, and (3) giant cell [47]. The tumor usually replaces a significant portion of the thyroid parenchyma, occasionally enough to cause thyroid failure (hypothyroidism). ATC is one of the most lethal human malignancies. It spreads aggressively and diffusely into the tissues of the neck. Distant dissemination usually occurs rapidly to lung, bone, liver, CNS, and other sites [44].

Clinical Features

Most pediatric patients with TC present with a solitary thyroid nodule, multinodular goiter, or cervical lymphadenopathy [35]. Single or multiple nodules of the thyroid gland are rather uncommon in pediatric patients, in contrast to their higher prevalence in adults. Furthermore, in children and adolescents, the implications of a solitary thyroid nodule are different from those of multiple nodules. The risk of malignancy is supposedly lower in a thyroid gland with discrete multiple nodules than in a solitary thyroid nodule. However, Garcia et al. [49] reported on 16 children and adolescents with multiple thyroid nodules; 4 (25%) of the patients had carcinoma. Of those 4, FTCs were found in 3 of the patients (1 of whom had a history of radiation therapy to the neck and upper chest), and 1 patient (with no history of exposure to radiation) had a PTC.

It is not always possible to define clinically that a single thyroid nodule is indeed solitary. In fact, more than 50% of thyroid glands, judged on physical examination to contain a single nodule, are found by ultrasonography (U/S) or surgical exploration to harbor more than one nodule. Table 23.1 lists the differential diagnosis of a solitary thyroid nodule in pediatric patients. Table 23.2 lists the underlying causes of multinodular goiter that develops during childhood and adolescence.

Table 23.1 Differential diagnosis of solitary thyroid nodules in children and adolescents

- Adenomas
  Follicular
  Colloid
  Toxic
- Carcinomas
  Papillary
  Follicular
  Mixed papillary-follicular
  Medullary
  Anaplastic
- Other tumorous conditions
  Chronic lymphocytic thyroiditis (pseudonodules)
  Cysts
  Abscesses
- Developmental anomalies
  Agenesis of one lobe
  Intrathyroidal thyroglossal duct cyst

Table 23.2 Differential diagnosis of multinodular thyroid disease in children and adolescents

- Chronic lymphocytic thyroiditis
- Thyrotoxicosis-associated
  Native (before medical therapy)
  Secondary to medical therapy
- Infections
  Bacterial
  Viral
- Multiple follicular adenomas
- Cysts
  Colloid
  Adenomatous
- Iodine deficiency
- Nodular hyperplasia
- Goitrogen-induced nodules
- Inborn errors of thyroid hormone synthesis
- Carcinoma secondary to radiation therapy
- Medullary thyroid carcinoma in the context of genetic syndromes
- Thyroid lymphoma (extremely rarely)

Initial Diagnosis

History-Taking and Physical Examination

The history-taking is important and should include questions about external irradiation to the head, neck, and upper chest. A history of goitrogen exposure should be also sought. Information regarding the rate of growth of the mass or masses, local or systemic symptoms, and hoarseness or dysphagia should be obtained. The family history should be explored for the presence of thyroid disease, hyperparathyroidism, and features compatible with pheochromocytoma. Rapid painless growth of a nodule suggests the presence of carcinoma. Pain or tenderness in the thyroid gland is an unusual complaint in the context of a malignancy but may be severe in postviral (subacute) or suppurative thyroiditis. A rapidly enlarging nodule with transient pain suggests hemorrhage into a cyst.

Careful palpation of a thyroid nodule helps define its nature. A soft, compressible nodule is less likely to be malignant, and more likely to be a cyst. However, some cysts can be quite firm on palpation. Conversely, some PTCs undergo cystic degeneration. Tenderness in a nodule suggests hemorrhage into a cyst or an inflammatory process. Malignancy should be suspected if the nodule is hard or if there is fixation to surrounding structures or vocal cord paralysis. Lymphadenopathy, particularly low in the neck and away from the midline, increases the likelihood of malignancy. In most pediatric patients with a malignant nodule, the surrounding thyroid tissue feels normal, and the gland is not globally enlarged.

Children with MTC generally have no clinical symptoms but are rather evaluated either because they have a thyroid nodule or palpable cervical lymphadenopathy, or – more commonly – because they are a member of a kindred affected with MTC and are found to have either a positive RET germline mutation or increased plasma calcitonin levels. Patients with MEN2A have a normal appearance; whereas those with MEN2B have marfanoid body build and demonstrate multiple neuromas of the lips, eyelids, and tongue. In MEN2B, slit-lamp examination of the cornea may show enlargement of the corneal nerves. Moreover, ganglioneuromas may be present throughout the gastrointestinal tract and cause symptoms, including constipation and diarrhea, the latter often beginning in infancy.

Biochemical Indices

In general, there is no blood test that is of value in the initial diagnosis of WDTC or ATC. Nevertheless, serum-free thyroxine (free T_4), total (or free) triiodothyronine (T_3), and TSH determinations are helpful in determining the functional status of the thyroid gland. It should be mentioned that the degree of hyperthyroidism due to a toxic nodule may not be sufficiently severe to allow diagnosis on clinical grounds alone. Hypothyroidism should be excluded because, if secondary to chronic lymphocytic (Hashimoto's) thyroiditis, it can be associated with solitary or multiple nodules. Serum thyroglobulin (Tg) levels can be elevated in patients with WDTC but are also elevated in a variety of benign thyroid disorders. Thus, the measurement of serum Tg is not helpful at the outset (unless of course one knows the diagnosis of TC); however, it is of great importance in the follow-up of patients with WDTC after initial therapy (see below).

Measurement of plasma calcitonin, both basally and in response to calcium with or without pentagastrin, permits the detection of MTC in some patients before the appearance of any clinical signs or symptoms of this malignancy, as it does in adults [50]. Until the recent advent of RET mutation genetic testing, stimulated calcitonin testing was of paramount importance in the screening of MTC family members who were at risk for C-cell disease. Unfortunately, this biochemical testing does not identify all patients at risk [51]. The stimulation test may be performed by giving the patient an infusion of calcium gluconate (2 mg/kg) and pentagastrin (0.5 μg/kg) over a period of 1 minute. The plasma calcitonin level is measured 1, 2, 3, 5, and 6 minutes after the infusion [50,52]. Abnormal basal and stimulated plasma calcitonin values must be obtained from the reference laboratory performing the study. Of note, pentagastrin is no longer available in the United States (internet site: http://www.fda.gov/cder/rxotcdpl/pdpl_200204.htm, last accessed 3 July 2004), although the National Institutes of Health

Drug Information Service is currently working closely with the Food and Drug Administration Gastrointestinal Diseases Division to facilitate its future availability.

Molecular diagnostic testing for the identification of mutations in the *RET* proto-oncogene allows the identification of patients who are gene carriers and are thus predisposed to CCH and MTC [51,53]. This knowledge allows prophylactic thyroidectomy to be performed before any neoplastic changes develop [54,55]. Molecular genetic testing is more specific than biochemical testing and should replace biochemical testing when possible.

Radionuclide Imaging

The traditional approach to evaluating patients with nodular thyroid disease has been radioisotope scintigraphy, aiming to classify nodules as "cold," "hot," or "warm," depending on their ability to concentrate the isotope. Scanning can be done with ^{123}I or technetium-99m pertechnetate (^{99m}Tc). Unfortunately, the value of such scans is limited by their inability to reliably differentiate between benign and malignant disease. However, scintigraphy can rule out the presence of developmental anomalies, such as agenesis of a lobe (with compensatory hypertrophy of the contralateral lobe), presenting clinically as a solitary nodule.

A solitary toxic nodule may be toxic or nontoxic and may or may not be autonomous in function. "Hot" (hyperfunctioning) nodules that do not lead to clinically apparent hyperthyroidism typically increase their secretion of thyroid hormones (THs) gradually and insidiously until symptoms emerge. In pediatric patients, there is a more rapid progression to hyperthyroidism and a higher incidence of hyperfunctioning TCs than in adults [56]. Therefore, it has been recommended that all "hot" solitary thyroid nodules in pediatric patients be removed surgically [56].

The above notwithstanding, in a study of 93 pediatric patients with solitary thyroid nodules, 77 of 93 nodules (82.8%) were scintigraphically "cold" (hypofunctioning) [57]. The most common solitary "cold" nodule in childhood is follicular adenoma, again in contradistinction to adulthood, in which "cold" nodules are usually due to nodular (colloid or hyperplastic) goiter. It is the patient with a "cold" nodule who presents the greatest clinical problem in differentiating a benign from a malignant nodule, because such nodules can underlie TCs, chronic lymphocytic thyroiditis, cysts, follicular adenomas, abscesses, hypofunctioning nodular goiter areas, or embryonic defects [57]. The highest incidence of TCs occurs in patients with "cold" solitary nodules, but certainly not all "cold" nodules represent TCs.

Ultrasonography

U/S examination of the thyroid provides an accurate means of assessing thyroid size and the presence, number, and size of thyroid nodules. U/S can also distinguish solid from cystic nodules and is more sensitive than radionuclide scintigraphy in detecting multiple nodules.

Cystic lesions are generally considered benign. Most cysts result from necrosis and degeneration of nodules. In a series of 12 pediatric patients with TC reported on by Desjardin and associates [58], nearly half had cystic nodules. Aspiration of all cystic nodules is recommended for both diagnosis and therapy [57]. Of note, cystic degeneration of PTCs is thought to occur more frequently in children and adolescents than in adults [59].

Response to Thyroid Hormone Suppression Therapy

The rationale for thyroid hormone suppression therapy (THST) is based on evidence that TSH is the main stimulator of thyroid growth and function, at least in normal thyrocytes [60]. It is not clear whether long-term levothyroxine (L-T_4) therapy to partially suppress TSH is effective in treating thyroid nodules, which are of course composed of neoplastic (not normal) thyroid tissue [61]. The use of high dose L-T_4 to fully suppress TSH in patients with benign thyroid disease is neither beneficial nor completely safe [62]. Therefore, THST for unknown nodular thyroid disease is not recommended for pediatric patients.

Biopsy

There has been increased and successful use of fine-needle aspiration biopsy (FNAB) in pediatric patients with thyroid nodules [63,64].

FNAB in pediatric patients must be performed by a person competent in aspirating thyroid nodules working closely with an experienced cytopathologist. FNAB is recommended if a solid solitary nodule is present and there is no suspicion of malignancy on the basis of the patient's history or physical findings. Even if there are telltale signs of malignancy (e.g. fixation, palpable lymph node metastases), FNAB is still indicated for the exact diagnosis of the type of malignancy, because initial surgical therapy approaches can differ depending on the type of carcinoma. If an experienced person to perform the FNA and cytopathologist are not available or repeated FNAB samples are unsatisfactory or nondiagnostic, open surgical biopsy (including a core tissue biopsy) or ipsilateral thyroid lobectomy is recommended.

Initial Treatment and Long-Term Management of Pediatric TC

Well-Differentiated Thyroid Carcinoma

There is continuing controversy regarding the optimal management of children and adolescents with WDTC because of the rarity of this malignancy and various almost unique features associated with it. These features include (1) more aggressive behavior with regard to locoregional extension than is seen in adults with TC; (2) a tendency to metastasize early; and (3) despite those factors, a usually good long-term prognosis with an overall 15-year survival rate exceeding 95% [65]. There are no prospective randomized clinical trials to guide the clinician in the management of pediatric patients with WDTC. It is unlikely that such trials will ever be conducted, given the small number of patients, the slow progression of the disease, and the overall good prognosis. The most controversial aspect of management is the extent and aggressiveness of treatment required, which mainly includes surgery and [131]I.

Surgery

Surgery is the primary therapy for WDTC in pediatric patients [66]. Controversy exists as to whether total (or near-total) thyroidectomy (T/NTT) or subtotal thyroidectomy should be the procedure of choice [67]. Although there is very seldom an indication for radical neck dissection in pediatric patients, extensive functional neck dissection for removal of infiltrated lymph nodes is certainly warranted in selected cases [68]. Regardless of the surgical procedure, surgery should be performed by an experienced thyroid surgeon, preferably one familiar with the anatomic vagaries of the pediatric neck. A few surgeons recommend subtotal thyroidectomy because they believe that the literature has not provided enough support for the conclusion that T/NTT leads to better survival than more conservative procedures [69]. This group of surgeons also makes the argument that T/NTT may increase the incidence of serious complications, such as permanent hypoparathyroidism and recurrent laryngeal nerve damage.

Most surgeons currently perform T/NTT in pediatric patients with WDTC on the basis of a favorable interpretation of the available data suggesting that this type of surgery reduces the rate of local recurrence [70,71]. In addition, they point to the well-known frequent occurrence of multiple, bilateral foci of papillary microcarcinoma in the glands of patients with PTC [72]. T/NTT increases the sensitivity of diagnostic RAI whole-body scanning (WBS) at the time of ablation therapy and improves the efficacy of subsequent ^{131}I therapy. This assumption is based on the fact that normal thyroid tissue concentrates RAI much more efficiently than WDTC tissue. Also, serum Tg levels are significantly lower after T/NTT than after more conservative procedures, thereby allowing this tumor marker to be used as a more sensitive indicator of residual or recurrent disease. After thyroidectomy and ^{131}I therapy, patients are typically placed on THST.

Radioactive Iodine

Depending on the amount of postoperative normal thyroid remnant, any coexisting WDTC metastases may or may not be detected at the time of a diagnostic RAI WBS [73]. Additionally, without ablation of the thyroid remnant, the treatment of metastases may be less effective, because normal thyroid tissue accumulates ^{131}I more efficiently than does WDTC. Therefore, we and others recommend the routine ablation of postoperative thyroid remnants [66,74]. Such ablative therapy has been successful in most pediatric patients after a single dose of [131]I [74]. Some clinicians recommend obtaining an RAI WBS 5 to 7 days after the ablation dose of [131]I [66,75]. Usually, this scan visualizes the thyroid remnant, but it may also reveal previously unsuspected areas of local or disseminated disease, which can be managed with further ^{131}I treatment [75].

After surgery and ^{131}I thyroid remnant ablation, a diagnostic WBS is recommended to assess the need for further RAI therapy; this should be performed 9–12 months after the remnant ablation and in conjunction with measurement of serum Tg [66]. In preparation for the diagnostic RAI WBS, patients are made hypothyroid over a period of 6 weeks. This is achieved through the implementation of various protocols to abrogate the deleterious effects of this prolonged iatrogenic hypothyroid state. We recommend the administration of L-triiodothyronine (liothyronine, $L-T_3$) at 1.0–1.2 µg/kg per day, divided into two or three doses, for the first 4 weeks of the 6-week treatment with the hypothyroid preparation. To increase the affinity of any thyroid tissue for RAI, a low iodine diet may be instituted (daily iodine content of about 50–75 µg) for the 2–3 weeks before the scan [66]. Patients who take $L-T_4$ after thyroidectomy should discontinue it and start $L-T_3$ for 4 weeks, as described above. $L-T_3$ is discontinued 2 weeks before the diagnostic RAI WBS. The serum TSH level should be higher than 25 µU/mL (as measured by a third-generation assay) to optimize iodine uptake by the thyroid tissue, if any exists at the time of the scan.

In an effort to bypass the need to induce hypothyroidism (with all its associated morbidities), an increasing number of adult endocrinologists administer recombinant human TSH (rhTSH) while the patients remain on $L-T_4$ therapy in preparation for a follow-up evaluation [76]. It has to be noted that, at present, the use of rhTSH in pediatric patients has not been approved by the US Food and Drug Administration.

The diagnostic RAI WBS can be performed using either [131]I (18–74 MBq; 0.5–2 mCi) or [123]I (5.6–37 MBq; 150–1000 µCi) as the tracer; quantitative uptakes can be measured at 24 h (and at 48 h and 72 h if ^{131}I is used) [77]. Some clinicians prefer to use larger doses of ^{131}I to increase the

sensitivity of the diagnostic WBS, but most WDTC metastatic lesions amenable to ^{131}I therapy are unlikely to be missed after T/NTT using the above-mentioned doses of diagnostic ^{131}I tracer, especially when the scan data are interpreted in combination with the measurement of serum Tg under hypothyroid conditions. Additionally, the use of larger ^{131}I scanning doses may result in thyroid stunning. This phenomenon occurs when the radiation dose from ^{131}I that has been administered for an imaging study results in a lower uptake of ^{131}I given subsequently for remnant ablation or WDTC therapy [78]. There is no well-documented evidence that ^{131}I tracer doses of less than 74 MBq (2 mCi) cause stunning, especially in WDTC tissue. Therefore, after thyroidectomy, it has been recommended that imaging be done with a maximum of 74 MBq (2 mCi) of ^{131}I in children and adolescents [73] or that ^{123}I be used instead.

Yeh and La Quaglia [74] have reported that most institutions treating pediatric patients with WDTC use empirically determined fixed doses of ^{131}I for therapy. The therapeutic dose of ^{131}I can be estimated on the basis of body surface or total body weight, as suggested by Reynolds [79], appropriately modifying the fixed ^{131}I dose protocols used in adults established by the University of Michigan group more than 25 years ago [80]. Maxon [81] proposed another approach to estimating the dose of ^{131}I administered for therapy in pediatric patients that involves the use of quantitative blood and whole body dosimetry. This method is more complicated than using the empirical, fixed-dose method and is not widely used.

The few reports of immediate side effects and complications in pediatric patients treated with ^{131}I have been reviewed by Yeh and La Quaglia [74]. Early side effects include painful swelling of the remnant tissue or metastases, nausea, vomiting, acute swelling of the salivary glands, and transient loss of taste and smell. Transient bone marrow suppression may occur, resulting in leukopenia or thrombocytopenia, with a blood count nadir occurring approximately 6–8 weeks after therapy. A complete blood count should be obtained at baseline and at 6–8 and 10–12 weeks after therapy. Pulmonary fibrosis can occur after therapy for pulmonary metastases, especially if doses exceed 118 MBq/kg body weight (3.2 mCi/kg) or if there is RAI retention in the lung parenchyma of more than

40 MBq/kg (1.1 mCi/kg) 48 h after RAI therapy [78]. There is a paucity of data regarding complications that may appear many years or even decades after therapy. The long-term complications reported to date have been reviewed by Wiersinga [82].

Total cumulative lifetime doses of ^{131}I are generally kept below 18.5 GBq (500 mCi) in children and about 30 GBq (800 mCi) in adolescents [83,84]. Larger cumulative lifetime RAI doses are more likely to be associated with serious long-term complications, including permanent bone marrow suppression and an increase in the subsequent development of leukemias, although the latter possibility has yet to be verified in the context of pediatric WDTC patients. Yet, even if the above relative thresholds have been reached, additional RAI therapies may be administered with great caution, depending on the individual patient's clinical status [66].

The risk of inducing secondary solid tumors after RAI therapy in children and adolescents is probably small, although primary data on this are not available. The most comprehensive study of the outcome of pregnancies in women who received ^{131}I for the treatment of WDTC was published by Schlumberger et al. [85]. Their data on 2130 pregnancies showed no evidence that such therapy affected the outcome of subsequent pregnancies, with the exception of a small increase in the frequency of miscarriages during the first year after therapy.

It should be noted that, although RAI therapy has been proven to reduce both recurrence and mortality in adults with WDTC [48,86], there has been no formal demonstration of equivalent benefits from this therapy in children and adolescents with these tumors [87]. This absence of solid proof of the efficacy of RAI therapy after initial surgery and remnant ablation is probably due to both the epidemiology of WDTC and its natural history features, possibly along with yet-unidentified factors. Nevertheless, most specialists still would consider treating unresectable, RAI-avid, residual/recurrent WDTC deposits with at least one high dose of RAI therapy and monitoring the degree of the resultant antitumor effect [66,74].

Thyroid Hormone Suppression Therapy

Many clinicians prescribe L-T_4 therapy immediately after thyroidectomy to prevent hypothy-

roidism and suppress TSH secretion. Other clinicians prefer that their patients become hypothyroid soon after surgery and, hence, forgo L-T_4 therapy to prepare for RAI diagnostic studies and serum Tg measurements [66]. THST is based on the assumption that the suppression of endogenous TSH deprives WDTC cells of the TSH-dependent stimulation of growth and proliferation. The dose of L-T_4 used to achieve THST is higher than that given for TH replacement in patients with spontaneously occurring primary hypothyroidism [88]. The *physiological* replacement dosage of L-T_4 during late childhood and adolescence is approximately 1–3 µg/kg per day or 100 µg/m^2 per day (or even higher in early childhood), and is typically given orally once daily. The L-T_4 dosage to *fully suppress serum TSH* in children and adolescents is approximately 2.5–5.0 µg/kg per day (150–175 µg/m^2 per day), which is usually higher than the corresponding weight-relative dose in adults.

In parallel with the lack of concrete evidence that RAI therapy has definite benefits in pediatric WDTC, there is lack of data regarding the formal demonstration of survival benefits and prevention of morbidity with THST [87]. On the other hand, THST is associated with fewer side effects (both short- and long-term) than RAI therapy, and has been proven beneficial in adults [86,89; unpublished data from the National Thyroid Cancer Treatment Cooperative Study Registry, Houston, TX]. Furthermore, there is a strong biological basis for its long-term use in the context of WDTC management [89]. Hence, THST remains a standard method of medical treatment after initial therapy of pediatric WDTC with surgery and RAI remnant ablation. Its degree and duration, especially in the low risk patient with PTC, remain controversial [66].

Other Therapies

External beam radiation therapy (EBRT) is rarely used in pediatric patients but may be indicated in select patients with advanced disease who are unresponsive to any other modalities, especially if there is a history of multiple prior neck dissections and the disease is imminently threatening the integrity of local structures. EBRT may slow rapid tumor growth but rarely leads to eradication of WDTC [90].

There has been very little experience with the use of chemotherapy in pediatric patients. However, combination chemotherapy (either with doxorubicin-based schemes or with a paclitaxel-carboplatin regimen) might be tried in select cases in rapidly growing, widely metastatic disease with no other means of clinical control [91; T. Fojo, National Cancer Institute, Bethesda, MD, personal communication; M. Kies, The University of Texas – M. D. Anderson Cancer Center, Houston, TX, personal communication]. Recent data from molecular pathology studies of pediatric PTC specimens have suggested that at least some refractory PTCs in children and adolescents may show responses to the novel fluoropyrimidine capecitabine [92]; however, this assumption has yet to be tested clinically. Chemotherapy should be performed under the guidance of a pediatric oncology specialist, preferably in a tertiary comprehensive cancer center.

Longitudinal Follow-up

Measurement of serum Tg is the most important test for the detection of disease persistence/recurrence in patients with WDTC after total thyroidectomy and ^{131}I thyroid remnant ablation [93,94]. The presumption is that, after thyroidectomy and RAI ablation and while the patient is receiving THST, the serum Tg should be undetectable. Serum Tg determinations are unreliable in the presence of serum antithyroglobulin (anti-Tg) antibodies [95], because those antibodies interfere with the Tg assay. Thus, it is essential to screen for the presence of these antibodies to avoid misinterpretation of the measured Tg levels. Serum Tg levels should be obtained both while on THST and under conditions of TSH stimulation, either after L-T$_4$ therapy has been withdrawn for 5–6 weeks or after rhTSH administration. Kirk et al. [93] have suggested that in the absence of residual/recurrent or metastatic WDTC, serum Tg levels measured under hypothyroid conditions should be less than 10.0 ng/mL, thus setting a threshold below which patients can be designated as having no evidence of disease (NED). We suggest the use of an even more sensitive cutoff Tg level of 8.0 ng/mL [66]. Although not specifically validated in children and adolescents, according to a recent consensus report in adults, the corresponding serum cutoff Tg level

after rhTSH stimulation, above which suspicion of residual/recurrent or metastatic disease is raised, is 2.0 ng/mL [94]. Conversely, patients with a history of WDTC (after primary therapy) who have post-rhTSH serum Tg levels lower than 2.0 ng/mL could be safely considered in NED status (in the absence of any other evidence of residual/recurrent disease).

Patients should be evaluated every 9–12 months for the first 18–24 months after the initial thyroid surgery and RAI therapy with serum Tg level determination, diagnostic RAI WBS, chest X-ray (CXR), and neck U/S [66]. Additionally, free thyroxine and TSH levels should also be obtained with the same frequency to ensure adequate (yet judicious) THST. During these serial follow-up evaluations, if a diagnostic RAI WBS is obtained, the necessity to repeat RAI therapy is determined by a synthesis of clinical and scintigraphic data and by the stimulated serum Tg level. If the diagnostic RAI WBS shows residual neck activity or extracervical disease, then repeat RAI therapy is usually indicated. If macroscopic, abnormal-appearing cervical lymph nodes are present, surgical removal is indicated, followed by repeat ^{131}I therapy. If the serum Tg levels or the diagnostic WBS are positive for disease, then repeat ^{131}I therapy is indicated (assuming an absence of macroscopic disease deposits detectable on neck U/S, which would be amenable to surgical extirpation) [96]. If the diagnostic RAI WBS is negative but the serum Tg level under hypothyroid conditions is higher than 8.0 ng/mL, there is a high probability that residual/recurrent WDTC is present. Some researchers recommend empiric treatment of such patients with the pattern of scan-negative/Tg-positive disease with RAI on the basis of observations in adults with a similar pattern of WDTC, in whom there is a 40–50% probability of obtaining a positive posttherapy RAI WBS. In such patients with a positive posttherapy scan, as many as 30% of them experienced subsequent further reductions in serum Tg levels, demonstrating at least a partial antitumor effect of the prior RAI therapy administered [95]. RAI therapy is usually repeated every 9–12 months, until the serum Tg level and diagnostic RAI WBS both indicate that functional thyroid tissue is no longer present or until a maximal cumulative dose of ^{131}I has been administered. If the maximal lifetime cumulative dose levels of RAI are reached, then further use of RAI needs to be very carefully evaluated on the basis of the patient's clinical status [66].

For patients who remain in NED status after the first 18 months, it has been recommended that three to four additional annual follow-up evaluations (with diagnostic RAI WBS, serum Tg assay, neck U/S, and CXR) be performed, followed by another thorough evaluation 3 years later (assuming that the patient continues to remain in NED status at all times) [66]. If the patient remains disease-free, the next evaluation should be 3–5 years later and, subsequently, every 5 years. Thyroid function and serum Tg levels while on THST should be monitored on a yearly basis for life.

Of note, CXRs typically have been obtained every 6 to 12 months after the initial surgery to detect pulmonary metastases. Unfortunately, CXRs are not sensitive in detecting lung parenchymal metastatic deposits early enough in most patients; these deposits may be detectable only on RAI WBS [97,98]. The role of neck and mediastinal magnetic resonance imaging and nuclear medicine scanning using radionuclides other than ^{131}I (including positron emitters, such as ^{18}F-fluorodeoxyglucose) in the follow-up evaluation of pediatric patients with WDTC has not been validated [66].

It must be emphasized that life-long follow-up is essential, because delayed recurrence is possible, even in the face of serial follow-up evaluations that deemed the patient "free-of-disease" prior to the time of the recurrence. Finally, it is extremely important to transfer care to an adult endocrinologist when the patient reaches adulthood. The suggested scheme for pediatric WDTC long-term follow-up is shown in Figure 23.1.

Medullary Thyroid Carcinoma

Total (or near-total) thyroidectomy with resection of the central cervical lymph node compartment (in multiple anatomical levels (II–VI)) is the procedure of choice for initial therapy in patients with MTC [39,99]. T/NTT is indicated because MTC is often multifocal. Life-long replacement L-T$_4$ therapy is necessary postoperatively. In addition to regional lymph nodes, other common sites of metastases include the lung, liver, bones, and CNS. Therefore, these sites of potential spread need to be screened using imaging methods at the time of initial presentation, as indicated by the clinical features and degree of elevation in plasma calcitonin levels in each case. All patients with MEN2 syndromes should be screened for pheochromocytoma. If pheochromocytoma is present, bilateral adrenalectomy may be necessary because of the multicentricity and bilaterality of these tumors in the context of MEN2 syndromes. Once a patient has been diagnosed as having MEN2A/MEN2B or FMTC through *RET* proto-oncogene mutation testing, such testing should be performed on all living relatives, to detect gene carriers who are predisposed to CCH and MTC [39]. Molecular genetic testing permits early identification of gene carriers before MTC becomes clinically apparent, thus allowing for prophylactic total thyroidectomy and additional surgical procedures as necessary [39,99]. *RET* germline mutation testing has replaced plasma calcitonin testing as the study of choice for the detection of gene carriers in MEN2 pedigrees [53].

The ideal age at which prophylactic T/NTT should be performed in children with *RET* germline mutations remains controversial. In the recent past, some clinicians have recommended surgery in carriers of *RET* mutations associated with MEN2B within the first year of life and for carriers of *RET* mutations associated with MEN2A by 5 years of age [100]. Heptulla et al. [54] proposed prophylactic T/NTT during the first decade of life in patients with FMTC.

A recent consensus conference suggested variable timing of the surgery depending on the actual codon of the *RET* gene where the mutation is located [39], as follows:

- Children with MEN2B and/or *RET* codon 883, 918, or 922 mutations are classified as having the highest risk for aggressive MTC development (level 3 risk) and should have T/NTT within the first 6 months – preferably within the first month – of life.
- Children with *RET* codon 611, 618, 620, or 634 mutations are classified as having a moderately high risk for aggressive MTC development (level 2 risk) and should have T/NTT performed before the age of 5 years.
- Children with *RET* codon 609, 768, 790, 791, 804, or 891 mutations are classified as having the lowest risk of aggressive MTC (level 1 risk). There is little consensus on the management of patients with these

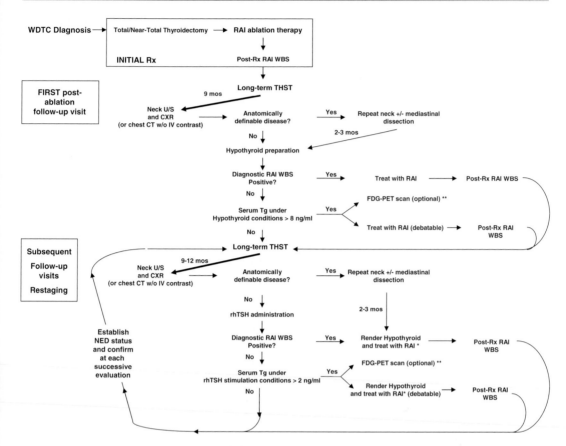

Figure 23.1 Algorithm for the follow-up of pediatric patients with well-differentiated thyroid carcinoma (WDTC) after total/near-total thyroidectomy and initial ^{131}I remnant ablation. In the proposed scheme, special emphasis is placed on the detection and erad-ication – whenever feasible – of persistent/recurrent metastatic disease in all patients who do not achieve no evidence of disease (NED) status. Different cutoff serum Tg values are used as corroborating evidence of residual/recurrent disease, depending on how TSH stimulation is achieved (thyroid hormone withdrawal versus recombinant human thyrotropin (rhTSH) administration). For more details, refer to the text. Abbreviations: CT: computed tomography, CXR: chest X-ray, FDG-PET: ^{18}F-fluorodeoxyglucose positron emis-sion tomography, IV: intravenous, RAI: radioiodine (^{131}I), Rx: therapy, TH: thyroid hormone, THST: thyroid hormone suppressive therapy, U/S: ultrasonography, WBS: whole-body scan, w/o: without; mos, months.
*RAI treatment can also be administered under stimulation with rhTSH. This is an "off-label" use of rhTSH, and should be preferably limited to tertiary center specialists with experience in the treatment of pediatric TC.
**The benefits of using FDG-PET for diagnostic purposes in pediatric TC patients should be balanced against the radiation exposure from the administration of FDG (a positron emitter). Hence, the use of FDG-PET scans in pediatric TC patients should be preferably limited to tertiary center specialists.

mutations. Some advocate T/NTT by the age of 5 years. Others suggest that thy-roidectomy by age 10 is appropriate. Still others recommended periodic pentagas-trin-stimulated calcitonin testing with surgery at the first occurrence of an abnor-mal test result.

The above guidelines were corroborated by the recent finding that the risk of age-related pro-gression from CCH to MTC is dependent upon the transforming potential of the individual *RET* mutation [101,102]. Postoperative EBRT may be offered to patients with high risk of recurrence in the thyroid bed and to those with cervical, supraclavicular, or mediastinal lymphadenopa-thy [103]. Of note, RAI ablative therapy has no role in the postoperative management of MTC.

Peripheral levels of calcitonin and carci-noembryonic antigen (CEA) are used for monitoring disease activity after the initial operation. Patients with persistently elevated or rising calcitonin levels have residual or recurrent metastatic disease, and, in these cases, additional imaging should be performed for localization of the disease, which could lead to further surgical treatment. Imaging is usually done with conventional modalities, such as neck U/S and CT/MRI, although ^{111}In-pentetrotide can also be of considerable help [104].

Anaplastic Thyroid Carcinoma

ATC typically presents clinically as a rapidly enlarging neck mass in the thyroid area. This is usually associated with compression signs, such as dyspnea and dysphagia. The duration of the disease is short, ranging from a few weeks to a few months. At the time of diagnosis, at least 50% of patients harbor metastases in the lung, bone, or brain [44]; these sites of potential disease spread should be carefully screened at the time of initial diagnosis. Surgical excision is the first line of therapy, although in most cases the tumor is so widespread or invasive that total removal is impossible. Nevertheless, surgery may be necessary to relieve compression symptoms. [131]I and THST are completely ineffective for ATC therapy, while multidrug chemotherapy (doxorubicin- or paclitaxel-based) has very minimal or no impact in prolonging survival [105]. The disease is universally lethal within a few months of diagnosis, regardless of the application of aggressive multimodality treatment [106].

Prognosis of Pediatric TC

Well-Differentiated Thyroid Carcinoma

The prognosis for pediatric patients with WDTC is better than for adults with same disease stage. The survival of children and adolescents until 1970 was approximately 82% at 20 years [106], but in four series published in the late 1980s, survival rates of more than 95% at 15–20 years were reported [86,107–109]. The presence of distant metastases does not necessarily portend a poor prognosis. In a series of young patients who presented with distant metastases (reported in 1988 from the Mayo Clinic), only 14% died by 15 years, compared with 68% of adults with disseminated WDTC [109]. It is important to remember that WDTC can recur very late. Indeed, in the Mayo Clinic series, 33% of metastases were detected 5 years after the initial therapy, and 15% were diagnosed more than 15 years later [109].

According to multivariate Cox regression analysis of prognostic factors in 109 children 6–17 years of age with WDTC, disease-free survival is longer in children older than 10 years than in younger children [110]. Disease-free survival is also longer after T/NTT than after less extensive surgery and longer after ^{131}I therapy than after no ^{131}I therapy. In another pediatric WDTC cohort study, age was identified as the major determinant of time to recurrence [111]. In this series, younger patients (younger than 10 years) experienced recurrences more frequently and earlier than patients 10 to 17 years old [110]. Mortality from WDTC in pediatric patients is low, and in many series no malignancy-induced deaths were reported [112]. At the same time, it should be remembered that the majority of disease-specific deaths in patients with WDTC occur years to decades after diagnosis, and, hence, that such incidents are reported only in studies carried out over very long follow-up periods.

Medullary Thyroid Carcinoma

The prognosis in patients with residual/metastatic MTC is overall poorer than that of patients with WDTC [101,113]. There is an early tendency for MTC to metastasize to the lungs and bone. Treatment of patients with persistent MTC remains controversial. Van Heerden et al. [114] reported a study of 31 patients with MTC who had 5- and 10-year survival rates of 90% and 86%, respectively. It is hoped that vigorous screening of MEN2A/B and FMTC family members will lead to early surgical intervention with T/NTT and rigorous life-long follow-up in *RET* mutation-carrying pedigree members, thus leading to increased survival for patients with these tumors [102,115].

Anaplastic Thyroid Carcinoma

As mentioned above, ATC in children and adolescents is fatal in almost all cases, despite occasional partial responses to chemotherapy, which are typically short-lived. Only anecdotal experience exists in the management in such cases. Once again, the extreme rarity of this type of TC in childhood should be emphasized [43,113].

Acknowledgment. We extend our most sincere thanks to Drs Rena Vassilopoulou-Sellin and Steven G. Waguespack, both at The University of Texas M.D. Anderson Cancer Center, Houston, TX, for their thorough review of the manuscript and constructive comments and suggestions. Our gratitude goes to Dr Jacob Robbins, Scientist Emeritus, National Institute of Diabetes and Digestive and Kidney Diseases, National Institutes of Health, Bethesda, MD, for stimulating discussions on the subject over many years.

References

1. Miller RW, Young JL Jr, Novakovic B. Childhood cancer. Cancer 1995; 75:395–405.
2. Harach HR, Williams ED. Childhood thyroid cancer in England and Wales. Br J Cancer 1995; 72:177–783.
3. Belfiore A, LaRosa GL, Padove G, et al. The frequency of cold thyroid nodules and thyroid malignancies in patients from an iodine deficient area. Cancer 1987; 60:3096–3102.
4. Aghini-Lombardi A, Antonangeli L, Martino E, et al. The spectrum of thyroid disorders in an iodine-deficient community: the Pescopagano survey. J Clin Endocrinol Metab 1999; 84:561–566.
5. Quimby EH, Werner SC. Late radiation effects in roentgen therapy for hyperthyroidism. JAMA 1949; 140: 1046–1047.
6. Yoshida A, Noguchi S, Fukuda K, et al. Low-dose irradiation to head, neck, or chest during infancy as a possible cause of thyroid carcinoma in teenagers: a match case-control study. Jpn J Cancer 1987; 78:991–994.
7. Prentice RL, Kato H, Mason M, et al. Radiation exposure and thyroid cancer incidence among Hiroshima and Nagasaki residents. National Cancer Institute Monograph 62, 1982: 207–212.
8. US Nuclear Regulatory Commission. Report on the accident at the Chernobyl power station. NUREG-1250. Washington, DC: US Government Printing Office, 1987.
9. Robbins J. Lessons from Chernobyl: the event, the aftermath fallout: radioactive, political, social. Thyroid 1997; 7:182–192.
10. Antonelli A, Miccoli P, Derzhitski VE, et al. Epidemiological and clinical evaluation of thyroid cancer in children corning from the Gomel region (Belarus). World J Surg 1996; 20:867–871.
11. Baverstock K, Egloff B, Pinchera A, et al. Thyroid cancer after Chernobyl. Nature 1992; 359:21–22.
12. Leehardt L, Aurengo A. Post-Chernobyl thyroid carcinoma in children. Baillière's Clin Endocrinol Metab 2000; 14:667–677.
13. Bounacer A, Wicker R, Caillou B, et al. High prevalence of activating ret proto-oncogene rearrangements in thyroid tumors from patients who had received external radiation. Oncogene 1997; 15:1263–1273.
14. Tuttle RM, Becker DV. The Chernobyl accident and its consequences: update at the millennium. Semin Nucl Med 2000; 30:133–140.
15. Mulligan LM, Kwok JBJ, Healy CS, et al. Germline mutations of the RET proto-oncogene in multiple endocrine neoplasia type 2A. Nature 1993; 363:458–460.
16. Nikiforov YE, Koshoffer A, Nikiforova M, et al. Chromosomal breakpoint positions suggest a direct role for radiation in inducing illegitimate recombination between the ELE1 and RET genes in radiation-induced thyroid carcinomas. Oncogene 1999; 18:6330–6334.
17. Ichihara M, Murakumo Y, Takahashi M. RET and neuroendocrine tumors. Cancer Lett 2004; 204:197–211.
18. Fugazzola L, Pilotti S, Pinchera A, et al. Oncogenic rearrangements of the RET proro-oncogene in papillary thyroid carcinomas from children exposed to the Chernobyl nuclear accident. Cancer Res 1995; 55:5617–5620.
19. Santoro M, Carlomagno F, Hay ID, et al. RET oncogene activation in human thyroid neoplasms restricted to the papillary subtype. J Clin Invest 1992; 89:1517–1522.
20. Bongarzone I, Fugazzola L, Vigneri P, et al. Age-related activation of the tyrosine kinase receptor proto-oncogene RET and NTRKl in papillary thyroid carcinoma. J Clin Endocrinol Metab 1996; 81:2006–2009.
21. Rabes HM, Demidchik EP, Sidorow JD, et al. Pattern of radiation-induced RET and NTRKl rearrangements in 191 post-Chernobyl papillary thyroid carcinomas: biological, phenotype, and clinical implications. Clin Cancer Res 2000; 6:1093–1103.
22. Nikiforov YE, Rowland JM, Bove KE, et al. Distinct pattern of ret oncogene rearrangements in morphological variants of radiation-induced and sporadic thyroid papillary carcinomas in children. Cancer Res 1997; 57:1690–1694.
23. Smida J, Salassidis K, Hieber L, et al. Distinct frequency of ret rearrangements in papillary thyroid carcinomas of children and adults from Belarus. Int J Cancer 1999; 80:32–38.
24. Beimfohr C, Kl.ugbauer S, Demidchik EP, et al. NTRKl re-arrangement in papillary thyroid carcinoma of children after the Chernobyl reactor accident. Int J Cancer 1999; 80:842–847.
25. Santoro M, Thoas G, Williams GH, et al. Gene rearrangement and Chernobyl related thyroid cancers. Br J Cancer 2000; 82:315–322.
26. Namba H, Rubin SA, Fagin JA. Point mutations are an early event in thyroid tumorigenesis. Mol Endocrinol 1990; 4:1474–1479.
27. Lemoine NR, Mayall ES, Wyllier FS, et al. High frequency of RAS oncogene activation in all stages of human thyroid tumorigenesis. Oncogene 1989; 4:159–164.
28. Kroll TG, Sarraf P, Pecciarini L, et al. PAX8-PPAR-gamma-1 fusion oncogene in human thyroid carcinoma. Science 2000; 289:1357–1360.
29. Nikiforova MN, Lynch RA, Biddinger PW, et al. RAS point mutations and PAX8-PPAR gamma rearrangement in thyroid tumors: evidence for distinct molecular pathways in thyroid follicular carcinoma. J Clin Endocrinol Metab 2003; 88:2318–2326.

30. Saez E, Rosenfeld J, Livolsi A, et al. PPAR-gamma signaling exacerbates mammary gland tumor development. Genes Dev 2004; 18:528–540.
31. Grigsby PW, Gal-or A, Michalski JM, et al. Childhood and adolescent thyroid carcinoma. Cancer 2002; 95: 724–729.
32. Sarlis NJ. Expression patterns of cellular growth-controlling genes in non-medullary thyroid cancer: basic aspects. Rev Endocr Metab Disord 2000; 1:183–196.
33. Blatt J, Gishan A, Gula MJ, et al. Second malignancies in very long term survivors of cancer. Am J Med 1992; 93:57–60.
34. Gow KW, Lensing S, Hill DA, et al. Thyroid carcinoma presenting in childhood or after treatment of childhood malignancies: an institutional experience and review of the literature. J Pediatr Surg 2003; 38:1574–1580.
35. De Keyser LFM, Van Herle AJ. Thyroid cancer in children. Head Neck Surg 1985; 8:100–114.
36. Pal T, Vogl FD, Chappuis PO, et al. Increased risk for nonmedullary thyroid cancers in the first degree relatives of prevalent cases of nonmedullary thyroid cancer: a hospital-based study. J Clin Endocrinol Metab 2001; 86:5307–5312.
37. Steiner AL, Goodman AD, Powers SR. Study of a kindred with pheochromocytoma, medullary thyroid carcinoma, hyperparathyroidism and Cushing's disease: multiple endocrine neoplasia, type 2. Medicine (Baltimore) 1968; 47:371–409.
38. Schimke RN, Hartmann WH, Prout TE, et al. Syndrome of bilateral pheochromocytomas, medullary thyroid carcinoma and multiple neuromas: a possible regulatory defect in differentiation of chromaffin tissue. N Engl J Med 1968; 279:1–7.
39. Brandi ML, Gagel RF, Angeli A, et al. Guidelines for diagnosis and therapy of MEN Type 1 and Type 2. J Clin Endocrinol Metab 2001; 86:5658–5671.
40. Farndon JR, Leight GS, Dilley WG, et al. Familial medullary thyroid carcinoma without associated endocrinopathies: a distinct clinical entity. Br J Surg 1986; 73:278–281.
41. Donis-Keller H, Dou S, Chi D, et al. Mutations in the RET proto-oncogene associated with MEN 2A and FMTC. Hum Mol Genet 1993; 2:851–856.
42. Komminoth P, Roth J, Muletta-Feurer S, et al. RET proto-oncogene point mutations in sporadic neuroendocrine tumors. J Clin Endocrinol Metab 1996; 81: 2041–2046.
43. Bucsky P, Parlowsky T. Epidemiology and therapy of thyroid cancer in childhood and adolescence. Exp Clin Endocrinol Diabetes 1997; 105(Suppl 4):70–73.
44. Ain KB. Anaplastic thyroid carcinoma: behavior, biology, and therapeutic approaches. Thyroid 1998; 8: 716–726.
45. Fagin JA, Matsuo K, Karmakar A, et al. High prevalence of mutations of the p53 gene in poorly differentiated human thyroid carcinomas. J Clin Invest 1993; 91:179–184.
46. Hundahl SA, Fleming ID, Fremgen AM, et al. A National Cancer Data Base report on 53,856 cases of thyroid carcinoma treated in the US, 1985–1995. Cancer 1998; 83:2638–2648.
47. Wenig BM, Heffess CS, Adair CF. Atlas of endocrine pathology. Philadelphia: WB Saunders, 1997.
48. Sherman SI. Thyroid carcinoma. Lancet 2003; 361:501–511.
49. Garcia CJ, Daneman A, Thorner P, et al. Sonography of multinodular thyroid gland in children and adolescents. Am J Dis Child 1992; 146:811–816.
50. Telander RL, Zimmerman D, Sizemore GW, et al. Medullary carcinoma in children: results of early detection and surgery. Arch Surg 1989; 124:841–843.
51. Ledger GA, Khosla S, Lindor NM, et al. Genetic testing in the diagnosis and management of multiple endocrine neoplasia type II. Ann Intern Med 1995; 122: 118–124.
52. Wells SA Jr, Donis-Keller H. Current perspectives on the diagnosis and management of patients with multiple endocrine neoplasia type 2 syndromes. Endocrinol Metab Clin North Am 1994; 23:215–228.
53. Marsh DJ, Robinson BG, Andrew S, et al. A rapid screening method for the detection of mutations in the RET proto-oncogene in multiple endocrine neoplasia type 2A and familial medullary thyroid carcinoma families. Genomics 1994; 23:477–479.
54. Heptulla RA, Schwartz RP, Bale AE, et al. Familial medullary thyroid carcinoma: presymptomatic diagnosis and management in children. J Pediatr 1999; 135:327–331.
55. Lips CJM, Landsvater RM, Hoppener JWM, et al. 1994 Clinical screening as compared with DNA analysis in families with multiple endocrine neoplasia type 2A. N Engl J Med 1994; 331:828–835.
56. Croom RD IIIrd, Thomas CG Jr, Reddick RL. Autonomously functioning thyroid nodules in childhood and adolescence. Surgery 1987; 102:1101–1108.
57. Hung W. Solitary thyroid nodules in 93 children and adolescents: a 35-years experience. Horm Res 1999; 52:15–18.
58. Desjardin JG, Khan AH, Montupet P, et al. Management of thyroid nodules in children: a 20-year experience. J Pediatr 1987; 22:736–739.
59. Lugo-Vicente H, Ortiz VN, Irizarry H, et al. Pediatric thyroid nodules: management in the era of fine needle aspiration. J Pediatr Surg 1998; 33:1302–1305.
60. Gharib H, Mazzaferri EL. Thyroxine suppressive therapy in patients with nodular thyroid disease. Ann Intern Med 1998; 128:386–394.
61. Csako G, Byrd D, Wesley RA, et al. Assessing the effects of thyroid suppression on benign solitary thyroid nodules. A model for using quantitative research synthesis. Medicine (Baltimore) 2000; 79:9–26.
62. Singer PA, Cooper DS, Daniels GH, et al. Treatment guidelines for patients with thyroid nodules and well-differentiated thyroid cancer. American Thyroid Association. Arch Intern Med 1996; 156:2165–2172.
63. Corrias A, Elnaudi S, Chiorboli E, et al. Accuracy of fine-needle aspiration biopsy of thyroid nodules in detecting malignancy in childhood: comparison with conventional clinical, laboratory and imaging approaches. J Clin Endocrinol Metab 2001; 86:4644–4648.
64. Al-Shaikh A, Ngan B, Daneman A, et al. Fine-needle aspiration biopsy in the management of thyroid nodules in children and adolescents. J Pediatr 2001; 138:140–142.

65. Gorlin JB, Sallen SE. Cancer in childhood. Endocrinol Metab Clin North Am 1990; 19:649–662.

66. Hung W, Sarlis NJ. Current controversies in the management of pediatric patients with well-differentiated nonmedullary thyroid cancer: A review. Thyroid 2002; 12:683–702.

67. Friedman M, Pacella BC Jr. Total versus subtotal thyroidectomy: arguments, approaches, and recommendations. Otolaryngol Clin North Am 1990; 23:413–427.

68. De Jong SA, Demeter JG, Lawrence AM, et al. Necessity and safety of completion thyroidectomy for differentiated thyroid carcinoma. Surgery 1992; 112:734–739.

69. Robie DK, Dinauer CW, Tuttle RM, et al. The impact of initial surgical management on outcome in young patients with differentiated thyroid cancer. J Pediatr Surg 1998; 33:1134–1140.

71. Dottorini ME, Vignati A, Mazzucchelli L, et al. Differentiated thyroid carcinoma in children and adolescents: a 37-year experience in 85 patients. J Nucl Med 1997; 38:669–675.

72. Hallwirth U, Flores J, Kaserer K, et al. Differentiated thyroid cancer in children and adolescents: the importance of adequate surgery and review of the literature. Eur J Pediatr Surg 1999; 9:359–363.

72. Katoh R, Sasaki J, Kurihara H, et al. Multiple thyroid involvement in intraglandular metastases in papillary thyroid carcinoma. Cancer 1992; 70:1585–1590.

73. Paryani SB, Chobe RJ, Scott W, et al. Management of thyroid carcinoma with radioactive [131]I. Int J Radiat Oncol Biol Phys 1996; 36(Suppl):S83–S86.

74. Yeh SD, La Quaglia MP. 131-I therapy for pediatric cancer. Semin Pediatr Surg 1997; 6:128–133.

75. Sherman SI, Tielens ET, Sostre S, et al. Clinical utility of posttreatment radioiodine scans in the management of patients with thyroid cancer. J Clin Endocrinol Metab 1994; 78:629–634.

76. Mazzaferri EL, Kloos RT. Using recombinant human TSH in the management of thyroid cancer: current strategies and future direction. Thyroid 2000; 10:767–778.

77. Mandel SJ, Shankar LK, Benard F, et al. Superiority of iodine-123 compared with iodine-131 scanning for thyroid remnants in patients with differentiated thyroid cancer. J Nucl Med 2001; 26:6–9.

78. Park HM, Perkins OW, Edmondson JW, et al. Influence of diagnostic radioiodine in the uptake of ablative dose iodine-131. Thyroid 1994; 4:49–54.

79. Reynolds JC. Comparison of I-131 absorbed radiation doses in children and adults: a tool for estimating therapeutic I-131 doses in children. In: Robbins J (ed.) Treatment of thyroid cancer in childhood. Washington, DC: Department of Energy (Publication DOE/EH-0406), 1993: 127–135.

80. Beierwaltes WH. Radioiodine therapy of thyroid disease. Int J Rad Appl Instrum B 1987; 14:177–181.

81. Maxon HR IIIrd Quantitative radioiodine therapy in the treatment of differentiated thyroid cancer. Q J Nucl Med 1999; 43:313–323.

82. Wiersinga WM. Thyroid cancer in children and adolescents – consequences in later life. J Pediatr Endocrinol Metab 2001; 14:1289–1296.

83. Menzel C, Grunwald P, Schomburg A. "High-dose" radioiodine therapy in advanced differentiated thyroid carcinoma. J Nucl Med 1996; 37:1496–1503.

84. Sisson JC. Medical treatment of benign and malignant thyroid tumors. Endocrinol Metab Clin North Am 1989; 18:359–387.

85. Schlumberger M, De Vathaire P, Ceccarelli C. Exposure to radioactive iodine-131 for scintigraphy or therapy does not preclude pregnancy in thyroid cancer patients. J Nucl Med 1996; 37:606–611.

86. Mazzaferri EL, Young RL, Oertel JE. Papillary thyroid carcinoma: the impact of therapy in 576 patients. Medicine (Baltimore) 1977; 56:171–196.

87. Vassilopoulou-Sellin R, Goepfert H, Raney B, et al. Differentiated thyroid cancer in children and adolescents: clinical outcome and mortality after long-term follow-up. Head Neck 1998; 20:549–555.

88. Burmeister L, Goumaz MO, Mariash CN, et al. Levothyroxine dose requirements for thyrotropin suppression in the treatment of differentiated thyroid cancer. J Clin Endocrinol Metab 1992; 75:344–350.

89. McGriff NJ, Csako G, Gourgiotis L, et al. Effects of thyroid hormone suppression therapy on adverse clinical outcomes in thyroid cancer. Ann Med 2002; 34:554–564.

90. Brierley JD, Tsang RW. External-beam radiation therapy in the treatment of differentiated thyroid cancer. Semin Surg Oncol 1999; 16:42–49.

91. Bonadonna G, Beretta G, Tancini G, et al. Adriamycin as a single agent in various forms of advanced neoplasia of adults and children. Tumori 1974; 60:373–391 [in Italian].

92. Patel A, Pluim T, Helms A, et al. Enzyme expression profiles suggest the novel tumor-activated fluoropyrimidine carbamate capecitabine (Xeloda) might be effective against papillary thyroid cancers of children and young adults. Cancer Chemother Pharmacol 2004; 53:409–414.

93. Kirk JMW, Mort C, Grant DB, et al. The usefulness of serum thyroglobulin in the follow-up of differentiated thyroid carcinoma in children. Med Pediatr Oncol 1992; 20:201–208.

94. Mazzaferri EL, Robbins RJ, Spencer CA, et al. A consensus report of the role of serum thyroglobulin as a monitoring method for low-risk patients with papillary thyroid carcinoma. J Clin Endocrinol Metab 2003; 88:1433–1441.

95. Spencer CA. Serum thyroglobulin measurements: clinical utility and technical limitations in the management of patients with differentiated thyroid carcinoma. Endocr Pract 2000; 6:481–484.

96. Robbins J. Management of thyroglobulin-positive, body-scan negative thyroid cancer patients: evidence for the utility of I-131 therapy. J Endocrinol Invest 1999; 22:808–810.

97. Samuel AM, Rajashejharrao B, Shah DH. Pulmonary metastases in children and adolescents with well-differentiated thyroid cancer. J Nucl Med 1998; 39:1531–1536.

98. Vassilopoulou-Sellin R, Libshitz HI, Haynie TP. Papillary thyroid cancer with pulmonary metastases beginning in childhood: clinical course over three decades. Med Pediatr Oncol 1995; 24:119–122.

99. Telander RL, Moir CR. Medullary thyroid carcinoma in children. Semin Pediatr Surg 1994; 3:188–193.

100. Skinner MA, DeBenedetti JF, Norton JA, et al. Medullary thyroid endocrine neoplasia type 2A and 2B. J Pediatr Surg 1996; 31:177–181.

101. Machens A, Niccoli-Sire P, Hoegel J, et al. Early malignant progression of hereditary medullary thyroid cancer. N Engl J Med 2003; 349:1517–1525.

102. Cote GJ, Gagel RF. Lessons learned from the management of a rare genetic cancer. N Engl J Med 2003; 349:1566–1568.

103. Brierley J, Tsang R, Simpson WJ, et al. Medullary thyroid cancer: analyses of survival and prognostic factors and the role of radiation therapy in local control. Thyroid 1996; 6:305–310.

104. Krausz Y, Rosler A, Guttmann H, et al. Somatostatin receptor scintigraphy for early detection of regional and distant metastases of medullary carcinoma of the thyroid. Clin Nucl Med 1999; 24:256–260.

105. McIver B, Hay ID, Giuffrida DF, et al. Anaplastic thyroid carcinoma: a 50-year experience at a single institution. Surgery 2001; 130:1028–1034.

106. Winship T, Rosvoll R. Thyroid carcinoma in childhood: final report on a 20 year study. Clin Proc Child Hosp Washington DC 1970; 26:327–349.

107. Zimmerman D, Hay ID, Gough IR, et al. Papillary thyroid carcinoma in children and follow-up of 1039 patients conservatively in one institution during three decades. Surgery 1988; 104:1157–1166.

108. La Quaglia MP, Corbally MT, Heller G. Recurrence and morbidity in differentiated thyroid carcinoma in children. Surgery 1988; 104:1149–1156.

109. Powers PA, Dinauer CA, Tuttle RM, et al. Treatment of recurrent papillary thyroid carcinoma in children and adolescents. J Pediatr Endocrinol Metab 2003; 16:1033–1040.

110. Jarzab B, Junak DH, Wloch J, et al. Multivariate analysis of prognostic factors for differentiated thyroid carcinoma in children. Eur J Nucl Med 2000; 27:833–841.

111. Alessandri AJ, Goddard KJ, Blair GK, et al. Age is the major determinant of recurrence in pediatric thyroid carcinoma. Med Pediatr Oncol 2000; 35:41–46.

112. Dottorini ME. Differentiated thyroid carcinoma in childhood. Rays 2000; 25:245–255.

113. Parlowsky T, Bucsky P, Hof M, et al. Malignant endocrine tumours in childhood and adolescence – results of a retrospective analysis. Klin Paediatr 1996; 208:205–209.

114. van Heerden A, Grant CS, Gharib H, et al. Long-term course of patients with persistent hypercalcitoninemia after curative primary surgery. Ann Surg 1990; 212:395–400.

115. Gill JR, Reyes-Mugica M, Lyengar S, et al. Early presentation of metastatic medullary carcinoma in multiple endocrine neoplasia, type IIA: implications for therapy. J Pediatr 1996; 129:459–464.

24

Radiation-Induced Thyroid Cancer: Lessons from Chernobyl

James A. Fagin and Yuri E. Nikiforov

Epidemiology of Thyroid Cancer Induced by Ionizing Radiation

The association between ionizing radiation and thyroid cancer was first suggested in 1950 in children who received X-ray therapy in infancy for an enlarged thymus [1]. More conclusive evidence for a causal relationship between external radiation exposure in childhood and thyroid cancer was obtained from pooling the data from several large studies following radiation treatment to the thymus, tonsils, or scalp, and showing a dose-dependent increase in relative risk for development of thyroid cancer [2]. Since the early 1960s, when the use of radiotherapy for benign conditions was abandoned, the incidence of radiation-associated thyroid malignancy in children has gradually decreased [3]. Currently, radiation therapy for other malignancies continues to be a source of radiation-associated thyroid cancer [4,5]. However, this association has been more difficult to establish, in part because radiation is used more often for adults where the thyroid is less sensitive to its effects [6].

An increased risk of thyroid cancer has also been linked to environmental irradiation and documented in survivors of the atomic bomb explosions in Japan in 1945 [7], and in residents of the Marshall Islands exposed to fallout after detonation of a thermonuclear device on the Bikini atoll in 1954 [8]. On 26 April 1986, an accident at the Chernobyl nuclear power station in northern Ukraine produced one of the most serious environmental disasters ever recorded and led to a dramatic increase in the frequency of childhood thyroid cancer in contaminated areas of Belarus, Ukraine, and western Russia. The accident released huge amounts of radioactive materials into the atmosphere, including 1.8×10^{18} Bq of ^{131}I, 2.5×10^{18} Bq of ^{133}I, and 1.1×10^{18} Bq of ^{132}Te, which decays to ^{132}I [9]. More than 10 million people were exposed to significant levels of radiation. It has been estimated that more than 80% of thyroid dose came from internal exposure to ^{131}I, and the dose was 3–10 times higher in children than in adults. Due to the weather conditions immediately after the accident, the most contaminated areas were in southern Belarus, where estimated thyroid doses in children under 7 were among the highest, and ranged between <0.05 and 4 Gy, with an average absorbed thyroid dose of 0.7 Gy [9]. Other areas of significant contamination included regions of northern Ukraine and western Russia.

Beginning in 1990, a dramatic increase in the incidence of pediatric thyroid cancer was noted in Belarus, and one or two years later in northern Ukraine and western areas of Russia. In Belarus, the incidence of thyroid cancer in children in 1995 was almost 30-fold higher than before Chernobyl, and compared to the incidence in other countries. In Gomel oblast, the region closest to Chernobyl, the incidence reached 100/million children/year, a 100-fold increase. Overall, the geographical distribution of cases corresponded to the fallout distribution. In some areas thyroid cancer risk in children was found to be linear in the dose interval 0.07–1.2 Gy [10]. There was a strong inverse correlation between the age at exposure and risk of thyroid cancer [11], a trend that has been documented previously in other populations of radiation-associated thyroid cancer [2]. In Belarus, children under the age of one year at the time of exposure had a relative risk of 237, whereas those aged 10 showed a relative risk of 6 [12]. Higher susceptibility to radiation-induced thyroid cancer in young children may reflect a higher thyroid dose, or other factors that have not been established conclusively. The thyroid cancers in these children were not incidental microcarcinomas discovered because of increased surveillance, but rather represented clinically significant disease, at least in the first few years. There are also reports of a two- to fourfold increase in thyroid carcinoma in adults from exposed areas [12], although it is not clear to what extent this represents a true increase in prevalence versus a higher detection rate of preclinical cancers.

Clinical Characteristics of Radiation-Induced Thyroid Cancers from Chernobyl

The average latency between radiation exposure and cancer diagnosis was 6.9 years in a series of 472 patients from Belarus reported by Pacini et al. [11]. Prior to Chernobyl, the latency period for radiation-induced thyroid cancer was considered to be at least 5 years, typically 5–10 years. However, the Chernobyl experience has clearly demonstrated that it can be as short as 4 years. The clinical characteristics of thyroid cancers arising in children exposed to radiation after Chernobyl differed in significant respects from those arising in children without known radiation exposure treated in Italian and French centers [11]. The vast majority of post-Chernobyl pediatric thyroid cancers were papillary carcinomas (94%) [11], which is consistent with what was found in other populations exposed to ionizing radiation. Although papil-

lary carcinomas were also the dominant tumor type in the sporadic Western European pediatric cases, the prevalence was significantly lower (82%). When compared with sporadically occurring thyroid cancers in children from Western Europe, the post-Chernobyl cancers affected younger subjects, and were less affected by gender [11]. A distinguishing histopathological feature of radiation-associated post-Chernobyl tumors is a high prevalence of solid growth pattern, which appears as sheets of malignant epithelial cells surrounded by varying amounts of fibrotic stroma [13,14]. About 37% of post-Chernobyl tumors had solid variant histology, which is relatively uncommon in sporadic pediatric cases. In the latter, >70% of papillary carcinomas have a classic papillary appearance. Almost half of the pediatric tumors from Belarus extended beyond the thyroid gland, compared to ~25% of sporadic cases. They also had a somewhat higher frequency of lymph node involvement (65% versus 54%). Thus, post-radiation cancers were clinically more aggressive at presentation. A younger age at exposure was associated with more extensive disease, manifesting as greater extrathyroidal tumor extension and frequency of lymph node involvement [15]. The frequency of distant metastases in post-Chernobyl cancers compared to sporadic cases could not be properly determined because, unlike the children from Western Europe, most pediatric patients from Belarus did not undergo postsurgical radioiodine scans, which are required for sensitive detection of distant lesions [11].

Molecular Pathogenesis of Radiation-Induced Thyroid Cancer

Genetic analysis of papillary cancers in children exposed to radiation following Chernobyl implicated the *RET* oncogene in the pathogenesis of these tumors [16–18]. RET is a tyrosine kinase receptor primarily expressed in cells of neural crest derivation. RET is normally not expressed or present at very low levels in thyroid follicular cells. RET activation in papillary carcinomas occurs through chromosomal recombination resulting in illegitimate expression of a fusion protein consisting of the intracellular tyrosine kinase (TK) domain of RET coupled to the N-terminal fragment of a heterologous gene, giving rise to the RET/PTC oncoproteins. Several forms have been identified, which differ according to the 5′ partner gene involved in the rearrangement. The two most common are RET/PTC1 and RET/PTC3. RET/PTC1 is formed by an intrachromosomal inversion of the long arm of chromosome 10 leading to fusion of *RET* with the *H4/D10S170* gene [19]. RET/PTC3 is also a result of an intrachromosomal inversion, in this case with the *RFG/ELE1* gene [20]. The fusion proteins generated by these chimeric genes dimerize in a ligand-independent manner and constitutively activate the tyrosine kinase function of RET. In post Chernobyl tumors, RET/PTC rearrangements are highly prevalent and have been found in 66–87% of all tumors [18,21]. *RET/PTC* oncogenes are not specific to radiation-induced cancers, since they are also found frequently in sporadic pediatric papillary thyroid cancers (~40%). In papillary carcinomas from adults RET/PTC rearrangements are found in 15–20% of cases, with considerable regional variability (range of 5–40%). There is now strong evidence implicating RET/PTC as a key first step in thyroid cancer pathogenesis [22–27]. More specifically, intrachromosomal recombination events, particularly paracentric inversions, appear to be a fundamental mechanism of radiation-induced thyroid carcinogenesis. Another rearrangement that contributes to about 7% of radiation-induced papillary carcinomas involves the nerve growth factor gene *NTRK1* and results from paracentric inversion of chromosome 1q [28,29]. Recently, a new thyroid oncogene arising through recombination of the *BRAF* gene was discovered in a small fraction of radiation-induced papillary thyroid cancers. A paracentric inversion of chromosome 7q results in an in-frame fusion between exons 1–8 of the *AKAP9* gene and exons 9–18 of *BRAF*. The fusion protein contains the protein kinase domain and lacks the autoinhibitory N-terminal portion of *BRAF*. It has elevated kinase activity and transforms NIH3T3 cells, confirming its oncogenic properties [30]. A unique feature of papillary thyroid cancers is that oncogenes thought to be involved in tumor initiation activate effectors that signal along the MAP kinase pathway. Mutation of these oncogenes is mutually exclusive, with very few if any cancers harboring mutations of more than one

of the oncogenes. In radiation-induced cancers they are activated by intrachromosomal recombination events, whereas in sporadic cancers point mutations predominate.

Genotype–Phenotype Correlations in Radiation-Induced Thyroid Cancer

The overall prevalence of *RET/PTC* was found to be significantly higher in radiation-induced tumors occurring after a short latency period, with *RET/PTC3* as the most common type. By contrast, tumors arising after a longer latency have a lower prevalence of *RET/PTC* and the predominant type was *RET/PTC1*. The *AKAP-BRAF* was also more prevalent in cancers appearing after a short latency. RET/PTC1 is associated with papillary carcinomas with a classical histological architecture. By contrast, RET/PTC3 is associated with solid variant papillary carcinomas. The latter appear to have a slightly more aggressive biological behavior.

Radiation-Induced Thyroid Autoimmunity

Children and adolescents living in the most heavily contaminated regions of Belarus were found to have a markedly higher prevalence of thyroid autoantibodies than age-matched controls residing in Braslav, a village in Belarus that was largely spared from radioactive fallout [31]. The increase in prevalence of plasma antithyroglobulin and antiperoxidase antibodies was already apparent in individuals who were in utero or newborn at the time of the accident. In children who were >9 years, the prevalence of autoantibodies was striking, reaching 35%. At the time of the study, there was no evidence of thyroid dysfunction, as serum free T_4, free T_3, and TSH levels were unaffected. Similar findings were reported in a smaller study of children from two iodine-deficient areas of western Russia, one of which received significant radioactive contamination [32]. Despite the fact that in these early studies there was no evidence of thyroid dysfunction in the exposed populations, there is well-founded concern that many of the affected children may develop hypothyroidism later in life.

Approaches to Reduce Exposure of the Thyroid Gland to Radiation

After release of large amounts of radioactive iodine isotopes into the atmosphere, prompt measures need to be taken to minimize thyroid exposure, particularly in children [33]. First and foremost the population needs to be alerted about the risk immediately. Although this is an obvious measure, it is sobering that for various reasons this was not appropriately implemented in some of the most notorious environmental disasters to date, such the Marshall Islands and Chernobyl. People should be instructed to remain indoors and keep doors and windows closed to minimize exposure by inhalation. Because >90% of radioiodine exposure is through contaminated food, and the half-life of the most prevalent iodine radioisotopes is less than 9 days, consumption of fresh milk from local dairies and fresh vegetables should be avoided for several weeks after the accident. Because stable iodine reduces radioiodine uptake, administration of potassium iodide is recommended to saturate the iodine transport mechanism and prevent uptake and incorporation of radioiodine into thyroid cells. In adults, a single dose of 100 mg of iodine reduces uptake in the thyroid to ≤1% at 24 hours [34], whereas in children lower doses are required. Time is of the essence, because when stable iodine is administered within 1 hour of the contamination, thyroid uptake is reduced by 90%. After 3 hours, only 60% reduction is possible. Nevertheless, even if not administered immediately after contamination iodine prophylaxis is still indicated since uptake levels can still be substantially reduced, and will protect the thyroid from continued exposure. Repeated daily administration for 1–2 weeks is advisable. A large potassium iodide (KI) distribution program was implemented in Poland after the Chernobyl nuclear disaster [35]. A single dose of KI was given to ~18 million Poles. When given 3 days after the accident, radioiodine uptake was reduced by 40%, whereas those that received KI

after 4 days had a reduction of 25%. The Polish experience also demonstrated the relative safety of population-wide treatment with KI. Very mild and transient changes in thyroid function were seen in 0.37% of newborn babies, with no apparent long-term consequences. A small proportion of children and adults developed nausea and vomiting, and a few individuals developed respiratory distress due to a presumed allergic reaction to the iodine preparation.

Clinical Management of Radiation-Induced Cancer in Children

The treatment recommendations for children with radiation-induced thyroid cancer do not differ in significant respects from those used for children with sporadic forms of the disease. The first line of treatment is surgery. There is consensus that a total or near-total thyroidectomy is required, but the extent of lymph node dissection is a subject of some controversy, heightened in this population because of the high prevalence of lymph node involvement. This should be followed by radioiodine ablation after withdrawal of thyroid hormone to allow TSH levels to reach a level ≥30 mIU/mL. The usual dose administered is about 1–2 mCi/kg (37–74 MBq/kg). A 3–7-day posttreatment whole-body scan (WBS) is performed to obtain a more sensitive assessment of potential local and distant metastases. A radioiodine WBS is repeated at 8–12 month-intervals after withdrawal of thyroid hormone, and treatment is repeated if significant uptake is observed. Thyroglobulin immunoassays are used as an independent sensitive marker of disease persistence or recurrence. There usefulness in the post-Chernobyl population may be limited because of the high prevalence of antithyroglobulin antibodies. The published experience after treatment of post-Chernobyl thyroid cancer cases shows that they appear to be relatively resistant to ablation, although it is unclear if this due to less radical surgery, or other factors. To our knowledge there are no reports of use of recombinant human TSH for surveillance or treatment in this patient population. Children are maintained on supraphysiological doses of thyroid hormone to achieve appropriate suppression of TSH. They appear to tolerate this moderate degree of iatrogenic hyperthyroidism quite well, with no deleterious consequences on growth. Despite their advanced disease at presentation, most children have responded well to therapy [36]. The long-term prognosis for these children appears favorable, but more time will be needed to fully understand the entire range of consequences of this environmental disaster.

References

1. Duffy BJ Jr, Fitzgerald PJ. Cancer of the thyroid in children: a report of 28 cases. J Clin Endocrinol Metab 1950; 10:1296–1308.
2. Ron E, Lubin JH, Shore RE, et al. Thyroid cancer after exposure to external radiation: a pooled analysis of seven studies. Radiat Res 1995; 141:259–277.
3. Mehta MP, Goetowski PG, Kinsella TJ. Radiation induced thyroid neoplasms 1920 to 1987: a vanishing problem? Int J Radiat Oncol Biol Phys 1989; 16:1471–1475.
4. Hancock SL, Cox RS, McDougall IR. Thyroid diseases after treatment of Hodgkin's disease. N Engl J Med 1991; 325:599–605.
5. Tucker MA, Jones PH, Boice JD Jr, et al. Therapeutic radiation at a young age is linked to secondary thyroid cancer. The Late Effects Study Group. Cancer Res 1991; 51:2885–2888.
6. Schneider AB, Robbins J. Ionizing radiation and thyroid cancer. In: Fagin JA (ed.) Thyroid cancer. Norwell, MA: Kluwer Academic Publishers, 1998: 27–57.
7. Nagataki S, Shibata Y, Inoue S, et al. Thyroid diseases among atomic bomb survivors in Nagasaki. JAMA 1994; 272:364–370.
8. Cronkite EP, Bond VP, Conard RA. Medical effects of exposure of human beings to fallout radiation from a thermonuclear explosion. Stem Cells 1995; 13(Suppl 1):49–57.
9. UNSCEAR. 2000 Report, Vol. 2. Annex J. New York and Geneva: United Nations, 2000.
10. Jacob P, Goulko G, Heidenreich WF, et al. Thyroid cancer risk to children calculated. Nature 1998; 392:31–32.
11. Pacini F, Vorontsova T, Demidchik EP, et al. Post-Chernobyl thyroid carcinoma in Belarus children and adolescents: comparison with naturally occurring thyroid carcinoma in Italy and France. J Clin Endocrinol Metab 1997; 82:3563–3569.
12. Williams D. Cancer after nuclear fallout: lessons from the Chernobyl accident. Nat Rev Cancer 2002; 2:543–549.
13. Furmanchuk AW, Averkin JI, Egloff B, et al. Pathomorphological findings in thyroid cancers of children from the Republic of Belarus: a study of 86 cases occurring between 1986 ("post-Chernobyl") and 1991. Histopathology 1992; 21:401–408.
14. Nikiforov Y, Gnepp DR. Pediatric thyroid cancer after the Chernobyl disaster. Pathomorphologic study of 84 cases (1991–1992) from the Republic of Belarus. Cancer 1994; 74:748–766.
15. Farahati J, Demidchik EP, Biko J, Reiners C. Inverse association between age at the time of radiation exposure and extent of disease in cases of radiation-induced childhood thyroid carcinoma in Belarus. Cancer 2000; 88:1470–1476.
16. Fugazzola L, Pilotti S, Pinchera A, et al. Oncogenic rearrangements of the RET proto-oncogene in papillary thyroid carcinomas from children exposed to the Chernobyl nuclear accident. Cancer Res 1995; 55:5617–5620.
17. Klugbauer S, Lengfelder E, Demidchik EP, Rabes HM. High prevalence of RET rearrangement in thyroid tumors of children from Belarus after the Chernobyl reactor accident. Oncogene 1995; 11:2459–2467.
18. Nikiforov YE, Rowland JM, Bove KE, Monforte-Munoz H, Fagin JA. Distinct pattern of ret oncogene rearrangements in morphological variants of radiation-induced and sporadic thyroid papillary carcinomas in children. Cancer Res 1997; 57:1690–1694.
19. Grieco M, Santoro M, Berlingieri MT, et al. PTC is a novel rearranged form of the ret proto-oncogene and is frequently detected in vivo in human thyroid papillary carcinomas. Cell 1990; 60:557–563.
20. Santoro M, Dathan NA, Berlingieri MT, et al. Molecular characterization of RET/PTC3; a novel rearranged version of the RET proto-oncogene in a human thyroid papillary carcinoma. Oncogene 1994; 9:509–516.
21. Rabes HM, Demidchik EP, Sidorow JD, et al. Pattern of radiation-induced RET and NTRK1 rearrangements in 191 post-Chernobyl papillary thyroid carcinomas: biological, phenotypic, and clinical implications. Clin Cancer Res 2000; 6:1093–1103.
22. Viglietto G, Chiappetta G, Martinez-Tello FJ, et al. RET/PTC oncogene activation is an early event in thyroid carcinogenesis. Oncogene 1995; 11:1207–1210.
23. Sugg SL, Ezzat S, Rosen IB, Freeman JL, Asa SL. Distinct multiple RET/PTC gene rearrangements in multifocal papillary thyroid neoplasia. J Clin Endocrinol Metab 1998; 83:4116–4122.
24. Corvi R, Martinez-Alfaro M, Harach HR, Zini M, Papotti M, Romeo G. Frequent RET rearrangements in thyroid papillary microcarcinoma detected by interphase fluorescence in situ hybridization. Lab Invest 2001; 81:1639–1645.
25. Mizuno T, Kyoizumi S, Suzuki T, Iwamoto KS, Seyama T. Continued expression of a tissue specific activated oncogene in the early steps of radiation-induced human thyroid carcinogenesis. Oncogene 1997; 15:1455–1460.
26. Nikiforov YE, Koshoffer A, Nikiforova M, Stringer J, Fagin JA. Chromosomal breakpoint positions suggest a direct role for radiation in inducing illegitimate recombination between the ELE1 and RET genes in radiation-induced thyroid carcinomas. Oncogene 1999; 18:6330–6334.
27. Nikiforova MN, Stringer JR, Blough R, Medvedovic M, Fagin JA, Nikiforov YE. Proximity of chromosomal loci that participate in radiation-induced rearrangements in human cells. Science 2000; 290:138–141.
28. Greco A, Miranda C, Pagliardini S, Fusetti L, Bongarzone I, Pierotti MA. Chromosome 1 rearrangements involving the genes TPR and NTRK1 produce structurally different thyroid-specific TRK oncogenes. Genes Chromosomes Cancer 1997; 19:112–123.
29. Beimfohr C, Klugbauer S, Demidchik EP, Lengfelder E, Rabes HM. NTRK1 re-arrangement in papillary thyroid

carcinomas of children after the Chernobyl reactor accident. Int J Cancer 1999; 80:842–847.

30. Ciampi R, Knauf JA, Kerler R, et al. Oncogenic *AKAP9-BRAF* fusion is a novel mechanism of MAP kinase pathway activation in radiation-induced and sporadic thyroid cancer. J Clin Invest 2005; 115(1):94–101.

31. Pacini F, Vorontsova T, Molinaro E, et al. Prevalence of thyroid autoantibodies in children and adolescents from Belarus exposed to the Chernobyl radioactive fallout. Lancet 1998; 352:763–766.

32. Vermiglio F, Castagna MG, Volnova E, et al. Post-Chernobyl increased prevalence of humoral thyroid autoimmunity in children and adolescents from a moderately iodine-deficient area in Russia. Thyroid 1999; 9:781–786.

33. Schlumberger M, Pacini F. Measures to reduce exposure of the thyroid gland to radiation. In: Thomas G, Karaglou A, Williams ED (eds) Radiation and thyroid cancer. Singapore: World Scientific Publishing, 1999: 363–368.

34. Sternthal E, Lipworth L, Stanley B, Abreau C, Fang SL, Braverman LE. Suppression of thyroid radioiodine uptake by various doses of stable iodide. N Engl J Med 1980; 303:1083–1088.

35. Nauman J, Wolff J. Iodide prophylaxis in Poland after the Chernobyl reactor accident: benefits and risks. Am J Med 1993; 94:524–532.

36. Ferdeghini M, Boni G, Grosso M, et al. Outcome of post-Chernobyl papillary thyroid carcinomas treated by surgery, radioiodine and TSH-suppressive therapy. In: Thomas G, Karaglou A, Williams ED (eds) Radiation and thyroid cancer. Singapore: World Scientific Publishing, 1999: 481–486.

25

The Use of Stable Potassium Iodide (KI) in the Event of a Nuclear Emergency

Christoph Reiners

The Board on Radiation Effects Research of the National Academy of Sciences of the United States of America set up a Committee in 2003 to draw up recommendations to the President of the United States regarding:

1. the benefits and harmful effects of a potassium iodide (KI) distribution program as part of a nuclear incident preparedness program;
2. the most effective and safe way to distribute and administer KI on a mass scale to prevent radiation effects;
3. the populations that should be included in the KI distribution program.

These recommendations have been recently published by the National Academies Press as a book [1] and are available for download on the internet (http://books.nap.edu/catalog/10868.html). This report has provided the main source for this chapter.

The Thyroid and Iodine

Physiological Need for Stable Iodine

Iodine is an essential component of the iodine-containing thyroid hormones thyroxine (T_4) and triiodothyronine (T_3). Severe iodine deficiency (intake less than 50 µg/day) causes mental retardation, cretinism, and endemic goiter. Even in developed countries such as Germany endemic goiter with thyroid enlarge-

ment and/or nodules is still prevalent in approximately 30% of the adult population [2]. The daily supply of iodine should amount to 90 µg in children aged 0–7 years, 120 µg in children aged 7–12 years, 150 µg in adolescents and adults, and 200 µg in pregnant and nursing women ([3], http://www.ICCIDD.org). In cases of iodine deficiency, the thyroid enlarges and more actively transports iodine from the bloodstream, thus allowing uptake of sufficient iodine for the maintenance of normal thyroid function. In contrast, when the iodine supply is excessive (more than 500 µg/day) the sodium iodide symporter (NIS) of thyrocytes is downregulated, thus inhibiting iodide transport from the bloodstream into the thyroid gland (Wolff–Chaikoff effect, [4]). This effect leads to a transient decrease in thyroid hormone synthesis for about 48 hours; shortly thereafter, normal thyroid hormone synthesis resumes.

Exposure to Radioiodine

Medical Use

For more than 60 years, radioactive isotopes of iodine (mainly ^{131}I as a β- and γ-emitter with a physical half-life of 8 days) have been used for the diagnosis and treatment of thyroid disorders. Moreover, ^{131}I has been employed extensively to study the biokinetics of iodine in healthy people and patients with disturbances of thyroid function. Thyroid radioiodine uptake is elevated in patients with hyperthyroidism and decreased in hypothyroid patients. In addition, it correlates inversely with the nutritional supply of stable iodine. Thus radioiodine uptake is high in iodine deficiency and low in case of iodine excess. In patients with hyperthyroidism, "toxic" nodular goiter, and differentiated thyroid cancer, ^{131}I has been used effectively to normalize thyroid function and to ablate tumor tissue because high activities of ^{131}I can cause cell death.

Nonmedical Use

Radioactive iodine is a byproduct of the fusion of uranium atoms. Minimal radioiodine is normally released into the environment from operating nuclear reactors, whether such reactors are operated for power production, for production of radioisotopes, for material testing or for research. In the case of nuclear power plants, the uranium fuel is contained in sealed metal tubes (fuel rods) and placed inside a steel reactor containment several inches thick, which itself is located inside a thick (several feet) concrete reactor building [1]. Before radioactive iodine from the nuclear fuel of a nuclear power plant can reach the environment, the fuel rods in the reactor core must be damaged, with additional damage to the containment enclosing the reactor. However, if the reactor construction does not fulfill usual safety standards, radioiodine may be released into the environment if there is a nuclear emergency, such as the Chernobyl reactor catastrophe. On the other hand, radioiodine may be released into the environment when uranium is used as an explosive material in atomic bombs or if iodine isotopes were to be used as radioactive components of "dirty bombs" [1].

Radioiodine can exist in particulate form as sodium iodide or as radioiodine vapor. Radioiodine in the gaseous state can be inhaled into the lungs and enter the bloodstream thus reaching the thyroid gland. With normal nutritional iodine supply, a normally functioning thyroid gland will take up and store between 15% and 30% of the radioiodine to which it is exposed. After the Chernobyl reactor catastrophe, most of the dose to the thyroid of people living in the vicinity to the reactor plant was caused by the consumption of radioactive iodine-contaminated water and food, including milk [1].

Harmful Effects of Radioiodine

Deterministic Effects

High doses of radioiodine (more than 5 Gy) may lead to necrosis and apoptosis of thyroid cells thus inducing hypothyroidism. In the case of a nuclear reactor emergency, exposure to high radiation doses sufficient to cause hypothyroidism may only occur in people within very close proximity to the nuclear power plant. After the Chernobyl reactor catastrophe, hypothyroidism occurred in very few people, only those working at the nuclear power plant at the time of the incident.

Stochastic Effects

Smaller doses of radiation (in the range of less than 1 Gy), however, may induce thyroid cancer, especially in vulnerable populations such as unborn or young children. Radiation from any source – including ingested or inhaled radioisotopes – can damage DNA and thus induce tumors. The health effects of the use of radioactive iodine isotopes for diagnosis and treatment of thyroid diseases in adults have been well studied, showing no significant consequences with respect to the induction of thyroid cancer [5]. However, after the Chernobyl reactor accident, the incidence of thyroid cancer in children increased considerably. By the year 2000, about 2000 cases of thyroid cancer had been reported from Belarus, northern Ukraine and the western parts of the Russian Federation [6]. A very important observation is that the relative risk for induction of thyroid cancer in children 0–1 years of age at the time of exposure is 40 or more times higher than that of children 10 years of age or older [7]. The thyroid gland of the fetus begins to concentrate iodine starting with the third month of pregnancy so that the risk for thyroid cancer is increased in unborn children as well. In contrast, the risk of radiation-induced thyroid cancer in adults is extremely low, close to zero [8].

In summary, exposure to radiation from radioactive iodine may lead to a dose-dependent increase of thyroid cancer incidence. Young children are by far the most sensitive group, whereas the risk of thyroid cancer after radiation exposure in adults is very low, and there is assumed to be no risk in adults over 40 years of age [1].

Potassium Iodide (KI) Prophylaxis

Mode of Action

Excess iodine supply downregulates NIS on the surface of thyroid cells, thus inhibiting the uptake of iodine (stable or radioactive) into the gland. In addition, excess iodide administration competes with radioactive iodine, diluting the amount available for uptake into the gland. In the case of radioiodine release from a nuclear incident, the uptake of radioactive iodine from inhalation or ingestion of contaminated foods may be blocked for at least 24 hours if 30–200 mg of KI is administered just before or shortly after exposure. The inhibitory effect of a single dose of 130 mg of KI amounts to 98%, 80%, and 40% if KI is given at the time of exposure, 2 or 8 hours afterwards, respectively (Table 25.1).

Recommended Use

According to the WHO *Guidelines for Iodine Prophylaxis Following Nuclear Accidents* [9] 130 mg of KI corresponding to 100 mg of stable iodine is recommended as a single dose in the event of a nuclear emergency to block radioiodine uptake in adults and adolescents over 12 years of age (Table 25.2). Tablets with a KI content of 130 mg or 65 mg should be available for protection (the latter being more convenient for dosing in children). As an alternative, 170 mg of potassium iodate (KIO_3) may be used. In neonates, infants, and children, lower doses of stable iodine have to be administered (Table 25.2).

Table 25.1 Percent thyroid protection from ^{131}I after a single 130 mg dosage of KI

Time of KI administration with respect to ^{131}I exposure (hours)	Protection provided by 130 mg of KI (% of control)
−96	Very little
−48	~80
−1	~80
0	98
2	80
3	60
8	40
24	16

According to the International Atomic Energy Agency (IAEA) *International Basic Safety Standards,* the generic optimized intervention level for iodine blockade is 100 mGy (10 rad) of avertable committed absorbed dose to the thyroid. Iodine prophylaxis is recommended when this projected dose is exceeded [10].

The life-time thyroid cancer risk in exposed children is estimated by WHO at 1% per Gy (1% per 100 rad) and, conversely the risk of severe side effects from a single administration of stable iodine is estimated at 10^{-7} [9]. WHO therefore recommends an *age-specific intervention level* of 10 mGy (1 Rad) for children and adolescents below the age of 18 years and for pregnant and for lactating women. WHO considers this to be justified because – even with the lower intervention level – some 2 to 5 extra thyroid cancer cases are expected to occur per 1 million children exposed per year [9]. For adults up to 40 years old, WHO follows the recommendation of IAEA for an intervention level of 100 mGy (10 Rad). Because the risk of thyroid cancer is very small in adults over the age of 40, WHO recommends iodine blockade only in the event of very high exposure with more than 5 Gy (500 rad) that may lead to hypothyroidism.

The Food and Drug Administration Guidance of the Unites States of America [11] recom-

Table 25.2 Recommended single dosage of stable iodine to block radioiodine uptake according to age group

Age group	Mass of iodine (mg)	Mass of KI (mg)	Mass of KIO_3 (mg)	Fraction of KI 130 mg tablet
Adults and adolescents (over 12 years old)	100	130	170	1
Children (3–12 years old)	50	65	85	$^1/_2$
Infants (1 months to 3 years old)	25	32	42	$^1/_4$
Neonates (birth to 1 month old)	12.5	16	21	$^1/_8$

mends a single directive for the entire population which should be adopted at an interventional level that is protective for the most susceptible population groups: 50 mGy (5 rad) of predicted thyroid dose for infants, children, adolescents, adults under 40 years of age, and pregnant and lactating women.

In the event of direct exposure to radioiodine in a nuclear emergency, evacuation and sheltering are the preferred methods to protect the population. In addition, the population has to be advised not to consume contaminated foods or drinks. Iodine blockade will rarely be used as a stand-alone protective action. It normally is combined with sheltering or evacuation. In the case of ingestion of contaminated food, however, restricting the production and consumption of foodstuffs will be more effective [9].

Adverse Effects

People with preexisting thyroid diseases – for example nontoxic nodular goiter or autoimmune thyroiditis – are at risk for iodine-induced thyroid dysfunction leading to hypothyroidism. In contrast to iodine-induced hypothyroidism, especially in regions of iodine deficiency, excess iodine ingestion may induce hyperthyroidism as toxic nodular goiter or Jod–Basedow disease [12]. In the most radiation-vulnerable groups of the population (young children) such effects are very rare, as has been observed after KI administration to a large population in Poland after the Chernobyl accident [13].

Additionally, a number of non-thyroidal side effects of iodine have to be mentioned. These may be gastrointestinal (stomach pain, nausea, vomiting, and diarrhea), allergy related (angioedema, arthralgia, eosinophilia, lymphadenopathy, urticaria), or skin rashes. However, such non-thyroidal side effects are very rare. Extremely rare disorders reported to be caused by excess iodine ingestion include dermatitis herpetiformis (Duhring's disease), iododerma tuberosum, and hypocomplementemic vasculitis and myotonia congenita [1].

Distribution Programs

First of all, it has to be mentioned again that iodine blockade is supplemental only to evacuation, sheltering, and restriction of contaminated milk and foodstuffs. Because KI is most effective when taken within a few hours of exposure to radioiodine, pre-distribution programs have been elaborated worldwide. Local, rapid access to KI is accomplished through stockpiling and pre-distribution. However, the effectiveness of pre-distribution programs depends strongly on educating the public. So even with the most efficacious pre-distribution programs, well-developed programs for local stockpiling and renewing pre-distributed tablets are required to ensure protection [1].

Conclusions

Potassium iodide (KI) should be available to everyone at risk of significant health consequences from thyroidal accumulation of radioiodine in the event of a radiological incident (i.e. infants, children, adolescents, adults up to the age of 40 years, and pregnant or lactating women), because it can prevent subsequent thyroid cancer. Providing KI to adults over 40 years of age is of very little benefit. To be most effective, KI must be taken within a few hours before or after exposure to inhaled or ingested radioiodine.

Generally, 130 mg of KI are recommended as a single dose in adults and adolescents over 12 years of age. The recommended dose of KI is 16 mg in neonates, 32 mg in children 1 month to 3 years of age, and 65 mg in children 3–12 years old. In combination with the protective measures of sheltering, evacuation, and restriction of contaminated food, a single level of 50 mGy predicted thyroid dose for infants, children, adolescents, adults under 40 years of age, and pregnant and lactating women seems to be justified for KI intervention.

Distribution of KI tablets should be included in the planning for comprehensive radiological incident response programs for nuclear power plants. KI distribution programs should consider pre-distribution, local and central stockpiling as well as educational and tablet renewing programs.

References

1. National Research Council of the National Academies. Distribution and administration of potassium iodide in the event of a nuclear incident. Washington, DC:

National Academy of Sciences, National Academies Press, 2003.

2. Reiners C, Wegscheider K, Schicha H, et al. Prevalence of thyroid disorders in the working population of Germany: ultrasonography screening in 96 278 unselected employees. Thyroid 2004; 14(11):926–932.
3. World Health Organization: Progress towards the elimination of iodine deficiency disorders. Geneva: WHO/NHD/99.4, 1999.
4. Wolff J, Chaikoff IL, Rosenfeld S: Inhibiting effects of inorganic iodide on the formation in-vitro of thyroxine and diiodotyrosine by surviving thyroid tissue. J Biol Chem 1944; 154:381–387.
5. Holm LA, Hall P, Wiklund K, et al. Cancer risk after iodine-131 therapy for hyperthyroidism. J Natl Cancer Inst 1991; 83:1072–1077.
6. Williams ED: Cancer after nuclear fallout: lessons from the Chernobyl accident. Nature Rev Cancer 2002; 2:543–549.
7. Cardis, Amoros E, Kesminiene A, et al. Observed and predicted thyroid cancer incidence following the Chernobyl accident. Evidence for factors influencing susceptibility to radiation induced thyroid cancer. In: Thomas G, Karaoglou A; Williams ED (eds) Radiation and cancer. Singapore: World Scientific Publishing, 1999: 395–405.
8. Ron E, Lubin JH, Shore RE, et al. Thyroid cancer after exposure to external radiation, a pooled analysis of 7 studies. Radiat Res 1995; 141:259–277.
9. Word Health Organization. Guidelines for iodine prophylaxis following nuclear accidents, Report No. WHO/SDE/PHE99.6, Update 1999. Geneva: World Health Organization, 1999.
10. IAEA (International Atomic Safety Agency). International basic safety standards for protection against ionising radiation and for the safety of radiation sources. Vienna: International Atomic Energy Agency, IAEA Safety Series No. 115, 1996.
11. FDA (Food and Drug Administration). Guidance potassium iodide as a thyroid blocking agent in radiation emergencies. Rockville, MD: US Department of Health and Human Services, Food and Drug Administration, Center for Drug Evaluation and Research, 2001.
12. Roti E, Colzani R, Braverman LE. Adverse effects of iodine on the thyroid. Endocrinologist 1997; 7:245–254.
13. Naumann J, Wolff J. Iodide prophylaxis in Poland after the Chernobyl reactor accident: benefits and risks. Am J Med 1993; 94:524–532.

Section VIII

Diagnostic Imaging Studies for Thyroid Cancer

26

Ultrasound of the Thyroid

David L. Richardson

Modern ultrasound (US) has improved dramatically with the advent of high resolution scanners operating in real time, with high frequencies and the facility to observe blood flow using Doppler.

Technique

Ultrasound as used for medical diagnosis relies on the reflection of sound from interfaces within the body. Use of high frequency sound (7–20 MHz) generates high resolution images over a short depth of tissue. This is ideal for US of the thyroid as it lies superficially under the skin. (Scanning of deeper structures, such as the pancreas, requires a lower frequency of sound to obtain sufficient penetration to visualize the organ. As a consequence the resolution is lower.)

The US probe is placed on the skin of the neck, using coupling gel. This allows transmission of the sound waves into the patient as well as acting as a lubricant. A linear array probe is generally used. This produces clear close images in a rectangular field of view, ideal for imaging the thyroid.

Normal Appearances

The normal thyroid gland has a uniform appearance slightly brighter than the surrounding muscles (Figure 26.1). Vessels and fibrous bands may be seen within it.

Any alteration in its appearance is easily demonstrated and US is therefore very sensitive for the detection of cysts, nodules, and malignancy. More nodules are usually apparent than are discovered by clinical examination [1–4]. There is no consensus how these asymptomatic nonpalpable nodules should be managed. They are often discovered during neck US when the thyroid is not the specific organ being examined. The rate of malignancy in incidentally detected thyroid nodules has been found to be as high as 12% [5], although most series suggest the rate is much lower [4,6].

Nodule Characterization [7]

Although US examination of the thyroid is very sensitive it is not very specific for identifying the cause of solid nodules. The appearances of benign and malignant nodules themselves can be similar. Examination of the surrounding structures for additional features of malignancy can be helpful. Local invasion (Figure 26.2) or large lymph nodes within the neck clearly indicate malignancy.

The majority of malignant nodules (approximately 90%) have a lower echo return than the normal thyroid without distal enhancement.

Hyperechoic nodules (Figure 26.3) are usually benign (malignancy rate less than 1%) but this only accounts for approximately 20% of benign nodules. Around 50–60% of benign

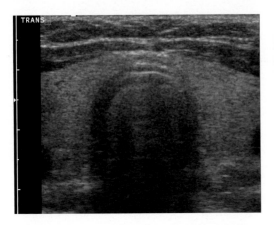

Figure 26.1 Normal transverse US image of the thyroid crossing the trachea.

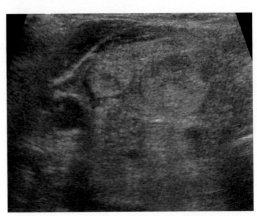

Figure 26.3 Hyperechoic nodules in a benign multinodular goiter.

nodules are hypoechoic, causing clear confusion with malignant nodules.

Cysts are usually benign and easily seen as very echo poor regions within the thyroid generally with thin walls and septa. Post cystic enhancement (a region of brighter echo return behind the cyst) confirms the fluid content (Figure 26.4). The liquid can be echo free (black) or contain floating echogenic "dots" indicating a benign lesion. Hemorrhage into a cyst, which may cause clinical enlargement of the thyroid nodule, shows as echogenic liquid of varying density and appearance when compressed or moved with respect to gravity. A solid element within the cyst wall should be looked for as this increases the probability of malignancy.

The appearance of the margins of a nodule can help in the differentiation of benign from malignant: benign generally have well-defined margins and malignant have poorly defined and irregular margins, sometimes with a thick hypoechoic halo. The difference, however, is often unclear in practice.

Tiny areas of calcification (microcalcification) are suggestive (30%) of malignancy (medullary and papillary carcinomas) but larger regions of calcification are less specific (Figure 26.5). The finding of calcification in a solitary nodule, however, indicates malignancy in 55% [8].

The blood flow pattern within the nodule as seen using Doppler (color and "power" – Figure 26.6) has been used to help in the differentiation between benign and malignant. An intranodular vascular pattern is more sugges-

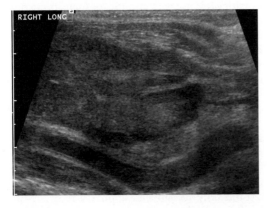

Figure 26.2 Malignant thyroid displacing the common carotid artery.

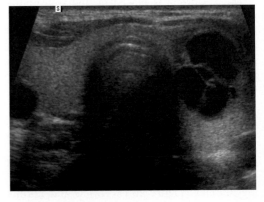

Figure 26.4 Normal right lobe and isthmus. Cysts are shown on the patient's left side, demonstrating post cystic enhancement.

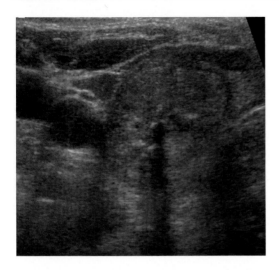

Figure 26.5 Calcification shown as bright echoes with shadowing beyond.

tive of malignancy than a peripheral pattern or no visible vessels [9,10].

Studies are currently under way to investigate whether the new US contrast can improve the benign/malignant differentiation. Promising early results show that contrast arrives within the nodule (from an arm intravenous injection) quicker in malignant nodules than benign (8 seconds versus 20 seconds) [11].

Nodule size can be easily measured with the calipers on modern US machines. Size has been used as a criterion for risk of malignancy but this view has recently been questioned [7,12]. Similarly, single or multiple nodules, easily determined by US, was considered an important risk factor, as the risk of malignancy was thought to be lower in multinodular goiters. The difference is now thought not to be significant [13].

Obtaining Cytological/ Histological Diagnosis

Fine-needle aspiration sampling (FNA) for cytological diagnosis is a standard procedure for palpable nodules. Traditionally this is performed by inserting a green needle on a syringe into the palpated nodule. It is safe and accurate for most head and neck masses [14,15].

Ultrasound is now increasingly being used to position the needle more accurately by selecting a particular part of the nodule, for example the solid component of the wall in a mainly cystic nodule [16,17] or into impalpable nodules (Figure 26.7). A particular nodule can be chosen

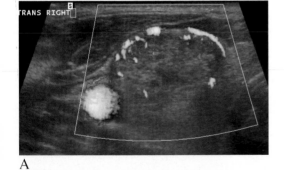

A

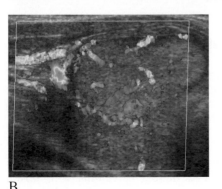

B

Figure 26.6 Power Doppler (**A**) showing peripheral flow in a benign nodule (and the common carotid artery) and color Doppler (**B**) showing central intranodular flow in a malignant nodule.

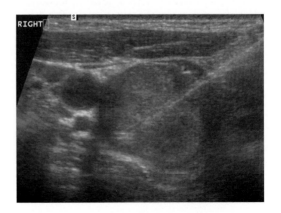

Figure 26.7 Cutting needle biopsy of thyroid nodule.

where the features are suggestive of malignancy. This is often not the palpable nodule. The needle is advanced through the tissues with US visualization in real time. The nondiagnostic sample rate is significantly reduced [18,19]. Deeper and smaller nodules can easily be sampled [20,21]. As a result the availability of US-guided biopsy is seen as important in centers treating thyroid disease [6,18,22–27].

Although historically cutting needles have not been used in the neck due to the theoretical risk of damage to other tissues, when used with US guidance the dangers are extremely small. As such this is the routine method in our hospital for impalpable nodules, where there has been a failed previous FNA or for recurrent disease, that is, for the most difficult cases. There have been no major complications. A double spring action needle is preferred (the inner stylette and the outer cutting sheath are both fired by spring action) as the size of the sample obtained is maximized. The needle is fired on the touch of a button on the handle for a fixed distance (either 2.2 or 1.1 cm). Under local anesthetic and ultrasound vision the needle is advanced to the target nodule and the path of the needle once fired can be considered to hit the target and miss important structures. Cutting needles significantly improve the quality of the sample obtained for the cytologist, reducing the nondiagnostic sample rate to less than 10% [27–29; Richardson et al., unpublished]. It is also a safe method of sampling neck lymphadenopathy [30]. Most patients who have had sampling performed using both methods ("blind" FNA and US-guided cutting biopsy) prefer the latter, in our experience.

Being able to position a needle precisely within the thyroid makes local injection of ethanol possible in the treatment of autonomous nodules and symptomatic cysts [31,32].

Staging Thyroid Malignancy

The International Union Against Cancer staging system [33] is the most widely used: T (tumor), N (node), M (metastasis).

T Stage

The size of the lesion is usually easily and accurately measured using US. Smaller than or equal to 2 cm is T1, 2–4 cm is T2 and greater than 4 cm is T3 for tumors confined to the thyroid. Confusion arises when there are multiple nodules in contact with each other. The differentiation between the nodules may be indistinct, making measurement of individual nodules difficult.

Local extension beyond the thyroid can be identified but again this can be unclear with large multinodular goiters.

Local invasion of the major vessels is seen if present but invasion into the larynx or esophagus is not reliably demonstrated.

N Stage

Nodal spread can be easily seen within the neck. Unfortunately the differentiation between benign and malignant nodes can be difficult. Malignant nodes are generally larger, more hypoechoic than benign nodes, and lose their internal nodal structure. They tend to be well defined when malignant.

M Stage

Metastatic spread to the liver can be demonstrated with ultrasound but generally computerized tomography, magnetic resonance and nuclear medicine imaging are used for the M stage.

Ultrasound therefore remains very important in the local staging of the disease within the neck [34].

Postoperative Patients

Ultrasound can also be used in the detection of recurrent thyroid malignancy (Figure 26.8). Local recurrence appears as a hypoechoic mass within the neck. It is usually ill defined. US-guided biopsy is usually possible and accurate [35].

Studies have also shown in the follow-up of differentiated thyroid carcinoma with serum thyroglobulin measurement that ultrasound

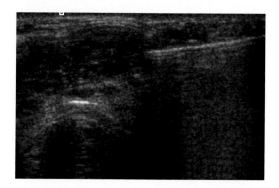

Figure 26.8 Needle biopsy of recurrent thyroid cancer.

significantly increases the sensitivity of tumor detection and may show lymph node metastases despite low thyroglobulin levels [36,37].

Occult Tumors

In high risk patients (family history or post neck irradiation) and in patients with carcinoma of unknown origin ultrasound is very sensitive in detecting occult thyroid primary disease. Metastases to the thyroid can also be seen, most commonly from lung, breast, and renal carcinomas as well as malignant melanoma [38,39]. They are seen as hypoechoic nodules, occasionally with cystic change, but without microcalcification [40].

Cytological sampling of metastases is performed as safely as for primary thyroid malignancy.

Key Points in Ultrasound of Thyroid

- Ultrasound is highly sensitive at detecting thyroid malignancy.
- Differentiation of benign from malignant on the appearances alone is not reliable.
- By using US to direct cytological sampling, high sensitivity and specificity can be achieved.

References

1. Wiest PW, Hartshorne MF, Inskip PD, et al. Thyroid palpation versus high-resolution thyroid ultrasonography in the detection of nodules. J Ultrasound Med 1998; 17(8):487–496.
2. Lee HK, Hur MH, Ahn SM. Diagnosis of occult thyroid carcinoma by ultrasonography. Yonsei Med J 2003; 44(6): 1040–1044.
3. Hegedus L, Bonnema SJ, Bennedbaek FN. Management of simple nodular goiter: current status and future perspectives. Endocr Rev 2003; 24(1):102–132.
4. Nabriski D, Ness AR, Brosh TO, et al. Clinical relevance of non-palpable thyroid nodules as assessed by ultrasound-guided fine needle aspiration biopsy. J Endocrinol Invest 2003; 26(1):61–64.
5. Nam GIS, Kim HY, Gong G, et al. Ultrasonography-guided fine needle aspiration of thyroid incidentaloma: correlation with pathological findings. Clin Endocrinol 2004; 60(1):21–28.
6. Hatada T, Okada K, Ishii H, et al. Evaluation of ultrasound-guided fine-needle aspiration biopsy for thyroid nodules Am J Surg 1998; 175(2):133–136.
7. Papini E, Guglielmi R, Bianchini A, et al. Risk of malignancy in nonpalpable thyroid nodules: predictive value of ultrasound and color-Doppler features. J Clin Endocrinol 2002; 87(5):1941–1946.
8. Kakkos SK, Scopa CD, Chalmoukis AK, et al. Relative risk of cancer in sonographically detected thyroid nodules with calcifications. J Clin Ultrasound 2000; 28(7):347–352.
9. Lebkowska UM, Dzieciol J, Lemancewicz D, et al. The influence of the vascularisation of the follicular thyroid nodules on the proliferative activity of the follicular cells. Folia Morphol 2004; 63(1):79–81.
10. Holden A. The role of colour and duplex Doppler ultrasound in the assessment of thyroid nodules. Australas Radiol 1995; 39(4):343–349.
11. Spiezia S, Farina R, Cerbone G, et al. Analysis of color Doppler signal intensity variation after Levovist injection: a new approach to the diagnosis of thyroid nodules. J Ultrasound Med 2001; 20(3):223–231.
12. Hagag P, Strauss S, Weiss M. Role of ultrasound-guided fine-needle aspiration biopsy evaluation in the evaluation of nonpalpable thyroid nodules. Thyroid 1998; 8(11):989–995.
13. Tollin SR, Mery GM, Jelveh N, et al. The use of fine-needle aspiration biopsy under ultrasound guidance to assess the risk of malignancy in patients with multinodular goiter. Thyroid 2000; 10(3):235–241.
14. Carroll CM, Nazeer U, Timon CI. The accuracy of fine-needle aspiration biopsy in the diagnosis of head and neck masses. Ir J Med Sci 1998; 167(3):149–151.
15. Ammedee RG, Dhurandhar NR. Fine-needle aspiration biopsy. Laryngoscope 2001; 111(9):1551–1557.
16. Court PM, Nygaard B, Horn T, et al. US-guided fine-needle aspiration biopsy of thyroid nodules. Acta Radiol 2002; 43(2):131–140.
17. Braga M, Cavalcanti TC, Collaco LM, et al. Efficacy of ultrasound-guided fine-needle aspiration biopsy in the

diagnosis of complex thyroid nodules. J Clin Endocrinol Metab 2001; 86(9):4089.

18. Leenhardt L, Hejblum G, Franc B, et al. Indications and limitations of ultrasound-guided cytology in the management of nonpalpable thyroid nodules. J Clin Endocrinol Metab 1999; 84(1):24–28.

19. Morgan J, Serpell JW, Cheng MSP. Fine-needle aspiration cytology of thyroid nodules: how useful is it? Aust N Z J Surg 2003; 73(7):480–483.

20. Multanen M, Haapianinen R, Leppaniemi A, et al. The value of ultrasound-guided fine-needle aspiration biopsy (FNAB) and frozen section examination (FS) in the diagnosis of thyroid cancer. Ann Chir Gynaecol 1999; 88(2):132–135.

21. Tambouret R, Szyfelbein WM, Pitman MB. Ultrasound-guided fine-needle aspiration biopsy of the thyroid. Cancer 1999; 87(5):299–305.

22. Carmeci C, Jeffrey RB, McDougall IR, et al. Ultrasound-guided fine-needle aspiration biopsy of thyroid masses. Thyroid 1998; 8(4):283–289.

23. Danese D, Sciacchitano S, Farsetti A, et al. Diagnostic accuracy of conventional versus sonography-guided fine-needle aspiration biopsy of thyroid nodules. Thyroid 1998; 8(1):15–21.

24. Yokozawa T, Fukata S, Kuma K, et al. Thyroid cancer detected by ultrasound-guided fine-needle aspiration biopsy World J Surg 1996; 20(7):848–853.

25. Newkirk KA, Ringel MD, Jelinek J, et al. Ultrasound-guided fine-needle aspiration and thyroid disease. Otolaryngol Head Neck Surg 2000; 123(6):700–705.

26. Deandrea M, Mormile A, Veglio M, et al. Fine-needle aspiration biopsy of the thyroid: comparison between thyroid palpation and ultrasonography. Endocr Pract 2002; 8(4):282–286.

27. Alexander EK, Heering JP, Benson CB, et al. Assessment of nondiagnostic ultrasound-guided fine needle aspirations of thyroid nodules. J Clin Endocrinol Metab 2002; 87(11):4924–4927.

28. Taki S, Kukuda K, Kakuma K, et al. Thyroid nodules: evaluation with US-guided core biopsy with an automated biopsy gun. Radiology 1997; 202(3):874–877.

29. Elvin A, Sundstrom C, Larsson SG, et al. Ultrasound-guided 1.2 mm cutting-needle biopsies of head and neck tumours. Acta Radiol 1997; 38(3):376–380.

30. Screaton NJ, Berman LH, Grant JW. Head and neck lymphadenopathy: evaluation with US-guided cutting-needle biopsy. Radiology 2002; 224(1):75–81.

31. Del PS, Russo D, Caraglia M, et al. Percutaneous ethanol injection of autonomous thyroid nodules with a volume greater than 40 ml: three years of follow-up. Clin Radiol 2001; 56(11):895–901.

32. Braga BM, Basaria S, Mesa C, et al. Sonographically guided percutaneous ethanol treatment of a symptomatic complex nodule with a large cystic component in a patient with thyroid hemiagenesis. J Clin Ultrasound 2002; 30(7):445–449.

33. International Union Against Cancer (UICC). TNM classification of malignant tumors, 6th edn. New York: Wiley-Liss, 2002:52–56.

34. King AD, Ahuja AT, To EWH, et al. Staging papillary carcinoma of the thyroid: magnetic resonance imaging vs ultrasound of the neck. Clin Radiol 2000; 55(3):222–226.

35. Krishnamurty S, Bedi DG, Caraway NP. Ultrasound-guided fine-needle aspiration biopsy of the thyroid bed. Cancer 2001; 93(3):199–205.

36. Pacini F, Molinaro E, Castagna MG, et al. Recombinant human thyrotropin-stimulated serum thyroglobulin combined with neck ultrasonography has the highest sensitivity in monitoring differentiated thyroid carcinoma. J Clin Endocrinol Metab 2003; 88(8):3668–3673.

37. Torlontano M, Crocetti U, D'Aliso L, et al. Serum thyroglobulin and ^{131}I whole body scan after recombinant human TSH stimulation in the follow-up of low-risk patients with differentiated thyroid cancer. Eur J Endocrinol 2003; 148(1):19–24.

38. Lin SY, Sheu WHH, Chang MC, et al. Diagnosis of thyroid metastasis in cancer patients with thyroid mass by fine needle aspiration cytology and ultrasonography. Zhonghua Yi Xue Za Zhi (Taipei) 2002; 65(3):101–105.

39. Ahuja AT, King W, Metreweli C. Role of ultrasonography in thyroid metastases. Clin Radiol 1994; 49:627–629.

40. Chung SY, Kim JH, Oh KK, et al. Sonographic findings of metastatic disease to the thyroid. Yonsei Med J 2001; 42(4):411–417.

27

Diagnostic Nuclear Medicine Investigations in the Management of Thyroid Cancer

Susan E.M. Clarke

Introduction

Whilst radionuclide imaging of the thyroid has long been used in the management of patients with thyroid cancer, its proven role is the subject of discussion. ^{131}I iodine has a clearly established place in the imaging and treatment of histologically proven differentiated papillary and follicular thyroid cancer but the role of radionuclide imaging in diagnosis remains controversial. Similarly, in patients with medullary thyroid cancer, radionuclide imaging is utilized very variably. It is in the centers where there is a close collaboration between the thyroid oncology service and the nuclear medicine department that the contribution of radionuclide imaging is most frequently recognized.

Diagnostic nuclear medicine techniques may be used in the detection of metastatic spread to the skeleton. The ^{99m}Tc diphosphonate bone scan remains a sensitive method for screening for bone metastases and investigating bone pain. ^{99m}Tc pertechnetate salivary gland imaging will identify patients with unilateral or bilateral salivary gland dysfunction including obstruction.

Radionuclide imaging must be considered in conjunction with other imaging modalities. In particular, ultrasound has been demonstrated to be sensitive in detecting cervical lymph nodes and liver metastases in medullary thyroid cancer, computed tomography (CT) will detect macroscopic lung metastases, brain and liver metastases, and magnetic resonance imaging (MRI) has proven sensitivity for detecting marrow involvement.

Although ^{131}I iodine has been used for over 50 years to image and treat thyroid cancer, it is in the last 20 years that there has been the development of many new radiopharmaceuticals that are now being used to image patients with thyroid cancer. Whilst many of these remain of research interest only, ^{18}fluorodeoxyglucose (^{18}FDG) is rapidly becoming established as a valuable agent in patients with ^{131}I iodine scan negative disease.

Whilst radionuclide imaging is a complementary imaging technique to other anatomical imaging methods, it has two main advantages. The first is the provision of whole-body information that facilitates accurate staging at the time of diagnosis and restaging following treatment. The second is the potential for therapy with the exchange of a gamma-emitting radionuclide for a beta or Auger electron emitter. Uptake of a diagnostic radiopharmaceutical will identify those patients who may benefit from therapy. This is particularly relevant in patients with recurrent inoperable medullary thyroid cancer in whom treatment options are extremely limited with no significant responses reported to external beam radiotherapy or chemotherapy.

Radionuclide Imaging

Facilities

Nuclear medicine diagnostic investigations for the investigation of thyroid cancer require appropriate equipment, trained authorized staff, and a supply of appropriate radiopharmaceuticals.

A gamma camera with tomographic capabilities is essential if high quality studies with appropriate sensitivity are to be achieved. Studies for small volume recurrent disease will be nondiagnostic if only planar views are obtained. High resolution, low, medium and high energy collimators will be required if the full range of radionuclide investigations is to be performed. Although gamma cameras with positron emission tomography (PET) capabilities are currently used for ^{18}FDG-PET imaging, the dedicated PET systems yield better results with small volume disease.

Nuclear medicine studies require a team of staff. This should include trained technologists, medical physicists to ensure that equipment is functioning optimally and address radiation protection issues for patients, staff and the public, appropriately trained doctors and radiopharmacists.

Many radiopharmaceuticals may be purchased directly from the manufacturer but some, such as ^{99m}Tc(V)-dimercaptosuccinic acid (DMSA), must be manufactured in-house, requiring an approved radiopharmacy facility and experienced radiopharmacist.

The legislation covering departments of nuclear medicine varies across the world but in some countries, such as the UK, nuclear medicine imaging may only be undertaken with appropriate certification of facilities and staff.

Radiopharmaceuticals

^{99m}Tc Pertechnetate

^{99m}Tc pertechnetate is the most commonly used radiopharmaceutical for routine thyroid imaging with a 6.4h half-life. It combines the advantages of good imaging characteristics (140 keV), availability, and low cost. Unlike the isotopes of iodine, however, it is trapped but not organified by thyroid follicular cells and its biological half-life within the thyroid is therefore significantly shorter than the isotope of iodine that is used for imaging, ^{123}I (Table 27.1). Imaging is performed 20 minutes after intravenous injection. ^{99m}Tc pertechnetate is also taken up by the salivary glands and dynamic studies of salivary gland function before and after stimulation with a sialogogue will identify glands that have been damaged by the radiation dose from therapeutic administration of ^{131}I sodium iodide and those that are functioning but obstructed.

^{123}I Sodium Iodide

^{123}I sodium iodide is an alternative agent for imaging the thyroid. Like ^{99m}Tc pertechnetate it has good imaging characteristics with a gamma energy of 159 keV and a half-life of 13.5h. It is both trapped and organified by the thyroid follicular cells and has a marginally higher sensitivity for detecting nonfunctioning nodules

Table 27.1 Radiopharmaceuticals used in thyroid disease

Radiopharmaceutical	Abbreviation	Clinical use
^{99m}Tc pertechnetate	^{99m}Tc	Thyroid nodules, goiter, thyrotoxicosis, ectopic thyroid
^{123}I iodide	^{123}I	Thyroid nodules, goiter, ectopic thyroid thyrotoxicosis, dyshormonogenesis
^{131}I iodide	^{131}I	Carcinoma of the thyroid, diagnosis and treatment
^{99m}Tc isonitrile	^{99m}Tc-MIBI	Thyroid nodules, Ca thyroid MTC
^{201}Thallous chloride	^{201}Tl	Thyroid nodules, Ca thyroid, MTC
^{18}Fluorodeoxyglucose	^{18}FDG	Ca Thyroid, MTC, Hürthle cell Ca
^{99m}Tc (V) dimercaptosuccinic acid	^{99m}Tc(V)-DMSA	MTC
^{123}I metaiodobenzylguanidine	$^{123/131}$I-MIBG	MTC diagnosis and treatment
^{111}In octreotide	^{111}In Oct	MTC, lymphoma, Hürthle cell Ca
^{67}Gallium gitrate	^{67}Ga	Lymphoma

than ^{99m}Tc pertechnetate. It is, however, significantly more expensive than ^{99m}Tc pertechnetate and is not routinely available. In combination with perchlorate it can be used to assess the organification capabilities of nodules.

^{124}I Sodium Iodide

^{124}I sodium iodide is a positron-emitting isotope of iodine and has been used in a limited number of dosimetric studies. With its ultrashort half-life and limited availability, its main use is in dosimetry research as it provides excellent data on functional volumes [1].

^{131}I Sodium Iodide

^{131}I iodine in the form of ^{131}I sodium iodide has been used for over 40 years to diagnose and treat thyrotoxicosis and differentiated thyroid carcinoma. It is produced by the fission of uranium-236 and by the neutron bombardment of stable tellurium in a nuclear reactor. It decays by emissions of gamma radiations 364 keV (81%), 337 keV (7.3%), and 284 keV (6%) with beta radiation of E_{max} 0.606 MeV to stable xenon-131. ^{131}I iodine has a half-life of 8.04 days. Imaging is performed using a high energy collimator on the gamma camera. Imaging is performed 24–130 hours after oral administration of the radiopharmaceutical, either in liquid form or as a capsule.

The main advantage of ^{131}I sodium iodide as a diagnostic and therapeutic radiopharmaceutical is its low cost and availability while its main disadvantage is the high energy gamma emissions, which has radiation protection implications for staff, relatives, and other patients. The normal biodistribution includes the salivary glands, stomach, and bladder. The bowel is also visualized on delayed studies (Table 27.2). An awareness of the normal biodistribution is essential for the accurate interpretation of whole-body images. Contamination of the skin and hair with saliva or urine may cause false-positive scans and care must be taken in image interpretation.

^{201}Tl Thallium

^{201}Tl thallium is a potassium analogue and crosses the cell membrane via the sodium-potassium ATPase pump. ^{201}Tl has been recog-

Table 27.2 Biodistribution of ^{131}I

Normal sites of ^{131}I accumulation	Nontumor sites of ^{131}I uptake
Salivary glands	Hepatic cysts
Saliva in mouth	Psoriasis
Stomach	
Intestine	
Bladder	

nized as a tumor-imaging agent since 1976, when Cox et al. [2] first demonstrated ^{201}Tl uptake in a bronchial carcinoma included inadvertently in the field of view during a myocardial stress study. Since then, ^{201}Tl uptake has been described in thyroid and breast carcinomas, lymphomas, osteosarcomas, Ewing's sarcomas, and esophageal cancers [3]. It has poor imaging characteristics, however, and nonspecific uptake in the myocardium, liver, and muscles limits its usefulness outside the neck.

^{99m}Tc Sestamibi (MIBI)

^{99m}Tc sestamibi (MIBI) uptake is proportional to blood flow and mitochondrial concentration. Although originally developed as a myocardial perfusion imaging agent, its role in tumor imaging is well proven, with uptake in parathyroid adenomas, breast tumors, and thyroid malignancies.

^{99m}Tc(V) Dimercaptosuccinic Acid

^{99m}Tc(V) dimercaptosuccinic acid (DMSA) was initially developed in Japan as a general tumor-imaging agent [4]. It rapidly became apparent that its main clinical use is in patients with medullary thyroid cancer (MTC). Sensitivities ranging from 50% [5] to 80% [6,7] have been reported in patients with primary and recurrent MTC. Images should be acquired 2–3 h after injection and uptake may be observed in both soft-tissue and bone metastases. The isomeric mix of ^{99m}Tc(V)-DMSA varies when it is prepared using different commercial kits [8,9]. It is suspected that the poor sensitivity results reported by some workers may be a result of the isomeric composition of their manufactured product. A further explanation for some of the poor results reported may be the patient selection. There is a well-recognized subset of patients in whom the calcitonin level is elevated but stable and in whom no focal disease can be demonstrated for several years. Imaging with ^{99m}Tc(V)-DMSA in this subset will yield a significantly lower sensitivity for tumor detection.

Single photon emission computed tomography (SPECT) imaging will increase the sensitivity of lesion detection and will also define the extent of the primary tumor more accurately [10].

The normal biodistribution of ^{99m}Tc(V)-DMSA is seen at 2 h to be in the nasal mucosa and faintly in the skeleton. Breast uptake may be noted in women. Blood pool activity persists at 2 h and the blood pool of the heart, liver, and spleen may be identified on whole–body imaging. There is no nonspecific tracer uptake observed in the liver, making ^{99m}Tc(V)-DMSA one of the few tumor-imaging agents that is able to reliably detect liver metastases. Pituitary uptake may be seen in some patients.

Uptake in sites of MTC ranges from intense to faint, with uptake ratios of greater than 30:1 observed in some patients with neck recurrence. Uptake in soft-tissue sites appears more intense than is observed in sites of bone metastases. Image quality is generally good, although the lack of nonspecific uptake may make localization of an identified lesion difficult. Studies using the principle of image registration have permitted the merger of image data from the ^{99m}Tc(V)-DMSA image with the data from an anatomically precise MRI image. This merged image gives clinically useful information to the surgeon prior to surgery. Image registration also raises the sensitivity of both imaging modalities by increasing the confidence with which small lesions may be diagnosed [9].

^{111}I Indium Octreotide

Like many neuroendocrine tumors, MTC tumors express somatostatin receptors [11]. Somatostatin is a neuropeptide that was discovered in 1978 [12] and has been found to have an inhibitory effect on growth hormone receptors. In animals this peptide appears to inhibit the growth of various malignant tumors [13].

^{123}I/^{131}I Iodine Metaiodobenzylguanidine

Following successful imaging of the adrenal medulla by Wieland et al. [14] in 1980, many groups have studied the uptake of the guanethidine analogue metaiodobenzylguanidine (MIBG) in neuroectodermally derived tumors including MTC. MIBG is commercially available in many countries labeled with either ^{123}I iodine or ^{131}I iodine. Tomographic imaging as well as planar imaging should be performed to optimize sensitivity. Although not routinely used for diagnostic purposes, a positive scan will indicate a possible therapeutic option. A number of commonly prescribed drugs interfere with the uptake of MIBG and should be avoided or discontinued in patients being considered for diagnostic or therapeutic uses of MIBG (Table 27.3).

^{18}FDG-PET

Radiolabeled fluorodeoxyglucose [^{18}FDG] is the most widely used tracer in PET tumor imaging. A structural analogue of 2-deoxyglucose, FDG is transported into and trapped by tumor cells. ^{18}F is a positron emitter with a 20-minute half-life. The emitted positrons interact with matter with release of two 511 KeV gamma photons and it is these that are imaged. A dedicated PET camera and appropriate staff are required for imaging and the short half-life of the tracer together with the high cost of equipment limits availability in many areas of the world. ^{18}FDG accumulation is a marker of metabolic activity and therefore reflects proliferative activity and the number of viable tumor cells.

Monoclonal Antibodies

Several monoclonal antibodies have been used to image patients with MTC. These include ^{123}I-, ^{131}I-, and ^{111}In-CEA [15,16], both whole anti-

Table 27.3 Drugs that interfere with MIBG uptake

| Tricyclic antidepressants |
| Labetalol |
| Reserpine |
| Sympathomimetics |
| Antipsychotics |
| Calcium channel blockers |
| Cocaine |

body and fragments, and ^{111}In-anticalcitonin antibody. These various monoclonal antibodies are currently only available on a research basis.

Cholecystokinin (CCK)-B/Gastrin Receptor Imaging

Amiri-Mosavi et al. in 1999 demonstrated that MTC expressed cholecystokinin-B/gastrin receptors [17]. Behr et al. have demonstrated that CCK-B/gastrin receptors can be detected in the biopsy specimens of patients with MTC but are not found in normal thyroid tissue [18]. This agent is only available on a research basis.

Papillary and Follicular Thyroid Cancer

Diagnosis

The role of imaging in the investigation of patients with suspected thyroid cancer is controversial, reflecting the high incidence of nodules in the normal population and low prevalence of thyroid malignancy.

In a patient with a palpable nodule in the thyroid, the simple technique of imaging the thyroid using ^{99m}Tc pertechnetate will identify whether the palpable nodule is functioning or nonfunctioning. Thyroid cancer typically appears as a hypofunctioning "cold" nodule on ^{99m}Tc pertechnetate thyroid imaging but this is a nonspecific finding (Figure 27.1A). Specificity varies with the iodine status of the population studied. In Austria, prior to iodine supplementation, the incidence of thyroid cancer in cold thyroid nodules was 3.5% [19] compared with 21% in the iodine-replete USA [20].

In 1978, Tonami et al. [21] described the use of ^{201}Tl in investigating patients with cold thyroid nodules. However, Harada et al. [22] demonstrated that ^{201}Tl could not distinguish between benign and malignant nodules. Alternative tumor-seeking radiopharmaceuticals such as ^{99m}Tc sestamibi, ^{99m}Tc tetrofosmin and [18]fluorodeoxyglucose have proved unreliable in differentiating benign and malignant thyroid nodules. In practice, many centers now proceed to fine-needle aspiration cytology under ultrasound guidance without prior imaging. A combined scintigraphy/ultrasound approach

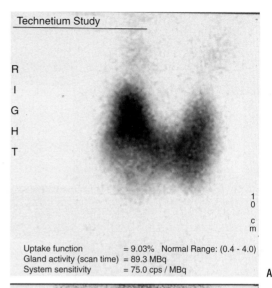

Technetium Study

Uptake function	= 9.03% Normal Range: (0.4 - 4.0)
Gland activity (scan time)	= 89.3 MBq
System sensitivity	= 75.0 cps / MBq

A

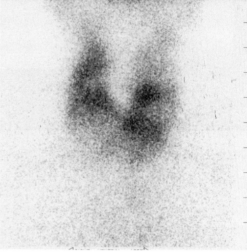

B

Figure 27.1 A ^{99m}Tc pertechnetate scan of a patient with toxic diffuse goiter (Graves' disease). Clinically nonpalpable cold nodule detected which was proven to be papillary thyroid cancer on fine-needle aspiration. **B** [99m]Tc pertechnetate scan of a patient with a multinodular goiter diagnosed on palpation. The dominant cold nodule was investigated with fine-needle aspiration and a colloid nodule was diagnosed.

reduces the number of unnecessary fine-needle aspirations performed on functioning nodules and improves sampling accuracy in dominant, nonfunctioning nodules arising from multinodular glands (Figure 27.1B).

[18]FDG-PET has been able to detect thyroid cancer during studies for other pathologies. An

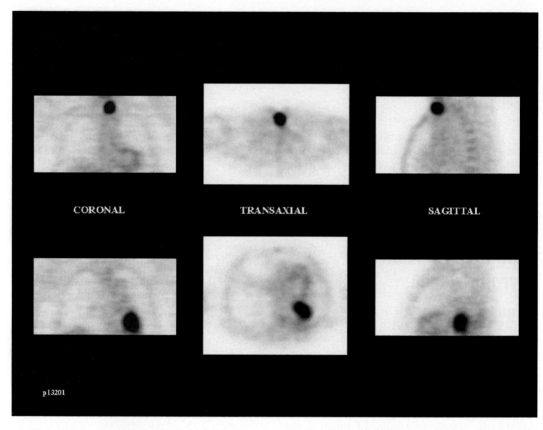

Figure 27.2 Sixty-two-year-old man undergoing staging investigations for carcinoma of the bronchus with ^{18}FDG-PET. The primary lung lesion was visualized but an additional area of high uptake in the lower left neck was identified. Further investigation confirmed a follicular carcinoma of thyroid.

intense area of focal uptake in the thyroid region warrants further evaluation as a number of such identified lesions have been proven to be thyroid cancer on fine-needle aspiration and surgery (Figure 27.2). Uptake of ^{18}FDG in a thyroid nodule, however, is not specific for thyroid cancer. Adler et al. in a study of 9 thyroid nodules demonstrated uptake in 2 of 3 nodules that were malignant but also in 3 out of 4 benign adenomas [23].

Uematsu et al. demonstrated standardized uptake values (SUVs) greater than 5 in proven cancers, differentiating them from benign nodules with lower SUVs. A patient with chronic thyroiditis had an SUV of 6.3, however [24].

Management Following Surgery

Radionuclide imaging is used following surgery to establish the presence of remnant thyroid tissue thereby identifying patients who require ^{131}I ablation therapy. Following successful ablation of remnant thyroid tissue, ^{131}I imaging is routinely used to identify patients with biochemical evidence of remnant or recurrent tumor and may also be used to plan the amounts of radioiodine to be administered.

Whilst the use of imaging with tracer doses of ^{131}I to establish the presence of remnant thyroid tissue following surgery for differentiated thyroid carcinoma has been an established practice for many decades, recent concerns that the tracer dose of ^{131}I may influence the efficacy of the subsequent therapy dose of ^{131}I-iodine have been raised.

Standard practice has been to undertake an ^{131}I tracer study using administered activities ranging from 74 to 370 MBq (2 to 10 mCi). The tracer study permits identification of residual thyroid tissue and also may identify metastatic disease. Whole-body imaging plus local views of the head and neck area are routinely performed, with imaging taking place 48 hours after administration of the tracer dose. As it is essential that TSH levels are elevated to ensure good uptake of the tracer dose, imaging should not be performed less than 4 weeks after surgery or 4 weeks after discontinuing thyroxine (T_4) or 2 weeks after discontinuing triiodothyronine (liothyronine, T_3). An awareness of the normal biodistribution of ^{131}I is essential in interpreting tracer images, and regions of normal biodistribution are listed in Table 27.2. Artifacts due to urine contamination and saliva must also be recognized.

Numerous authors have raised the issue of "stunning" which results in the reduction of uptake of a therapy dose of ^{131}I iodine following a high dose diagnostic tracer scan. The concept of the "stunned" thyroid has raised controversy as to the dose of ^{131}I to be used for these diagnostic studies. Many believe that a large dose is essential, Waxman et al. [25], for example, having shown that identification of an increasing number of remnants was associated with increasing the tracer dose up to 100 MBq (30 mCi) or more. However, several authors have observed that the uptake of a therapeutic dose may be less than that of a preceding diagnostic dose. Even a dose of 5 mCi was found sufficient to reduce the uptake of a therapeutic dose by 54% [26]. Various strategies have been proposed to overcome the problem of stunning. These include using low tracer scan doses of [131]I (<185 MBq, 5 mCi). Whilst data confirms that this strategy reduces the problem of stunning, lower tracer scan doses will reduce the sensitivity of imaging for detecting metastatic disease. Reporting that the induction of the "stunned" thyroid by 370 MBq (10 mCi) diminished thyroidal uptake of a 3.7 GBq (100 mCi) treatment dose, Park et al. [27] recommended that pretherapy scanning should be undertaken with [123]I. Murphy et al. [28] have shown that ^{123}I has a sensitivity of 75% compared with ^{131}I if activities of 74 MBq (2 mCi) are used.

If only an estimate of the amount of remaining normal tissue is required, ^{99m}Tc can be used (Figure 27.3A, B)[29], but when, in follow-up studies, identification of possible metastases is sought, an iodine isotope is essential because of the relatively poor trapping avidity of neoplastic tissue for [131]I.

Another proposed strategy is to assume that the majority of patients undergoing total thyroidectomy for differentiated thyroid cancer will have small remnants of thyroid tissue and patients are therefore treated with an ablation therapy dose of ^{131}I without prior imaging. Whilst this strategy avoids the problem of stunning, it prevents therapy dose adjustment on the

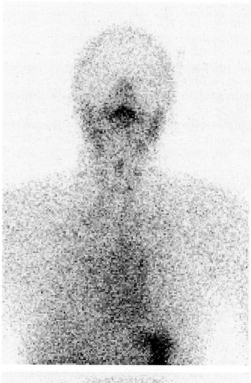

A

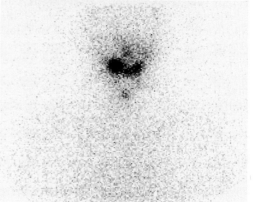

B

Figure 27.3 A ^{99m}Tc pertechnetate scan of a patient's neck after surgical ablation of thyroid for papillary cancer. A small remnant is demonstrated (arrow). **B** ^{131}I-iodine tracer scan in same patient showing identical pattern of uptake.

basis of the size of the thyroid remnant or dosimetric calculations to be performed.

Selection of Ablation Dose

Many centers opt for a fixed ^{131}I ablation dose,
but others opt for a varied ^{131}I dose based on the
size of the thyroid remnant and retention of the
tracer dose of [131]I. If an ^{131}I tracer study is performed, data may be used to determine an
appropriate ablation dose using the following
formula. There are few data to suggest that dosimetric calculations improve the first time ablation rate following a first therapy dose.

A posttherapy ^{131}I scan should be performed
in all patients, particularly those who have not
undergone an ^{131}I tracer scan prior to ablation
therapy. The posttherapy high activity scan has
a higher sensitivity for detecting unsuspected
metastatic disease compared with the low activity ^{131}I tracer scan (Figure 27.4).

Postablation Management

Following the successful ablation of remnant
thyroid tissue, the ^{131}I whole-body scan will
show no abnormal foci of uptake in the absence
of metastatic disease. It is appropriate to
monitor these patients subsequently with thyroglobulin measurements and to utilize the [131]I
tracer scan in patients whose thyroglobulin
measurements become elevated. Patients who
have metastatic disease at the time of diagnosis
will require regular ^{131}I tracer scans between
treatments to determine the efficacy of [131]I
therapy (Figure 27.5A, B, C). Tracer scans with
[131]I should be undertaken using doses of 185
MBq (5 mCi) or less to avoid effects of stunning,
although stunning has been only clearly proven
as a problem with remnant thyroid tissue.
Tracer scans using ^{131}I are not normally performed in less than 6 months following [131]I
treatment and as the TSH levels must be elevated to optimize the sensitivity of the [131]I
tracer scan, patients should discontinue thyroid
replacement hormone for an appropriate interval or receive human recombinant TSH used to
transiently elevate TSH levels [30].

A percentage of patients will be found to have
elevated thyroglobulin levels with negative
iodine tracer scans. This is a particular issue in
patients with Hürthle cell carcinomas in whom
only 10% of tumors are iodine avid. Patients

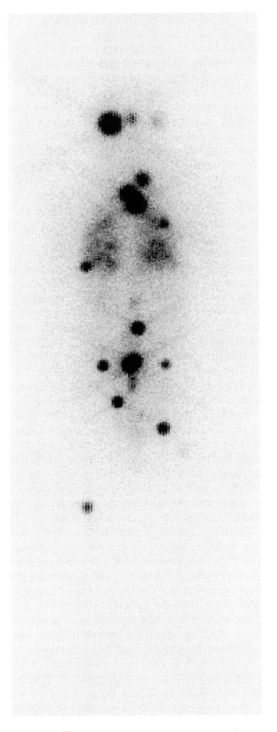

Figure 27.4 ^{131}I iodine postablation scan in a patient demonstrating unsuspected widespread metastases from papillary
thyroid cancer.

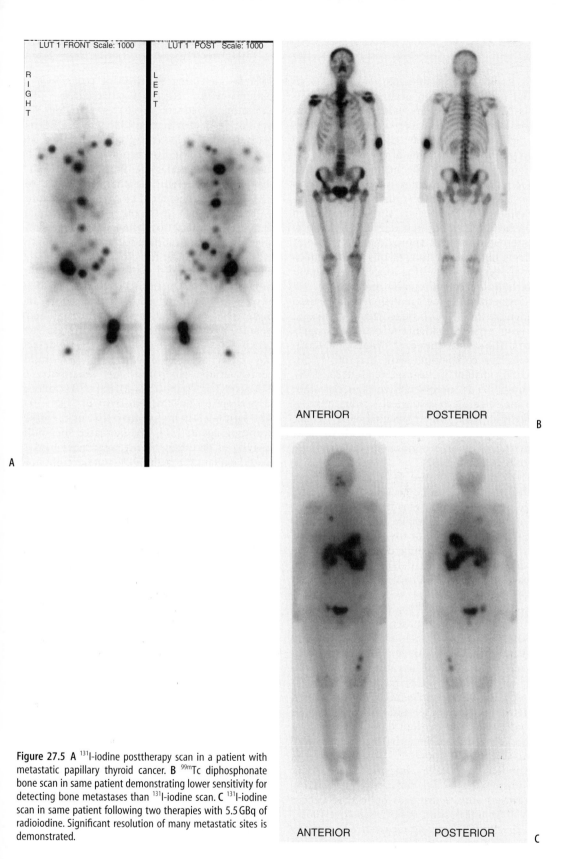

Figure 27.5 A ^{131}I-iodine posttherapy scan in a patient with metastatic papillary thyroid cancer. **B** [99m]Tc diphosphonate bone scan in same patient demonstrating lower sensitivity for detecting bone metastases than ^{131}I-iodine scan. **C** ^{131}I-iodine scan in same patient following two therapies with 5.5 GBq of radioiodine. Significant resolution of many metastatic sites is demonstrated.

with papillary and follicular carcinomas in whom dedifferentiation occurs may also continue to have raised thyroglobulin levels, but become iodine tracer scan negative as a feature of dedifferentiation. Various strategies have been proposed in patients in whom dedifferentiation is suspected. These include a proposal to use to retinoic acid to cause tumor redifferentiation and restoration of tumor iodine uptake capabilities. A number of studies have been published confirming that retinoids will cause redifferentiation in approximately 30% of patients but the duration of this redifferentiation appears short and the longer-term benefit of retinoid treatment remains unclear.

Alternative imaging agents may also be used to identify the location of recurrent disease in ^{131}I scan negative patients to determine operability. The sensitivities of ^{201}Tl and ^{99m}Tc tetrofosmin are comparable with that of ^{131}I for detecting distant metastases (0.85, 0.85, 0.78), although ^{131}I is more sensitive than the other two for detecting postsurgical residual thyroid tissue [31]. Scintigraphic imaging with ^{201}Tl has been thought to reflect the abnormal DNA characteristic of poor prognosis in differentiated thyroid carcinoma [32].

MIBI has been proved to be clinically more useful than ^{201}Tl in detecting lung, lymph node, and bone metastases from differentiated thyroid carcinoma, as image quality was better. The overall sensitivity of the two techniques is not, however, significantly different [33]. The superiority of MIBI in detecting lymph node disease before initial ^{131}I treatment has also been described by Ng et al. [34], who noted that MIBI is not as sensitive as ^{131}I scanning for thyroid remnants or lung metastases.

Both MIBI and ^{201}Tl yield high specificity and positive predictive value for residual thyroid cancer in patients with negative ^{131}I scans who have an increased risk of recurrence after ^{131}I therapy. Both imaging agents have been shown to detect residual cancer and cause a change in management in more than half the patients in whom conventional imaging techniques were unreliable [35].

Another myocardial imaging agent, ^{99m}Tc tetrofosmin, has a high sensitivity in detecting metastases and recurrences of thyroid cancer [36]. ^{99m}Tc tetrofosmin is both sensitive (86%) and specific for detecting recurrence in patients taking thyroxine and also has a sensitivity of

74% for detecting the sites of recurrence in patients with ^{131}I scan negative disease [37]. Preliminary reports suggest a role for ^{111}In octreotide in this setting [38]. ^{18}FDG-PET has proved useful in detecting cervical nodes and can direct surgical intervention. It can also be used to identify metastases in the mediastinum, thorax, and skeleton. The main value of ^{18}FDG-PET in the management of thyroid carcinoma patients, like that of the other methods above, lies in its ability to demonstrate metastatic sites after negative iodine scanning. Its accuracy is high, particularly for cervical lymph nodes where it has proved particularly helpful for directing surgical management. It can also identify metastases in the mediastinum, thorax, and bone. Studies on patients with thyroglobulin positive and iodine scan negative disease gave sensitivities of between 70% and 90% for detecting iodine negative disease [39,40]. A multicenter study compared the sensitivity of ^{18}FDG-PET, ^{201}Tl, and ^{99m}Tc-MIBI in ^{131}I scan negative disease. The 90% sensitivity of ^{18}FDG-PET was significantly higher than that of the other scanning agents [41]. The increased metabolic activity of dedifferentiating, aggressive tumors would explain the high ^{18}FDG uptake compared with much lower uptake seen in iodine avid tumors. The 3-year survival of patients with ^{18}FDG positive scans is markedly reduced compared with patients whose scans are negative [42].

Recently, the importance of TSH stimulation in the uptake of ^{18}FDG has been appreciated. In a number of studies, patients have been imaged whilst on TSH suppressive dose of thyroxine and when off thyroxine with a high endogenous TSH. Several studies have confirmed the increased sensitivity of tumor detection in patients off thyroxine [43]. A recent study by Petrich et al. [44] has confirmed that the use of recombinant human TSH prior to imaging with ^{18}FDG increases imaging sensitivity.

In patients with iodine negative, thyroglobulin positive disease, these studies, in conjunction with anatomical imaging, will assist in patient management decisions by identifying whether the recurrence is operable or inoperable due to location or multifocality. ^{18}FDG-PET scanning has the highest sensitivity for detecting dedifferentiating recurrent disease, particularly with the patient off thyroxine or after recombinant TSH administration.

Hürthle Cell Cancer

The Hürthle cell variant of follicular thyroid cancer is characterized by oxyphilic follicular cells. They are more aggressive than follicular carcinomas and metastasize more frequently. Unlike standard follicular cancers, only 10% of Hürthle cell cancers take up iodine and this fact, together with their aggressive behavior, results in a 20-year survival of 65% compared with 81% for follicular cancers.

Imaging Hürthle cell cancers has been attempted with a variety of radiopharmaceuticals. Yen et al. [45] have explored the role of ^{99m}Tc-MIBI in diagnosing metastatic disease and shown a significantly better sensitivity than with ^{131}I. Vergara et al. [46] have studied 99mTc(V)-DMSA in Hürthle cell tumors and have shown that although uptake is seen in some tumors, the sensitivity is not adequate for clinical purposes. ^{111}I indium octreotide uptake has been demonstrated in some Hürthle cell tumors but, again, the uptake is not reliably sensitive for routine clinical use [47].

The role of ^{18}FDG-PET has been explored in a number of studies. Intense uptake in sites of recurrent disease has been demonstrated, changing management in 50% of the patients who were so studied [48,49].

Insular Carcinoma

This rare variant of follicular cancer is poorly differentiated and highly aggressive. Local invasion and distant metastases at the time of diagnosis are common. Poor results have been observed with most radionuclide imaging methods including ^{131}I, ^{111}In octreotide [50], ^{99m}Tc-MIBI [51], and ^{99m}Tc(V)-DMSA [52].

The aggressive nature of insular carcinomas with negative ^{131}I uptake makes it probable that ^{18}FDG-PET uptake will be seen and this has been confirmed by Diehl et al. [53] in a retrospective study of five patients.

Medullary Thyroid Cancer

Diagnosis and Follow-Up

In a patient undergoing investigation for thyroid nodules, the identification of bilateral nonfunctioning nodules on the ^{99m}Tc pertechnetate thyroid scan raises the possibility of MTC associated with familial MTC (FMTC), multiple endocrine neoplasia type 2A (MEN2A), or MEN2B [54].

Parthasarathy et al. [55] first described the accumulation of ^{201}Tl in an MTC primary lesion, and subsequently uptake has been reported in both primary and recurrent lesions[56–58] with sensitivities of up to 91% and specificities of 100% reported. The poor imaging characteristics of ^{201}Tl are not a problem in visualizing neck recurrence, but limit the value of this agent in detecting distant metastases. The nonspecific uptake of this tracer in the liver and lungs and its uptake in the myocardium reduce its sensitivity in detecting liver and lung metastases.

The main role for ^{99m}Tc(V)-DMSA imaging is in the follow-up of patients after surgery [56]. In primary MTC, ^{99m}Tc(V)-DMSA can confirm a clinical suspicion of MTC while the calcitonin results are awaited. Papillary and follicular tumors of the thyroid do not take up ^{99m}Tc(V)-DMSA and positive uptake in a cold nodule on a ^{99m}Tc pertechnetate scan is strongly suggestive of MTC. ^{99m}Tc(V)-DMSA whole-body imaging is also useful when planning surgery to stage the disease. It is probably the most effective imaging agent for demonstrating soft-tissue and bone metastases.

Immediately following surgery, ^{99m}Tc(V)-DMSA imaging may be useful in determining whether residual tumor is present (Figure 27.6A). It is essential that the patient is imaged prior to surgery when there is bulky disease in order to assess whether the primary tumor takes up the agent. In longer-term follow-up, ^{99m}Tc(V)-DMSA imaging can be used to determine the site of recurrence in patients in whom the postoperative calcitonin levels start to rise. Again SPECT imaging will increase the sensitivity of lesion detection, particularly in patients with small-volume recurrent mediastinal deposits.

(V)-DMSA may also be labeled with rhenium-186 [57]. Clinical experience with this radiopharmaceutical confirms that its biodistribution resembles that of ^{99m}Tc(V)-DMSA, although renal retention is greater [58]. Limited therapy experience is available The availability of ^{186}Re is limited, however. ^{188}Re produced from a generator is now available and studies using ^{188}Re (V)-DMSA are in progress.

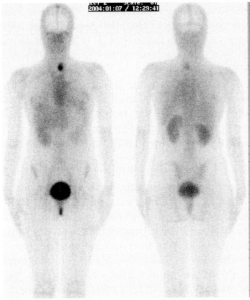

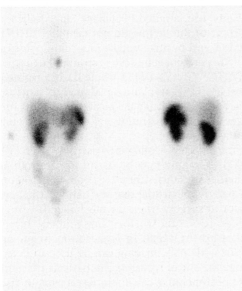

Figure 27.6 A ^{99m}Tc(V)-DMSA whole-body scan following surgery for medullary thyroid cancer demonstrating residual tumor in lower left neck. **B** ^{111}I indium octreotide scan in same patient showing lower uptake in remnant tumor.

The role of ^{99m}Tc-MIBI has been investigated as an imaging agent in patients with recurrent MTC. Learoyd et al. [59] compared the uptake of ^{99m}Tc-MIBI with CT in patients with recurrent

MTC and demonstrated that ^{99m}Tc-MIBI is more sensitive than CT for detecting recurrence in the head, neck, and chest, but CT was more sensitive for detecting disease in the liver. The ^{99m}Tc bone scan was more sensitive for detecting bone metastases than ^{99m}Tc-MIBI. Ugur et al. [60] compared the sensitivities of ^{99m}Tc-MIBI, ^{201}Tl, and ^{99m}Tc(V)-DMSA and showed them to be 47%, 19%, and 95%, respectively. These data confirm that at present ^{99m}Tc(V)-DMSA is the most sensitive radionuclide imaging agent available. Juweid et al. have used ^{99m}Tc-MIBI to explore the multidrug resistance of MTC [61].

Following successful imaging of the adrenal medulla by Wieland et al. [14] in 1980, the role of $^{123/131}$I-MIBG in MTC has been investigated in MTC. Nakajo et al. [62] in 1983 studied a number of patients with neuroectodermal tumors, including one patient with MTC. They reported no uptake in MTC. The first positive case of ^{131}I-MIBG uptake in a patient with MEN2A was reported by Endo et al. [63] in 1984. Uptake in both the primary MTC and the coexistent pheochromocytoma was observed. In the same year Connell et al. [64] also described ^{131}I-MIBG uptake in a primary tumor of a patient with familial MTC. The first report of uptake in metastatic MTC was made by Sone et al. [65] in 1985, who studied a nonfamilial case of MTC with bone and liver metastases. Uptake was seen in all sites of known disease.

Following the publication of these case reports a number of series of cases have been reported. Poston et al. [66] in 1985 studied six patients, three with sporadic MTC, two with MEN2A, and one with MEN2B. Although all patients studied were postoperative with calcitonin evidence of recurrence, only one patient had a positive study. The results of many series of MTC patients studied with MIBG have been published [5,67–71]. The later series have been performed with ^{123}I-MIBG that has increased resolution, but none of the studies have utilized SPECT. In most studies a sensitivity of 30% is reported, and this is confirmed when the cumulative experience is reviewed.

Several studies have been undertaken to compare the sensitivities of different radiopharmaceuticals in MTC. Clarke et al. [72] in 1988 compared the uptake of ^{99m}Tc(V)-DMSA, ^{131}I-MIBG, and ^{99m}Tc-MDP in patients with MTC and showed that ^{99m}Tc(V)-DMSA was the most sensitive agent for detecting sites of MTC. Verga et al. [5] in 1989 compared ^{99m}Tc(V)-DMSA and ^{123}I- or ^{131}I-MIBG and again confirmed that ^{99m}Tc(V)-DMSA was the more sensitive agent.

The technical aspects of ^{123}I- or ^{131}I-MIBG imaging in MTC need to be considered. In patients with primary disease or suspected neck recurrence who have not undergone total thyroidectomy, it is essential to block the thyroid prior to administration of MIBG. Unless adequate blockade with potassium iodate is achieved, interpretation of uptake in the neck will be extremely difficult. Whole-body images at 4 and 24 hours should be acquired, and SPECT imaging of the neck and liver at 24 hours will increase lesion detection in patients imaged with ^{123}I-MIBG. The role for ^{131}I-MIBG in diagnostic imaging is debated. The slow tumor accumulation of MIBG may indicate that the later imaging possible with ^{131}I-MIBG compared with ^{123}I-MIBG may increase the sensitivity of lesion detection.

Although ^{131}I- and ^{123}I-MIBG have been shown to have an unacceptably low sensitivity for diagnostic imaging, the therapeutic potential of ^{131}I-MIBG in those patients in whom good uptake is demonstrated should be recognized.

A number of patients with MTC have now been treated with ^{131}I-MIBG and a palliative response has been achieved in about 50% of patients so treated [73]. Partial response has been observed in a further 25% of patients, with response times lasting up to 18 months [74,75] (Figure 27.7).

^{111}In octreotide is also used to detect recurrence in patients with rising calcitonin levels indicating recurrent MTC. SPECT imaging will enhance lesion detection in the neck and liver. Sensitivities of 65% have been reported in detecting MTC lesions, although the sensitivity is lower in the liver as a result of nonspecific uptake (Figure 27.6B) [76].

Since some therapeutic responses in MTC have been reported using a somatostatin analogue [77], the ability to demonstrate which MTC patients may respond to this agent should prove of great benefit given the high cost of treatment. Therapy has been undertaken with high doses of ^{111}In octreotide utilizing the radiation effect of Auger electrons [78]. Various ^{90}Y-labeled compounds have been evaluated although some studies have reported renal toxicity as a dose limiting factor [79].

The importance of detecting recurrent disease to facilitate surgery and prolong symptom-free survival has been emphasized earlier. Numerous studies have been undertaken with ^{18}FDG in patients with calcitonin elevations indicating the site of recurrent MTC (Figure 27.8). A multicenter study by Diehl et al. [80] concluded that ^{18}FDG is sensitive in detecting recurrent disease and compares favorably with other radionuclide and non-radionuclide imaging techniques. Other studies have suggested that ^{18}FDG-PET imaging is more sensitive in patients with rapidly progressive disease than in patients with slowly rising calcitonin levels [81].

Results from imaging with monoclonal antibodies have been varied, ranging from 0% with anticalcitonin antibody to 78% with ^{131}I-anti-CEA antibody. The results of imaging with monoclonal antibodies in patients with MTC have been compared with imaging with other radiopharmaceuticals by a number of groups. Cabezas et al. [16] compared imaging with ^{131}I-anti-CEA antibody and ^{131}I-MIBG and showed

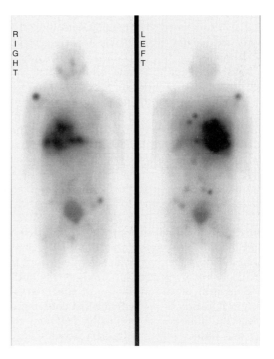

Figure 27.7 ^{131}I-MIBG posttherapy scan in a patient with metastatic medullary thyroid cancer. Good uptake of therapy dose at metastatic sites is identified.

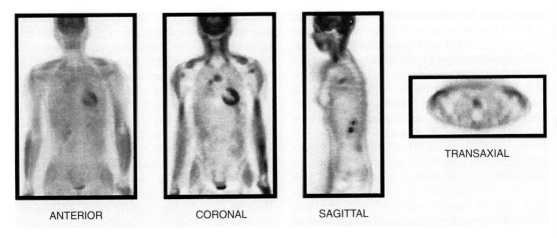

Figure 27.8 [18]FDG-PET scan in patient with history of medullary thyroid cancer and a rising calcitonin. Other imaging investigations failed to identify the location of recurrence but the [18]FDG-PET scan demonstrated uptake in bihilar nodes. As recurrence was inoperable, patient was referred for chemotherapy.

significantly higher lesion detection with the antibody. They also compared the relative sensitivity of CT imaging with the two radionuclide techniques and showed that CT imaging was also inferior to ^{131}I-anti-CEA imaging. Sandrock et al. [71] compared the results of imaging with ^{131}I-MIBG, ^{201}Tl, and ^{111}In-anti-CEA antibody and also concluded that imaging with the antibody yielded the best results. Troncone et al. [70] evaluated [99m]Tc(V)-DMSA, ^{131}I-MIBG, and ^{131}I-anti-CEA antibody and showed that the sensitivity of imaging with [99m]Tc(V)-DMSA and ^{131}I-anti-CEA antibody was far superior to imaging with MIBG. As the target to background ratio of anti-CEA antibody is low, the Marseille group have developed a two-step targeting technique of a bispecific antibody. The first arm (Fab fragment) recognizes the CEA tumor expression and the second arm (Fab fragment) is specific for the bivalent di-DTPA–indium hapten. In the first step of the process the non-labeled antibody is injected and binds to the tumor cells expressing CEA, Four to 5 days later, the bivalent hapten which is radiolabeled is injected and binds to the anti-hapten arm of the antibody. In the interval before injection of the radiolabeled compound bispecific antibody is gradually degraded by normal tissues [82]. Preliminary studies have been encouraging in a French multicenter study in patients with MTC and preliminary results of a phase I/II clinical trial been published [83].

Juweid et al. [84] explored high dose ^{131}I-MN-[14]F(ab)(2) anti-CEA antibody and autologous hemopoietic stem cell rescue in patients with rapidly progressive disease, with all patients achieving disease stabilization and some showing tumor regression. The same group has also undertaken animal studies using combinations of ^{90}Y-labeled CEA antibody with doxorubicin and Taxol. The efficacy of the combined treatments was greater than either treatment given alone [85].

Imaging studies in patients with MTC using ^{111}In diethylenetriamine pentaacetic acid-Dglu(1)-minigastrin have demonstrated a 91% sensitivity for detecting tumor, even in patients with occult disease. Dose escalation studies are now being undertaken to assess the efficacy and toxicity of ^{90}Y-minigastrin in patients with advanced metastatic disease. Initial results are reported as promising although nephrotoxicity is a major concern [22]. A summary of the advantages and disadvantages of the various radiopharmaceuticals used to image patients with MTC is given in Table 27.1.

Conclusion

Nuclear medicine imaging continues to have an established role in the management of patients with papillary and follicular thyroid cancers, with ^{131}I scanning remaining the routine imaging technique for localizing remnant and recurrent disease. The development of recombinant human TSH offers increased flexibility for imaging and treatment, whilst reducing the side effects of thyroxine withdrawal. The newer radionuclide imaging techniques remain under-utilized, despite good evidence for their sensitivity in detecting tumor recurrence. The development of new agents continues with the potential for new therapeutic agents. The importance of the development of evidence-based strategies for the optimal integration of radionuclide imaging in the diagnosis and follow-up of patients with thyroid cancers needs to be recognized.

References

1. Flower MA, al-Saadi D, Harmer CL, McCready VR, Ott RJ. Dose response study on thyrotoxic patients undergoing positron emission tomography and radioiodine therapy. Eur J Nucl Med 1994; 21:531–536.

2. Cox PH, Belfer AJ, Van der Pompe WB. Thallium 201 uptake in tumours, a possible complication in heart scintigraphy. Br J Radiol 1976; 49:767–768.

3. Hisada K, Tonami N, Miyamae T, et al. Clinical evaluation of tumour imaging with 201-Tl chloride. Radiology 1978; 129:497–500.

4. Ohta H, Yamamoto K, Endo K. A new imaging agent for medullary thyroid cancer. J Nucl Med 1984; 25:323–325.

5. Verga V, Muratori F, Sacco G, Ban F, Libroia A. Role of ^{131}iodine MIBG and ^{99m}Tc (V)DMSA in the diagnostic value of MTC. Henry Ford Hosp Med J 1989; 37:175–177.

6. Clarke SEM, Fogelman I, Lazarus CR, Edwards S, Maisey MN. A comparison of ^{131}iodine-MIBG and ^{99m}Tc-pentavalent-DMSA for imaging patients with medullary carcinoma of the thyroid. In: Schmidt HAE, Emrich D (eds) Nuklearmedizin – nuclear medicine in research and practice. Stuttgart: Schattauer, 1987: 375–378.

7. Guerra UP, Pizzocara C, Terzi A. New tracers for imaging MTC. Nucl Med Comm 1989; 10:285–295.

8. Blower P, Singh J, Clarke SEM, Bisnnaden M, Went M. Pentavalent ^{186}rhenium DMSA: a possible tumour therapy agent. J Nucl Med 1990; 31:768–770.

9. Blower PJ, Singh J, Clarke SEM. The chemical identity of pentavalent technetium 99m-dimercaptosuccinic acid. J Nucl Med 1991; 32:845–849.

10. Chaudhuri AR, Lewis MK, Bingham JB, Clarke SEM. Registration of MR and SPECT images in medullary thyroid carcinoma. Nucl Med Comm 1993; 14:256.

11. O'Brien DS, DeLellis RA, Wolfe HJ, Tashjian AH, Reichlin S. Somatostatin immunoreactivity in human C-cell hyperplasia and medullary thyroid carcinoma. J Lab Clin Med 1987; 109:320–326.

12. Guillemin R. Peptides in the brain: the new endocrinology of the neuron. Science 1978; 202:390–402.

13. Lamberts SWJ, Koper JW, Reubi JC. Potential role of the somatostatin analogues in the treatment of cancer. Eur J Clin Invest 1987; 17:281–287.

14. Wieland DM, Win JL, Brown LE. Radiolabelled adrenergic neuroblocking agents: adrenomedullary imaging with Iodine-131 meta iodobenzylguanidine. J Nucl Med 1980; 21:349–353.

15. Reiners C, Eilles C, Spiegel W, Becker W, Boerner W. Immunoscintigraphy in MTC using ^{123}I or ^{111}In labelled monoclonal anti CEA antibody fragment. J Nucl Med 1986; 25:227–231.

16. Cabezas RC, Berna L, Estorch M, Carrio I, Garcia-Ameijeiras A. Localisation of metastases from medullary thyroid carcinoma using different methods. Henry Ford Hosp Med J 1989; 37:169–172.

17. Amiri-Mosavi A, Ahlman H, Tisell LE, Wangberg B, Kolby L, Forsell-Aronsson E. Expression of cholecystokinin–B/gastrin receptors in MTC. Eur J Surg 1999; 165:628–631.

18. Behr TM, Behe MP. Cholecystokinin–B/gastrin receptor targeting peptides for staging and therapy of MTC and other cholecystokinin-B receptor expressing malignancies. Sem Nucl Med 2002; 32:97–109.

19. Ricabonna G. In: Thyroid cancer. Berlin: Springer, 1987: 8.

20. Oberdisse K, Klein E, Reinwein D. Die Krankheiten der Schilddrusse. Stuttgart: Thieme, 1980.

21. Tonami N, Bunko H, Mishigishi T, Kuwajima A, Hisada K. Clinical application of ^{201}Tl scintigraphy in patients with cold thyroid nodules. Clin Nucl Med 1978; 3:217–221.

22. Harada T, Ito Y, Shimaoka K, Taniguchi T, Matsudo A, Senoo T. Clinical evaluation of ^{201}Tl-chloride scan for thyroid nodule. Eur J Nucl Med 1980; 5:125–130.

23. Adler LP, Bloom AD. Positron emission tomography of thyroid nodules. Thyroid 1993; 3:195–200.

24. Uematsu H, Sadat N, Ohtsubu T. Fluorine-18 fluoro-deoxyglucose PET versus thallium-201 scintigraphy evaluation of thyroid tumours. J Nucl Med 1998; 39:453–459.

25. Waxman A, Ramanna L, Chapman N, et al. The significance of I-131 scan dose in patients with thyroid cancer: determination of ablation (concise communication). J Nucl Med 1981; 22:861–865.

26. Jeevanram RK, Shah DH, Sharma SM, Ganatra RD. Influence of initial large dose on subsequent uptake of therapeutic radioiodine in thyroid cancer patients. Nucl Med Biol 1986; 13:277–279.

27. Park HM, Perkins OW, Edmonson JW, Schnute RB, Manatunga A. Influence of diagnostic radioiodines on the uptake of ablative doses of iodine 131. Thyroid 1994; 4: 49–54.

28. Murphy EJ, Almeida F, Lull R, et al. ^{123}I scanning for follow-up of thyroid cancer. J Invest Med 2000; 70A.

29. Blake G.

30. rTSH scans.

31. Ünal S, Menda Y, Adalet I, Boztepe H. Ozbey N, et al. Thallium-201, technetium-99m-tetrofosmin and iodine-131 in detecting differentiated thyroid carcinoma metastases. J Nucl Med 1998; 39:1897–1902.

32. Nakada K, Katoh C, Morita K, et al. Relationship among ^{201}Tl uptake, nuclear DNA content and clinical behavior in metastatic thyroid carcinoma. J Nucl Med 1999; 40: 963–967.

33. Miyamoto S, Kasagi K, Misaki T, Alam MS, Konshi J. Evaluation of technetium-99m-MIBI scintigraphy in metastatic differentiated thyroid carcinoma. J Nucl Med 1997; 38:352–356.

34. Ng DCE, Sundram FX, Sin AE. ^{99m}Tc-Sestamibi and ^{131}I whole-body scintigraphy and initial serum thyroglobulin in the management of differentiated thyroid carcinoma. J Nucl Med 2000; 41:631–635.

35. Seabold JE, Gurll N, Schurrer ME, Aktay R, Kirchner PT. Comparison of ^{99m}Tc-methoxyisobutyl isonitrile and ^{201}Tl scintigraphy for detection of residual thyroid cancer after ^{131}I ablative therapy. J Nucl Med 1999; 40: 1434–1440.

36. Gallowitsch H-J, Mikosch P, Kresnik E, et al. Thyroglobulin and low-dose iodine-131 and technetium-99m-tetrofosmin whole-body scintigraphy in differentiated thyroid carcinoma. J Nucl Med 1998; 39:870–875.

37. Lind P, Gallowitsch H-J, Langsteger W, et al. Technetium-99m-tetrofosmin whole-body scintigraphy in the follow-up of differentiated thyroid carcinoma. J Nucl Med 1997; 38:348–352.

38. Baudin E, Schlumberger M, Lumbroso J, et al. Octreotide scintigraphy in patients with differentiated thyroid carcinoma: contribution for patients with negative radio-iodine scan. J Clin Endocrinol Metab 1996; 81:2541–2544.

39. Chung J-K, So Y, Lee JS, et al. Value of FDG PET in papillary thyroid carcinoma with negative ^{131}I whole-body scan. J Nucl Med 1999; 40:986–992.

40. Wang W. [^{18}F]-2-Fluoro-2-deoxy-D-glucose positron emission tomography localizes residual thyroid cancer in patients with negative diagnostic ^{131}I whole body scans and elevated serum thyroglobulin levels. J Clin Endocrinol Metab 1999; 84:2291–2302.

41. Grunwald F, Kalicke T, Feine U, et al. Fluorine-18 fluorodeoxyglucose positron emission tomography in thyroid cancer: results of a multicentre study. Eur J Nucl Med 1999; 26:1547–1552.

42. Wang W, Larson SM, Fazzari M. Prognostic value of ^{18}FDG PET scanning in patients with thyroid cancer. J Clin Endocrinol Metab 2000; 85:1107–1113.

43. van Tol KM, Jager PL, Piers DA, et al. Better yield of 18-fluoro deoxyglucose positron emission tomography in patients with metastatic differentiated thyroid carcinoma during thyrotropin stimulation. Thyroid 2002; 12: 381–387.

44. Petrich T, Borner AR, Otto D, et al. Influence of rhTSH on 18-F fluorodeoxyglucose uptake by differentiated thyroid cancer. J Nucl Med Mol Imaging 2002; 29: 641–647.

45. Yen TC, Lin HD, Lee CH, Chang SL, Yeh SH. The role of ^{99m}Tc MIBI whole body scans in diagnosing metastatic Hurthle cell carcinoma of the thyroid gland after total thyroidectomy: a comparison with ^{131}I iodine and ^{201}Tl thallium whole body scans. Eur J Nucl Med 1994; 21: 980–983.

46. Vergara E, Lastoria S, Varella P, Lapenta L, Salvatore M. Technetium-99m pentavalent dimercaptosuccinic acid uptake in Hurthle cell tumour of the thyroid, J Nucl Biol Med 1993; 37:67–68.

47. Forsell-Aronsson EB, Nilsson O, Bejegard SA, et al. ^{111}I Indium–DTPA-D-Phe1-octreotide binding and somatostatin receptor subtypes in thyroid tumours. J Nucl Med 2000; 41:636–642.

48. Lowe VJ, Mullan BP, Hay ID, McIver B, Kasperbauer JL. ^{18}F FDG PET of patients with Hurthle cell Ca. J Nucl Med 2003; 44:1402–1406.

49. Plotkin M, Hautzel H, Krause BJ, et al. Implication of ^{18}F FDG PET in the follow up of Hurthle cell thyroid cancer, Thyroid 2002; 12:155–161.

50. Tenenbaum, FR, Lumbroso J, Schlumberger M, et al. Radiolabelled somatostatin scintigraphy in differentiated thyroid cancer. J Nucl Med 1999; 36:807–810.

51. Zak IT, Seabold JE, Robinson RA, et al. ^{99m}Tc MIBI. Scintigraphic detection of metastatic insular thyroid cancer. Clin Nucl Med 1995; 20:31–36.

52. Yen TC, King KL, Yang AH, et al. Comparative radionuclide imaging of metastatic insular carcinoma of the thyroid: value of ^{99m}Tc(V)-DMSA. J Nucl Med 1996; 37: 78–80.

53. Diehl M, Graichen S, Menzel C, Lindhorst C, Grunwald F. ^{18}F FDG PET in insular thyroid cancer. Clin Nucl Med 2003; 28:728–731.

54. Anderson RJ, Sizemore GW, Wahner HW. Thyroid scintigraphy in familial medullary carcinoma of the thyroid gland. Clin Nucl Med 1978; 3:148.

55. Parthasarathy KL, Shimaoka K, Bakshi SP, Razack MS. Radiotracer uptake in medullary carcinoma of the thyroid. Clin Nucl Med 1980; 5:45–48.

56. Clarke SEM, Lazarus CR, Maisey MN. Experience in imaging medullary thyroid carcinoma using 99mTc (V) dimercaptosuccinic acid (DMSA). Henry Ford Hosp Med J 1989; 37:167–168.

57. Singh J, Powell AK, Clarke SEM, Blower PJ. Crystal structure and isomerism of a tumour targeting radiopharmaceutical: [ReO(DMSA)2] – (H2DMSA = meso-2, 3-dimercapto succinic acid). J Chem Soc Chem Commun 1991; 16:1115.

58. Allen S, Blake GM, McKenney DB, et al. ^{186}Re-V-DMSA: dosimetry of a new radiopharmaceutical for therapy of medullary carcinoma of the thyroid. Nucl Med Commun 1990; 11:220–221.

59. Learoyd LA, Roach PJ, Briggs GM, Delbridge LW, Wilmshurst EG, Robinson BG. ^{99m}Tc-sestamibi scanning in recurrent MTC. J Nucl Med 1997; 38:227–230.

60. Ugur O, Kostakoglu L, Guler N, et al. Comparison of ^{99m}Tc (v) DMSA, ^{201}Thallium, and ^{99m}Tc MIBI imaging in the follow up of patients with MTC. Eur J Nucl Med 1996; 23:1367–1371.

61. Juweid M, Blumenthal RD, Hajjar G, Yeldell D, Stein R, Goldenberg DM. Use of 99(m) Tc-Sestamibi for imaging and assessment of multidrug resistance (MDR) of MTC. Eur J Nucl Med 1999; 26:OS 172.

62. Nakajo M, Shapiro B, Copp J. The normal and abnormal distribution of the adrenomedullary imaging agent M-[I-131] re Meta [I-131] iodobenzylguanidine in man: evaluation by scintigraphy. J Nucl Med 1983; 24: 672.

63. Endo K, Shiomi K, Kasagi K, et al. Imaging of medullary thyroid carcinoma with ^{131}iodine-MIBG. Lancet 1984; ii:233–235.

64. Connell JMC, Hilditch TE, Elliott A, Semple PF. ^{131}I-MIBG and medullary carcinoma of the thyroid. Lancet 1984; ii:1273–1274.

65. Sone T, Fukunaga M, Otsuka N, et al. Metastatic medullary thyroid cancer: localization with ^{131}iodine metaiodobenzylguanidine. J Nucl Med 1985; 26:604–608.

66. Poston GJ, Thomas AM, Macdonald DW, et al. Imaging of the medullary carcinoma of the thyroid with [131]iodine metaiodobenzylguanidine. Nucl Med Commun 1986; 7:215–221.

67. Hoefnagel CA, deKraker J, Marcuse HR, Voûte PA. Detection and treatment of neural crest tumours using ^{131}I MIBG. Eur J Nucl Med 1985; 11:A73.

68. Hilditch TE, Connell JMC, Elliot AT, Murray T, Reed NS. Poor results with ^{99m}Tc-V-DMS and [131]iodine MIBG in the imaging of medullary thyroid carcinoma. J Nucl Med 1986; 27:1150–1153.

69. Clarke SEM, Lazarus CR, Edwards S. Scintigraphy and treatment of MTC with [131]iodine MIBG. J Nucl Med 1987; 28:1820–1825.

70. Troncone L, Rufni V, De Rosa G, Testa A. Diagnostic and therapeutic potential of new radiopharmaceutical agents in medullary thyroid carcinoma. Henry Ford Hosp Med J 1989; 37:178–184.

71. Sandrock D, Blossey HC, Bessler MJ, Steinroder M, Muntz D. Contribution of different scintigraphic techniques to the management of MTC. Henry Ford Hosp Med J 1989; 37:173–174.

72. Clarke SEM, Lazarus CR, Wraight P, Sampson C, Maisey MN. Pentavalent ^{99m}Tc DMSA, ^{131}I MIBG, and ^{99m}Tc MDP – an evaluation of three imaging techniques in patients with medullary carcinoma of the thyroid. J Nucl Med 1988; 29:33–38.

73. Clarke SEM. [131]I Meta iodobenzylguanidine therapy in MTC: Guy's Hospital experience. J Nucl Med Biol 1991; 35:323–327.

74. Hoefnagel CA, Delprat CC, Valdes Olmes RA. Role of metaiodobenzylguanidine therapy in MTC. J Nucl Med Biol 1991; 35:334–336.

75. Proceedings of Fourth International Workshop on 131 I MIBG Therapy. Barcelona, 2000 (in press).

76. Krenning EP, Lamberts SWJ, Reubi JC, et al. Somatostatin receptor imaging in medullary thyroid carcinoma. Thyroid 1991; 1(Suppl 1):564.

77. Libroia A, Verga U, Di Sacco G, Piolini M, Muratori F. Use of somatostatin analog SMS 201–995 in MTC. Henry Ford Hosp Med J 1989; 37:151–153.

78. Krenning EP, Valkeme R, Kooij PPM, et al. Radionuclide therapy with ^{111}In-DTPA-octreotide. Eur J Nucl Med 1996; 29:1118.

79. Waldherr C, Schumacher T, Pless M, Crazzolara A, Maecke HR, Nitzsche EU. Radiopeptide transmitted internal irradiation of non-iodophil thyroid cancer and conventionally untreatable MTC using [Y-90]-DOTA-D-Phe(1)-Tyr(3)-octreotide: a pilot study. Nucl Med Comm 2001; 22:673–678.

80. Diehl M, Risse JH, Brandt-Mainz K, Dietlin M, Bohuslav-izki KH, Matheja P. Fluorine-18 fluorodeoxyglucose PET in MTC: results of a multicentre study Eur J Nucl Med 2001; 28:1671–1676.

81. Brandt-Mainz K, Muller SP, Gorges R, Saller B, Bockisch A. The value of fluorine-18 fluorodeoxyglucose PET in patients with medullary thyroid cancer Eur J Nucl Med 2000; 27:490–496.

82. Peltier P, Curtet C, Chatal JF, et al. Radioimmunodetection of MTC using a bispecific antiCEA/anti indium-DTPA antibody and an [111]Indium labeled DTPA dimer. J Nucl Med 1993; 34:1267–1273.

83. Kraeber-Bodere F, Bardet S, Hoefnagel CA, et al. Radioimmunotherapy in MYC using bispecific antibody and iodine 131-labeled bivalent hapten: Preliminary results of Phase I/II clinical trial. Clin Cancer Res 1999; 5:3190S–198S.

84. Juweid ME, Hajjar G, Stein R, Sharkey RM, Herskovic T, Swayne LC. Initial experience with high dose radioimmunotherapy of metastatic MTC using I-131-MN-14F(ab)(2)anti- CEA antigen Mab and AHSCR. J Nucl Med 2000; 41:93–103.

85. Stein R, Juweid M, Zhang CH, Goldenberg DM. Assessment of combined radioimmunotherapy and chemotherapy for the treatment of MTC Clin Cancer Res 1999; 5:199S–206S.

28

CT and MRI in Thyroid Cancer

Julian E. Kabala

Technique and Normal Appearances

Images in computed tomography (CT) are reconstructed mathematically from data derived from multiple X-ray projections through the region of interest in the patient [1]. Originally data were acquired one slice at a time; after each exposure the patient would move a specific distance along the scanner table and the procedure would be repeated. Numerous technical advances have dramatically increased the speed and quality of the technique since its announcement in 1972 (for example improvements in detector sensitivity and efficiency, power of the X-ray beam, computational power and speed). Probably the most important innovation has been the development of slip ring technology, which allows the continuous rotation of the X-ray source as the patient moves through the scanner. This is the basis of spiral (helical) scanning, named after the helical pattern the X-ray beam traces around the patient. This has been followed by the development of CT scanners employing more than one bank of detectors (multislice or multidetector CT) [2]. This technique has permitted substantial increase in speed and quality of scanning. Thin slices (1 mm or less) can be obtained over large areas and patients can be scanned in a matter of seconds (for example the entire chest during suspended inspiration). It also facilitates high quality reconstruction in any plane or as a three-dimensional representation. These advantages can be further enhanced by increasing the number of detectors. Initial experience was with four banks of detectors (four slice scanners). Currently 16 and 32 slice scanners are commercially available; 64 and 128 slice scanners are being developed. The rapid acquisition of good quality images is especially useful in patients who are unwell and restless or with bulky tumors which cause them to swallow continuously.

The protocol for CT scanning will vary between centers, relating to local experience and equipment. The underlying principle for any head and neck tumor is to obtain high quality images of the primary tumor and adjacent areas of potential direct spread and to extend the scan to screen the area of predicted lymph node drainage. Conventionally CT protocols could be described in terms of slice thickness, which would correspond to the actual thickness of the slice that was exposed at the time of the investigation. So relatively thin slices would therefore be obtained following contrast through the primary tumor, say 3–5 mm [3], while thicker slices of the order of 8–10 mm were recommended for the rest of the neck. Some authorities would also suggest a relatively thick slice scan (8–10 mm) through the area of interest before contrast was administered. Axial scans are routinely obtained but coronal images should also be generated to demonstrate particular features such as contiguous extension into the mediastinum. When considering multislice scanners (which are likely to become universally available in the not too distant future) the principle of obtaining relatively thin slices through the area of interest is retained but is derived in a more virtual way. It is more useful to think in terms of the scanner acquiring a volume of data which can be displayed in a variety of ways. If the table on which the patient lies moves rapidly through the scanner as the X-ray tube rotates, then the effective slice thickness increases. Conversely if the table movement is slower, then the effective slice thickness falls. If a 16 slice scanner is considered; each row of detectors is around 0.75 mm thick. Therefore the thinnest effective slice thickness that can be acquired is 0.75 mm. This would only be acquired if the scanner is set so that the table on which the patient lies moves forward 12 mm for each rotation of the tube (this can be referred to as a pitch of 1). This would be associated with a considerable radiation dose to the patient but would produce high quality data through the area examined. In practice for head and neck work a larger effective slice thickness of 1.5 mm is recommended [4]. This still permits excellent quality reconstructions in any plane but involves half the radiation dose (obtained by having the scanner set so that the table advances 24 mm per tube rotation; pitch of 2). In routine clinical use axial reconstructions plus coronal and (for specific questions) sagittal reconstructions are sufficient. Iodinated material used for CT contrast will reduce subsequent ^{131}I uptake by thyroid tissue for 4 to 8 weeks [5]. Therefore the timing of the sequence of examinations should be thought out in advance or the alternative modality of MRI considered. In most circumstances where CT is performed for thyroid cancer it would appear logical to extend the examination to include the chest to search for pulmonary metastases.

The principles underlying magnetic resonance imaging (MRI) are relatively simple, although the applications can be extremely complex [6]. The following summary merely attempts to give some idea of the underlying concepts. All nuclei carry a positive charge (by virtue of the protons present) and are known to spin. A spinning positive charge behaves like a small magnet. In biological tissue by far the most numerous and important nucleus is hydrogen, containing a single proton. Although functional MRI (largely experimental) may

image different nuclei (notably phosphorus), clinical MRI is essentially concerned with producing images that reflect the distribution of hydrogen nuclei and to a certain extent their environment (what sort of chemical bonds and structures they are involved in). Normally the spinning protons are randomly aligned, as are the small magnetic fields they produce, and therefore there is no net magnetic effect. If, however, the patient is placed within a huge magnetic field (from 0.15 to 3.0 tesla or more in some experimental scanners) there will be a predominant alignment along the axis of the field. This is referred to as the magnetization of the sample. In order for an MRI signal to be produced the magnetization must be deflected from this parallel state. This can be achieved by the application of a second magnetic field perpendicular to the original field. This deflects the magnetization. As soon as the net magnetization is deflected from its initial state it starts to precess like a spinning top, due to the angular momentum of the spinning protons. In order to produce a deflection of the net magnetization the deflecting field is made to vary sinusoidally at the same frequency as the magnetization precesses. This can be regarded as a resonance phenomenon. The frequency of sinusoidal variation is in the radiofrequency range and hence the deflecting field may be referred to as a radiofrequency field. The coil that produces the deflecting field is often referred to as the radiofrequency (RF) coil. When the deflecting pulse is switched off there is a tendency for the magnetization to return to the original axis. As it moves towards its original alignment it induces an electric current in the RF coil. This current is the basis for one of the major components of the resultant MR image and is often referred to as the free induction decay (FID). Three important parameters affect the FID, namely T1, T2, and spin (proton) density. Before the deflecting pulse is transmitted the spinning protons are in a low energy state. After the pulse they have been deflected to a high energy state. They will gradually lose energy as they return to their initial state, a change that shows an exponential time course and has a constant referred to as the T1 relaxation time. This may also be called the spin–lattice relaxation time, indicating it is related to energy transfer from excited protons to the environment. There is also a tendency for the numerous components of the magnetization (the spinning protons) to dephase with respect to each other. This dephasing shows an exponential pattern over time, with a time constant of T2. The T2 relaxation time is a property of the tissue under investigation and it generally increases with disease. Alternatively it may be called the spin–spin relaxation time, the name indicating it is related to interactions between the spinning protons. The FID is proportional to the spin density, that is, the FID is related to the number of protons involved in the MR process per unit volume.

Utilization of these parameters to form an MR image becomes quite complex since the above account considered only a single deflecting pulse. The production of images usually involves a sequence of pulses. Varying the strength and timing of the transmitted pulses, the timing of reception of the induced signals (time to echo, TE) and the rate of repetition of the whole sequence (time to repetition, TR) determine the characteristics of the resultant image. Generally sequences with short TEs and TRs are T1 weighted (T1W), sequences with long TEs and TRs are T2 weighted (T2W). Various designer sequences have evolved including fat suppression sequences, which are particularly useful to induce lymph nodes and other areas of pathology to stand out against background fat.

An intravenous contrast agent has been evolved for use in MRI. This is based on gadolinium which is chelated (Gd-DTPA) to make it safe to administer [7]. Gadolinium is a paramagnetic material that shortens the T1 and T2 relaxation times. At the normal doses used (0.1–0.2 mm per kg body weight) only T1 shortening is observed. Areas that take up Gd-DTPA therefore appear of increased signal intensity (brighter) on T1W scans. Tissue uptake of gadolinium is related to perfusion (avascular structures will not significantly increase their signal) and the integrity of the small vessels. Tissues that enhance include intensely vascular tissues such as nasal mucosa and diseased tissues such as areas of tumor and inflammation.

MRI and CT are powerful imaging tools and the choice of which modality to use is not always straightforward. MRI shows exquisite soft-tissue contrast [8] and will therefore better demonstrate tumor invasion of structures such as strap muscle, larynx, and esophagus. It does not involve ionizing radiation and this may

be important, especially in younger patients. Traditionally it had the disadvantage of lower resolution and higher susceptibility to motion-induced degradation of images. However, although these problems have not been entirely overcome, each generation of scanner continues to improve image resolution and reduce scanning time. MRI offers imaging in any plane, which was an advantage over CT, but with the advent of multislice CT scanners this is equally offered by CT. MRI scanners are generally more claustrophobic than CT scanners and some individuals are unable to tolerate the procedure. Fine bone detail is not seen on MRI, although this may not matter in most situations and MRI is very sensitive to tumour infiltration of marrow. However, areas of calcification are much better seen on CT, which may be helpful in assessing thyroid carcinoma (although since the diagnosis is still histological this may not matter that much). Some foreign bodies are potentially dangerous in the powerful magnetic field of the MR scanner [9,10]. These include pacemakers, spinal dural electrodes, some shrapnel, heart valves, intradural clips and cochlear implants, and some intraorbital foreign bodies [11]. The biggest advantage that CT has currently is the ease with which the chest can be assessed at the same time as scanning the neck. However, given the constant and rapid advance of these fields of technology this is likely to be a fleeting situation.

MRI scanning protocols vary considerably between centers, partly related to the availability of scanning time, the preferences of the radiologist and the capabilities of the MRI scanner (which may vary in field strength and software). As with CT, high quality images of the primary tumor and its potential sites of direct invasion should be obtained and the area of predicted lymph node drainage should be included [12]. Scanning should be performed in multiple planes and in some centers will include sagittal as well as coronal and axial images. A T1W sequence is routine in most institutions, often repeated in two planes after intravenous contrast. A sequence in which signal from fat is largely absent is useful; either a STIR sequence or a post contrast fat suppression sequence is useful to facilitate demonstration of abnormal lymph nodes.

MRI scanners continue to improve in terms of speed and image quality. Scans used for radiotherapy planning are generally in the 0.2 to 1.0 T (tesla) range and based on resistive magnets. Most diagnostic scanners are based on a super-conducting magnetic field of 1.0 to 1.5 T. Larger field strengths, generally 3 T (but up to 9 T or more in some research situations), may be utilized. There are potential safety problems (nerve stimulation, for example, with very high field strengths) and a current lack of evidence to suggest routine imaging will be of better quality (brain imaging possibly excepted). However, scanning at this strength does facilitate the performance of magnetic resonance spectroscopy. This technique has largely been a research tool in neurological conditions but is also being used to assess tumor metabolism. Relatively low field spectroscopy (1.5 T) is also becoming technically feasible. Potentially this technique may detect malignancy in difficult situations (low volume and/or within previously treated sites) and offer a potentially extremely useful tool in oncology, especially in the detection of recurrent tumor and the effects of treatment [13].

The normal thyroid gland has homogeneous high density on CT due to the high iodine content. On MRI it appears as an intermediate signal on T1 weighted sequences and intermediate to low on T2 weighted sequences. It shows intense diffuse enhancement with intravenous contrast on both CT and MRI.

Thyroid Cancer

The use of CT and MRI in the management of thyroid cancer can be considered in two situations: preoperative assessment and the follow-up of treated disease. The commonest situation preoperatively is that of a solitary or a dominant thyroid nodule. Cytology, ultrasound, and the clinical picture may indicate a likely diagnosis but often a definitive diagnosis is not available until formal histology can be performed on the operative specimen. In this situation CT and MRI have little to add and are not routinely indicated. However, one of these modalities may be useful when the limits of an enlarged thyroid cannot be determined with ultrasound or if there is evidence of a locally advanced tumour, for example clinically fixed in the neck or associated with hemoptysis [14].

In these patients the function of the imaging modality is not diagnosis but staging; particularly to advise the surgeon about extension into critical areas and structures, notably the adjacent muscles, the carotid arteries, the trachea, larynx, pharynx, esophagus, and the mediastinum. Small tumours visible on ultrasound (less than 10 mm diameter) may be completely overlooked on CT and MRI; ultrasound is preferred therefore if preoperative assessment of the presence of a multifocal tumor is required [15]. The appearance of thyroid malignancies is variable but generally they are intermediate signal on T1 weighted and high signal on T2 weighted sequences [16]. They may be ill defined but at least as often are well defined when they cannot confidently be distinguished from benign thyroid nodules. Different forms of thyroid malignancy cannot be confidently distinguished on imaging although some suggestive features have been described and may be observed (Table 28.1).

Papillary carcinoma is usually relatively small, well defined, and localized. A minority, however, are locally invasive and may invade throughout both lobes of the thyroid or out of the thyroid into adjacent structures, including the larynx and trachea and, less often, the esophagus. Areas of cystic necrosis are often present within the tumor (Figure 28.1). Punctate or cloudy calcific areas (psammoma bodies) may be apparent on CT and multifocal deposits are not uncommon (Figure 28.2). Lymph node

Table 28.1 Imaging features of thyroid carcinoma on CT and MRI

	Calcification	Necrosis	Invasive
Papillary	+/−, punctate, cloudy	+++/−	−−/+
Follicular	−−−/+	−−−−−/+	−−/+
Medullary	+/−, coarse	−−−−/+	−−/+
Undifferentiated	+++/−, amorphous	+++/−	+++/−
Lymphoma	−−−−−/+	−−−−/+	+/−

Rare −−−−−/+, uncommon −−−/+, occasionally −−/+, sometimes +/−, often +++/−.

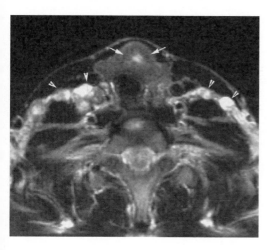

Figure 28.1 Transverse MRI scan through the thyroid (T2 weighted image) showing a relatively centrally placed papillary carcinoma of the thyroid (arrows) with central cystic change. Multiple abnormal lymph nodes are seen bilaterally (arrowheads) in the internal jugular and posterior cervical chains, also showing cystic change and representing metastatic disease.

metastases are extremely common, up to 50% of cases at presentation, and may be bilateral. Lymph nodes may show calcification and vary from entirely solid and hypervascular to largely or entirely cystic.

Follicular carcinoma is also occasionally aggressive and locally invasive. They are rarely cystic and are much less commonly associated

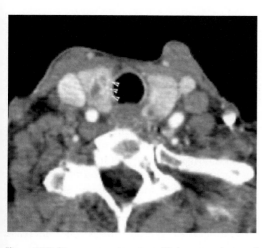

Figure 28.2 Transverse post-contrast CT demonstrating small bilateral papillary carcinomas, both showing substantial cystic change centrally. Small calcific foci are also discernible (arrowheads).

with lymph node metastases (roughly 10%). Anaplastic carcinomas are classically locally invasive into a variety of structures including the great vessels of the neck and the trachea and larynx (Figure 28.3). They often show substantial cystic necrosis and hemorrhage. Amorphous calcification is common. Lymph node metastases are common and up to a quarter involve the mediastinum. Medullary cell carcinoma is usually solid and may show coarse or psammomatous calcifications and local invasion [17]. Up to 50% are associated with neck and mediastinal lymph node involvement. Around one third of these tumours are familial and may be associated with multiple endocrine neoplasia, in which case they are often bilateral. Thyroid lymphoma is almost always primary and often associated with hashimoto's disease. It usually appears as a solitary mass, occasionally as multiple nodules. It rarely necroses (Figure 28.4).

Metastases to the thyroid constitute around 2% of thyroid cancer (although some series report up to 17% [18]). They most commonly arise from primary bronchial or breast carcinoma, sometimes from elsewhere including malignant melanoma and renal cell carcinoma. They have nonspecific malignant appearances and may demonstrate local extraglandular invasion. If they arise from squamous cell carcinoma then they may reflect the tendency of that tumor to demonstrate substantial necrosis (Figure 28.5).

Conventional tnm staging of thyroid cancer is primarily clinical, supported by ultrasound and other imaging findings. In day-to-day practice the radiologist is probably serving the surgeon best if he adequately describes the areas involved by tumor and indicates the degree of confidence he feels. Ultrasound appears to be the superior modality for the assessment of tumor extent within the thyroid gland but once extracapsular extension has occurred MRI or CT is indicated, particularly for the diagnosis of invasion of the aerodigestive tract (Figure 28.6) Which has been reported in around 6.5% of patients [15].

The British Thyroid Association recommends that all lymph nodes within the central compartment of the neck including the pre- and paratracheal nodes should be removed [14] (level VI node dissection) and that lymph nodes lying along the carotid sheath and internal

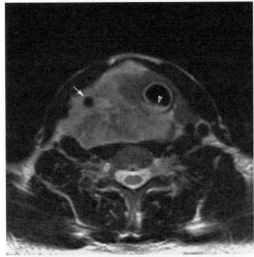

A

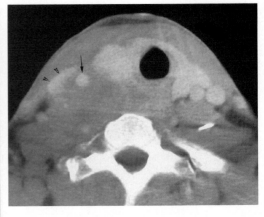

B

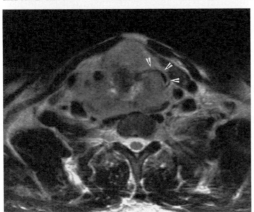

C

Figure 28.3 Transverse MRI scan (T2 weighted) through the thyroid and neck. The remaining normal thyroid gland is seen as relatively low signal compared with the ill-defined mass of anaplastic carcinoma arising from the posterior aspect of the right lobe (**A**). The tumor extends posteriorly, coming to lie against the prevertebral muscles and laterally to encase the carotid artery (arrow). Posteromedially the tumor extends round the back of the trachea, which it invades posteriorly (arrowhead), and abuts the esophagus (arrowhead), which is also probably invaded. For comparison a transverse post-contrast CT scan (**B**) on the same patient demonstrates the irregular tumor enhancing poorly compared with the intensely enhancing normal thyroid. Once again carotid artery encasement is seen (arrow) and also invasion of the sternocleidomastoid muscle (arrowheads). Further inferiorly at the level of the thoracic inlet (**C**) the trachea is grossly narrowed by extensive tumor, the airway (arrowheads) reduced to a narrow slit.

jugular vein (levels II to IV) should be palpated; suspicious nodes should be sent for frozen section with a view to selective neck dissection of levels proving positive. Radical neck dissection is therefore not routinely recommended. As indicated above, routine preoperative CT or MRI is only recommended for clinically advanced disease and then principally to stage the primary tumor. Ultrasound should have been performed and neither CT or MRI is likely to improve the detection of lymph node metastases substantially, except arguably for some relatively inaccessible lymph nodes, particularly inferior to the thyroid and beyond, into the superior mediastinum. Normal lymph nodes are routinely visible on CT and MRI and may have a maximum diameter anywhere between 2 and 25 mm. Lymph node metastases are common with thyroid cancer, especially papil-

lary carcinoma, being present in up to 50% or more in papillary carcinoma at presentation. The lymph nodes, however, will often remain small. Therefore conventional size criteria for abnormal nodes (greater than 10 mm transverse diameter in the upper neck, 9 mm elsewhere) are insensitive for the detection of metastases. Attempts to increase sensitivity by reducing the accepted upper limit of normal to 7 mm in the jugulodigastric and 6 mm at other levels in the neck leads to substantial numbers of false positives. Nodes may change shape with involvement, becoming rounded instead of the normal well-defined elliptical/bean-shape, and the number of lymph nodes may increase substantially. These signs, however, can be subjective and give rise to considerable overlap with benign lymph nodes. There does appear to be a strong tendency for the normal

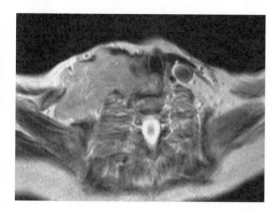

Figure 28.4 Transverse MRI (T2 weighted image) demonstrating a homogeneous mass of lymphoma arising from the right lobe of an atrophic thyroid (long-standing Hashimoto's disease) and extending widely in the right supraclavicular fossa and posterior to the thyroid. The patient was elderly and has a marked thoracic kyphosis, hence the appearance of the upper ribs in this plane.

architectural pattern (focal fat at the hilum; appearing on CT as low density and on MRI as high signal on T1 and T2 weighted sequences, low signal on fat suppression sequences) to disappear early. Cystic change in the lymph nodes is common (Figure 28.7), reported in

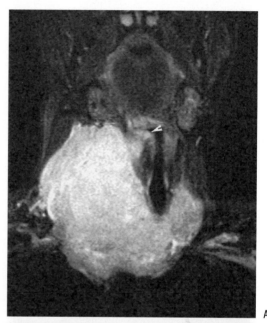

A

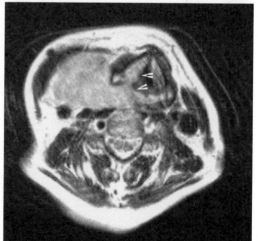

B

Figure 28.6 Coronal MRI scan (STIR sequence) showing enormous enlargement of the thyroid gland by lymphoma (**A**). Tumor extends in all directions, including into the mediastinum but also superomedially into the larynx and pharynx (arrowhead). Tumor can be seen on the transverse T2 weighted image (**B**) extending into the posterior aspect of the right vocal cord and the hypopharynx (arrowheads).

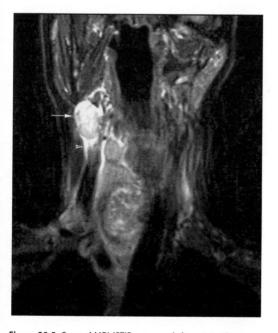

Figure 28.5 Coronal MRI (STIR sequence) demonstrating squamous cell carcinoma metastasis to the right lobe of thyroid showing the characteristic necrotic appearance of this process. There is a large right upper cervical nodal metastasis (arrow) showing similar necrosis and a halo of high signal edema (arrowhead) indicating extranodal extension.

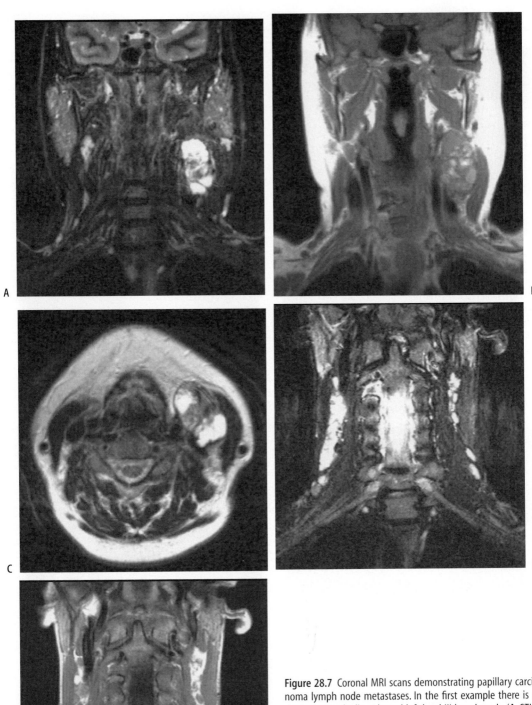

Figure 28.7 Coronal MRI scans demonstrating papillary carcinoma lymph node metastases. In the first example there is a dominant markedly enlarged left level III lymph node (**A**, STIR sequence) showing loss of normal architectural pattern and considerable heterogeneity. The T1 weighted sequence (**B**) shows the classic high signal cystic areas within the diseased node mass; heterogeneous appearances with high signal cystic areas are also demonstrated on the T2 weighted sequence (**C**). The second patient shows more extensive bilateral lymph node metastases, especially on the right. They are easily visible on the STIR sequence (**D**) while the T1 weighted sequence (**E**) once again demonstrates the high signal cystic areas characteristic of this condition.

around 50% of patients on MRI [15]. These changes are likely to be due to thyroid protein (colloid or thyroglobulin), hemorrhage, or tumor necrosis. Papillary thyroid carcinoma may also give rise to calcification within involved lymph nodes, best seen on ultrasound or CT.

Following treatment life-long follow-up is required. This will be primarily clinical and biochemical with an appropriate isotope scan if recurrence or metastatic disease is suspected (radioactive iodine for papillary or follicular thyroid cancer) [18]. Ultrasound, potentially with guided aspiration biopsy, is likely to be first line for clinically or isotopically evident local recurrence. CT or MRI is indicated to evaluate local recurrence in the neck if this is inadequately delineated with ultrasound or if it extends into the thorax. They may also be used to evaluate thoracic metastases, CT being the modality of choice for this purpose.

In contrast to most other head and neck cancer surgery, there is usually only modest postsurgical change in the neck on scanning. Often a neat scar at the thyrodectomy site is seen on CT or MRI. In the acute stage this will have a fairly active appearance. Loss of tissue planes, edema, distortion/swelling of normal structures, and engorgement of lymphatics can be identified on CT and MRI. High signal on T2W and STIR sequences is seen in edematous fat and other tissues on MRI. Tissue that has been traumatized by surgery will also show enhancement with gadolinium. However, it is rare that the neck needs to be imaged in the first few weeks after surgery and most of these acute changes will resolve by 6 weeks, although in some patients a stable postoperative appearance may not be apparent until 12–18 months following intervention. As the tissue matures the signal spectrum will generally fall towards intermediate to low on all sequences with the disappearance of enhancement. The stereotypical scar tissue of more than 6 months' age is therefore fairly inert in appearance on MRI. By comparison deposits of recurrent tumor have a more active appearance (Figure 28.8) with enhancement following intravenous contrast and elevation of signal on the T2 weighted sequence [5].

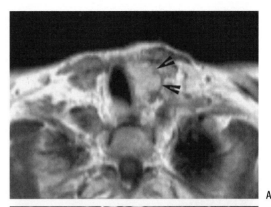

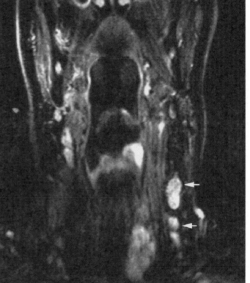

Figure 28.8 MRI scan 4 years after thyroidectomy for medullary thyroid carcinoma. The post-contrast transverse T1 weighted image (**A**) demonstrates a substantial enhancing mass of recurrent tumour (arrowheads) lying against the trachea at the thoracic inlet. This is seen as a heterogeneous but predominantly high signal mass on the STIR sequence (**B**), which also demonstrates recurrent disease in the lymph node drainage (arrows).

Key Points in MRI and CT of Thyroid

- MRI and CT have very little role in the detection and assessment of thyroid cancer confined to the thyroid gland, a situation much better assessed with ultrasound.

- MRI or CT is indicated where there is a suspicion of a locally advanced tumor or in the assessment of recurrent disease.
- In the context of staging, both MRI and CT will demonstrate local invasion of critical structures (such as the aerodigestive tract) by thyroid cancer, although MRI is likely to be more accurate.
- CT is still the investigation of choice for the assessment of pulmonary metastases.

References

1. Dendy PP, Heaton B. Computed axial transmission tomography. In: Physics for diagnostic radiology, 2nd edn. Bristol: Institute of Physics Publishing, 1999: 254–271.
2. Dawson P, Lees WR. Multidetector computed tomography. Clin Radiol 2001; 56:302–309.
3. The use of computed tomography in the initial investigation of common malignancies. London: The Royal College of Radiologists, 1994.
4. Henrot P, Blum A, Toussaint B, Troufleau P, Stines J, Roland J. Dynamic maneuvers in local staging of head and neck malignancies with current imaging techniques: Principles and clinical applications. Radiographics 2003; 23(5):1201–1215.
5. Weber AL, Randolph G, Aksoy FG. The thyroid and parathyroid glands: CT and MR Imaging and correlation with pathology and clinical findings. Radiol Clin North Am 2000; 38(5):1105–1130.
6. Dendy PP, Heaton B. Magnetic resonance imaging. In: Physics for diagnostic radiology, 2nd edn. Bristol: Institute of Physics Publishing, 1999: 378–407.
7. Gibby WA. MR contrast agents. Radiol Clin North Am 1988; 26:1047–1058.
8. Dillon WP. Magnetic resonance imaging of head and neck tumours. Cardiovasc Intervent Radiol 1986; 8(5–6): 275–282.
9. Shellock FG. MRI of metallic implants and materials: a compilation of the literature. Am J Radiol 1988; 151:811–814.
10. Kanal E, Shellock FG. The value of published data on MR compatibility of metallic implants and devices. Am J Neuroradiol 1994; 15:1394–1396.
11. Oliver C, Kabala J. Air gun pellet injuries: the safety of MR imaging. Clin Radiol 1997; 52:299–300.
12. Royal College of Radiologists' working party. A guide to the practical use of MRI in oncology. London: Royal College of Radiologists, 1999: 18–23.
13. Rabinov JD, Lee PL, Barker FG. In vivo 3T MR spectroscopy in the distinction of recurrent glioma versus radiation effects: initial experience. Radiology 2002; 225(3):871–879.
14. The National Thyroid Cancer Guidelines Group. Guidelines for the management of thyroid cancer in adults. 2004. www.british-thyroid-association.org.
15. King AD, Ahuja AT, To EWH, et al. Staging papillary carcinoma of the thyroid: magnetic resonance imaging vs ultrasound of the neck. Clin Radiol 2000; 55(3):222–226.
16. Nakahara H, Noguchi S, Murakami N, et al. Gadolinium enhanced MR imaging of thyroid and parathyroid masses. Radiology 1997; 202:765–772.
17. Naik KS, Bury RF. Imaging the thyroid. Clin Radiol 1998; 53:630–639.
18. Keston Jones M. Management of papillary and follicular thyroid cancer. J R Soc Med 2002; 96(7):325–326.

Section IX

Papillary Microcarcinoma

29

Papillary Microcarcinoma of the Thyroid

William D. Drucker and Richard J. Robbins

Introduction

Papillary thyroid carcinoma is the most common type of differentiated thyroid carcinoma [1]. The majority of these lesions are small [2]; those whose diameters measure ≤1 cm have been designated by the World Health Organization as papillary microcarcinoma of the thyroid (PMCT) [3]. In the older literature, they were frequently referred to as occult thyroid cancers since most were first discovered at autopsy; others, now usually designated as incidentalomas, were identified in operative specimens submitted for nonmalignant diseases of the thyroid [4]. One conclusion drawn from these discoveries is that PMCT seldom constitutes a clinically significant problem [5] and, therefore, may not require a therapeutic response. One group [6] has even proposed that solitary PMCT be renamed as "papillary microtumor" to reflect its benignity and to eliminate the emotionally charged diagnosis of cancer [6].

Today, many PMCTs are no longer occult or incidental, but are discovered in life and prior to head and neck surgery [7]. This change results from the expanded use of high resolution neck imaging [8] and from the expanding application of ultrasound-guided fine-needle aspiration biopsy (FNAB) of eventing thyroid nodules [9]. Despite the fact that not all PMCTs are without complications [10], the prognosis of PMCT remains excellent, and the disease is seldom fatal. Because of this, there is no consensus con-

cerning the management of PMCT. Controversy persists regarding the extent of appropriate intervention or whether any intervention is necessary at all beyond follow-up. A review of the literature suggests, however, that reasonable guidelines can be developed to aid in decision-making.

In this chapter, we will use the term *incidental* to refer to a PMCT found at autopsy or in an operative specimen removed for other than known thyroid malignancy. *Non-incidental* will refer to lesions diagnosed by palpation or by another technique such as ultrasound (US) prior to any therapeutic intervention. *Occult* PMCTs will refer to those that are unsuspected by history or physical examination but are known to exist because of some distant manifestation, usually a metastasis.

Prevalence

Autopsy studies are a major source of information regarding the prevalence of PMCT. Numbers depend, undoubtedly, on how finely thyroid glands are sectioned [11], how thoroughly they are reviewed, and the criteria used for the diagnosis of malignancy. Differences in prevalence may also be due to factors such as geography, diet, and exposure to radiation. In a study of 408 consecutive autopsies from Tokushima, Japan, Yamamoto et al. found 64 papillary carcinomas in 46 individuals, an incidence of 11.3% [12]. They cite other Japanese studies using different methods of examination in which incidences were reported to be between 8.0% and 28.4%. In the Yamamoto study, there was no significant difference in incidence between males and females; however, multiple foci were observed in 38% of the men but only 20% of the women. Of the 14 cases with multiple foci, 10 involved both lobes. The overall incidence of PMCT was not related to age. Most tumors were less than 4 mm in diameter and tumor size likewise did not correlate with age. There was a high incidence of malignancy in subjects who also had adenomatous goiters. Based upon their histologic observations the authors postulate that PMCTs arise initially as minute lesions showing mainly a follicular pattern and, as they grow, they develop fibrosis, capsules, and a more papillary pattern. Metastases to cervical lymph nodes were noted in only two cases, both males ages 16 and 53. Their tumors were non-encapsulated, had psammoma bodies, and showed intrathyroidal metastatic foci.

A lower incidence of PMCT was found in an autopsy study from a rural area of Greece not known for a high incidence of endemic goiter or iodine deficiency [13]. Thyroid glands from 160 subjects who died following accidents, suicide, or sudden death were examined. Twelve papillary tumors were discovered, nine of which were smaller than 1 cm, yielding a PMCT incidence of 5.6%. There was no preponderance of either sex in these nine. A much higher incidence of PMCT was found by Harach et al. [14] in a meticulous study of 101 consecutive autopsies in Finland. They found that 35.6% of thyroid glands had one or more PMCTs; 66.7% were in nodular specimens and 64% measured less than 6 mm. There was no correlation between tumor size and age. Sixteen of the 36 glands containing tumors had multiple foci, many bilateral, and were found predominantly in males. In fact, 64% of the PMCTs in this series were discovered in males. Since clinical papillary carcinomas are much more common in women, the authors suggest that promoting factors are more important for their development than the mere existence of a PMCT. PMCTs were so common that the authors regarded them as normal findings and concluded that detection of a PMCT without regional metastases should not result in any treatment.

Lang et al. [15] evaluated thyroid glands from 1020 sequential autopsies in Germany. Sixty-two papillary carcinomas were discovered, a 6% incidence, with a slightly greater number in males, a striking difference again, from the female predominance in clinically apparent thyroid cancer. There was no significant peak age incidence. About one half of the PMCTs were multifocal, with 65.5% of these being found in both lobes. Regional lymph node metastases were found in 14%, all but one from the multifocal group. Of the 62 PMCTs, 41 (65%) were designated as invasive, the remainder being well circumscribed with or without a capsule. It is from the invasive group that the lymph node metastases were noted. The authors concluded that since these incidental tumors showed no tendency to progress and become clinically apparent with age, therapeutic intervention would not be warranted when discovered in life. In the United States, a study from Memorial Sloan-Kettering of 5636 consecutive autopsies on patients dying of cancer found the rate of incidental, independent, primary thyroid cancer to be only 6.4 per 1000 autopsies, although histologic examinations were not so thorough and not all tumors were necessarily papillary [16].

Nishyama and colleagues in Michigan discovered PMCTs in 13 thyroid glands (7 from males) culled from 100 consecutive autopsies [17]. In 7 of the specimens, lesions were multiple. In Olmstead County, Minnesota, a meticulous study by Sampson et al. [18] revealed 9 occult thyroid carcinomas from 157 autopsies (5.7% incidence). Eight of the 9 malignancies were papillary, with 3 being multifocal. Male sex predominated in this study and there was no suggestion that prevalence was associated with advancing age.

Lastly, Fukunaga and Yatani [19] collected 1167 thyroid glands from autopsies performed in different parts of the world: Canada, Japan, Poland, Colombia, and Japanese living in Hawaii. They sectioned the glands at 2–3 mm intervals, and applied stringent criteria for the diagnosis of thyroid carcinoma. They discovered a total of 139 incidental malignancies, all papillary save one, (11.9% total incidence), women predominating 1.7/1, but not significantly. Only two PMCTs were associated with lymph node metastases. In spite of the fact that the incidence of PMCTs in native Japanese and those resident in Hawaii far exceeded those from other countries, the incidence of clinical cancers in this population was not significantly different from those of the other countries. The authors proposed that the Japanese experienced a greater exposure to initiating factors than the other groups, but not to promoting factors.

Another measure of the incidence of PMCT can be gleaned from study of thyroid glands removed surgically for benign indications. Fink et al. [20] from Toronto collected 425 consecutively resected thyroids between 1991 and 1995. Seventy-one of these contained 118 PMCTs, 22 being multifocal. Fifty-one tumors from 343 women and 20 tumors from 82 men, an incidence of 14.9% and 24.4% respectively, barely missed significance statistically. Total thyroidectomy specimens yielded more PMCTs than lobectomies. The authors cite three other studies, collectively equaling 3546 surgically resected specimens for benign disease, with PMCT prevalence of 5.5% in Japan, of 10.5% in Italy, and of 10% from Canada. The peak occurrene of PMCTs in this study was between 40–70 years suggesting that these tumors took some time to develop, and with aging, may have involuted, supporting the notion that carcinogens may incite tumor development, but promoters are necessary for their uncontrolled growth. In the Italian study cited above, Pelizzo and co-workers examined serial 3 mm sections of thyroids from 277 consecutive patients operated for euthyroid and hyperthyroid multinodular goiter, Graves' disease, and functioning adenomas [4]. Females predominated 3.4/1 and the age range was 16–80 years. Twenty-nine PMCTs were discovered (2–10 mm). They were found in all patients except those with hyperthyroid multinodular goiters (22/277 patients). PMCTs were present in 17.1% of euthyroid multinodular goiters, 5.7% of the Graves' patients, 2.5% of patients with autonomous adenomas, and none of those with toxic nodular goiters.

Interestingly, Delides et al. [21] the prevalence of PMCT in Greek autopsy specimens compared to 611 thyroids resected for benign indications. The prevalence rate for the resected glands was 1.8% and for the autopsy specimens, 1.5%. Ignoring the fact that the population of patients for the resected gland group was on average younger and predominantly female, and frequently only one thyroid lobe could be examined, the authors' conclusion that PMCTs in the resected thyroid glands were coincidental and not associated etiologically with the underlying thyroid disease seems reasonable. However, a question remains concerning the relationship between thyrotoxicosis and papillary cancer.

When considering the prevalence of PMCT, one cannot ignore its increasing recognition by serendipity owing to the increasing use of high resolution US of the neck for a variety of indications. Once identified, a nodule of very modest size can often be biopsied successfully under US-guided FNAB. Recognition of these non-incidental lesions is a contributing factor to the apparent rise in papillary thyroid cancer incidence. However, these lesions may be the very same tumors formerly identified only in autopsy and postsurgical studies.

In summary, multiple studies reveal significant geographic disparities in the prevalence of PMCT. With a few exceptions, most find that the female predominance characteristic of clinically apparent papillary thyroid carcinoma does not apply to microcarcinomas. Further, the incidence and progression of the latter is not age dependent. In short, one postulate drawn from the data is that PMCTs may be biologically different from clinically apparent lesions.

Etiology

The nature of the apparent geographic disparities in the prevalence of PMCT remains to be defined. Purely technical matters such as the stringency of the histological criteria used to diagnose cancer, or the thickness of histological sections do not adequately explain the differences. Dietary iodine, exposure to radiation, the association of PMCT with Graves' disease, and genetic influences have all been explored.

Iodine

Iodine deficiency remains a worldwide problem, especially in Africa, Europe, and the eastern Mediterranean [22]. In these three areas, up to 56% of the general population, including children, are deficient (urinary iodine less than 100 μg/L). Iodine deficiency may shift the histological type of thyroid malignancy from follicular to papillary. For example, in a formerly iodine-deficient area of Argentina with a stable population, the ratio of papillary to follicular carcinoma rose from 2.5 : 1 to 6.2 : 1 following the introduction of iodine prophylaxis [23]. The shift was noted in tumors both less than and greater than 1 cm in diameter.

Further, the incidence of papillary vs. follicular lesions increased over time, the ratio being greater in the second 10 years after the introduction of iodine prophylaxis than in the first decade. After iodine repletion both micropapillary lesions and tumors greater than 1 cm showed a decrease in psammoma bodies, ground-glass nuclei, and calcifications.

In 1963, Austria, with a historically high incidence of goiter, mandated the addition of 10 mg of potassium iodide to each kilogram of table salt, which later was doubled to 20 mg [24]. After the 10 mg supplementation, the ratio of papillary to follicular carcinoma shifted from 0.2 to 1.1 [25]. After the 20 mg supplement, the ratio rose to 2.6 in the period 1985–1989, and increased sill further to 4.0 between the years 1990–1995. When iodine prophylaxis was introduced into Switzerland, another region of endemic goiter, a shift from undifferentiated to papillary carcinoma was noted as well [26]. While the overall incidence of thyroid carcinoma appears to be on the increase, enhanced iodine intake is not generally regarded as responsible [27]. Iodine's influence seems mainly restricted to the determination of histological type.

A change in dietary iodine cannot always be seen as an isolated, uncomplicated factor promoting an observed change in tumor subtype. Burgess describes how Tasmania and the eastern coast of Australia were iodine-deficient areas until, in 1966, potassium iodate was added to the bread-making process and, around the same time, dairymen began using an iodophor-containing disinfectant which resulted in a rise in the iodine content of milk [28]. Between 1974 and the mid-1980s both forms of iodine were discontinued rendering the region iodine-deficient once again. The predicted effect would be a decrease in the ratio of papillary to follicular cancer. In fact, there was both an increase in the total prevalence of thyroid cancer and a significant rise in papillary tumors including microscopic lesions. Follicular cancer incidence stayed relatively flat. Burgess concluded that greater identification of non-incidental lesions could account for some but not all of the observed increases in total and papillary tumors. The area of the world in question was exposed to radioactive fallout from the frequent testing of nuclear devices in the 1950s and 1960s, a time when the population was iodine deficient. Radiation may have induced tumor formation, especially in the young, and when iodine was sufficient, it may well have favored the development of papillary cancer.

Another complex situation is that of Iceland and Hawaii, both of which have high endogenous iodine intake and a high prevalence of thyroid carcinoma. In these two active volcanic regions, natural radiation was suspected as being responsible rather than iodine abundance [29]. While unproven, the high dietary iodine of this region may play some role by protecting against the effects of radiation and thereby modulating the overall incidence of thyroid malignancy.

Ionizing Radiation

That radiation exposure favors the development of thyroid carcinoma including the papillary variety, and that the very young are especially vulnerable, is unquestioned. Duffy and Fitzgerald called attention to this as far back as 1950 in their study from Memorial Hospital in New York of 28 cases ranging in age from 4 to 18 years [30]. Ten of their patients had had prior exposure to X-ray irradiation of the head and neck and the authors drew attention to this as an etiological factor. Forty-six percent of the tumors examined were papillary, but all were papillary from the 10 that had been irradiated. Ron et al. [31] summarized seven studies on thyroid cancer incidence after the exposure of children to external radiation administered as therapy, often at low doses, for benign conditions such as tinea capitis. They found that the diagnosis of thyroid carcinoma was frequently not made until 25–35 years after exposure.

The atomic bombs that exploded in Hiroshima and Nagasaki, resulting in mainly neutron and gamma irradiation in 1945 and the subsequent testing of nuclear weapons, exposing unprotected populations from radiation and fallout, afforded the opportunity to study the issue of ionizing radiation and thyroid cancer. Sampson et al. [32] examined the thyroid glands at autopsy of 3067 Japanese survivors who had lived in proximity to the atomic detonations. They discovered 536 thyroid carcinomas, a combined incidence rate of 17.5% for both men and women. Ninety-seven percent of the tumors were PMCTs although tumors as large as 1.5 cm were included in the series. Thompson et al. [33]

summarized data on the incidence of solid tumors diagnosed between 1958 and 1987 as part of the extended Life Span Study Cohort of atomic bomb survivors of Hiroshima and Nagasaki. In regard to the thyroid, they found that age at exposure was critical to the subsequent development of cancer and the data also suggested a strong dose–response effect. The risk of thyroid cancer was threefold higher in those <10 years than in those who were 10–19 years old at the time of exposure. Persons older than age 40 incurred no increased risk. Lund and Galanti [34] reported on the incidence of thyroid malignancy in Sweden and Norway, countries exposed to fallout from Russian nuclear testing during the years 1951–1952. They found that exposure to radioactive fallout in early childhood posed an increased risk of papillary thyroid carcinoma. Furthermore, the disease became manifest the earliest in those with the highest level of exposure. Young adults exposed at ages 20–24 did not manifest an increase in papillary carcinoma.

In 1954, a high yield thermonuclear bomb was detonated on the Bikini Atoll in the Pacific. Because of a wind shift, fallout exposed inhabitants on several atolls in the Marshall Islands, to high levels of short-lived, very energetic iodine isotopes as well as I-131 [35]. Twenty-two years later, 40 of 243 exposed Marshall Islanders, 75% of whom were exposed as children, manifested palpable thyroid nodules. Of the 31 patients who went to surgery, 7 (22.6%) had malignant lesions, mainly papillary or mixed papillary/follicular. Two of the tumors were less than 1 cm in size and 4 demonstrated localized metastases or blood vessel invasion. Perhaps additional small, nonpalpable tumors would have been discovered had high resolution ultrasound examination been available.

The accident at the Chernobyl nuclear power station in April 1986, which released unprecedented quantities of radioactivity including short-lived isotopes of iodine, I-131, gamma radiation, and other long-lived isotopes, resulted in worldwide concern regarding its potential damaging effects on the thyroid, both locally and beyond Ukraine. Children received the highest doses of I-131 by drinking cow's milk contaminated with the isotope [36]. Kazakov et al. reported in 1990, only four years after the explosion, a sudden increase in thyroid carcinoma in children in several regions of

southern Belarus, downwind to Chernobyl [37]. By mid-1992 they had diagnosed 131 cases of thyroid cancer, 128 of which were papillary, 55% of which were aggressive. Twenty-three percent of the tumors were PMCT [38]. By 1991–1992, the annual increase in thyroid carcinoma in children and adolescents was 62 times greater than in the 10 years preceding the Chernobyl accident [38]. Baverstock et al. [39] corroborated the findings of Kazakov in Belarus and noted that the 8 youngest victims of the explosion diagnosed with thyroid carcinoma were *in utero* past 3-months of fetal age at the time of the disaster. A rise in the I-131 content of milk immediately after the Chernobyl accident has been documented in some key cities in the United States. In Connecticut, about 4320 miles from Chernobyl, a small but statistically significant increase in thyroid carcinoma was documented 4–7 years after the Chernobyl catastrophe [39a]. The rise in incidence was similar for both males and females. Although the size and type of the tumors was not mentioned, a previous study done in Connecticut on the effects of ionizing radiation showed the predominant type to be papillary [40]. A future silent but significant source of external radiation may be cosmic in origin caused by the current progressive weakening of the earth's magnetic field, which ordinarily deflects such radiation [41].

Benign Thyroid Disorders Associated with PMCT

Many papers have been written concerning the coexistence of thyroid cancer and Graves' disease. Some conclude that there is an increased incidence of malignancy and speculate that thyroid-stimulating immunoglobulins may act to promote and sustain thyroid cancer. Others conclude that the incidence of thyroid carcinoma in patients with Graves' disease may not be greater than in the general population. Valana et al. published a retrospective study of 1853 hyperthyroid patients, 512 of whom went to surgery [42]. Of this number, 108 had Graves' disease, 251 had toxic multinodular goiters, and 153 had a single toxic nodule. Papillary carcinoma was discovered in 24 (4.7%) of the 512 patients, 7 of whom had Graves' disease. Three of the 7 tumors were non-incidental and diagnosed by US and FNAB preoperatively. All 7 were papillary and none were larger than 1.5 cm. Fourteen of the remaining patients in the other groups had papillary lesions as well, 10 of which were less than 1 cm in diameter. In their paper, the authors also summarized the findings from 13 published studies dealing with the coexistence of hyperthyroidism and thyroid malignancy. The incidence ranged from 0.5% to 21%, papillary lesions predominating.

In 1990, Belfiore et al. highlighted an increased aggressiveness of thyroid cancer occurring in patients with Graves' disease [43]. Compared to patients with thyroid cancer associated with non-autoimmune, autonomously functioning thyroid nodules or euthyroid nodular goiters, the tumors of Graves' disease patients were more locally invasive, more often multifocal, and more often associated with lymph node and distant metastases. Granted that those going to surgery were preselected, it is noteworthy that patients treated with radioiodine (RAI) did not develop clinically apparent disease in follow-up, although the length of that follow-up was not stated. It is possible, however, that RAI therapy had a destructive effect on malignant cells. In response to this and other papers in the literature, Mazzaferri concluded that the high prevalence of thyroid malignancy associated with Graves' disease was not solely because thyroidectomy exposed the presence of incidental tumors [44]. While large papillary lesions are uncommonly aggressive in the setting of Graves' disease, many carcinomas in Graves' patients are less than 5 mm in diameter. The management of these usually indolent tumors is debatable, but Mazzaferri pointed out that they might prove troublesome in the setting of high titers of thyroid-stimulating immunoglobulins.

Pellegriti et al. reported on 950 patients with Graves' disease [45]. Of the 450 who went to surgery, 35 had thyroid cancer. Fifteen of the tumors measured less than 1.5 cm. and 91% were papillary thyroid carcinoma. Sixty percent of the patients had a high risk of recurrence and new distant metastases, and three manifested pulmonary metastases at the time of diagnosis. The 15 subjects with small-size cancers did not exhibit aggressive behavior in long-term follow-up. Hales et al. reported on 16 cases of thyroid cancer associated with Graves' disease [46]. The mean tumor diameter was 0.9 cm. Hales et al.

found no difference in disease progression in these patients with small tumors compared to a sex- and age-matched euthyroid papillary cancer group.

Since thyroid nodules are frequently encountered in Graves' disease patients, should thyroid ultrasound become routine and an FNAB be performed if a nodule of any size is detected? Cantalamessa and associates addressed this question in 315 consecutive patients with Graves' disease [47]. They detected nodules in 128 subjects, 22 of which were less than 8 mm in diameter. These nodules were not biopsied. Forty-nine of the larger lesions were present at the time Graves' disease was diagnosed; the rest developed during follow-up and were associated with increased levels of thyroid-stimulating immunoglobulins. One hundred and six of the patients had FNABs; just two suspicious lesions were found and only one had a confirmed malignancy. The authors concluded that if FNAB cytology is neither suspicious nor diagnostic of malignancy, thyroid nodules in Graves' disease do not warrant an aggressive approach.

Familial Thyroid Cancer

In 1997, Loh reviewed 15 studies of non-medullary thyroid carcinoma performed between 1975 and 1996, excluding all patients with Gardner or Cowden syndrome or a history of radiation exposure in monozygotic twins [48]. He found that 2.5–6.3% of the cases were familial and 91% of the tumors were papillary. There were 178 affected individuals in 87 kindreds; females predominated over males, 2.2/1. The peak incidence was in the fourth decade. Six of the 15 series found that disease in the familial cohorts was more aggressive than usually observed in sporadic disease. They had a higher incidence of multifocality, local invasiveness, and locoregional recurrence. The incidence of PMCT in familial PTC could not be accurately determined.

In 1997, Burgess et al. [48a] published two kindreds with familial PTC. The index case had PTC in a multinodular thyroid gland as did four of her six children. Tumor size was not recorded in all instances, but at least two of the sibs had PMCTs. Another branch of the same family had multinodular goiters and PTCs. The index case, a 49-year-old man, had a monozygotic twin with multinodular goiter and lymph node metastases. Both men had daughters in their twenties with thyroid cancer, a sclerosing PMCT in one and a 1.2 cm lesion in the other.

In 1999, Lupoli and associates brought attention to "a new clinical entity" by publishing a retrospective study of 119 patients with PMCT, 7 of whom were from 6 different families with papillary thyroid carcinomas [49]. The largest tumor measured 1 cm. All of the patients underwent a total or near-total thyroidectomy except one, a 29-year-old woman, who had only a lobo-isthmusectomy. Local invasion through the thyroid capsule was found in this gland and, about $3^1/_2$ years after surgery, the patient developed a locoregional recurrence. A 49-year-old woman developed lung metastases 4 years after surgery and succumbed 11 months later. A 22-year-old woman with initial local invasion experienced a local recurrence 6 years postoperatively. All except two sisters had multifocal disease and three of the seven had bilateral disease. Five of the seven patients had lymph node metastases. The three patients who experienced recurrent disease also had evidence of vascular invasion at the time of surgery. The authors concluded that an aggressive therapeutic approach to patients with a family history of differentiated thyroid carcinoma was warranted. In response to the foregoing study another case report appeared concerning a 58-year-old woman with a diffuse goiter and an uncomplicated 7 mm PMCT [50]. Two years later her 33-year-old daughter appeared with a 7 mm, well-encapsulated PMCT. The index case ultimately died of bronchoalveolar carcinoma, not thyroid carcinoma.

Marchesi et al. have reported papillary carcinoma in nine first-degree relatives from four families [51]. At least one family had a strong history of hypothyroidism and multinodular goiter. Four of the nine tumors found measured 1 cm or less and 44% were multifocal. Rios et al. discovered 59 thyroid carcinomas in a series of 672 patients operated on for multinodular goiter in Spain [52]. Thirty-seven (62.7%) of the tumors were microcarcinomas, the vast majority papillary. By multivariate analysis, a family history of thyroid pathology, type unspecified, was one of the significant variables with a relative risk of 1.6. Musholt et al. reviewed the English literature on familial PTC covering

the period 1958 to 1999 [53]. They collected about 160 kindreds with 2 or more related individuals some with, and some without, concomitant multinodular goiters. In addition, they unearthed from their own clinic, 12 new kindreds by chart review of 282 documented cases of PTC. In the 6 kindreds they studied in depth, many had multinodular goiters or other non-malignant thyroid diseases. In these kindreds only four patients had microcarcinomas, one of which was invasive and one of which had spread to lymph nodes. Four of the 13 patients in these kindreds had microcarcinomas; one was invasive and one had spread to lymph nodes. The authors offered prediction criteria for the identification of PTC/multinodular goiter families: autosomal dominant inheritance with partial penetrance, a fairly early age of onset and, not uncommonly, a more aggressive behavior than the course seen in sporadic disease. Total thyroidectomy, microdissection of the central compartment, and postoperative ablation with RAI was recommended for familial PTC.

Papillary Microcarcinoma in Childhood and Adolescence

Data in the literature concerning incidental PTC in children is limited. From Finland, Fransilla and Harach carefully studied 93 thyroid glands from 56 medicolegal and 37 medical autopsies of children and young adults [54]. Of 58 glands from individuals below age 20, only one had a PMCT. Thirteen thyroid glands in all yielded PMCTs; only two were greater than 1 mm in diameter. In four thyroids, there were multiple foci.

Chow et al. have reported on 60 patients from Hong Kong with papillary thyroid carcinoma who were less than 21-years-old [55]. Tumor size was described in 43 of the 60; but only 2 were PMCT. Compared to the authors' adult patients, the younger had a higher ratio of females, higher incidences of lymph node metastases, pulmonary metastases at presentation, and relapse. Fortunately, in spite of considerable morbidity, the mortality rate is very low in childhood papillary disease, especially for those with smaller lesions [56]. Collins et al. studied papillary carcinoma in patients who were irradiated between 1939 and 1962 for benign conditions as children [57]. Years later, they were able to locate 3083 individuals from a group of 4296. Thyroid carcinoma had developed in 357 (11.6%) of them. From these cases, the authors were able to evaluate 30 paraffin blocks that were well enough preserved to warrant study. They selected paraffin blocks from non-irradiated children with PTC matched as closely as possible to the age and sex of the radiation-exposed group. The tumors in the irradiated group were smaller (mean size of the largest, 1.29 cm) than those in the control group (mean size of the largest, 2.49 cm). The irradiated group may have had tumors of smaller size because closer surveillance of this cohort made earlier detection possible. However, despite their smaller tumor size, lymph node metastases and multifocality were more frequently encountered in the radiated patients than in the non-irradiated control cohort. The authors found that in childhood PTC associated with prior radiation, RET immunoreactivity was more frequently positive than in the non-radiated group. Tumors associated with positive RET immunoreactivity did not demonstrate any unique characteristics, however.

In a retrospective study culled from 15 children's hospitals or cancer centers, Newman et al. analyzed 329 patients 21 years of age or younger with differentiated thyroid cancer excluding medullary lesions [58]. Ninety percent of the tumors were either papillary or papillary-follicular. Thirteen percent of the children had a history of irradiation and 6% had a positive family history of PTC. Regarding tumor size, some were as small as 0.4 cm but the number of tumors less than 1 cm was not stated. Unexpectedly, neither tumor size nor prior radiation exposure were deemed determinants of progression. Age at diagnosis was the most significant factor: younger patients were the ones most likely to experience disease progression. This conclusion is fully supported in a retrospective study of 38 patients from the province of British Columbia [59].

Ultrasound, Color Doppler Imaging, and FDG-PET

High resolution ultrasound (US) is a powerful tool for the description and detection of micronodules of the thyroid and, when com-

bined with FNAB, is a potential means to distinguish benign from malignant lesions. Thus, US contributes significantly to the management of clinical problems but, its very power is revealing a high rate of previously undetected thyroid nodules. Having discovered an impalpable nodule or multiple nodules of very small size by US for whatever indication, what is the appropriate action? In his Commentary concerning thyroid incidentalomas, Topliss raises several questions [60]. Are there size criteria or US criteria to determine which nodules should be biopsied? Are the cytological results of FNAB reliable and what does one do if the pathological report is indeterminate or nondiagnostic? If malignancy is detected in an incidental nodule, does it have the same biological significance as a clinically apparent tumor? A few studies contribute useful data concerning these issues, but none give final answers to the questions.

Chan et al. reviewed the sonographic and color Doppler imagining characteristics of 55 proven PTCs they collected from 1995–2003 without regard to size [61]. The typical appearance was that of a hypoechoic, solid, round, smooth nodule with internal hypervascularity and microcalcifications. However, one half of the lesions incorporated at least one uncommon feature: a partially or predominantly cystic structure, an irregular shape and sharp angulations, a halo, an intrinsically hypovascular pattern, coarse or peripheral calcifications, or a hyperechoic or a mixture of hyper- and isoechoic sonographic signals. The authors did not find any papillary cancers that had a predominantly cystic pattern, a halo, or a non-hypoechoic texture to be associated with a hypovascular flow pattern on Doppler imaging; those that were non-hypoechoic demonstrated intrinsic or at least perinodular flow. Thus, color Doppler sonography is an important adjunct to US examination if one is to target suspicious lesions for further study.

Papini and co-workers correlated the ultrasonographic features of nonpalpable thyroid nodules (8–15 mm) with pathological diagnoses [62]. This prospective study involved 402 consecutive patients with nonpalpable thyroid nodules and adequate FNAB cytology. Surgery was performed in 96 patients who had abnormal or suspicious cytological findings. Those subjects with benign pathology were reevaluated at 6 months. If their nodules grew, US-guided biopsy was repeated. Eleven additional patients had thyroidectomy based on enlarging nodules or goiter growth. Histological examination of the 107 resected thyroids revealed 31 cases of carcinoma (28.9%) of which 87% were papillary. The prevalence of cancer was the same in nodules of 8–10 mm as in those of 11–15 mm. Irregular or blurred nodular margins, microcalcifications, and an intranodular vascular pattern were independent risk factors for malignancy on US/Doppler imaging. A solid hypoechoic pattern was seen more frequently in malignant than in benign lesions. If this pattern was combined with any one of the independent risk factors, only 4 of the 31 cases of cancer in the series and only 1 of the 11 specimens that demonstrated local invasion would have been missed. Malignancy risk could not be predicted by the number of nodules, nodule size, or the coexistence of a multinodular goiter. The authors recommended that FNAB be performed on all nonpalpable nodules greater than 8 mm that are both hypoechoic and demonstrate one or more of the independent risk factors. All others should be followed in 6–12 months with a repeat US examination.

Leenhardt et al. published on the limits of US-guided cytology in the management of nonpalpable thyroid nodules [63]. They performed US-guided biopsies of 450 nonpalpable nodules ranging in size from 0.57 to 2.6 cm. Adequate cytological material was obtained in 81% of the cases, the larger the lesion the more likely it was to obtain an adequate sample. Ninety-four of the 450 patients were referred for surgery. Forty-seven of them (43%) had a FNAB diagnosis of malignancy or a suspicious lesion while others had some additional feature such as a palpable nodule in a multinodular gland, a supracentrimetric or cold nodule, or an enlarging nodule, etc. Twenty carcinomas, 16 of which were papillary, were found in the surgical specimens, 8 measuring 0.63–1 cm on US. In 16 of the 20 cases, US-FNAB had correctly diagnosed a likely malignancy but 4 were missed. A solid hypoechoic lesion on US was found to be a useful predictor of malignancy. Of the 450 nodules assessed, 115 were below 1 cm in size; 45 (39%) of these were both hypoechoic and solid. Sixteen of these were operated upon; 7 proved to be carcinoma. By contrast, 77 of the 115 micronodules were cystic or hyperechoic; from this group, only 1, a hyperechoic nodule, was found to be malignant. Diagnosis at final histology was not associated significantly with size, presence of

calcifications, or blurred margins of the nodules, however, either calcifications or blurred margins were found in half of the malignant nodules and both were present in 7 of the malignancies. This was true for 11 benign nodules as well. The authors suggested restricting US-FNAB to lesions 1 cm or greater, or to those that are solid and hypoechoic, in order to avoid operating on an unwarranted number of patients. Using these criteria, however, 84% of the patients in this study would have been biopsied and 25% of the overall carcinomas would have been missed. If only solid hypoechoic nodules were biopsied, intervention would have been limited to just 31% of the patients but at the expense of missing 35% of the malignancies. Interestingly, using either criterion, 7 of the 8 microcarcinomas would have been correctly identified.

Nam-Goong et al. studied retrospectively thyroid incidentalomas measuring between 0.2 and 1.5 cm by US-guided FNAB [64]. They aspirated 317 nodules from 267 patients. Forty-two (13%) were interpreted as consistent with or suspicious of PTC. Based upon cytology, 8% of nodules measuring less than 0.5 cm by US were judged to be malignant; the rate was 15% for nodules between 0.5 and 1.0 cm and 14% for those between 1.0 and 1.5 cm. Age, sex, and multiplicity of nodules had no bearing on these rates. However, the malignancy rate was significantly higher in solid than in cystic or mixed cystic/solid nodules, in hypoechoic than in isoechoic or hyperechoic nodules, in lesions with punctate calcifications than in those without this feature, and in those with ill-defined rather than well-defined margins. Nodules that demonstrated increased vascularization on color Doppler examination had a significantly higher rate of malignancy than lesions showing decreased intranodular vascularization. Of 48 patients with suspicious cytology, 40 went to surgery. Preoperative cytological diagnoses of PTC were confirmed in all by histology. In PTC patients, extrathyroidal extension was observed in 15 cases (43%), regional lymph node metastases in 17 (49%), and multifocal tumors in 13 (37%). The incidence of these findings was not significantly different between nodules measuring less than 1 cm and those measuring 1–1.5 cm. Eleven of the 22 patients with microcarcinomas had extrathyroidal invasion. Only long-term prospective studies can determine the natural history of these lesions with or without surgical intervention, and whether search for nonpalpable thyroid nodules would be of benefit to patients and at what cost.

The increasing use of high resolution US and its identification of thyroid nodules never before suspected is not the only modality causing conundrums in the appropriate management of these discoveries. Now ^{18}F-fluorodeoxyglucose positron emission tomography (FDG-PET) is unearthing unsuspected thyroid nodules. In one study, as many as 2.3% of patients without known thyroid disease had PET-positive thyroid lesions, 47% of which were malignant [65]. Kang et al. have published a retrospective review of their experience in patients undergoing FDG-PET for metastatic evaluation of non-thyroidal cancer (999 patients) versus a second group of healthy volunteers without known malignancy, undergoing cancer screening (331 subjects) [66]. Twenty-one focal type lesions were identified in this group of 1330 subjects (1.6%). Thirteen were from the cancer patients and 8 from the volunteers. Fifteen of the 21 focal type lesions were evaluated by either US-guided core biopsy or surgical histology. Four of the nodules proved to be PTCs, 3 from the cancer cohort. The rest were benign.

Clinical Presentation of PMCT

PMCTs are frequently discovered as incidental findings on neck imaging for indications other than thyroid cancer. Unsuspected PMCTs also appear in surgical specimens from operations for benign thyroid disease or in search of a parathyroid adenoma. Occasionally, however, the patient notes a cervical mass that proves to be a metastatic lymph node. In the older literature, these lesions, often cystic, were referred to as lateral aberrant thyroid tissue. Sugitani et al. reviewed 34 patients with PMCTs, who presented with cervical nodes of 1 cm or greater [67]. Four of these patients later developed distant metastases and died of their disease. These observations contrasted with 156 patients with PMTC who presented without clinically apparent lymph node metastases. None of this latter group developed distant metastases and rarely had local recurrence. Factors associated with worse outcomes were lymph nodes greater than 3 cm in size and thyroid cancers that were

non-encapsulated or sclerosing. Patient age, sex, maximum tumor size, extrathyroidal invasion, multifocality, and the number of lymph node metastases were not statistically significant. Sugitani et al. recommended not treating asymptomatic PMCTs by surgery. For clinically apparent PMCTs they recommended a more aggressive approach. Since total thyroidectomy and RAI did not improve final outcome in their high risk patients, the authors concluded that prognosis is little influenced by therapy and is more likely determined by the inherent biological aggressiveness of the tumor.

Verge et al. reported seven cases of PMTC presenting as enlarged cervical cystic lymph nodes [68]. The primary thyroid tumors identified subsequently varied in size from 2 to 8 mm. All patients had conservative cervical neck dissection as part of their thyroidectomy procedure and received postoperative RAI. None of the patients suffered a recurrence or metastasis in follow-up that extended 1–7 years. In another report, Coleman and co-workers described 12 patients whose initial manifestation of occult thyroid carcinoma was a long-standing neck mass and 2 patients whose cervical metastases were discovered during neck dissection for diseases unrelated to the thyroid [69]. Nine of these 14 relatively young individuals had microcarcinomas, 4 of which were less than 4 mm in size. In many instances, CT scans, MRI, and US failed to identify the thyroid primary. Open biopsy of the involved lymph node was more successful than FNA in establishing the correct pathology of the cervical lesion. All 14 patients had total thyroidectomy except for one who had hemithyroidectomy/isthnusectomy; 12 of 14 also had postoperative RAI. Most of the thyroid tumors were unilateral and unifocal but 4 had multiple, bilateral disease and 2 were multifocal on the same side. None of the patients had evidence of disease on relatively brief follow-up that extended from 2 to 48 months.

Monchik et al. added another eight cases of lateral neck cystic nodes associated with PMCTs. The primary tumors ranged from 2 to 9 mm [70]. Therapy consisted of total thyroidectomy and RAI. Tumors were found to be multicentric in three cases and all but one patient had metastatic disease in paratracheal nodes or thymic nodes, or both. During follow-up lasting 8–10 years, two patients who had had modified cervical neck dissections experienced nodal recurrence within 1–2 years.

Additional data from these publications also demonstrate that PMCT, manifest initially by enlarged cervical lymph node metastases, is associated with a younger than average age, male gender, multifocal and bilateral thyroid tumors, and recurrent disease. Distant metastases may develop and patients may die of their disease despite thyroidectomy and radiation. Even the smallest of the microcarcinomas may give rise to complications. Nevertheless, the majority of patients treated by total thyroidectomy and RAI experienced good outcomes for the period of follow-up. PMCTs presenting with lymph node metastases may represent a more aggressive form of the disease and the application of both bilateral surgery and postoperative radiation may have offered real benefit to most patients.

Management Options and Outcomes

Several large series have been published describing a variety of surgical procedures and other modalities for the management of PMTC. The largest is that of Hay et al., who studied retrospectively 535 patients seen over a 50-year period [71]. Tumor size ranged from 1 to 10 mm (median 8 mm) with 22% measuring less than 5 mm. Patient ages ranged from 6 to 85 years (mean 47) and the mean follow-up was 17.5 years (median 16.1). The mode of diagnosis varied over time mainly owing to the introduction of FNAB in 1980. The initial pathological diagnosis was then made more often (40% of the cases) by FNAB than by the histology of operative specimens. The diagnosis was made as an incidental finding in 18% of the cases. In approximately 20% of the patients the initial presentation was by open biopsy of a cervical lymph node. Apparently none of the patients' tumors were discovered as an incidental or occult lesion by US. All FNABs were performed on patients with palpable nodules. No mention was made as to how many patients might have been exposed to external radiation. Over the period of study, patients underwent unilateral lobectomy, bilateral subtotal thyroidectomy, or total, and near-total thyroidectomy (74%). Fifty-

six percent of them did not undergo any node removal and only 30% of those who did had a modified neck dissection. The rest just had "node picking." Ten percent had remnant ablation with RAI. Only 2 of the 535 patients died of disease and both had had their initial diagnosis made by neck node biopsy. One had a grade 1, 0.1 mm primary tumor, but despite remnant ablation, experienced loco-regional recurrences and finally osseous spread 16 years post surgery. While no other patients died of their disease, 6% developed a recurrence within the neck or at a distant site by 20 years. Neck nodal recurrences occurred in 4% of the patients by 10 years and in 5% by 20 years. Those with neck node metastases at initial diagnosis had a much greater incidence of locoregional recurrence than those without this finding (1% versus 18%). The type of surgery had a very significant impact on both locoregional and nodal recurrence rates. Patients who had bilateral lobar resection, subtotal, total, or near-total resections experienced lower rates of recurrence than those who underwent unilateral lobectomy. Meaningful data concerning the impact of postoperative remnant ablation by RAI came from a cohort of 153 patients who had initial lymph node metastases. Of these, 45 received RAI and 108 did not. Their rates of locoregional recurrence did not differ significantly either at 2, 5, or 10 years postoperatively. At the most, the patients treated solely by surgery had a recurrence rate of 12% versus a 9% rate for the radiated group. Among the conclusions drawn from the study were that PMCTs generally do not present a significant biological threat and hemithyroidectomy does not compromise survival since recurrences, should they occur, can be dealt with successfully and pose little risk. The major risk factors for recurrence were lymph node metastases at the time of initial diagnosis and the extent of thyroid surgery. The authors stated a preference for bilateral lobar resection, especially near-total thyroidectomy with modified neck dissection when neck nodes were palpable. They were not partial to RAI adjunctive therapy or repeat isotope scans for follow-up in those who received RAI because of the negative effects of thyroxine withdrawal, necessary at that time, and the small risk of recurrences with or without isotope administration.

From 1962 to 1995, investigators at the Institut Gustave Roussy in France treated and followed 281 patients with microcarcinomas, 247 of whom had PMCTs [72]. Forty-nine percent of the tumors measured less than 5 mm. Patient demographics were similar to those in the Mayo Clinic report by Hay et al. [71]. Treatment was highly individualized, but all patients received thyroid suppression postsurgically, and 124 of the 195 patients treated by total thyroidectomy received an ablative dose of 100 mCi of I-131 plus a total body scan 4 days later. They also underwent a 2 mCi I-131 scan 6 months after initial therapy. Ultrasonography, thyroid-stimulating hormone (TSH), and thyroglobulin measurements were utilized in follow-up when available. Seventeen patients had a history of prior external radiation. Microcarcinomas were incidentally found in operative specimens for benign adenomas in 186 patients and in 3 for Graves' disease. Surgery was performed in 89 patients because of clinically apparent lymph node metastases and in 3 for distant metastases. These 92 subjects with equal numbers of both sexes, were younger than the others, and they had a higher frequency of bilaterality, multicentricity, lymph node metastases, and extrathyroidal involvement. Multivariate analysis of the outcomes in the total cohort of 281 patients found only two parameters that influenced recurrence rates: the extent of initial surgery (lobectomy alone having higher recurrences than bilateral surgery), and the number of foci on pathological examination. Only 11 patients (3.9%), all with PMCTs, experienced locoregional recurrences within 10 years, either in the thyroid bed, in lymph nodes, or in both sites. Initially, 9 had had multifocal and only 2 had had unifocal tumors. Some of them had received RAI, total thyroidectomy and/or lymph node dissection as initial therapy. Conservative therapy, which included lobectomy, was recommended for patients with unifocal tumors. This was based on the fact that only two recurrences were documented in patients so treated, and contralateral disease was discovered in only 19.8% of patients with supposedly unifocal lesions who were treated by bilateral thyroidectomy. In the presence of multifocal disease, bilaterality was found in greater than 50% of the cases and the recurrence rate was reduced from 20% to 5% when total thyroidectomy was the procedure of choice. Thus, total or subtotal thyroidectomy was recommended for multifocal disease with the addition of central compartment nodal dis-

section. RAI was a possible option although the authors could not make a strong case for its inclusion.

In a retrospective series of 120 patients ranging in age from 23 to 77 years, Appetecchia et al. identified factors associated with recurrence in PMTC [73]. Microcarcinomas were incidental findings from operative specimens in 80 patients; surgery in 40 patients was for a suspicious FNAB of either a thyroid nodule (34 patients) or a regional lymph node (6 patients). Total thyroidectomy was performed in 92 of the 120 patients; 74 of them had a unifocal tumor and 18 had multiple tumor foci. All patients with positive nodes had systematic lymph node dissection. For 28 of the 120 patients, lobo-isthmusectomy was the primary procedure. Two of them demonstrated multiple neoplastic foci. Fourteen others went on to have completion thyroidectomy; and another 2 were shown to have multifocal disease. Thus, 108 patients in all underwent total thyroidectomy of which 60 were given ablative therapy with 75–100 mCi of I-131 including all 26 patients who had nodal metastases or multifocal disease. No patient was documented with distant metastases but extracapsular invasion was found in 16.7% of the patients. Follow-up extended from 5 to 15 years. In that period, only 2 patients who had been treated initially by total thyroidectomy, lymph node dissection, and RAI experienced a recurrence, both in lymph nodes. After therapy for the recurrence, both had undetectable thyroglobulin levels upon thyroid hormone withdrawal. Lymph node metastases were highly correlated with tumors that exceeded 5 mm in diameter and occurred in association with both unifocal and multifocal lesions. Despite lymph node metastases in 26 patients and thyroid capsular invasion in 20, only 1.7% of the 120 subjects experienced local recurrent disease. The authors concluded that patient outcomes were favorable whether they had lobectomy or total thyroidectomy even in the presence of extrathyroidal invasion. One can speculate that the low rate of recurrence in this study may be due to the fact that a majority of the patients had been treated quite aggressively and those recommended for completion thyroidectomy were well chosen, based upon operative findings and histology. While the authors make the point that PMCTs should not be overtreated, their rather aggressive approach may have been responsible for limiting instances of recurrence.

Chow et al. reported a retrospective analysis of 203 PMCT patients seen in Hong Kong from 1960 to 1999 [74]. The mean tumor size was 0.72 cm. Most of the patients with incidental PMCTs apparently accepted completion thyroidectomy, so that around 90% eventually had the equivalent of a total thyroidectomy. Of the 203 patients, 63 had multifocal disease, 42 had extrathyroidal extension, and 50 had lymph node metastases. Fifty-five patients had either lymph node excision/sampling ($n = 35$) or lymph node dissection ($n = 20$). RAI was given to 137 patients. Locoregional recurrences, 2 in the thyroid bed and 10 in lymph nodes appeared, within 8 years of diagnosis. Distant metastases were found in 5 patients. Multivariate analysis revealed that locoregional recurrences were higher in those with cervical node metastases at presentation, multifocal disease, and not having received RAI ablation. Tumor size had no significant influence on patient outcome but those with the smaller tumors presented at a younger age and none in this group had distant metastases. The authors recommended bilateral thyroidectomy for patients whose PMCTs are detected non-incidentally and RAI ablation for those with positive lymph nodes or multifocality.

The findings of Chow are essentially borne out in a retrospective study of 299 patients by Pellegriti et al. [75]. Included in this report are tumors measuring up to 1.5 cm, 18 patients with familial thyroid cancer, 122 with familial thyroid disease, 36 with concurrent Graves' disease, and 25 from an iodine-deficient area. Patient demographics were the same as in other studies. For purposes of comparison, the patients were placed into two groups: those with non-incidental carcinoma (148 patients) mainly diagnosed by FNAB and those with incidental carcinomas (151 patients) after thyroidectomy for benign thyroid disorders. Two hundred and ninety-two patients underwent near-total or total thyroidectomy either as primary therapy ($n = 269$) or as completion thyroidectomy ($n = 15$) within 8 months of diagnosis. Seven patients had a lobectomy. The major findings in both groups were a surprisingly high incidence of multifocality, bilaterality, lymph node metastases, and extrathyroidal extension. Except for bilaterality, they occurred more frequently sta-

tistically in the non-incidental group. Eight patients had distant metastases (seven from the non-incidental group). Five of the eight with metastases occurred in patients with small tumors. Ten in the non-incidental group also had vascular invasion compared with only 4 in the incidental group. Patients judged to be low risk and who had near-total or total thyroidectomy received an ablative dose of 30 mCi of I-131 and those with a TNM rating of T4 or N1 received 100 mCi. The follow-up period ranged from 1.2 to 16.2 years. At the end of the study, 256 were disease free while 43 had either disease in lymph nodes ($n = 17$), distant metastases ($n = 6$), or an elevated thyroglobulin level. By multivariate analysis, persistent disease was associated with neck lymph node metastases at presentation, bilateral tumors, and a non-incidental status. The sclerosing variant of papillary carcinoma and lymph node metastases were associated with distant metastases. Tumor size did not predict relapse. Of 18 with familial thyroid carcinoma, 12 were incidental and 15 were less than 1 cm. Only 1/18 had distant metastases, and 4/18 had lymph node metastases. The purported aggressiveness of familial thyroid carcinoma was not supported by this study. However, concomitant Graves' disease was positively associated with relapse while patients from an endemic goiter area had a negative association with relapse. Patients with a stimulated thyroglobulin <1 ng/mL had only a 1% probability of a locoregional recurrence and none had distant metastases. The authors suggested that total thyroidectomy should be the surgical therapy of choice. In an editorial accompanying this article, Pearce and Braverman advocate near-total or total thyroidectomy with central compartment node dissection for patients with non-incidental tumors and recommend RAI ablation in those with positive lymph nodes, multicentricity, or vascular or extracapsular invasion [76]. They also recommend similar surgery for patients with multinodular goiter or documented benign nodules to obviate the need for later completion thyroidectomy.

Pelizzo et al. reported on 149 consecutive patients with PMCT who were operated on by a single surgeon over a 12-year period [77]. Patient demographics were very similar to those of other reports. The series consisted of incidental, non-incidental, and occult PMCTs diagnosed by US-guided FNAB. Seven patients (4.7%) had positive lymph node presentation. They had total thyroidectomy, lymphadenectomy, and RAI ablation. Of the other 142 patients, 119 had a total thyroidectomy whereas 23 underwent partial thyroidectomy. Seventy-three of the patients diagnosed with PMCT or metastatic lymph nodes preoperatively had lymphadenectomy as part of their surgery. Lymph node metastases were found in 20 of the 73. All with a total thyroidectomy also had RAI ablation and whole body scans; 95 of the 125 patients scanned demonstrated thyroid remnants, and in 3, previously unrecognized lymph node metastases. Patients ≥45 years with multifocality, extrathyroidal extension, or positive lymph nodes received 100–150 mCi of RAI. During a 1–12-year follow-up, only three manifested locoregional recurrence by US examination. These three patients did not have total thyroidectomy or I-131 therapy. Their primary tumors were greater than 5 mm in size, were unifocal, showed no evidence of extracapsular invasion or lymph node metastases, and lacked a peritumoral capsule. These patients were operated on again and subsequently received 150 mCi of I-131. They had no evidence of disease 3–4 years later. The authors believe that RAI whole-body scintigraphy is worth doing in patients who have had total thyroidectomy in order to detect unrecognized metastatic deposits and that I-131 therapy may benefit patients with acknowledged risk factors. For patients whose PMCT is discovered incidentally, reoperation might not be necessary if their lesions are unifocal, thyroid capsular invasion is absent, and US examination of residual thyroid tissue is negative for any nodules.

Regarding this study, one could argue that the infrequency of recurrence came at the price of extensive surgery and the liberal use of RAI ablation. Did the three patients who had a recurrence require another operation? Has high resolution US created as many problems as it has solved by revealing recurrences that might never have become clinically significant? Would adverse consequences have occurred if patients lacking other compelling reasons for surgery received no intervention?

Ito et al. have attempted to answer these questions in part by offering their 732 patients, all of whose PMCTs were diagnosed by FNAB, the option of immediate surgery versus observation by US [78]. This cohort did not include patients with occult or incidental papillary tumors. The only patients assigned to surgery without choice had tumors invading the recurrent laryngeal nerve or trachea, had a high grade malignancy by cytology, or had positive lymph node metastases. One hundred and sixty-two patients initially chose observation by US. Follow-up extended for this group from 1.5 to 9.5 years. The surgical treatment group comprised 571 patients who were either assigned surgery, chose the surgical option, or underwent surgery after a period of observation in the former group (56 patients). The two groups were otherwise very close in almost all respects. Average tumor size increased significantly by ≥2 mm in about 30% of the observation group after 3 and 4 years of follow-up; in the rest it did not increase or actually decreased. Some tumors actually decreased in size. No difference in size was noted between the patients taking thyroxine and those on no TSH suppression. In 18 patients, tumors grew to >10 mm; 7 of them were recommended for surgery. After one year, the size in the 11 other subjects had not changed. Of the 162 in the observation group, 11 were suspected of having lymph node metastases and in another 9 patients, they appeared during follow-up. Of these 20 patients, 18 were suspected of having central compartment involvement only and surgery was not performed. In the other 2, suspicious lateral nodes appeared and they were referred for surgery. After 19–56 months, a total of 56 patients in the observation group converted to surgery by choice or for some change in the status of their benign thyroid disease.

The surgical group had 626 patients. A total or near-total thyroidectomy was performed in 276 because they had disease (malignant or not) in both lobes. For 350 patients, less than total thyroidectomy was performed. Central compartment node dissection was carried out in 594 subjects with metastases confirmed in 258. Lateral neck dissection was carried out in 317 patients; metastases were found in 141 (55 had been detected preoperatively). More than 40% of the patients had both positive lymph nodes and multicentricity. Follow-up time averaged 48.7 months extending out as far as 10 years. In that period, 16 (2.6%) of the 626 patients had a recurrence of disease, 12 in lymph nodes.

Four with thyroid bed recurrence had not had total thyroidectomy. No patient had distant metastases. The use of RAI whole-body scanning or RAI therapy was not mentioned in the report.

Given the findings in the operative group, it is likely that many patients in the observation group lived with undetected microscopic lymph node metastases yet did not show any progression of clinical disease. The authors themselves questioned how necessary some of their referrals for surgery were. They suggested that surgery could be delayed until signs of progression appear. For those chosen to have surgery however, routine central lymph node dissection was recommended to avoid possible future, more difficult, re-operation. Lateral neck dissection was favored only for those with a preoperative diagnosis of metastasis. The outcomes in this large series were excellent in spite of no or limited surgery and the absence of adjunctive RAI.

Wada et al. published a retrospective study dealing with the implications of lymph node dissection at initial surgery and its influence on recurrence [79]. They compared the impact of lymph node dissection in 259 patients with PMCTs diagnosed preoperatively because of a palpable nodule or through US screening with the outcome in 155 patients whose PMCTs were discovered incidentally after thyroidectomy for benign disease. None of the latter patients, therefore, had lymph node dissection. In the first group, 24 had palpable nodes at presentation and underwent modified neck dissections – the "therapeutic" node dissection group. The other 235 patients had a "prophylactic" node dissection either of the central compartment or a modified neck dissection. Surgery was mostly lobectomy or subtotal thyroidectomy. In the non-incidental group, 64% of the patients without palpable nodes at presentation had positive nodes in the central and/or lateral compartments by histology. Only one patient from the prophylactic node dissection group had a nodal recurrence after 1.3–12 years. Five patients with preoperative palpable nodes manifested recurrences. Only one of 155 patients in the incidental group who did not have a node dissection had a recurrence. Most patients were placed on thyroid suppression but none received RAI ablation. Five of the patients had familial carcinoma but none had distant metas-

tases or died of disease. The authors concluded that prophylactic node dissection conferred no benefit. Therapeutic lymph node dissection was recommended for those presenting with palpable lymphadenopathy at diagnosis.

Summary and Recommendations

The problem of PMCT continues to engage the interest of endocrinologists and surgeons, but in spite of an extensive literature addressing various aspects of the problem, diversity of opinion predominates over consensus. However, there are several points upon which most investigators would probably agree: (i) PMCT appearing at any age, no matter how treated or even not treated, carries an excellent prognosis; (ii) distant metastases and death due to disease are rare; (iii) fatal outcomes do occasionally occur, but there is no reliable way to predict, at the time of diagnosis, which tumors will behave so aggressively; (iv) tumor size is not a reliable predictor of biological behavior; (v) lymph node metastases at the time of diagnosis are frequently associated with tumor recurrence; (vi) multifocality has a significant association with tumor recurrence and bilateral disease; (vii) high resolution US and FNAB is increasing the recognition of PMCT and they are creating many management conundrums as well; (viii) external radiation plays a significant role in promoting PMCTs and may be associated with a biologically aggressive course; (ix) from autopsy data and some of the studies quoted, most PMCTs are indolent and harmless, suggesting that promoting factors are necessary for the expression of significant clinical disease; (x) just about everything else is controversial.

Given the foregoing, it seems reasonable that the initial step to be taken is to establish the aim of therapy with the patient. If the goal is to eliminate all disease possible and reduce to a minimum the likelihood of recurrence, then near-total thyroidectomy, node dissection, and RAI ablative therapy should be recommended. If PMCTs were found incidentally, completion thyroidectomy should be recommended if initial surgery was only partial. On the other hand, if the goal is to keep intervention to a minimum while accepting some degree of risk of recurrence, then many options, including nothing more than careful follow-up, are possible. The final approach requires individualization and the realization that much of the data in the literature is conflicting. What follows seems reasonable to us.

Management of Incidental PMCT

Most likely, incidental PMCTs will be discovered in patients undergoing thyroid surgery for benign thyroid disorders or, occasionally, hyperparathyroidism. If none of the lesions show vascular invasion, thyroid capsular invasion, or high histological grade, and there are no suspicious cervical nodes, patients should be informed and reassured. Further surgery need not be considered. Follow-up should include periodic physical examination and high resolution US of the neck. Unless there are other indications, TSH suppression need not be undertaken. If any suspicious nodules or nodes are found subsequently, US-guided FNAB should be attempted. A positive lymph node should be dealt with by completion thyroidectomy, node dissection, RAI ablation, and TSH suppression. The presence of a positive thyroid nodule. We generally recommend ultrasound surveillance alone, with an FNAB if significant growth is documented. While size does not necessarily predict behavior of PMCTs, this conservative approach seems to be for tumors less than 5 mm in diameter.

If the final pathological analysis reveals high histological grade, vascular or extrathyroidal invasion, or positive cervical nodes, completion thyroidectomy should be considered coupled with RAI ablation and TSH suppression. However, we cannot lose sight of the fact that autopsy studies have revealed PMCTs that are all of the above, went undiagnosed, and were without sequelae in life. Thus, in the absence of any practical means to predict future tumor behavior, one could adopt the attitude that the likely outcome of doing nothing except follow-up might not differ from intervention. We are doubtful, however, that many patients would embrace this approach once they learn they were harboring a malignancy with some risk factors, and in the litigious environment in which medicine is practiced, at least in the United States, we are doubtful many physicians

would encourage it. Yet, on the evidence, it is a reasonable option.

Management of Occult PMCT

The very notion that an occult PMCT exists suggests that it has called attention to itself in some unfavorable way, either as a cervical lymph node metastasis or, much more rarely, a distant metastasis. Should the latter be the case, there is no question that it should be treated as one would treat any papillary carcinoma. In the absence of distant metastases, high-resolution and color-Doppler examinations of the thyroid and neck to find and define any non-palpable nodules or other pathology should be undertaken. If a single thyroid nodule is found and FNAB identifies it as a PMCT, one could limit surgery to lobo-isthmusectomy with central compartment and ipsilateral regional lymph node dissection. If the surgeon observes or palpates any nodules in the contralateral lobe or frozen section identifies multicentricity, bilateral thyroidectomy should be completed. RAI ablation might be optional after total thyroidectomy remembering that some studies did not find this of benefit. However, having achieved removal of almost all thyroid tissue, it seems reasonable to try to eliminate micrometastases and residual thyroid tissue and take advantage of future thyroglobulin monitoring. If preoperative US identifies multiple and/or bilateral nodules, whether or not they are proved by FNAB to be PMCTs, the situation should be treated as one would any larger-size papillary carcinoma.

Management of Non-Incidental PMCT

The discovery of PMCTs in life when one is not seeking them, or finding an isolated small nodule by palpation that proves to be a papillary carcinoma by FNAB, is an increasing problem. We would encourage a patient with a unifocal lesion <5 mm in diameter to delay intervention unless new foci appear, there is sustained tumor enlargement, or there is suspicion of lymph node involvement. For solitary lesions between 5 and 10 mm, we recommend a simple lobectomy or lobo-isthmusectomy with central compartment node dissection with additional lymph node dissection being left to the discretion of the surgeon. Any suspicion of bilaterality or lymph node involvement should prompt a near-total thyroidectomy, lymph node dissection, and RAI ablation.

Any patient with an incidental, occult, or non-incidental PMCT who has a history of significant prior radiation exposure, no matter when, or a documented history of familial papillary carcinoma, should probably have a near-total thyroidectomy rather than a more conservative operation. The latter applies especially to children and adolescents as age alone in this group constitutes a risk factor for recurrence and distant metastases. These individuals require RAI ablation and very close follow-up.

Until we can distinguish the indolent microcarcinomas, likely in the majority, from the trouble-makers, difficult and uncertain choices in managing PMCTs will continue to be made. Prospective randomized studies to test the recommendations presented here will probably never be undertaken since the clinical outcome in most patients with a PMCT is so favorable and since superiority of one approach would require follow-up of impracticable length. What we have suggested regarding management of PMCTs, although rather conservative, may nonetheless, result in some unnecessary surgery. On the positive side, it may also reduce recurrent disease to a minimum. That is as much a hope as a certainty.

References

1. Schlumberger M, Filetti S, Hay ID. Non-toxic goiter and thyroid neoplasia. In: Williams RH, Larsen PR (eds) Williams textbook of endocrinology, 10th edn. Philadelphia, PA: Saunders, 2003: 457–490.
2. Hazard JB. Small papillary carcinoma of the thyroid. A study with special reference to so-called nonencapsulated sclerosing tumor. Lab Invest 1960; 9:86–97.
3. Hedinger C, Williams ED, Sobin LH. The WHO histological classification of thyroid tumors: a commentary on the second edition. Cancer 1989; 63:908–911.
4. Pelizzo MR, Piotto A, Rubello D, Casara D, Fassina A, Busnardo B. High prevalence of occult papillary thyroid carcinoma in a surgical series for benign thyroid disease. Tumori 1990; 76:255–257.
5. Edis A. Natural history of occult thyroid cancer. In: DeGroot LJ, Frohman L, Kaplan E, Refetoff S (eds) Radiation-associated thyroid carcinoma. New York: Grune & Stratton, 1977: 155–160.
6. Rosai J, LiVolsi VA, Sobrinho-Simoes M, Williams ED. Renaming papillary microcarcinoma of the thyroid gland: the Porto proposal. Int J Surg Pathol 2003; 11:249–251.

7. Tan GH, Gharib H. Thyroid incidentalomas: management approaches to nonpalpable nodules discovered incidentally on thyroid imaging. Ann Intern Med 1997; 126:226–231.
8. Ross DS. Nonpalpable thyroid nodules – managing an epidemic. J Clin Endocrinol Metab 2002; 87:1938–1940.
9. Yang GC, LiVolsi VA, Baloch ZW. Thyroid microcarcinoma: fine-needle aspiration diagnosis and histologic follow-up. Int J Surg Pathol 2002; 10:133–139.
10. Strate SM, Lee EL, Childers JH. Occult papillary carcinoma of the thyroid with distant metastases. Cancer 1984; 54:1093–1100.
11. Sampson RJ. Prevalence and significance of occult thyroid cancer. In: DeGroot LJ, Frohman L, Kaplan E, Refetoff S (eds) Radiation-associated thyroid carcinoma. New York: Grune & Stratton, 1977: 137–153.
12. Yamamoto Y, Maeda T, Izumi K, Otsuka H. Occult papillary carcinoma of the thyroid. A study of 408 autopsy cases. Cancer 1990; 65:1173–1179.
13. Mitselou A, Vougiouklakis T, Peschos D, Dallas P, Agnantis NJ. Occult thyroid carcinoma. A study of 160 autopsy cases. The first report for the region of Epirus-Greece. Anticancer Res 2002; 22:427–432.
14. Harach HR, Franssila KO, Wasenius VM. Occult papillary carcinoma of the thyroid. A "normal" finding in Finland. A systematic autopsy study. Cancer 1985; 56: 531–538.
15. Lang W, Borrusch H, Bauer L. Occult carcinomas of the thyroid. Evaluation of 1,020 sequential autopsies. Am J Clin Pathol 1988; 90:72–76.
16. Schottenfeld D, Gershman ST. Epidemiology of thyroid cancer – part I. Clin Bull 1977; 7:47–54.
17. Nishyama R, Ludwig G, Thompson NW. The prevalence of small papillary thyroid carcinomas in 100 consecutive necropsies in an American population. In: DeGroot LJ, Frohman L, Kaplan E, Refetoff S (eds) Radiation-associated thyroid carcinoma. New York: Grune & Stratton, 1977: 123–135.
18. Sampson RJ, Woolner LB, Bahn RC, Kurland LT. Occult thyroid carcinoma in Olmsted County, Minnesota: prevalence at autopsy compared with that in Hiroshima and Nagasaki, Japan. Cancer 1974; 34:2072–2076.
19. Fukunaga FH, Yatani R. Geographic pathology of occult thyroid carcinomas. Cancer 1975; 36:1095–1099.
20. Fink A, Tomlinson G, Freeman JL, Rosen IB, Asa SL. Occult micropapillary carcinoma associated with benign follicular thyroid disease and unrelated thyroid neoplasms. Mod Pathol 1996; 9:816–820.
21. Delides GS, Elemenoglou J, Lekkas J, Kittas C, Evthimiou C. Occult thyroid carcinoma in a Greek population. Neoplasma 1987; 34:119–125.
22. de Benoist B, Andersson M, Takkouche B, Egli I. Prevalence of iodine deficiency worldwide. Lancet 2003; 362:1859–1860.
23. Harach HR, Escalante DA, Onativia A, Lederer Outes J, Saravia Day E, Williams ED. Thyroid carcinoma and thyroiditis in an endemic goitre region before and after iodine prophylaxis. Acta Endocrinol (Copenh) 1985; 108:55–60.
24. Bacher-Stier C, Riccabona G, Totsch M, Kemmler G, Oberaigner W, Moncayo R. Incidence and clinical characteristics of thyroid carcinoma after iodine prophylaxis in an endemic goiter country. Thyroid 1997; 7:733–741.

25. Lind P, Langsteger W, Molnar M, Gallowitsch HJ, Mikosch P, Gomez I. Epidemiology of thyroid diseases in iodine sufficiency. Thyroid 1998; 8:1179–1183.

26. Langsteger W, Koltringer P, Wolf G, et al. The impact of geographical, clinical, dietary and radiation-induced features in epidemiology of thyroid cancer. Eur J Cancer 1993; 29A:1547–1553.

27. Feldt-Rasmussen U. Iodine and cancer. Thyroid 2001; 11:483–486.

28. Burgess JR, Dwyer T, McArdle K, Tucker P, Shugg D. The changing incidence and spectrum of thyroid carcinoma in Tasmania (1978–1998) during a transition from iodine sufficiency to iodine deficiency. J Clin Endocrinol Metab 2000; 85:1513–1517.

29. Arnbjornsson E, Arnbjornsson A, Olafsson A. Thyroid cancer incidence in relation to volcanic activity. Arch Environ Health 1986; 41:36–40.

30. Duffy BJ Jr, Fitzgerald PJ. Thyroid cancer in childhood and adolescence; a report on 28 cases. Cancer 1950; 3:1018–1032.

31. Ron E, Lubin JH, Shore RE, et al. Thyroid cancer after exposure to external radiation: a pooled analysis of seven studies. Radiat Res 1995; 141:259–277.

32. Sampson RJ, Key CR, Buncher CR, Iijima S. Thyroid carcinoma in Hiroshima and Nagasaki. I. Prevalence of thyroid carcinoma at autopsy. JAMA 1969; 209:65–70.

33. Thompson DE, Mabuchi K, Ron E, et al. Cancer incidence in atomic bomb survivors. Part II: Solid tumors, 1958–1987. Radiat Res 1994; 137:S17–S67.

34. Lund E, Galanti MR. Incidence of thyroid cancer in Scandinavia following fallout from atomic bomb testing: an analysis of birth cohorts. Cancer Causes Control 1999; 10:181–187.

35. Conrad R. Summary of thyroid findings in Marshallese 22 years after exposure to radioactive fallout. In: DeGroot LJ, Frohman L, Kaplan E, Refetoff S (eds) Radiation-associated thyroid carcinoma. New York: Grune & Stratton, 1977: 241–257.

36. Becker DV, Robbins J, Beebe GW, Bouville AC, Wachholz BW. Childhood thyroid cancer following the Chernobyl accident: a status report. Endocrinol Metab Clin North Am 1996; 25:197–211.

37. Kazakov VS, Demidchik EP, Astakhova LN. Thyroid cancer after Chernobyl. Nature 1992; 359:21.

38. Nikiforov Y, Gnepp DR. Pediatric thyroid cancer after the Chernobyl disaster. Pathomorphologic study of 84 cases (1991–1992) from the Republic of Belarus. Cancer 1994; 74:748–766.

39. Baverstock K, Egloff B, Pinchera A, Ruchti C, Williams D. Thyroid cancer after Chernobyl'. Nature 1992; 359:21–22.

39a. Mangano JJ. A post-Chernobyl rise in thyroid cancer in Connecticut, USA. Eur J Cancer Prev 1996; 5:75–81.

40. Pottern LM, Stone BJ, Day NE, Pickle LW, Fraumeni JF Jr. Thyroid cancer in Connecticut, 1935–1975: an analysis by cell type. Am J Epidemiol 1980; 112:764–774.

41. Simpson S. Headed south? Earth's fading field could mean a magnetic flip soon. Sci Am 2002; 287:24.

42. Valana R, Cappelli C, Perini P, et al. Hyperthyroidism and concurrent thyroid cancer. Tumori 1999; 85:247–252.

43. Belfiore A, Garofalo MR, Giuffrida D, et al. Increased aggressiveness of thyroid cancer in patients with Graves' disease. J Clin Endocrinol Metab 1990; 70:830–835.

44. Mazzaferri EL. Thyroid cancer and Graves' disease. J Clin Endocrinol Metab 1990; 70:826–829.

45. Pellegriti G, Belfiore A, Giuffrida D, Lupo L, Vigneri R. Outcome of differentiated thyroid cancer in Graves' patients. J Clin Endocrinol Metab 1998; 83:2805–2809.

46. Hales IB, McElduff A, Crummer P, et al. Does Graves' disease or thyrotoxicosis affect the prognosis of thyroid cancer. J Clin Endocrinol Metab 1992; 75:886–889.

47. Cantalamessa L, Baldini M, Orsatti A, Meroni L, Amodei V, Castagnone D. Thyroid nodules in Graves disease and the risk of thyroid carcinoma. Arch Intern Med 1999; 159:1705–1708.

48. Loh KC. Familial nonmedullary thyroid carcinoma: a meta-review of case series. Thyroid 1997; 7:107–13.

48a. Burgess JR, Duffield A, Wilkinson SJ, et al. Two families with an autosomal dominant inheritance pattern for papillary carcinoma of the thyroid. J Endocrinol Metab 1997; 82:345–348.

49. Lupoli G, Vitale G, Caraglia M, et al. Familial papillary thyroid microcarcinoma: a new clinical entity. Lancet 1999; 353:637–639.

50. Fernandez-Real JM, Ricart W. Familial papillary thyroid microcarcinoma. Lancet 1999; 353:1973–1974.

51. Marchesi M, Biffoni M, Biancari F, et al. Familial papillary carcinoma of the thyroid: a report of nine first-degree relatives of four families. Eur J Surg Oncol 2000; 26:789–791.

52. Rios A, Rodriguez JM, Canteras M, Galindo PJ, Balsalobre MD, Parrilla P. Risk factors for malignancy in multinodular goitres. Eur J Surg Oncol 2004; 30:58–62.

53. Musholt TJ, Musholt PB, Petrich T, Oetting G, Knapp WH, Klempnauer J. Familial papillary thyroid carcinoma: genetics, criteria for diagnosis, clinical features, and surgical treatment. World J Surg 2000; 24:1409–1417.

54. Franssila KO, Harach HR. Occult papillary carcinoma of the thyroid in children and young adults. A systemic autopsy study in Finland. Cancer 1986; 58:715–719.

55. Chow SM, Law SC, Au SK, et al. Changes in clinical presentation, management and outcome in 1348 patients with differentiated thyroid carcinoma: experience in a single institute in Hong Kong, 1960–2000. Clin Oncol (R Coll Radiol) 2003; 15:329–336.

56. Welch Dinauer CA, Tuttle RM, Robie DK, et al. Clinical features associated with metastasis and recurrence of differentiated thyroid cancer in children, adolescents and young adults. Clin Endocrinol (Oxf) 1998; 49:619–628.

57. Collins BJ, Chiappetta G, Schneider AB, et al. RET expression in papillary thyroid cancer from patients irradiated in childhood for benign conditions. J Clin Endocrinol Metab 2002; 87:3941–3946.

58. Newman KD, Black T, Heller G, et al. Differentiated thyroid cancer: determinants of disease progression in patients <21 years of age at diagnosis: a report from the Surgical Discipline Committee of the Children's Cancer Group. Ann Surg 1998; 227:533–541.

59. Alessandri AJ, Goddard KJ, Blair GK, Fryer CJ, Schultz KR. Age is the major determinant of recurrence in pediatric differentiated thyroid carcinoma. Med Pediatr Oncol 2000; 35:41–46.

60. Topliss D. Thyroid incidentaloma: the ignorant in pursuit of the impalpable. Clin Endocrinol (Oxf) 2004; 60:18–20.

61. Chan BK, Desser TS, McDougall IR, Weigel RJ, Jeffrey RB Jr. Common and uncommon sonographic features of papillary thyroid carcinoma. J Ultrasound Med 2003; 22:1083–1090.

62. Papini E, Guglielmi R, Bianchini A, et al. 2002 Risk of malignancy in nonpalpable thyroid nodules: predictive value of ultrasound and color-Doppler features. J Clin Endocrinol Metab 87:1941–1946.

63. Leenhardt L, Hejblum G, Franc B, et al. Indications and limits of ultrasound-guided cytology in the management of nonpalpable thyroid nodules. J Clin Endocrinol Metab 1999; 84:24–28.

64. Nam-Goong IS, Kim HY, Gong G, et al. Ultrasonography-guided fine-needle aspiration of thyroid incidentaloma: correlation with pathological findings. Clin Endocrinol (Oxf) 2004; 60:21–28.

65. Cohen MS, Arslan N, Dehdashti F, et al. Risk of malignancy in thyroid incidentalomas identified by fluorodeoxyglucose-positron emission tomography. Surgery 2001; 130:941–946.

66. Kang KW, Kim SK, Kang HS, et al. Prevalence and risk of cancer of focal thyroid incidentaloma identified by 18F-fluorodeoxyglucose positron emission tomography for metastasis evaluation and cancer screening in healthy subjects. J Clin Endocrinol Metab 2003; 88:4100–4104.

67. Sugitani I, Yanagisawa A, Shimizu A, Kato M, Fujimoto Y. Clinicopathologic and immunohistochemical studies of papillary thyroid microcarcinoma presenting with cervical lymphadenopathy. World J Surg 1998; 22:731–737.

68. Verge J, Guixa J, Alejo M, et al. Cervical cystic lymph node metastasis as first manifestation of occult papillary thyroid carcinoma: report of seven cases. Head Neck 1999; 21:370–374.

69. Coleman SC, Smith JC, Burkey BB, Day TA, Page RN, Netterville JL. Long-standing lateral neck mass as the initial manifestation of well-differentiated thyroid carcinoma. Laryngoscope 2000; 110:204–209.

70. Monchik JM, De Petris G, De Crea C. Occult papillary carcinoma of the thyroid presenting as a cervical cyst. Surgery 2001; 129:429–432.

71. Hay ID, Grant CS, van Heerden JA, Goellner JR, Ebersold JR, Bergstralh EJ. Papillary thyroid microcarcinoma: a study of 535 cases observed in a 50-year period. Surgery 1992; 112:1139–1146; discussion 1146–1147.

72. Baudin E, Travagli JP, Ropers J, et al. Microcarcinoma of the thyroid gland: the Gustave-Roussy Institute experience. Cancer 1998; 83:553–559.

73. Appetecchia M, Scarcello G, Pucci E, Procaccini A. Outcome after treatment of papillary thyroid microcarcinoma. J Exp Clin Cancer Res 2002; 21:159–164.

74. Chow SM, Law SC, Chan JK, Au SK, Yau S, Lau WH. Papillary microcarcinoma of the thyroid – prognostic significance of lymph node metastasis and multifocality. Cancer 2003; 98:31–40.

75. Pellegriti G, Scollo C, Lumera G, Regalbuto C, Vigneri R, Belfiore A. Clinical behavior and outcome of papillary thyroid cancers smaller than 1.5 cm in diameter: study of 299 cases. J Clin Endocrinol Metab 2004; 89:3713–3720.

76. Pearce EN, Braverman LE. Papillary thyroid microcarcinoma outcomes and implications for treatment. J Clin Endocrinol Metab 2004; 89:3710–3712.

77. Pelizzo MR, Boschin IM, Toniato A, et al. Natural history, diagnosis, treatment and outcome of papillary thyroid microcarcinoma (PTMC): a mono-institutional 12-year experience. Nucl Med Commun 2004; 25:547–552.

78. Ito Y, Uruno T, Nakano K, et al. An observation trial without surgical treatment in patients with papillary microcarcinoma of the thyroid. Thyroid 2003; 13:381–387.

79. Wada N, Duh QY, Sugino K, et al. Lymph node metastasis from 259 papillary thyroid microcarcinomas: frequency, pattern of occurrence and recurrence, and optimal strategy for neck dissection. Ann Surg 2003; 237:399–407.

Section X

Aggressive Thyroid Cancers

30

Rare Thyroid Cancers

Masud S. Haq and Clive Harmer

While the relatively low mortality rate of thyroid cancer in general is due to the preponderance of well-differentiated carcinoma, a subset of rare thyroid tumors exist that exhibit aggressive behavior and poor prognosis. These require careful consideration and different treatment paradigms to optimize clinical outcome. Extremely rare types of thyroid cancer include thymus-like tumors, mucoepidermoid carcinoma, spindle cell tumor, mixed medullary follicular cancers, and teratoma. In view of the limited literature on their management these extremely rare types are not covered in this chapter.

Thyroid Lymphoma

Primary thyroid non-Hodgkin's lymphoma (NHL) is uncommon, representing 4% of all thyroid cancers [1]. Only 2% of extranodal lymphomas arise within the thyroid. Secondary involvement is more frequent as a manifestation of generalized disease, which occurs in 10% of all lymphomas and leukemias [2]. The mean age at presentation is 60–70 years with a female : male predominance of 3:1. Presentation before age 40 is rare. Preexisting Hashimoto's thyroiditis is a significant risk factor [3] and may be the result of chronic antigen stimulation. Radiation exposure is not associated with an increased risk.

Primary thyroid lymphoma is usually of B-cell type and CD20 positive [4]; T-cell lymphoma is very rare. Approximately 80% of tumors are of the diffuse large-cell type (histiocytic) and the majority of these are high grade. The remainder comprise follicular (nodular), mixed, plasmacytoid, and lymphocytic subtypes. NHL of the thyroid is classified into MALT (mucosa-associated lymphoid tissue) positive and MALT negative characterized by the presence of lymphoepithelial lesions with cytokeratin staining. The frequency of MALT-positive thyroid lymphoma varies between 10% and 80% and is associated with improved prognosis [5]. The REAL (Revised European-American Lymphoma) and WHO (World Health Organization) classifications designate these as extranodal marginal zone B-cell lymphomas of MALT type.

Typical presentation is with a rapidly enlarging thyroid mass; associated compressive symptoms comprise dysphagia, dyspnea, stridor, hoarseness, and superior vena caval obstruction. A preceding history of goiter in association with hypothyroidism is characteristic. The thyroid mass is often fixed to underlying structures, with confluent cervical lymphadenopathy occurring in up to 50% of cases. Only 10% of patients report B symptoms of fever, night sweats, or weight loss.

Lymphoma should enter the differential diagnosis of a solitary thyroid nodule, a dominant nodule in a multinodular goiter, or any patient with rapid enlargement of a goiter associated with Hashimoto's thyroiditis. Diagnosis may be made from fine-needle aspiration cytology

(FNAC) but immunocytochemistry is necessary to demonstrate the type of lymphocyte monoclonality, achieved by core biopsy. Large B-cell lymphoma has to be distinguished from undifferentiated carcinoma and MALT lymphoma from Hashimoto's thyroiditis.

The Ann Arbor classification is used to stage lymphoma. Over 90% of patients with primary lymphoma present with disease confined to the thyroid (stage I$_E$) or limited to the thyroid and regional neck nodes (stage II$_E$). More widespread disease (stages III and IV) makes up the remainder, with affected sites including the gastrointestinal tract, bone marrow, lungs, or liver. Initial staging investigations (Figure 30.1) should therefore comprise a full blood count, serum biochemistry including thyroid function, lactate dehydrogenase and uric acid, CT scan of the neck thorax abdomen plus pelvis, and bone marrow aspirate plus trephine. Lactate dehydrogenase, uric acid, and antithyroid antibody titers (antimicrosomal) are often raised. CT imaging often demonstrates invasion of the trachea, retrosternal extension, or involvement of mediastinal lymph nodes.

As patients are often elderly and require urgent treatment to relieve airway obstruction, full staging may be impracticable until later. Aggressive surgery to debulk the tumor is neither feasible nor necessary [6]. For localized disease, external beam radiotherapy has been the standard practice for several decades, resulting in 5-year survival rates of approximately 35%. Local bulky disease and gross mediastinal involvement are significantly associated with failure distant from the irradiated volume [4]. Chemotherapy for high grade lymphoma has demonstrated better local and distant disease control with overall long-term disease-free survival of about 50%. The combination of radiotherapy preceded by chemotherapy has become standard practice in most institutions, improving 5-year survival rates to 65–90% [7]. Six cycles of cyclophosphamide, doxorubicin, vincristine, and prednisolone (CHOP) given over 4 months is usually recommended. If complete response has been achieved with drugs, external beam radiotherapy should follow with 35 Gy mid-plane dose given in 20 fractions, confined to the initial extent of disease.

Rituximab, an unconjugated anti-CD20 monoclonal antibody, has been designed to recognize cancer-forming B-cell lymphocytes [8]. The drug binds to CD20 receptors on the surface of B cells and initiates a series of reactions that result in cell death. It also appears to sensitize cells to conventional chemotherapy. It has been extensively evaluated and is now an integral component of chemotherapy [9]. The National Institute for Clinical Excellence (NICE) recommends that rituximab should be included (with CHOP) in the treatment of patients with moderate to advanced CD20-positive B-cell NHL stages II, III, and IV. Patients with stage I disease should be given the drug only as part of a clinical trial.

Lymphomas showing MALT characteristics present as localized extranodal tumor with favorable prognostic factors and follow a more indolent course. Radiotherapy as single modality treatment resulted in a complete response rate approaching 100%, a relapse rate of around 30%, a salvage rate of over 50%, and an overall cause-specific survival of almost 90% at 5 and 10 years [5]. Our policy is to treat stage I$_E$A MALT-positive lymphoma with radiotherapy only but to use initial chemotherapy for all other tumors. The radiotherapy volume includes both sides of the neck from the mastoid tips to the carina treated by opposed anterior and undercouched fields to a dose of 40 Gy in 20 fractions over 4 weeks. In addition to infraclavicular lung shielding, the mandible and submandibular salivary glands are protected, although there is no midline lead. Primary Hodgkin's disease of the thyroid is exceedingly rare and should be separated from primary Hodgkin's disease of the mediastinum or neck, involving the thyroid by direct spread. Treatment is similar to extranodal Hodgkin's disease at any other site [10].

Squamous Cell Carcinoma

Primary squamous cell carcinoma is very rare, accounting for less than 1% of thyroid cancers, usually occurring in middle-aged or elderly patients [11]. The clinical behavior has been reported to resemble that of anaplastic carcinoma [12]. Prognosis is poor, with the majority of tumors advanced at presentation. The diagnosis should be made only once metastasis from other sites (such as the lung) and direct local invasion from tumors in adjacent structures (such as trachea or esophagus) are excluded. Squamous carcinoma must also be distin-

Figure 30.1 Royal Marsden Hospital policy for the management of primary thyroid lymphoma. CXR, chest radiograph; MALT, mucosa-associated lymphoid tissue; R-CHOP, rituximab, cyclophosphamide, hydroxydaunomycin (doxorubicin), vincristine (Oncovin), and prednisone; MPD, mid-plane dose, Ann Arbor Classification: Stage I_E, disease in single extralymphatic site; Stage II_E, disease in extralymphatic site with its regional nodes; Stage III, disease in lymph node regions on both sides of the diaphragm affected; Stage IV, widespread disease, including multiple involvement at one or more extranodal (beyond the lymph node) sites, such as the bone marrow.

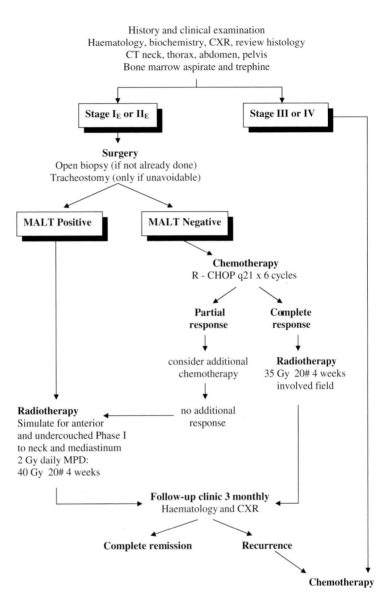

guished from squamous metaplasia seen in papillary carcinoma, which is of no prognostic significance, and areas of squamous differentiation seen in anaplastic tumors [13]. Etiology remains uncertain but it may arise from embryological remnants such as the thyroglossal tract or from areas of squamous metaplasia within the gland. Alternatively it may develop directly from undifferentiated follicular cells, which differentiate into squamous cells during neoplastic transformation. Histological diagnosis requires identification of keratin or intercellular bridge structures. Immunohistochemistry is helpful, with negative staining for thyroglobulin and calcitonin.

Squamous cell carcinoma of the thyroid follows an aggressive clinical course [13]. We have reported 16 patients of whom 12 had locoregional disease only at presentation and 4 had distant metastases [14]. Eight underwent surgery (5 complete and 3 incomplete resection) with 4 given postoperative radiotherapy. Radiotherapy alone was used in 6 patients unsuitable for surgery. Median survival was only 16 months, although there were 3 long-term survivors treated with complete resection followed by radiotherapy. Patients treated with surgery alone all developed local recurrence. Sarda et al. reported 8 patients, none of whom were amenable to radical surgery [15]; none displayed any significant response to either radiotherapy or chemotherapy. Similarly, Shimaoka et al. described 5 patients who failed to respond to chemotherapy or radiotherapy and all died of local disease [13].

Simpson and Carruthers suggested that early complete macroscopic excision followed by external beam radiotherapy can offer the best chance of cure and local control, having described two patients displaying long-term survival [16]. Our series supports this recommendation, with three patients treated in this fashion remaining disease-free, in contrast to two who underwent complete macroscopic resection without irradiation developing local recurrence.

We recommend radiotherapy after total thyroidectomy to a dose of at least 60 Gy in 30 fractions over 6 weeks [17]. The initial target volume should include potential areas of lymph node spread up to a dose of 46 Gy (spinal cord tolerance) with a further 14 Gy using 3D conformal planning. Our data support reports that radiotherapy alone or following incomplete resection results in poor local control. In seven patients treated with radiotherapy following biopsy alone, the median survival was only 6 months. However, high dose palliative irradiation for inoperable tumors may be beneficial. Consistent with other reports, chemotherapy is of little value and radioiodine is without benefit as these tumors are non-iodine avid.

Sarcoma

Primary sarcomas of the thyroid gland are extremely rare. They have mesenchymal (stromal) features and can resemble undifferentiated tumors, rendering differentiation from anaplastic carcinoma difficult. Previous case reports have described sarcomas when in fact these tumors were spindle cell variants of anaplastic carcinoma. This is of little practical significance, as the natural history and response to treatment remain similar. Most malignant thyroid tumors with a sarcoma-like appearance show signs of epithelial differentiation by morphological or immunohistochemical criteria and are therefore classified as undifferentiated tumors. The WHO committee states that diagnosis of thyroid sarcoma should be made only in tumors lacking all evidence of epithelial differentiation and showing definite evidence of specific sarcomatous differentiation [18,19]. Various subtypes have been described including liposarcoma, fibrosarcoma, angiosarcoma, osteosarcoma, chondrosarcoma, and leiomyosarcoma [20–23]. Sarcomas may rarely metastasize to the thyroid gland; primary sites other than the thyroid should first be excluded.

Angiosarcoma and hemangioendothelioma are very rare, affecting middle-aged or elderly patients [24]. These tumors are extremely aggressive, resembling the behavior of anaplastic cancer. Tumors are typically large with extensive areas of hemorrhage and necrosis (Figure 30.2) [25,26]. Microscopically, endothelial differentiation together with immunoreac-

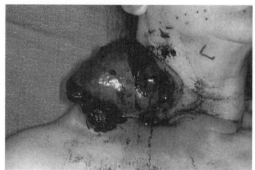

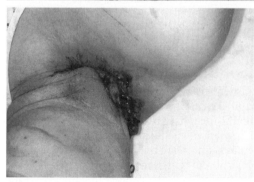

Figure 30.2 A Epithelioid angiosarcoma of thyroid. Massive recurrence in the right supraclavicular fossa extending into the superior mediastinum following total thyroidectomy. **B** Inoperable tumor threatened exsanguination despite chemotherapy but rapid shrinkage followed EBRT.

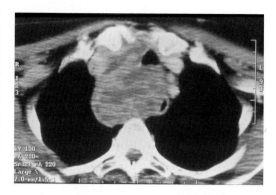

Figure 30.3 Thyroid liposarcoma: a large mixed attenuation retrosternal mass compressing the trachea and almost obliterating the lumen of the esophagus.

tivity to factor VIII-related antigen and keratin are common [27]. Cases have been described from the Alpine regions of Central Europe where iodine deficiency is common. An enlarging mass following a long history of goiter, with invasion of local structures and lymph node involvement (unusual with other sarcoma subtypes) is the typical presentation. Hemothorax from pleuropulmonary metastases may occur at presentation [24]. Prognosis is poor, with the majority dying of locoregional or metastatic disease. As with sarcoma at any site, surgery remains the definitive and potentially curative treatment comprising total thyroidectomy with excision of any locally involved tissue, along with neck dissection. This may be impossible in the majority of cases if tumor extends beyond the thyroid capsule and invades vital structures. Postoperative radiotherapy is indicated but the role of chemotherapy is yet to be established.

All other sarcomas are extremely rare, with only a limited number of reports in the literature [20,22,28–35]. We have reported two patients with liposarcoma (Figure 30.3) treated by macroscopic resection and external beam radiotherapy that achieved locoregional control; although one died of pulmonary metastases after 10 months the second remains alive with metastatic disease at 24 months.

Survival in sarcomas of the head and neck is shorter than that of limb sarcomas and local recurrence is more frequent. A series of 130 head and neck sarcomas treated at the Royal Marsden Hospital showed an overall 5-year survival of only 50%. Results with surgery alone

were poor, as were those with radiotherapy as sole treatment. However, surgery with radiotherapy improved survival. Radiotherapy is recommended pre- or postoperatively as curative management [36].

Metastases to the Thyroid

The majority of metastases to the thyroid remain undetectable in clinical practice [37]. However, incidence in postmortem studies varies between 1.2% and 24% in patients with widespread malignancy [2,38,39]. Based on these figures, thyroid metastases are 10 times more frequent than primary thyroid tumors [40]. This is not surprising given that the thyroid has a rich blood supply, second only to the adrenals. Involvement may arise by direct spread from adjacent structures, hematogenous spread, or retrograde lymphatic spread. Postmortem studies report breast (26%), lung (25%), and malignant melanoma (11%) to be the most frequent cancers to metastasize to the thyroid, with disease usually remaining clinically occult. In contrast, the largest clinical series [41] found that the kidney was the most common primary site (33%) followed by lung (16%), breast (16%), and esophagus (9%).

Metastasis may be the first presentation of a distant cancer treated several years previously; typically there is a long latent period between diagnosis of the primary tumor and the appearance of a thyroid mass, especially with breast and renal cell carcinoma [40,42]. Long-term survival is possible after total thyroidectomy for metastases from hypernephroma [43]. In contrast, appearance of metastatic disease may indicate a poor prognosis, with secondaries from lung, esophagus, and melanoma representing preterminal events.

A thyroid nodule detected in a patient with a previous history of malignancy poses a diagnostic challenge [41]. Differential diagnosis includes a benign thyroid nodule, multinodular goiter, and metastasis. Fine-needle aspiration cytology (FNAC) can provide accurate diagnosis and proves invaluable in patients with a poor prognosis unsuitable for thyroidectomy. Immunohistochemistry with demonstration of negative staining to antithyroglobulin and anticalcitonin antibodies favors metastatic involvement. Occasionally FNAC cannot determine whether tumor originates from the thyroid gland or not and open biopsy is required. Clear cell changes have been described in benign and malignant tumors of the thyroid, making the diagnosis of metastasis from renal cell carcinoma dependent on immunohistochemistry for thyroid transcription factor-1 (TTF1) and thyroglobulin. Diagnostic reevaluation of the primary site and restaging investigations may prove helpful, together with comparison of new cytology or histology with the original.

Previous reports have suggested thyroid metastasis to be associated with a poor prognosis [43]. However, surgical resection for an isolated metastasis can be curative. Overall management depends on the primary site of the original tumor, symptoms caused by the thyroid mass and involvement of other organs. Surgical excision may prolong survival provided that extensive disease is not present elsewhere. Irradiation of unresectable metastases may provide valuable palliation of symptoms but radioiodine is unhelpful.

In our report of 15 patients [44] the most common site of origin was the kidney (27%). The longest latent period between presentations of primary tumor to diagnosis of thyroid metastasis was 15 years. Eleven patients presented with a thyroid mass (74%), two complained of dysphagia (13%), and two were diagnosed incidentally (13%). Nine had evidence of metastatic disease elsewhere (60%). Five patients have survived longer than 24 months and one patient with metastatic paraganglioma remains disease free 84 months following lobectomy.

Insular Carcinoma

Insular carcinoma is a form of poorly differentiated tumor arising from follicular cells, with behavior intermediate between differentiated (papillary/follicular) and undifferentiated (anaplastic) carcinoma [18]. They usually retain some features of differentiated follicular thyroid cells with ability to produce thyroglobulin and retain radioiodine but display a more aggressive clinical behavior [45,46].

Macroscopic features are of an invasive solid tumor typically greater than 5 cm in diameter exhibiting areas of necrosis. Microscopically tumor is characterized by well-defined nests (insulae) of small uniform cells displaying

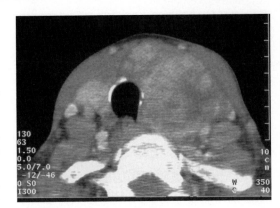

Figure 30.4 Inoperable insular thyroid carcinoma: CT scan demonstrating a large heterogeneous mass centered on the left lobe of thyroid with marked displacement and narrowing of the trachea. The tumor rapidly progressed and proved fatal despite palliative radiotherapy.

an infiltrative pattern of growth and vascular invasion.

Insular carcinoma is infrequent comprising 2–4% of all thyroid cancers. Patients are usually middle-aged or elderly, often with a preceding history of goiter. The usual presentation is an enlarging mass (Figure 30.4), although distant metastases at presentation are not uncommon. They have an aggressive behavior with a high recurrence rate of 20–60% and a 10-year cause-specific mortality of 13–41% [47,48]. Tumors with only an insular component do not appear to have such an adverse prognosis, a discrepancy relevant to treatment and outcome [48,49].

Due to its rarity, reports include only small numbers of patients. As many insular carcinomas occur in the elderly who frequently have large tumors it was previously uncertain whether their aggressive behavior was related to these variables rather than the actual histotype. Pellegriti et al. compared patients of similar age and tumor size of which 13 were insular, 18 follicular, and 26 papillary [50]. Those with insular carcinoma had the worst outcome with a cause-specific mortality rate of 62% compared with 17% and 15% in the follicular and papillary groups, respectively. Distant metastasis occurred in 85% of insular tumors compared with 50% and 19% of patients with follicular and papillary subtypes. All patients with metastases from insular carcinoma displayed radioiodine avidity but clinical benefit was seen in only one. Multivariate analysis revealed insular histotype as being the only variable related independently to cause-specific mortality.

Insular carcinoma demands initial aggressive treatment including total thyroidectomy, lymph node dissection, and radioiodine ablation. External beam radiotherapy may be required in addition and can also provide palliation of symptoms from unresectable disease. Radioiodine is recommended for treatment of distant metastases but may prove of limited value. Chemotherapy has no proven role.

Hürthle Cell Carcinoma

Hürthle cell carcinoma (HCC) is rare, comprising 3–5% of all differentiated thyroid tumors. Also known as oncocytic or oxyphilic tumors, they have previously been considered a variant of follicular thyroid cancer [51], although are now known to represent a distinct pathological entity [52].

Hürthle cells are rich in mitochondria and have a characteristic granular cytoplasm. They may occur in a variety of thyroid conditions including benign nodules, Hashimoto's thyroiditis, and Hürthle cell neoplasms. A true Hürthle cell neoplasm must consist of at least 75% Hürthle cells. The majority are benign Hürthle cell adenomas with only a minority being malignant. Fine-needle aspiration cytology fails to distinguish between them and surgical excision is mandatory for identification of capsular or vascular invasion indicative of HCC.

HCC has a more aggressive natural history than follicular carcinoma, with a higher rate of recurrence, distant metastasis, and mortality [53]. Stojadinovic et al. [54] reported a series of 56 HCCs with degree of invasion, tumor size greater than 4 cm, extrathyroidal extension, and initial nodal or distant metastasis all predictive of cause-specific mortality. No patient with minimally invasive HCC developed recurrence or died of disease. Recurrence and death were confined to patients with widely invasive carcinoma. Patients are usually female and older than 50 at presentation. They often have large multifocal tumors, lymph node metastases, and evidence of extrathyroidal extension. Tumors are poorly iodine avid, which in part explains their worse outcome.

For these reasons an aggressive initial approach comprising total thyroidectomy with selective neck dissection in the presence of pathological lymph nodes is recommended, although lobectomy alone may be adequate for low risk patients [54]. ^{131}I ablation may confer a survival benefit and is recommended if only to assist long-term follow-up with serum thyroglobulin (Tg) measurement. Tumors retain the ability to produce Tg and early warning of recurrence may enable potentially curative surgery. In the recently published series of 89 patients with HCC from the M.D. Anderson Cancer Center [55], those undergoing ablation had an improved outcome. Of the 37 patients with known metastases, only 38% showed radioiodine uptake in lymph nodes, bone, or lung.

Life-long follow-up in conjunction with appropriate thyroid-stimulating hormone (TSH) suppression is recommended. Further surgery remains the treatment of choice for recurrence but external beam radiotherapy (EBRT) offers locoregional control for inoperable disease and useful palliation of painful bone metastases. Foote et al. [56] reported on 16 HCC patients who received EBRT. Adjuvant irradiation was successful in preventing recurrence in 4 of 5 patients, 2 of whom had positive surgical margins. Salvage EBRT was successful in 3 of 5 patients, and palliative radiotherapy provided sustained symptomatic relief at 67% of irradiated sites in 6 patients.

Our unpublished series of 62 patients had a median age at diagnosis of 59 years and median follow-up of 5 years; a neck mass was the commonest mode of presentation (85%). Tumors were larger than 4 cm in 31%, displayed extrathyroidal extension in 20%, and distant metastasis at presentation in 15%. Overall survival at 10 and 20 years was 64% and 37%, respectively. Multivariate analysis identified nodal disease, distant metastasis, and tumor size to be associated with an increased cause-specific mortality ($P < 0.01$). Extent of surgery improved cause-specific survival, whereas radioactive ablation had no effect on survival but EBRT achieved symptomatic benefit in 11 of 14 distant metastases. None of 17 metastatic sites concentrated ^{131}I.

Metastatic HCCs often express somatostatin receptors that can be visualized with ^{111}In (indium) octreotide diagnostic imaging. Subsequent treatment with [90]Y (yttrium)-labeled DOTATOC (DOTA[0], Tyr[3]) may be beneficial. Our series of 18 patients with non-iodine-avid differentiated thyroid cancer included one patient with HCC extensively metastatic to bone [57]; prolonged symptomatic benefit together with limitation of further progression of disease was achieved following four ^{90}Y-DOTATOC therapies. Unfortunately, chemotherapy is of limited benefit in HCC and should be restricted to progressive symptomatic disease.

Diffuse Sclerosing Variant

The diffuse sclerosing variant of papillary cancer (DSPC) is rare, with an incidence of only 0.7–5.3% [58,59]. It commonly affects young adults, with a female preponderance, and is important in the differential diagnosis of Hashimoto's thyroiditis. Histologically it is characterized by diffuse involvement of one or both lobes, fibrosis, squamous metaplasia, numerous psammoma bodies, and extensive lymphatic infiltration.

A number of studies suggest DSPC to have an aggressive nature [58,60] but others [59] suggest a similar prognosis to classical papillary thyroid cancer (PTC). Chow et al. reported a series of 8 cases (6 female, 2 male) amongst 1086 PTCs with a mean follow-up of 8 years [59]. Patients displayed a younger age at presentation (mean 27 versus 45 years), larger tumor size (mean 6.9 versus 2.4 cm), higher incidence of lymph node metastasis (100% versus 32%), and more frequent antithyroglobulin antibodies (75% versus 11%). All underwent total thyroidectomy and ^{131}I ablation. One patient with distant metastasis at presentation was treated with additional radioiodine therapy. Two others received postoperative adjuvant external beam radiotherapy (EBRT). One patient developed locoregional recurrence, which was treated with salvage surgery and EBRT. At the time of last follow-up, all eight were alive and free of disease.

Although DSPC is associated with more advanced locoregional disease and a high rate of distant metastasis, prognosis remains comparable to classical PTC. An aggressive initial approach comprising total thyroidectomy, selective neck dissection, and radioiodine ablation results in a favorable outcome.

References

1. Souhami L, Simpson WJ, Carruthers JS. Malignant lymphoma of the thyroid gland. Int J Radiat Oncol Biol Phys 1980; 6(9):1143–1147.
2. Shimaoka K, Sokal JE, Pickren JW. Metastatic neoplasms in the thyroid gland. Pathological and clinical findings. Cancer 1962; 15:557–565.
3. Hyjek E, Isaacson PG. Primary B cell lymphoma of the thyroid and its relationship to Hashimoto's thyroiditis. Hum Pathol 1988; 19(11):1315–1326.
4. Tupchong L, Hughes F, Harmer CL. Primary lymphoma of the thyroid: clinical features, prognostic factors, and results of treatment. Int J Radiat Oncol Biol Phys 1986; 12(10):1813–1821.
5. Laing RW, Hoskin P, Hudson BV, et al. The significance of MALT histology in thyroid lymphoma: a review of patients from the BNLI and Royal Marsden Hospital. Clin Oncol (R Coll Radiol) 1994; 6(5):300–304.
6. Harrington KJ, Michalaki VJ, Vini L, et al. Management of non-Hodgkin's lymphoma of the thyroid: the Royal Marsden experience. Br J Radial 2005; 78:405–410.
7. Matsuzuka F, Miyauchi A, Katayama S, et al. Clinical aspects of primary thyroid lymphoma: diagnosis and treatment based on our experience of 119 cases. Thyroid 1993; 3(2):93–99.
8. Seymour JF. New treatment approaches to indolent non-Hodgkin's lymphoma. Semin Oncol 2004; 31(1 Suppl 2):27–32.
9. McLaughlin P, Grillo-Lopez AJ, Link BK, et al. Rituximab chimeric anti-CD20 monoclonal antibody therapy for relapsed indolent lymphoma: half of patients respond to a four-dose treatment program. J Clin Oncol 1998; 16(8):2825–2833.
10. Vini L, Harmer C. Thyroid. In: Price P, Sikora K (eds) Treatment of cancer. London: Arnold, 2002: 401–427.
11. Goldman R. Primary squamous cell carcinoma of the thyroid gland: report of a case and review of the literature. Am Surg 1964; 30:247–252.
12. Segal K, Sidi J, Abraham A, Konichezky M, Ben Bassat M. Pure squamous cell carcinoma and mixed adenosquamous cell carcinoma of the thyroid gland. Head Neck Surg 1984; 6(6):1035–1042.
13. Shimaoka K, Tsukada Y. Squamous cell carcinomas and adenosquamous carcinomas originating from the thyroid gland. Cancer 1980; 46(8):1833–1842.
14. Cook AM, Vini L, Harmer C. Squamous cell carcinoma of the thyroid: outcome of treatment in 16 patients. Eur J Surg Oncol 1999; 25(6):606–609.
15. Sarda AK, Bal S, Arunabh, Singh MK, Kapur MM. Squamous cell carcinoma of the thyroid. J Surg Oncol 1988; 39(3):175–178.
16. Simpson WJ, Carruthers J. Squamous cell carcinoma of the thyroid gland. Am J Surg 1988; 156(1):44–46.
17. Harmer C, Bidmead M, Shepherd S, Sharpe A, Vini L. Radiotherapy planning techniques for thyroid cancer. Br J Radiol 1998; 71(850):1069–1075.
18. Hedinger C, Williams E, Sobin L. World Health Organization histological typing of thyroid tumours. Berlin: Springer-Verlag, 1988: 9–11.
19. Sobin LH, Fleming ID. TNM Classification of Malignant Tumors, fifth edition (1997). Union Internationale

Contre le Cancer and the American Joint Committee on Cancer. Cancer 1997; 80(9):1803–1804.

20. Mitra A, Fisher C, Rhys-Evans P, Harmer C. Liposarcoma of the thyroid. Sarcoma. 2004; 8(2):91–96.

21. Sniezek JC, Holtel M. Rare tumors of the thyroid gland. Otolaryngol Clin North Am 2003; 36(1):107–115.

22. Tsugawa K, Koyanagi N, Nakanishi K, et al. Leiomyosarcoma of the thyroid gland with rapid growth and tracheal obstruction: A partial thyroidectomy and tracheostomy using an ultrasonically activated scalpel can be safely performed with less bleeding. Eur J Med Res 1999; 4(11):483–487.

23. Uygur K, Tuz M, Dogru H, Sari A. Chondrosarcoma of the thyroid cartilage. J Laryngol Otol 2001; 115(6):507–509.

24. Egloff B. The haemangioendothelioma. In: Hedinger C (ed.) Thyroid cancer. Berlin: Springer-Verlag, 1969:52–59.

25. Chan YF, Ma L, Boey JH, Yeung HY. Angiosarcoma of the thyroid. An immunohistochemical and ultrastructural study of a case in a Chinese patient. Cancer 1986; 57(12):2381–2388.

26. Eusebi V, Carcangiu ML, Dina R, Rosai J. Keratin-positive epithelioid angiosarcoma of thyroid. A report of four cases. Am J Surg Pathol 1990; 14(8):737–747.

27. Tanda F, Massarelli G, Bosincu L, Cossu A. Angiosarcoma of the thyroid: a light, electron microscopic and histoimmunological study. Hum Pathol 1988; 19(6):742–745.

28. Andrion A, Gaglio A, Dogliani N, Bosco E, Mazzucco G. Liposarcoma of the thyroid gland. Fine-needle aspiration cytology, immunohistology, and ultrastructure. Am J Clin Pathol 1991; 95(5):675–679.

29. Awad WI, Rhys Evans PH, Nicholson AG, Goldstraw P. Liposarcoma of the thyroid gland mimicking retrosternal goiter. Ann Thorac Surg 2003; 75(2):566–568.

30. Chetty R, Clark SP, Dowling JP. Leiomyosarcoma of the thyroid: immunohistochemical and ultrastructural study. Pathology 1993; 25(2):203–205.

31. Iida Y, Katoh R, Yoshioka M, Oyama T, Kawaoi A. Primary leiomyosarcoma of the thyroid gland. Acta Pathol Jpn 1993; 43(1–2):71–75.

32. Kawahara E, Nakanishi I, Terahata S, Ikegaki S. Leiomyosarcoma of the thyroid gland. A case report with a comparative study of five cases of anaplastic carcinoma. Cancer 1988; 62(12):2558–2563.

33. Ozaki O, Sugino K, Mimura T, Ito K, Tamai S, Hosoda Y. Primary leiomyosarcoma of the thyroid gland. Surg Today 1997; 27(2):177–180.

34. Takayama F, Takashima S, Matsuba H, Kobayashi S, Ito N, Sone S. MR imaging of primary leiomyosarcoma of the thyroid gland. Eur J Radiol 2001; 37(1):36–41.

35. Thompson LD, Wenig BM, Adair CF, Shmookler BM, Heffess CS. Primary smooth muscle tumors of the thyroid gland. Cancer 1997; 79(3):579–587.

36. Eeles RA, Fisher C, A'Hern RP, et al. Head and neck sarcomas: prognostic factors and implications for treatment. Br J Cancer 1993; 68(1):201–207.

37. Ivy HK. Cancer metastatic to the thyroid: a diagnostic problem. Mayo Clin Proc 1984; 59(12):856–859.

38. Berge T, Lundberg S. Cancer in Malmo 1958–1969. An autopsy study. Acta Pathol Microbiol Scand Suppl 1977; (260):1–235.

39. Silverberg SG, Vidone RA. Carcinoma of the thyroid in surgical and postmortem material. Analysis of 300 cases at autopsy and literature review. Ann Surg 1966; 164(2):291–299.

40. Haugen BR, Nawaz S, Cohn A, et al. Secondary malignancy of the thyroid gland: a case report and review of the literature. Thyroid 1994; 4(3):297–300.

41. Nakhjavani MK, Gharib H, Goellner JR, van Heerden JA. Metastasis to the thyroid gland. A report of 43 cases. Cancer 1997; 79(3):574–578.

42. Green LK, Ro JY, Mackay B, Ayala AG, Luna MA. Renal cell carcinoma metastatic to the thyroid. Cancer 1989; 63(9):1810–1815.

43. Chen H, Nicol TL, Udelsman R. Clinically significant, isolated metastatic disease to the thyroid gland. World J Surg 1999; 23(2):177–180.

44. Wood K, Vini L, Harmer C. Metastases to the thyroid gland: the Royal Marsden experience. Eur J Surg Oncol 2004; 30(6):583–588.

45. Flynn SD, Forman BH, Stewart AF, Kinder BK. Poorly differentiated ("insular") carcinoma of the thyroid gland: an aggressive subset of differentiated thyroid neoplasms. Surgery 1988; 104(6):963–970.

46. Papotti M, Botto MF, Favero A, Palestini N, Bussolati G. Poorly differentiated thyroid carcinomas with primordial cell component. A group of aggressive lesions sharing insular, trabecular, and solid patterns. Am J Surg Pathol 1993; 17(3):291–301.

47. Albareda M, Puig-Domingo M, Wengrowicz S, et al. Clinical forms of presentation and evolution of diffuse sclerosing variant of papillary carcinoma and insular variant of follicular carcinoma of the thyroid. Thyroid 1998; 8(5):385–391.

48. Carcangiu ML, Zampi G, Rosai J. Poorly differentiated ("insular") thyroid carcinoma. A reinterpretation of Langhans' "wucherndе Struma". Am J Surg Pathol 1984; 8(9):655–668.

49. Ashfaq R, Vuitch F, Delgado R, Albores-Saavedra J. Papillary and follicular thyroid carcinomas with an insular component. Cancer 1994; 73(2):416–423.

50. Pellegriti G, Giuffrida D, Scollo C, et al. Long-term outcome of patients with insular carcinoma of the thyroid: the insular histotype is an independent predictor of poor prognosis. Cancer 2002; 95(10):2076–2085.

51. Shaha AR, Loree TR, Shah JP. Prognostic factors and risk group analysis in follicular carcinoma of the thyroid. Surgery 1995; 118(6):1131–1136.

52. Masood S, Auguste LJ, Westerband A, Belluco C, Valderama E, Attie J. Differential oncogenic expression in thyroid follicular and Hurthle cell carcinomas. Am J Surg 1993; 166(4):366–368.

53. Watson RG, Brennan MD, Goellner JR, van Heerden JA, McConahey WM, Taylor WF. Invasive Hurthle cell carcinoma of the thyroid: natural history and management. Mayo Clin Proc 1984; 59(12):851–855.

54. Stojadinovic A, Hoos A, Ghossein RA, Urist MJ, et al. Hurthle cell carcinoma: a 60-year experience. Ann Surg Oncol 2002; 9(2):197–203.

55. Lopez-Penabad L, Chiu AC, Hoff AO, et al. Prognostic factors in patients with Hurthle cell neoplasms of the thyroid. Cancer 2003; 97(5):1186–1194.

56. Foote RL, Brown PD, Garces YI, McIver B, Kasperbauer JL. Is there a role for radiation therapy in the management of Hurthle cell carcinoma? Int J Radiat Oncol Biol Phys 2003; 56(4):1067–1072.

57. Christian JA, Cook GJ, Harmer C. Indium-111-labelled octreotide scintigraphy in the diagnosis and management of non-iodine avid metastatic carcinoma of the thyroid. Br J Cancer 2003; 89(2):258–261.

58. Carcangiu ML, Bianchi S. Diffuse sclerosing variant of papillary thyroid carcinoma. Clinicopathologic study of 15 cases. Am J Surg Pathol 1989; 13(12):1041–1049.

59. Chow SM, Chan JK, Law SC, et al. Diffuse sclerosing variant of papillary thyroid carcinoma – clinical features and outcome. Eur J Surg Oncol 2003; 29(5):446–449.

60. Soares J, Limbert E, Sobrinho-Simoes M. Diffuse sclerosing variant of papillary thyroid carcinoma. A clinicopathologic study of 10 cases. Pathol Res Pract 1989; 185(2):200–206.

31

Management of Anaplastic Thyroid Cancer

Jan Tennvall, Göran Lundell, and Göran Wallin

Introduction

Anaplastic (giant cell) thyroid carcinomas (ATC), in sharp contrast to differentiated thyroid carcinomas, confer a dismal prognosis with a median survival time after diagnosis of 3–6 months [1–3]. It is both a locally and systematically aggressive disease, with a better prognosis seen only in the few cases with a small tumor confined to the thyroid [2,4].

ATC is uncommon, accounting for less than 5% of all thyroid carcinomas [5,6]. Current epidemiological studies indicate that ATC has decreased over time [2] and this might be partly related to iodine prophylaxis and a decrease in endemic goiter, and also to more aggressive treatment of long-standing goiter [7].

Most patients suffering from ATC have until recently died due to uncontrolled local tumor invasion and mainly by suffocation [4,8]. ATC is a disease of the aged and the majority of patients are older than 60 years [2,9–11]. The treatment must consequently be influenced by conditions associated with high age. On the other hand, although patients with ATC can rarely be cured, every effort should be made to control the primary tumor and thereby improve the quality of remaining life.

At diagnosis, almost all patients have a rapidly enlarging thyroid mass. This mass is usually the main reason for seeking urgent medical consul-tation. Other symptoms at diagnosis, usually related to the local tumor growth, are dyspnea, dysphagia, local pain, and hoarseness. The duration of symptoms prior to diagnosis is usually very short. The tumor mostly extends into the surrounding tissues. Even if pulmonary metastases are observed as early as at diagnosis, the local growth is nonetheless mostly the dominating problem for these patients.

Surgical biopsy delays the initiation of therapy in patients with ATC due to poor healing of the surgical scar and in some cases even enhances tumor growth [12–14]. Furthermore, an open biopsy from only one part of an enlarged thyroid may be nondiagnostic if there is a coexisting nodular goiter or well-differentiated carcinoma. The diagnosis can instead be established by means of multiple fine-needle aspiration biopsies [15,16], which are neither harmful nor troublesome for the patient. The cytological diagnosis of this high grade malignant tumor is usually not difficult for a certified cytologist [15,16]. This technique leads to a rapid diagnosis, and treatment can usually start in our clinics the same or next day. In a few patients with unclear diagnosis, additional immunohistochemistry should be performed. It is especially important to rule out primary lymphomas of the thyroid (previously often diagnosed as small cell anaplastic carcinomas of the thyroid), which have a much better prognosis [17].

Local Tumor Control

Primary surgery of ATC is an uncertain and controversial issue due to the grossly invasive disease and poor prognosis. It might be justifiable in a few cases if cervical and mediastinal disease can be resected with reasonable morbidity, particularly to avoid upper airway obstruction [18]. Radical dissection of the tumor is difficult to achieve in these cases. In one series of 43 patients with distant metastases, it was stated that only one had virtually the entire tumor removed at the primary thyroidectomy [19]. Prophylactic tracheotomy should be avoided as it might enhance local tumor growth and delay scar healing [14].

In 32 ATC patients treated with tracheotomies (of which 45% were prophylactic against later respiratory complications), survival was significantly lower (2 months compared with 5 months) than for 45 patients who did not receive tracheotomies. Many of the patients had local wound complications that led to delays in postoperative radiation therapy [20].

Foci of ATC can sometimes be found in patients operated on for a differentiated thyroid carcinoma or a goiter. These patients have a better prognosis. They are sometimes included in retrospective analyses, which falsely improves the prognosis.

Primary radiotherapy alone of ATC has not been very successful as these large tumors are relatively resistant compared with other solid malignant tumors. Local control of the primary lesion (the neck and the upper mediastinum) is almost never accomplished with radiation doses of 60–65 Gy conventionally fractionated [8]. Hyperfractionated radiotherapy can reduce the early reaction in normal tissues [21,22]. As ACT is a rapidly growing tumor, it might be important to decrease the "overall treatment time" by accelerating the fractionation of the radiotherapy regimen, thereby reducing the opportunity for tumor cells to repopulate during the course of treatment [22].

Multimodal Therapy Regimens

Surgery, radiation therapy, or chemotherapy used alone is seldom adequate to control the disease [1,23], though a combination of these modalities might at least improve local control [23,24]. The rationale for combining radiotherapy and chemotherapy is that, as the toxicity of these modalities is not entirely overlapping, an enhanced tumoricidal effect might be obtained [25].

Regimens Employed

The first successful report of local control of ATC by radiotherapy and concomitant chemotherapy (5-fluorouracil and cyclophosphamide) was in 1973 by Wallgren and Norin [26]. A combination of dactinomycin and radiotherapy was in 1974 reported as successful in a small series [27]. However, when this material was enlarged [1] and more advanced cases were included, no obvious beneficial effects were observed with this additional chemotherapy. Simpson [28] reported complete local tumor regression in 6 out of 14 patients who had received hyperfractionated radiotherapy (1 Gy ×2) to a total dose of 36 Gy in combination with different cytostatic regimens (usually doxorubicin). More promising results were reported a few years later by Kim and Leeper [29], who used doxorubicin (1.6 Gy twice daily 3 days a week up to 57.6 Gy). Out of nine patients, eight had complete remissions. In 1987 Kim and Leeper [30] reported that 19 patients had received the same treatment and that 84% had a complete remission. However, these patients were younger than expected for having ATC (median age 60 years), the tumors were rather small, and none had disseminated disease at the start of therapy.

Our own experience dates back to the early 1970s. Since then, different treatment regimens have been used at Radiumhemmet, Stockholm and the Department of Oncology, University Hospital, Lund (Table 31.1). Since 1980 the same regimens have been used at both cancer centers and the patient materials have been pooled before assessment of the regimen employed. Almost all patients with ATC diagnosed in Stockholm and southern Sweden are referred and admitted to these two cancer centers. Thus, there is no obvious selection-bias in our patient materials.

At first, single-drug chemotherapy was used at Radiumhemmet in combination with concomitant radiotherapy (Table 31.1). Out of eight patients treated with methotrexate and radiotherapy (2 Gy, one fraction per day up to 30–40 Gy), seven showed a transient but objective

Table 31.1 Various regimens used for treatment of anaplastic thyroid carcinoma (since 1980 the patient materials from Lund and Stockholm have been pooled)

Stockholm: Period	Lund: Period	No. of patients	Regimen
1971–1973	–	8	RT + methotrexate [12]
1973–1975	1973–1975	9; 8	RT + BCF[a] [12; 31]
–	1975–1979	5	RT + BCF[a] + surgery[b] [32]
1975–1983	1980–1983	25	HRT + BCF + surgery[b] [33]
1984–1988 (A)	1984–1988	16	HRT + doxorubicin + surgery[b] [11]
1988–1993 (B)	1988–1993	17	HART (1.3 Gy × 2/d) + doxorubicin + surgery [11]
1994–1999 (C)	1994–1999	22	HART preoperatively only (1.6 Gy × 2/d) + doxorubicin + surgery [36]

[a] Bleomycin was not used in Lund during 1973–1979.
[b] Surgery if feasible.
RT, radiotherapy; HRT, hyperfractionated RT; HART, hyperfractionated accelerated RT; BCF, bleomycin +Sendoxan+ 5-FU.
Reference numbers are given in square brackets.

remission. As this combination carried severe side effects in all the patients, methotrexate was replaced by BCF (bleomycin, 5 mg/day, cyclophosphamide 200 mg/day, 5-fluorouracil, 500 mg every second day). This combination was less toxic. Seven of nine patients had a complete or partial remission. Of these nine patients, one was operated on after the combination treatment was terminated. This patient was still alive 20 years later.

The same regimen but without the bleomycin (CF – the regimen proposed by Wallgren and Norin) was used in Lund between 1973 and 1975 (Table 31.1). This regimen was adopted in eight patients [31] and arrested the local growth in six, but finally all patients except one died due to local failure. By adding debulking surgery to this regimen [32], four out of five patients achieved local control and died as a result of disseminated disease. Debulking surgery can consequently remove the large necrotic tumor mass, which may enhance the efficacy of the other treatment modalities [24,32].

In a study from our institutions, presented by Werner et al. [33] and reviewed by Ekman et al. [13], BCF was given pre- and postoperatively, and the radiotherapy was changed into two fractions per day. After the first course of radiotherapy (30 Gy) resectable parts of the tumor were removed as a debulking procedure. However, if surgery was considered not possible, the second course of radiotherapy was resumed within 3 weeks. The radiotherapy was preoperatively administered to a target dose of 30 Gy in 3 weeks and postoperatively an additional 16 Gy in 1.5 weeks, resulting in a total target dose of 46 Gy. It

was administered twice daily, with a target dose of 1 Gy per fraction with a minimum interval of 6 hours. The radiation target volume included the cervical nodes and the upper mediastinum. Only 36% (9/25 patients) died due to local failure. Three patients were cured, after a follow-up of 6 years without any recurrence. Several of these patients, however, suffered from severe related toxicity (epithelitis or mucosa ulcerations in the mouth and throat), which caused treatment interruptions.

Because ATC usually affects people of advanced age, a compromise between efficacy and toxicity must be accepted. An aggressive cytostatic regimen within a multimodal approach is probably infeasible [24]. The most effective and widely used single cytostatic agent against thyroid carcinomas is doxorubicin [13]. The combination of doxorubicin and radiation in mammalian tumor cells is synergistic, when a low dose of this cytostatic agent (<0.15 mg/kg) is used [34]. The mechanism responsible for the radiosensitizing effect of doxorubicin is still the subject of speculation [35]. The treatment recommended by Kim and Leeper in 1983 [29] was therefore used, replacing the BCF regimen with Adriamycin, administered once weekly 1–2 hours before the first radiotherapy session.

Between 1984 and 1999, we have prospectively treated 55 consecutive patients with ATC (Table 31.2) according to a combined regimen consisting of hyperfractionated radiotherapy, doxorubicin, and, when feasible, surgery [36].

Radiotherapy was carried out for 5 days a week. The daily fraction until 1988 was 1.0 Gy ×2 (protocol A) and 1989–1992 1.3 Gy ×2 (protocol

B) (Tennvall et al. 1994 [11]). Thereafter 1.6 Gy ×2 (protocol C) was administered [36] (Figure 31.1). Radiotherapy was administered to a total target dose of 46 Gy; of which 30 Gy was administered preoperatively in the first two protocols (A and B), while the whole dose was given preoperatively in the third protocol (C). Since the radiotherapy was accelerated, the minimum interval of 6 hours between the two fractions was even more important so as to prevent spinal cord myelopathy [37,38]. The therapy was otherwise identical. Twenty mg doxorubicin was administered intravenously weekly. Surgery was possible in 40 patients. No patient failed to complete the protocol due to toxicity. In only 13 cases (24%) death was attributed to local failure. Five patients (9%) had a "survival" exceeding 2 years. No signs of local recurrence were seen in 33 patients (60%); 5/16 (31%) patients in protocol A, 11/17 (65%) patients in protocol B, and 17/22 (77%) patients in protocol C (P = 0.017). In the 40 patients undergoing additional surgery, no signs of local recurrence were seen in 5/9 (~56%) patients, 11/14 (~79%) patients and 17/17 (100%) patients in groups A, B, and C, respectively (P = 0.005). On the other hand, in protocol A, two patients with pulmonary metastases at diagnosis did not undergo surgery and finally succumbed due to local failure.

The primary aim of preventing patients with ATC from dying due to suffocation caused by local tumor invasion was achieved in protocol C, which is also in accordance with our current recommendations for local therapy. The present multimodal treatment of ATC seems to be feasible and effective, despite the patients' age and locally advanced disease. There was a significant positive correlation between accelerated radiotherapy and local tumor control. None of the 17 patients in protocol C, that is, those receiving the most accelerated hyperfractionated radiotherapy and subsequent surgery, had a local remnant tumor or suffered local recurrence.

Macroscopically radical surgery is a prerequisite for local cure, since all 33 patients showing no signs of remnant or recurrent local tumor growth had radical surgery. It appears that the surgery does not need to be microscopically radical as only three patients fulfilled this criterion: one in protocol A, and two in protocol B. A conceivable alternative to a preoperative radiation dose of 46 Gy would be a dose of 68–70 Gy with the same fractionation (1.6 Gy ×2) but without succeeding operation. Such an alternative would probably not be feasible for this elderly patient population and furthermore the eradication of large thyroid tumours would probably be less effective than that of the present multimodal strategy [39].

Treatment of Disseminated Disease

Several studies have indicated that ATC is relatively resistant to chemotherapy. No response was observed in distant metastases in our recent study [36], or in another study employing doxorubicin (60 mg/m^2), cisplatin (90 mg/m^2), and local radiation [24]. The use of a more aggressive cytostatic regimen in a multimodal approach is therefore not justified, except possibly in younger subjects performing well upon termination of local therapy. Such a strategy would not compromise the completion of the local therapy, which, however, comes into conflict with starting the systemic therapy when the metastases are still small or not yet apparent.

In vitro assays on ATC from 14 patients, demonstrated chemoresistance to doxorubicin, etoposide, cisplatin, carboplatin, and cyclophosphamide in the majority of tumors [40]. The observed relative ineffectiveness of antineoplastic agents in ATC suggests an active role for one or more cellular mechanisms associated with

Table 31.2 Anaplastic giant cell carcinoma of the thyroid: Patient characteristics and tumor extent at start of therapy in the studies performed at Karolinska and Lund University Hospitals during 1984–1999 [36]

No. of patients	55
Sex (M/F)	17/38
Age: median	76
Age: range	46–94
Disease: limited to the neck	38
Disease: disseminated (=lung)	17
Extrathyroidal growth (T4, UICC)	51
Large intrathyroidal tumor (pT3)	4
Vocal cord paralysis	18
Estimated tumor volume:	
<50 cm^3	12
50–200 cm^3	22
>200 cm^3	21

Anaplastic Giant Cell Carcinoma of the Thyroid

Treatment protocol A

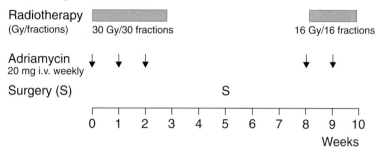

Treatment protocol B

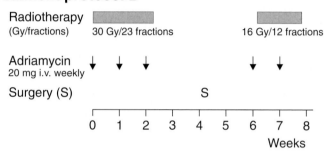

Treatment protocol C

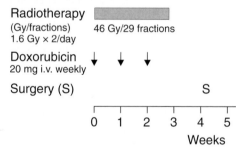

Figure 31.1 Treatment protocol for anaplastic carcinoma of the thyroid for the three consecutive protocols A, B, and C [36]. Our current recommendations for local therapy are according to protocol C. i.v., Intravenous. (Reprinted with permission from Tennvall J, Lundell G, Wahlberg P, et al. Anaplastic thyroid carcinoma: three protocols combining doxorubicin, hyperfractionated radiotherapy and surgery. *Br J Cancer* 2002; 86:1848–1853.)

chemotherapy resistance [3,41]. Apart from providing an explanation of the failure of systemic chemotherapy, such mechanisms might provide appropriate targets for inactivation in order to restore clinical response to standard chemotherapies [3].

Although no form of chemotherapy has yet been found to result in improvement in survival or to have a substantial effect on established metastases, new chemotherapeutic agents should be tested [3]. Paclitaxel has recently been shown to have activity both against tumor cell lines and tumor xenografts [42]. Furthermore a phase II study with 96-hour continuously administered paclitaxel every third week has demonstrated 50% objective remissions [43].

New modalities, such as inhibitors of angiogenesis, might in the future also prove to be useful tools for control of the growth of ATC [44]. One patient with ATC, who had exhausted all known treatment regimens used for this disease, responded completely to combretastatin (Oxigene) as a single-agent treatment. The patient has been disease free for more than 36 months [45]. This finding has initiated a new protocol in the USA with combretastatin in ATC. Combretastatin has also displayed significant cytotoxicity against ATC cell lines comparable to paclitaxel and these effects were long-lasting in two cell lines compared with the duration of paclitaxel [46]. However, as tumors grow, they begin to produce a wider array of angiogenic molecules. Therefore, if only one molecule is blocked, tumors may switch to another molecule [47]. Thus a cocktail of antibodies/inhibitors may be required.

There is increasing evidence that tumor removal alters the growth of minimal residual disease leading to perioperative growth [14]. These factors may be broadly classified as dissemination of tumor cells, postoperative immunosuppression, and accelerated residual tumor growth through, for example, reduced apoptosis and angiogenic switch. Because the patients seem to be at maximum risk during the immediate postoperative period this may represent a therapeutic window of opportunity during which novel paradigms aimed at reducing perioperative tumor growth may be used.

A large proportion of patients with ATC have had multinodular goiter for many years. Differentiated thyroid carcinoma is often found concomitantly in or adjacent to the ATC. The question whether all or some ATCs develop from differentiated thyroid carcinoma remains unclear. Multistep tumorigenesis has been proposed by several authors [48,49], but there is as yet no definite proof for that hypothesis. In the future, a major task will be to identify genetic markers in papillary or follicular thyroid carcinomas that eventually predisposed to anaplastic dedifferentiation. Sodium/iodide symporter (NIS) gene therapy is also being currently considered for dedifferentiated thyroid carcinomas with the ultimate aim of making radioiodine therapy possible [50,51]. Effective radioiodine therapy requires, however, more than a functional hNIS gene. There should be sufficient expression of TSH receptors and downstream signal transduction machinery to amplify hNIS expression when TSH levels rise. In addition, failure to organify radioiodine compromises ^{131}I residence time in thyroid carcinoma cells, permitting radioiodine reflux and insufficient radiation delivery [50,52].

References

1. Aldinger KA, Saaman NA, Ibanez M, Hill CS Jr. Anaplastic carcinoma of the thyroid: A review of 84 cases of spindle and giant cell carcinoma of the thyroid. Cancer 1978; 41:2267.
2. Tan RK, Finley RK, Driscoll D, Bakamjian V, Hicks WL, Shedd DP. Anaplastic carcinoma of the thyroid: A 24-year experience. Head Neck 1995; 17:41–47.
3. Ain KB. Anaplastic thyroid carcinoma: behavior, biology, and therapeutic approaches. Thyroid 1998; 9:715–726.
4. Jereb B, Stjernswärd J, Löwhagen T. Anaplastic giant-cell carcinoma of the thyroid: a study of treatment and prognosis. Cancer 1975; 35:1293–1295.
5. Akslen LA, Haldorsen T, Thoresen S, Glattre E. Incidence of thyroid cancer in Norway 1970–1985. APMIS 1990; 98:549–558.
6. Mazzaferri EL. Undifferentiated thyroid carcinoma and unusual thyroid malignancies. In: Mazzaferri EL, Samaan NA (eds) Endocrine tumors. Boston: Blackwell Scientific Publications, 1993; 98:378–398.
7. Demeter JG, De Jong SA, Lawrence AM, Paloyan E. Anaplastic thyroid carcinoma: risk factors and outcome. Surgery 1991; 100:956–961.
8. Junor EJ, Paul J, Nicholas SR. Anaplastic thyroid carcinoma: 91 patients treated by surgery and radiotherapy. Eur J Surg Oncol 1992; 18:83–88.
9. Nel CJ, van Heerden JA, Goellner JR, et al. Anaplastic carcinoma of the thyroid: a clinicopathologic study of 82 cases: Mayo Clin Proc 1985; 60:51–58.
10. Nilsson O, Lindeberg J, Zedenius J, et al. Anaplastic giant cell carcinoma of the thyroid gland – treatment and survival during 25 years. World J Surg 1998; 22:725–730.
11. Tennvall J, Lundell G, Hallquist A, et al. Combined doxorubicin, hyperfractionated radiotherapy and surgery in anaplastic thyroid carcinoma. Report on two protocols. Cancer 1994; 74:1348–1354.
12. Tallroth E, Wallin G, Lundell G, Löwhagen T, Einhorn J. Multimodality treatment in anaplastic giant cell thyroid carcinoma. Cancer 1987; 60:1428–1431.
13. Ekman E, Lundell G, Tennvall J, Wallin G. Chemotherapy and multimodality treatment in thyroid carcinoma. Otolaryngol Clin North Am 1990; 23:523–527.
14. Coffey JC, Wang JH, Smith MJF, Bouchier-Hayes D, Cotter TG, Redmond HP. Excisional surgery for cancer cure: therapy at a cost. Lancet Oncol 2003; 4:760–768.
15. Löwhagen T, Willems JS, Lundell G, Sundblad R, Granberg PO. Aspiration biopsy cytology in diagnosis of thyroid cancer. World J Surg 1981; 5:61–73.
16. Åkerman M, Tennvall J, Biörklund A, Mårtensson H, Möller T. Sensitivity and specificity of fine needle aspiration cytology in the diagnosis of tumors of the thyroid gland. Acta Cytol 1985; 29:850–855.
17. Tennvall J, Cavallin-Ståhl E, Åkerman M. Primary localized non-Hodgkin's lymphoma of the thyroid: a retro-

spective clinicopathological review. Eur J Sur Oncol 1987; 13:297–307.

18. Loré JM Jr. Surgery for advanced thyroid malignancy. Otolaryngol Clin North Am 1991; 24:1295–1319.

19. Levendag PC, DePorre PMZR, van Putten WLJ. Anaplastic carcinoma of the thyroid gland treated by radiation therapy. Int J Radiation Oncol Biol Phys 1993; 26:125–128.

20. Hötling T, Meyerbier H, Buhr H. Stellenwert der tracheotomie in der behandlung des respiratorischen notfalls beim anaplastichen schilddrusenkarzinom. Wien Klin Wochenschr 1990; 102:264–266.

21. Thames HD, Peters LJ, Rodney WH, Fletcher GH. Accelerated fractionation vs hyperfractionation: Rationales for several treatments per day. Int J Radiat Oncol Biol Phys 1982; 9:127–138.

22. Withers HR. Biologic basis for altered fractionation schemes. Cancer 1985; 55:2086–2095.

23. Venkatesh YSS, Ordonez NG, Schultz PN, Hickey RC, Goepfert H, Samaan NA. Anaplastic carcinoma of the thyroid. A clinicopathologic study of 121 cases. Cancer 1990; 66:321–330.

24. Schlumberger M, Parmentier C, Delisle MJ, Couette JE, Droz JP. Combination therapy for anaplastic giant cell thyroid carcinoma. Cancer 1991; 67:564–566.

25. Wendt TG, Chucholowski M, Hartensein R, Rohloff R, Willich N. Sequential chemo-radiotherapy in locally advanced squamous cell carcinoma of the head and neck. Int J Radiat Oncol Biol Phys 1985; 12:397–399.

26. Wallgren A, Norin T. Combined chemotherapy and radiation therapy in spindle and giant cell carcinoma of the thyroid gland. Report of a case. Acta Radiol Ther Phys Biol 1973; 12:17–20.

27. Rogers JD, Lindberg RD, Hill CS Jr, Gehan EG. Spindle and giant cell carcinoma of the thyroid: A different therapeutic approach. Cancer 1974; 34:1328–1332.

28. Simpson WJ. Anaplastic thyroid carcinoma: a new approach. Can J Surg 1980; 23:25–27.

29. Kim JH, Leeper RD. Treatment of anaplastic giant and spindle cell carcinoma of the thyroid gland with combination Adriamycin and radiation therapy. A new approach. Cancer 1983; 52:954–957.

30. Kim JH, Leeper RD. Treatment of locally advanced thyroid carcinoma with combination doxorubicin and radiation therapy. Cancer 1987; 60:2372–2375.

31. Andersson T, Biörklund A, Landberg T, Åkerman M, Aspegren K, Ingemansson S. Combined therapy for undifferentiated giant and spindle cell carcinoma of the thyroid. Acta Otolaryngol 1977; 83:372–377.

32. Tennvall J, Andersson T, Biörklund A, Ingemansson S, Landberg T, Åkerman M. Undifferentiated giant and spindle cell carcinoma of the thyroid. Report on two combined treatment modalities. Acta Radiol Oncol 1979; 18:408–416.

33. Werner B, Abele J, Alveryd A, et al. Multimodal therapy in anaplastic giant cell thyroid carcinoma. World J Surg 1984; 8:64–70.

34. Byfield JE, Lynch M, Kulhanian F, Chan PYM. Cellular effects of combined Adriamycin and X-irradiation in human tumor cells. Int J Cancer 1977; 19:194–204.

35. Rosenthal CJ, Rotman M. The development of chemotherapy drugs as radiosensitizers: an overview. In: Rotman M, Rosenthal CJ (eds) Concomitant continuous infusion and radiation. Berlin: Springer Verlag, 1991: 1–9.

36. Tennvall J, Lundell G, Wahlberg P, et al. Anaplastic thyroid carcinoma: three protocols combining doxorubicin, hyperfractionated radiotherapy and surgery. Br J Cancer 2002; 86:1848–1853.

37. Dische S, Saunders MI. Continuous, hyperfractionated, accelerated radiotherapy (CHART). An interim report upon late morbidity. Radiother Oncol 1989; 6:65–72.

38. Wong CS, Van Dyk J, Simpson J. Myelopathy following hyperfractionated accelerated radiotherapy for anaplastic thyroid carcinoma. Radiother Oncol 1991; 20: 3–9.

39. Mitchell G, Huddart R, Harmer C. Phase II evaluation of high dose accelerated radiotherapy for anaplastic thyroid carcinoma. Radiother Oncol 1999; 1:33–38.

40. Asakawa H, Kobayashi T, Komoike Y, et al. Chemosensitivity of anaplastic thyroid carcinoma and poorly differentiated thyroid carcinoma. Anticancer Res 1997; 17:2757–2762.

41. Satake S, Sugawara I, Watanabe M, Takami H. Lack of point mutation of human DNA topoisomerase II in multidrug-resistant anaplastic thyroid carcinoma cell lines. Cancer Lett 1997; 116:33–39.

42. Ain KB, Tofiq S, Taylor KD. Antineoplastic activity of Taxol against human anaplastic thyroid carcinoma cell lines in vitro and in vivo. J Clin Endocrinol Metab 1996; 81:3650–3653.

43. Ain KB, Egorin MJ, DeSimone PA. Treatment of anaplastic thyroid carcinoma with paclitaxel: phase 2 trial using ninety-six-hour infusion. Collaborative Anaplastic Thyroid Cancer Health Intervention Trials (CATCHIT) Group. Thyroid 2000; 10:587–594.

44. Hama Y, Shimzu T, Hosaka S, Sugenoya A, Usuda N. Therapeutic efficacy of angiogenesis inhibitor O-(chloroacetyl-carbamoyl) fumagillo (TNP-470;AGM-1470) for human anaplastic thyroid carcinoma in nude mice. Exp Toxicol Pathol 1997; 49:239–247.

45. Antiangiogenesis drugs target cancers, mechanisms. News. J Natl Cancer Inst 2000; 92:520–522.

46. Dziba JM, Marcinek R, Venkataraman GM, Robinson JA, Ain KB. Combretastatin A4 phosphate has primary antineoplastic activity against human anaplastic thyroid carcinoma cell lines and xenograft tumors. Thyroid 2002; 12:1063–1070.

47. Carmeliet P, Jain RK. Angiogenesis in cancer and other diseases. Nature 2000; 407:249–257.

48. Wynford-Thomas D. Molecular basis of epithelial tumorigenesis: the thyroid model. Crit Rev Oncog 1993; 4:1–23.

49. Dobashi Y, Sugimura H, Sakamoto A, et al. Stepwise participation of p53 gene mutation during dedifferentiation of human thyroid carcinomas. Diagn Mol Pathol 1994; 3:9–14.

50. Venkataraman GM, Yatin M, Marcinek R, Ain KB. Restoration of iodide uptake in dedifferentiated thyroid carcinoma: relationship to human Na$^+$/I$^-$ symporter gene methylation status. J Clin Endocrinol Metab 1999; 84:2449–2457.

51. Spitzweg C, Harrington KJ, Pinke LA, Vile RG, Morris JC. The sodium iodide symporter and its potential in cancer therapy. J Clin Endocrinol Metab 2001; 86:3327–3335.

52. Shimura H, Haraguchi K, Miyazaki A, Endo T, Onaya T. Iodide uptake and experimental ^{131}I. therapy in transplanted undifferentiated thyroid cancer cells expressing the Na$^+$/I$^-$ symporter gene. Endocrinology 1997; 138: 4493–4496.

32

Specialist Palliative Care for Anaplastic Thyroid Carcinoma

Mary Comiskey

Introduction

Palliative care aims to improve the quality of life of all patients with progressive life-threatening diseases including cancer. It focuses on the psychological, social, and spiritual as well as physical domains through a multidisciplinary approach and also encompasses care of family and friends. Problems caused by the disease and by its treatment are addressed.

Fortunately most patients presenting with thyroid cancer are cured. This chapter will focus on the management of physical problems encountered by patients with anaplastic thyroid cancer, which carries a poor prognosis in contrast to other forms of thyroid cancer. The principles of management discussed may be applied to the other diagnostic groups. The focus is on physical problems including end-of-life care as psychological issues are dealt with in Chapter 6. Timely referral to a palliative care service is advisable for this patient group.

Table 32.1 details the likely sites of metastases seen in the common types of thyroid cancer and the associated symptoms.

During the course of this chapter I shall use the case of Jane, who died from anaplastic thyroid cancer 6 months following presentation, to illustrate the typical palliative care problems encountered in patients with incurable thyroid cancer.

Jane was aged 47 years when she presented with a 6 × 4 cm rapidly growing inoperable anaplastic carcinoma of her thyroid gland causing stridor, fear, and pain. Her early pain was nociceptive in origin and easily controlled using a combination of oral codeine, titrated from 30 mg to 60 mg 6-hourly, high dose corticosteroids that also afforded a degree of upper airways protection, and paracetamol. She required immediate tracheal stenting for stridor. Her fear abated with relief of stridor and pain and also following a clear explanation of the cause of her problems and the treatment plan.

Pain

Most cancer patients fear pain yet in general 25% of patients with cancer have no pain [1] and 33% have three or more pains [2]. Approximately 15% of pains encountered in cancer patients [2] are not due to malignancy. Patients with recurrent and/or metastatic thyroid cancer more commonly suffer pain due to local tumor progression, bone metastases, and nerve compression or infiltration.

The key to successful pain management is:

- accurate diagnosis of the cause;
- appropriate analgesia including disease modifying treatment(s);

Table 32.1 Disease sites and symptoms associated with advanced thyroid cancer

Type	Problem	Symptom
Anaplastic Papillary Medullary	Local disease progression	Pain, tumor fungation, infection, bleeding, pressure symptoms
Papillary Anaplastic Medullary	Lymph node metastases	Pain, neuropathy, lymphedema
Follicular Anaplastic	Lung metastases	Dyspnea, cough, hemoptysis
Medullary	Bone metastases	Pain, fracture, immobility

- adequate explanation and empathy;
- regular monitoring of response.

World Health Organization Analgesic Ladder

More than 90% of cancer pains are relieved by following the World Health Organization's analgesic ladder (Figure 32.1) [3]. It provides a basis for the use of primary analgesics. The choice of primary analgesics is wide. Those commonly used and thus widely available are listed in Table 32.2. Analgesia should be given orally, regularly to prevent pain, and by the ladder. Thus if pain fails to respond to a non-opioid (step 1), a weak opioid (step 2) is added and should that fail, a strong opioid (step 3) substituted. Occasionally step 2 is bypassed in favor of using a small dose of strong opioid for convenience. If pain fails to respond to one weak opioid a strong opioid should be used rather than trying an alternative weak opioid. In addition to regular preventative analgesia, patients with ongoing pain should also be provided with a rapid-acting analgesic for breakthrough pain. This should be equivalent to 10–20% of their 24-hour dose.

Prescribing Morphine

Morphine is the oral strong opioid analgesic of choice [3]. A typical starting dose in patients switching from a weak opioid (e.g. codeine 240 mg daily) is 40–60 mg daily. Smaller starting doses (e.g. 10–20 mg daily) should be considered in the elderly, patients with renal impairment, and those who are opioid naïve. During the titration phase it may be given 4-hourly and the dose adjusted daily, for example from 5 to 10 to 15 to 20 to 30 to 40 mg 4-hourly and thereafter by increments of 25–33% in patients under close supervision or every 3 days in patients at home. Patients with renal impairment should be titrated slowly as they accumulate morphine-6-glucuronide (M6G) and morphine-3-glucuronide (M3G), which can

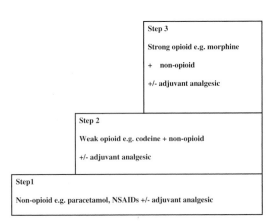

Step 3

Strong opioid e.g. morphine

+   non-opioid

+/- adjuvant analgesic

Step 2

Weak opioid e.g. codeine + non-opioid

+/- adjuvant analgesic

Step1

Non-opioid e.g. paracetamol, NSAIDs +/- adjuvant analgesic

Figure 32.1 The World Health Organization three-step analgesic staircase for cancer pain [3].

Table 32.2 Choice of primary analgesics

Analgesic class	First choice	Second choice
Non-opioid	Acetaminophen (paracetamol)	Nonsteroidal anti-inflammatory drugs (NSAIDs) Aspirin
Weak opioid	Codeine	Dihydrocodeine
Strong opioid	Morphine	Oxycodone Hydromorphone Fentanyl Methadone

cause respiratory depression, neurotoxicity, or excessive sedation. Once pain is controlled a modified release preparation given 12-hourly or once daily should be substituted for convenience. There is no ceiling dose for morphine.

Common side effects of all strong opioids include the following:

- *Chemically mediated nausea and vomiting* occurs in approximately 30% of patients, lasts 5–7 days, is mediated by dopamine and can be controlled by haloperidol 1.5–3 mg once daily. Haloperidol may be discontinued after one week. It may recur with subsequent opioid dose escalation.
- *Constipation* affects most patients. Laxative therapy should be prescribed for all patients commenced on opioids unless there is a contraindication. The laxative dose requirement increases with opioid dose increase and most patients on higher opioid doses require a combined softening and stimulating laxative such as codanthramer.
- *Transient drowsiness* lasts 3–5 days and may recur with subsequent dose increases. Patients should be should be advised of this and counseled not to drive or operate mechanical equipment while affected.

Morphine Intolerance

Some patients are intolerant of morphine. Our understanding of opioid pharmacogenetics is incomplete and as yet there is no way of predicting which opioid will suit an individual patient. In addition there is significant inter-individual variation in bioavailability (Table 32.3). Management strategies include:

1. morphine dose reduction;
2. switching the patient to an alternative strong opioid;

3. addition of drug treatment targeted at controlling the intolerable adverse effect.

If opioid dose reduction fails to resolve the problem or results in recurrence of pain, switching opioid is usually preferable to adding another pharmacological agent.

Clinical Presentation and Management of Morphine Intolerance

- *Gastric stasis* manifested by early satiation, large volume vomiting, flatulence, hiccups, and little nausea occurs in less than 5% of patients on opioids and can be relieved by the addition of a prokinetic agent such as metoclopramide or domperidone.
- *Cognitive impairment* presenting as delirium and hallucinations can be managed by opioid dose reduction, switching to an alternative strong opioid and/or addition of a major tranquilizer such as haloperidol.
- *Dysphoria* is rare and necessitates either dose reduction or switching to an alternative opioid.
- *Dry mouth* can be particularly troublesome for patients, affecting sleep, speech, and swallowing. Artificial salivas are of limited value. It is best managed by switching opioids.
- *Vestibular stimulation* – patients complain of movement-related nausea, vomiting, and dizziness. Switching opioids or adding an antihistamine such as cyclizine may control it.
- *Pruritus* is rare when opioids are administered orally. It may be relieved by oral ondansetron 4 mg 12-hourly or by switching opioids.
- *Myoclonus* presents as jerking and/or multifocal twitching. Patients will often com-

Table 32.3 Pharmacokinetics of oral strong opioids [10,11]

	Morphine	Hydromorphone	Oxycodone	Methadone
Oral bioavailability	16–68%	37–62%	60–87%	40–96%
Onset of action (min)	20–30	20–30	20–30	30
Duration of action (hours)	3–6	4–5	4–6	4–24
Plasma half-life (hours)	1.5–4.5	2.5	3.5	8–75
Active metabolites	Yes	Yes	Minor	No

plain of dropping items or spilling drinks. It can be a manifestation of toxicity, and thus the first step in management is opioid dose reduction. Low dose benzodiazepines are usually helpful [4].

- *Histamine release* causing bronchoconstriction and breathlessness requires immediate opioid switch together with short-term bronchodilator and antihistamine therapy.

Alternative Strong Opioids

The more frequently used strong opioid analgesics oxycodone, hydromorphone, transdermal fentanyl, and methadone are as effective as morphine [5–9]. They differ in their pharmacokinetic profiles (Table 32.3).

The recommended conversion ratios between some opioids vary between the UK and USA [10,11] (Table 32.4).

When switching opioids it is important to consider incomplete cross-tolerance and observe the patient closely for opioid toxicity. Choice depends on:

- patient-related factors, for example renal status, problems with constipation;
- disease treatment related factors, for example risk of mucositis or vomiting;
- cost – in the UK methadone is least expensive, fentanyl most expensive, and

Table 32.4 Recommended conversion ratios for strong opioids, USA and UK [10,11]

	Conversion ratio
Morphine → hydromorphone	5:1 USA
	7.5:1 UK
Hydromorphone → morphine	1:3.5–5 USA
Morphine → oxycodone	3:2 USA
	2:1 UK
Morphine → methadone	10:1
Morphine → TD/SC fentanyl	100–150:1
Oral morphine → SC diamorphine	3:1
Oral → SC morphine	2:1
Oral → SC hydromorphone	2:1
Oral → SC oxycodone	2:1

TD, transdermal; SC, subcutaneous.

oxycodone is 10% more expensive than hydromorphone.

Table 32.5 may help with making a rational choice.

Non-Oral Routes

Generally there is no analgesic benefit in giving strong opioids that are available in oral formulations by the parenteral route for chronic pain management. The indications for injectable analgesics are:

- vomiting;
- need for rapid analgesic effect;

Table 32.5 Advantages and disadvantages of alternative strong opioids [5–9,12,13]

Drug	Advantages	Disadvantages
Oxycodone	Less cognitive impairment, pruritus and sedation No major active metabolites Easy to calculate conversion rates Oral liquid available in UK	More constipating No potent injectable form in UK 5% of white people lack CYPD6 enzyme necessary for metabolism
Hydromorphone	Cheaper than oxycodone in UK Injectable form is highly soluble	May accumulate in renal failure Risk of error in calculating conversion dose No oral liquid form in UK
Transdermal fentanyl	Safe in renal impairment Useful in patients with dysphagia, vomiting or mucositis Less constipating and possibly less cognitive impairment	Unsuitable in unstable pain Patch allergy Most expensive – may save on laxative
Methadone	Least expensive Safe in renal and liver impairment NMDA receptor antagonist activity No active metabolites	Long half-life posing risk of fatal dose accumulation

- progressive or severe dysphagia;
- last hours or days of life where swallowing is inconvenient for the patient.

Adjuvant Analgesics

Some pains, typically neuropathic pain, skin pain, movement-related pain, and colic, are only partially responsive or do not respond to opioids. Adjuvant analgesics, also called secondary analgesics or co-analgesics, should be considered. They are usually used along with but may be considered instead of primary analgesics (i.e. paracetamol (acetaminophen), NSAIDs, and opioids).

- *Tricyclic antidepressants*, for example amitriptyline 10–75 mg at night, and/or *anticonvulsants*, for example sodium valproate 200–1000 mg at night or gabapentin 100–800 mg 8-hourly, are the mainstay of treatment for neuropathic pain. Both drug groups have similar efficacy, relieving neuropathic pain intensity by 50% in 30% of patients on average [14,15]. Some patients benefit from a combined approach.
- *Antispasmodics*, for example hyoscine butylbromide (not available in the USA) 20 mg subcutaneously (SC) as required or 40–180 mg by continuous infusion and glycopyrronium 200–400 μg SC as required or 600–1200 μg by continuous infusion, relieve colic.
- *Corticosteroids* may be used to reduce peritumor edema and thus relieve pain related to nerve compression or cerebral metastases.
- *Muscle relaxants*, for example diazepam or baclofen, are useful for muscle cramp and myofascial pain.
- *NMDA receptor channel blockers*, for example ketamine, for neuropathic, mucosal, skin, or incident pain should be used under specialist supervision.

Non-Drug Therapies

Some patients benefit greatly from physiotherapy including heat therapy, ultrasonic therapy, massage, and trancutaneous electrical nerve stimulation (TENS). Trigger point injection and acupuncture can be particularly useful for myofascial pain. Other useful treatments include relaxation therapy, lifestyle management advice, nerve blockade, cognitive behavioral therapy techniques, and hypnosis.

Persistent Pain

When pain persists it is important to reassess the patient. Common pitfalls in management include:

- failure to diagnose and treat coexisting anxiety and depression;
- onset of new pain or presence of previously undiagnosed pain;
- poor patient adherence to prescribed medications;
- inadequate analgesic dosing or inappropriate dosing intervals.

Jane commenced radiotherapy with palliative intent. Her course was complicated by painful mucositis, which responded to replacement of codeine 240 mg, originally initiated for neck pain, by morphine 40 mg daily (using a conversion ratio of 10:1) and subsequent dose titration to 120 mg daily. She also developed progressive dysphagia due to mucositis and preferred nasogastric intubation for feeding and delivery of medication rather than the alternative option of gastrostomy feeding.

The formulation of morphine was changed from modified release tablets to an equal dose of a modified release liquid formulation. She suffered a series of blackouts that were attributed to carotid sinus dysfunction secondary to tumor encroachment. They occurred without warning and required her to have constant companionship for safety. Their frequency was greatly reduced following reintroduction of corticosteroids, which presumably reduced peritumor edema. Four weeks following completion of treatment she complained of drowsiness and twitching, which was due to opioid toxicity. Her morphine requirement had fallen as a result of response to radiotherapy and improvement in mucositis.

Discussion Points

1. *Mucositis* – other treatment options include:
   - benzydamine 0.15% oral rinse 15 mL 2-hourly if required;
   - topical lidocaine as a 2% solution or made up as frozen or sugar-free lozenge;
   - alcohol-free liquid morphine 10 mg in 5 mL 4-hourly used as a mouth rinse or swallowed;
   - coating agents such as sucralfate suspension 10 mL 4–8-hourly as a rinse and swallowed 12-hourly;
   - ketamine transmucosal, oral or parenteral under specialist supervision.
2. *Changing opioid requirements:* It is important to monitor patients on opioids for toxicity following disease-modifying treatments or introduction of opioid-sparing drugs such as corticosteroids, NSAIDs and ketamine or nerve blockade. Signs of toxicity include pinpoint pupils, drowsiness, jerking, and respiratory depression. Their opioids including breakthrough medication should be reduced by 25–50%.
3. *Dysphagia:*
   - Consult a speech and language therapist for advice on swallowing techniques. If likely to be progressive or protracted consider percutaneous endoscopic gastrostomy (PEG) for feeding and administration of medication.
   - Rationalize medication and use non-oral preparations if practicable. Jane required a nasogastric tube and thus a change in opioid formulation. Transdermal fentanyl could have been used. Her anticipated requirement would have been 25–50 µg/hour starting with the lower option. In a randomized crossover study of oral morphine and transdermal fentanyl [6], most patients required a higher fentanyl dose than the manufacturers' recommendations when switched to fentanyl from morphine.
4. *Corticosteroids as interim palliation* may prove valuable in reducing tumor-associated edema pending response to radio-therapy. In fact, edema may be temporarily exacerbated by radiotherapy causing an increase in local neck symptoms.

Jane's disease progressed despite radiotherapy and Caelyx chemotherapy, with progression of local neck disease, widespread pulmonary, nodal and base of skull metastases. She complained of increasing neck pain and tenderness, facial pain with associated allodynia involving the mandibular division of the right trigeminal nerve and ondynophagia related to candidiasis and possibly glossopharyngeal neuralgia. Her neuropathic pains responded to introduction of gabapentin 100 mg 8-hourly with dose titration to tolerance – 400 mg 8-hourly – and supplementation with amitriptyline 10 mg at night. The inflammatory component of neck pain responded to NSAIDs and pain on swallowing resolved with treatment of candidiasis.

She also complained of dry cough, which was eventually controlled by nebulized lidocaine 2% 4 mL 6-hourly, occasional minor hemoptysis, which resolved with introduction of tranexamic acid 500 mg 8-hourly, breathlessness, which initially responded to relaxation techniques and a 25% increase in her daily opioid dose. She subsequently required re-stenting of her original tracheal stent for recurrence of upper airways obstruction. She felt particularly anxious and frightened that she would choke and was also troubled by excessive oropharyngeal secretions and drooling.

Discussion Points

1. *Breathlessness* is a particularly frightening, distressing, and challenging symptom. To manage:
   - correct reversible causes, for example bronchospasm or pleural effusion;
   - ensure optimal environmental conditions, for example cool ambient temperature and through airflow or fan;
   - position patient comfortably;

- explain the cause and treatment plan;
- involve a physiotherapist to teach breathing techniques;
- treat associated anxiety using relaxation and cognitive behavioral therapy techniques;
- prescribe oxygen for hypoxic patients;
- prescribe benzodiazepines for panic and anxiety;
- prescribe opioids to reduce the sensation of breathlessness – if patient is opioid naïve start with a low dose, for example morphine 2.5–5 mg 4-hourly, and titrate as required. If patient is already on opioids increase their 24-hour dose by 25% and continue to adjust according to response;
- prescribe helium 80% and oxygen 20% mixture, which is lighter than room air for upper airways obstruction.

2. *Dry cough* – if there is no underlying reversible cause it may be suppressed by:
   - oral antitussives such as simple linctus 10 mL as required, codeine linctus 15–30 mg 6-hourly or methadone linctus 1–2 mg 6-hourly;
   - inhaled or nebulized steroids;
   - lidocaine 2% 4 mL nebulized for troublesome cough where other measures have failed. Patients should be advised to avoid eating or drinking for 90 minutes following treatment to prevent aspiration.

3. *Fear and panic* (see also Chapter 6) are understandably common in patients with compressive symptoms related to neck disease and also in patients facing death. It is important to:
   - explore the underlying causes and deal with any irrational thoughts;
   - seek help from a clinical psychologist for patients with complex problems;
   - consider benzodiazepines, for example diazepam 2–5 mg 8-hourly or lorazepam 0.5–1 mg 12-hourly. Antidepressants with anti-panic actions such as the selective serotonin reuptake inhibitor (SSRI) sertraline 20 mg daily or the tricyclic antidepressant clomipramine 25 mg daily may also help.

4. *Excess oral secretions and salivary drooling* can be particularly frustrating and embarrassing. Drugs with anticholinergic activity such as hyoscine hydrobromide 1 mg transdermal (TD) patch or 150–300 µg sublingually (SL)/orally 6-hourly are effective. Glycopyrronium 200–400 µg SC or 400–1200 µg by continuous SC infusion (CSCI) and hyoscine butylbromide 20 mg orally or SC and 40–180 mg by CSCI are equally effective.

5. *Management of bleeding*
   - Identify and treat underlying cause if appropriate.
   - Consider referring patient for palliative radiotherapy.
   - Monitor patient for anemia and transfuse if indicated.
   - Prescribe tranexamic acid (avoid in hematuria) 500 mg 8-hourly or etamsylate 500 mg 6-hourly to reduce bleeding.
   - For patients at risk of a major bleed in the terminal phase ensure ready availability of sedative medication such as midazolam 10 mg injection buccal/intravenous (IV)/intramuscular (IM)/SC or diazepam 10 mg per rectum, and green towels or surgical cloths to minimize the visual impact of blood loss. If a major bleed occurs stay with and reassure the patient and family.

6. *Lymphedema* – the mainstay of management is:
   - good skin care;
   - regular exercise of the affected limb;
   - massage therapy;
   - compression therapy;
   - prevention and early treatment of infection in the lymphedematous area;
   - a short course of high dose corticosteroids, for example dexamethasone 16 mg daily for one week for acute lymphatic obstruction;
   - further radiotherapy or chemotherapy if appropriate.

Other Problems Seen in Advanced Thyroid Cancer

Fungating Malodorous Neck Tumor

This is fortunately rare. Affected patients often require continuous inpatient care to manage the associated anxiety and fear of bleeding or choking as well as frequent need for dressings. Specific management should include:

- radiotherapy if appropriate to reduce bleeding and discharge;
- regular change of occlusive dressings;
- use of topical metronidazole 0.75–1% gel with dressings, which will control malodor in most patients; some will require systemic metronidazole for deep-seated anaerobic infection;
- active management of aerobic infection.

Nausea and Vomiting

It is important to distinguish the cause(s) of nausea and vomiting and target antiemetic treatment at the appropriate receptor(s) [16,17]. Commonly overlooked causes in this patient group include constipation, excess pharyngeal secretions, cerebral metastases, oropharyngeal candidiasis, emetogenic drugs, and gastric stasis. It is often necessary to initiate parenteral antiemetic therapy to gain control, switching to oral therapy after 24–48 hours.

There are five main causes:

- *Chemical* causes include drugs such as opioids or metronidazole, or biochemical disturbances such as hypercalcemia and uremia. They act via the chemoreceptor trigger zone (CTZ), which in animals has a preponderance of dopamine receptors. Thus the treatment of choice is haloperidol, a dopamine (D_2) antagonist, 1.5–3 mg oral/SC once daily.
- *Impaired gastric motility*, which is characterized by epigastric fullness, early satiation, flatulence, reflux and large volume vomiting, may be treated with metoclopramide 10–20 mg 8-hourly or 30–90 mg by CSCI or domperidone 10–20 mg 8-hourly if extrapyramidal side effects are a risk.

- *Chemotherapy or radiotherapy* induced nausea and vomiting should be managed with oral or parenteral $5HT_3$ antagonists.
- *Vestibular or direct stimulation of the vomiting center* due to intracranial disease or radiotherapy and *vagal/autonomic afferent stimulation of the vomiting center* due to pharyngeal irritation, mediastinal, or subdiaphragmatic metastases are common in patients with advanced cancer. The main neurotransmitters implicated are histamine 1 (H_1), acetylcholine (AChm), and $5HT_2$. Cyclizine blocks H_1 and AChm receptors, hyoscine hydrobromide blocks AChm receptors and levomepromazine has broad-spectrum antiemetic activity blocking $5HT_2$, D_1, AChm, and possibly H_1. The respective doses are: cyclizine 50 mg oral/SC 8-hourly or 150 mg by CSCI; levomepromazine 5–12.5 mg oral/SC once daily; hyoscine hydrobromide 1 mg TD or 150–300 μg SL/oral 6-hourly or 600–1800 μg by CSCI over 24 hours.

> One month later Jane was admitted as an emergency from home with sudden onset of stridor and a large intrapulmonary hemorrhage. She was given midazolam 10 mg IM during transfer from home and remained calm until she died peacefully a few hours later surrounded by family and friends. On arrival she had marked halitosis that resolved within 20 min of receiving IV metronidazole.

End-of-Life Care [18]

- Ensure patient and family are aware that death is imminent.
- Address their fears and concerns; be mindful of spiritual needs.
- Stop all unnecessary drugs and interventions.
- Ensure that appropriate regular and breakthrough medications are prescribed for ongoing management of pain, nausea, excess retained respiratory secretions, and agitation. At this stage many patients are unable to reliably take oral medications

and require introduction of parenteral medication. See Table 32.4 for opioid conversion ratios.

Typical end-of-life drug regimens include:

1. parenteral opioid by CSCI;
2. cyclizine 100–150 mg or levomepromazine 5–12.5 mg by CSCI to prevent emesis;
3. midazolam 10–60 mg or levomepromazine 25–100 mg for terminal agitation;
4. glycopyrronium 600–1800 μg, hyoscine hydrobromide 600–1800 μg, or hyoscine butylbromide 60–180 mg to reduce troublesome respiratory secretions.

References

1. Bonica JJ. Cancer pain: Current status and future needs. In: Bonica JJ (ed.) The management of pain, 2nd edn. Philadelphia: Lea and Febiger, 1990: 400–445.
2. Grond S, Zech D, Diefenbach C, Radbruch L, Lehmann K. Assessment of cancer pain: a prospective evaluation in 2266 cancer patients referred to a pain service. Pain 1996; 64:107–114.
3. World Health Organization. Cancer pain relief with a guide to opioid availability, 2nd edn. Geneva WHO, 1996; available at http://whqlibdoc.who.int/publications/9241544821.pdf.
4. Mercadente S. Pathophysiology and treatment of opioid-related myoclonus in cancer patients. Pain 1998; 74:5–9.
5. Heiskanen T, Kalso E. Controlled-release oxycodone and morphine in cancer related pain. Pain 1997; 73:37–45.
6. Allan L, Hays H, Jensen N-K, et al. Randomised crossover trial of transdermal fentanyl and sustained release oral morphine for treating chronic non-cancer pain. BMJ 2001; 322:1154–1158.
7. Hagen N, Babul N. Comparative clinical efficacy and safety of a novel controlled-release oxycodone formulation and controlled release hydromorphone in the treatment of cancer pain. Cancer 1997; 79:1428–1437.
8. Mucci-Lo P, Berman BS, Silberstein PT, et al. Controlled-release oxycodone compared with controlled-release morphine in the treatment of cancer pain: a randomised, double-blind, parallel-group study. Eur J Pain 1998; 2:239–249.
9. Morley J, Makin M. The use of methadone in cancer patients poorly responsive to other opioids. Pain Rev 1998; 5:51–58.
10. Lawlor P, Turner K, Hanson J, Bruera E. Dose ratio between morphine and hydromorphone in patients with cancer pain: a retrospective study. Pain 1997; 72: 79–85.
11. Moriarty M, McDonald CJ, Miller AJ. A randomised crossover comparison of controlled release hydromorphone tablets with controlled release morphine tablets in patients with cancer pain. J Drug Assess 1999; 2: 1–8.
12. Twycross RG, Wilcock A, Charlesworth S. PCF2-Palliative care formulary, 2nd edn. Abingdon: Radcliffe Medical Press, 2003 (also available at http://www.palliativedrugs.com/).
13. Twycross R, Wilcock A. Symptom management in advanced cancer, 3rd edn. Abingdon: Radcliffe Medical Press, 2001.
14. McQuay HJ, Carroll D, Jadad A, Wiffen P, Moore A. Anticonvulsant drugs for management of pain: a systematic review. BMJ 1995; 311:1047–1052.
15. McQuay HJ, Tramer T, Nye BA, Carroll D, Wiffen P, Moore RA. A systematic review of antidepressants in neuropathic pain. Pain 1996; 68:217–227.
16. Peroutka SJ, Snyder SH. Antiemetic neurotransmitter receptor binding predicts therapeutic actions. Lancet 1982; i:658–659.
17. Mannix KA. Palliation of nausea and vomiting. In: Calman K, Doyle D, Hanks GWC (eds) Oxford textbook of palliative medicine, 3rd edn. Oxford: Oxford University Press, 2002.
18. Ellershaw J, Ward C. Care of the dying patient: the last hours or days of life. BMJ 2003; 326:30–34.

Further Reading

Calman K, Doyle D, Hanks GWC (eds) Oxford textbook of palliative medicine, 3rd edn. Oxford: Oxford University Press, 2002.
Regnard C, Hockley J. A guide to symptom relief in palliative care, 5th edn. Abingdon: Radcliffe Medical Press, 2004.
Twycross R, Wilcock A. Symptom management in advanced cancer, 3rd edn. Abingdon: Radcliffe Medical Press, 2001.

Useful Websites

http://www.palliativedrugs.com/ (Features a very useful palliative care formulary, a bulletin board for professionals together with monthly newsletter covering topical issues in palliative care.)
http://www.sign.ac.uk/guidelines/fulltext/44/ (Features evidence-based guidelines on pain management.)
http://www.cme.utoronto.ca/endoflife/default.htm (Features continuing medical education on end-of-life care.)

Section XI

Future Developments and Directions for Research in Thyroid Cancer

33

Emerging Therapies for Thyroid Cancer

Matthew D. Ringel

In comparison to many epithelial cancers, thyroid cancer therapy has long been rationally based on the specific characteristics of thyroid cancer cells; in particular, the retained expression and function of thyroid-specific proteins, such as the thyrotropin receptor (TSHR) and the Na, I symporter (NIS), that have created targets for therapies. Indeed, the use of TSH suppressive doses of levothyroxine (L-T_4) and radioiodine, in combination with surgery, has resulted in long-term survival rates for patients with localized thyroid cancers that approach 98% at 20 years [1–4]. However, some thyroid cancers lose expression and/or function of these two critical proteins, a feature that leads to poor responses to traditional therapies and a high incidence of cancer-related death. Alternative therapies, including cytotoxic chemotherapeutic agents, have yielded disappointing results with high morbidities. There has therefore been an effort to devise targeted therapies for aggressive thyroid cancers in a manner analogous to iodine-131 and TSH suppression therapy for typical thyroid cancers. Targeting therapy for these tumors requires identification of the pathways of tumor progression, and the mechanisms responsible for the loss of TSHR and NIS expression [5]. In this chapter, the emerging therapies based on defined molecular targets in progressive thyroid cancers will be discussed. Table 33.1 lists the main targets of thyroid cancer therapies.

Cell Signaling Inhibition

Over the past two decades, enormous gains have been made in our understanding of the genetic pathogenesis of thyroid cancers. The specific genetic alterations responsible for more than 50% of thyroid cancers have now been identified (Table 33.2). Overexpression or oncogenic rearrangements in tyrosine kinase receptors [6–8], activating mutations of downstream serine-threonine kinases, including RAS [9,10] and BRAF [11–17], and loss of tumor suppressor expression [18–20] resulting in pathway activation all have been identified. Several of these genetic abnormalities are specific for thyroid cancer (e.g. RET/PTC rearrangements), while others are common to a number of other malignancies (e.g. *RAS*, *BRAF*, and *PTEN* mutants). The identification of these specific abnormalities has created the opportunity to target therapies for more aggressive thyroid cancers in a manner analogous to the use of levothyroxine suppression and radioactive iodine for earlier stage tumors.

Several approaches have been taken to devise targeted therapies against receptor tyrosine kinases. Among the most successful has been inhibition of BCR/ABL and C-KIT in chronic myelogenous leukemia and gastrointestinal stromal tumors using STI-571 [21–23]. The

Table 33.1 Targets for thyroid cancer therapies

Tyrosine kinase receptor blockers
  RET
  CMET
  IGF-1
  VEGF
  EGF
Signaling molecule inhibitors
  BRAF
  RAS
  AKT
  RAP1
  PKC
Angiogenesis inhibitors
  VEGF
  Combretastatins
  Thalidomide
Apoptosis sensitizers
  TRAIL
  BCL-2 inhibition
  AKT inhibition
  Gene therapy
Enhancing iodine uptake
  Demethylating agents
  Histone deacetylase inhibitors
  Retinoids
  Gene therapy
Enhanced chemotherapy effects
  Drug resistance gene inhibitors
  Combination therapy
Immunotherapy
  Gene therapy
  Tumor vaccines
  BCG
Multimodality therapy including
  Radiation therapy and I-131

thyroid cancer and in many papillary thyroid cancers [24,25]. In addition, other agents that have activity against the family of vascular endothelial growth factor (VEGF) or epidermal growth factor (EGF) receptors are appropriate agents to consider as therapy for thyroid cancers.

Other approaches to inhibition of receptor tyrosine kinase functions include the use of antibodies that block ligand-induced receptor activity, as has been utilized for rheumatological disorders and some hematological malignancies. This approach has been utilized to block binding of VEGF to its receptors with preclinical success in vitro and in vivo for thyroid cancer [26,27].

Inhibition of downstream kinases, such as BRAF, RAS and AKT, has also been utilized. The use of small molecule inhibitors of these kinases, agents that block the mechanism of activation (e.g. farnesyl transferase inhibitors) [28,29], and agents that destabilize the proteins (heat shock protein binding agents) [30,31] are all in clinical trials currently. One concern about these inhibitors is the lack of cancer specificity. In comparison to agents that inhibit specific tyrosine kinase receptors, agents that block cell signaling pathways are more likely to induce non-tumor cell death. Surprisingly, several agents in this family have demonstrated excellent safety profiles in phase I studies, perhaps related to mechanism of action, or the relative degree of cancer cell pathway activation in comparison to normal cells.

Combination therapy using signaling inhibitors and traditional cytotoxic chemotherapy, or using inhibitors of several different pathways, is now under evaluation for several different types of cancer. For thyroid cancer, combinations including these agents have been used successfully in vitro and provide promise for future clinical trials.

success of this tumor-targeted therapy has led to the development of a number of tyrosine kinase inhibitors, each with their unique receptor specificity. Some have demonstrated ability to inhibit the function of RET, the tyrosine kinase that is activated both in medullary

Table 33.2 Common oncogenes in papillary (PTC) and follicular (FTC) thyroid cancer

Mutation/Rearrangement	PTC	FTC	Other
RET/PTC1–3	Yes (20–30%)	Rare	Associated with radiation and invasion (*RET/PTC3*)
BRAF	Yes (30–50%)	Rare	Tall cell variant
RAS	Rare	Yes (20–30%)	*N-RAS* most common
PPARγ/Pax8	Rare	Yes (20%)	Possibly more invasive
PTEN	Rare	Yes (10–15%)	Cowden syndrome

Antiangiogenesis Therapy

Cancer cells create a unique microenvironment that allows the growing malignant cell population to have access to nutrients and oxygen. Disruption of this microenvironment by targeting neovascularization is a goal of some new forms of therapy that have had success in vitro, in animal models, and in several patients with aggressive thyroid cancers. Perhaps the most promising agents in this class of drugs include VEGF receptor blockade (see above), combretastatins, and thalidomide. Each of these agents has a unique mechanism of action.

Of these targeted agents, combretastatin A4 phosphate appears to have the most promise in early clinical trials. Combretastatins are a family of tubulin-binding proteins derived from the African willow that target vascular endothelial cells and can also be cytotoxic to cancer cells. Partial or complete responses were noted in three of six patients with thyroid cancer, including one complete response in a patient with anaplastic thyroid cancer [32,33]. This response has resulted in a phase II study for patients with anaplastic thyroid cancer that is ongoing. The major toxicity of this agent is cardiac arrhythmia and ischemia; thus, patients need to be cleared for use of this agent.

Thalidomide (Celgene, Warren, NJ), and VEGF neutralizing antibodies, such as bevacizumab (Avastin, Genenetech, S. San Francisco, CA) or receptor blockers, such as Semaxanib (Sugen, S. San Francisco, CA) have shown promise in early clinical trials or in animal models of thyroid cancer [26,27]. The agents may be particularly useful in highly vascular cancers, such as anaplastic carcinoma, or those with osseous metastasis.

Enhancement of Iodine Uptake

As thyroid cancer cells dedifferentiate, they frequently display diminished iodine uptake or retention. Over the past several years, the mechanisms for this effect have been better characterized. The cloning of the gene encoding the Na, I symporter (NIS) has led to careful determination of the regulation of NIS gene expression, protein expression, and protein localization. Indeed, abnormalities in NIS gene and protein expression, and protein localization have been identified in thyroid cancers [34–36]. Reduced NIS expression, as reported by a number of investigators, appears to be an epigenetic event due to hypermethylation of the NIS promoter [37,38]. There has been significant interest in devising therapies to increase expression of endogenous NIS to enhance iodine uptake and, thus, the cytotoxic effect of radioiodine therapy.

In vitro, treatment of thyroid cancer cell lines with demethylating agents or histone deacetylase inhibitors, such as 5-azacytidine and depsipeptide, respectively, can enhance expression of NIS, induce iodine uptake, and induce apoptosis [37,38]. 5-Azacytidine is being used as a parent compound for other agents due to its rapid induction of resistance. Depsipeptide is in clinical trials as a therapy for thyroid cancer and neuroendocrine tumors, albeit not in combination with I-131 therapy.

Retinoid receptor agonists have also been used to enhance iodine uptake in thyroid cancers that do not respond to radioiodine. While there were promising results in vitro, and in initial studies [39,40], the use of more generalized retinoic acid receptor agonists appears to be limited [41]. However, studies using specific agonists of subtypes or retinoic acid receptors may hold promise and are ongoing [42].

A third approach to enhance iodine uptake is to utilize gene therapy to induce expression of an exogenous NIS gene to high levels in thyroid cancer cells. In vitro, gene therapy approaches are quite effective using viral vectors. Even in vitro, however, cancer cells demonstrate variable expression of receptors that are important proteins for cellular transport of viruses. In vivo experiments using gene therapy approaches by direct injection of the virus into tumors have been successful [43,44]. Systemic therapy has been more problematic due to a high hepatic first-pass effect and an immune response against the virus. Research using nonviral gene transporters is ongoing by several groups and holds promise for less antigenic delivery methods for future therapy.

Targeted Cytotoxic Agents

Many of the families of agents described earlier also induce cell death, either by inducing apoptosis (programmed cell death) or inhibition of anti-apoptotic pathways, or by causing cell necrosis. Several additional families of compounds have been targeted against cell survival pathways. These include activation of the TNF-related apoptosis-inducing ligand (TRAIL) receptor using recombinant TRAIL, inhibition of anti-apoptotic signaling molecules [45–47], such as BCL-2, using antisense RNA compound (e.g. olbermersen sodium, Genasense, Genta, Berkeley Heights, NJ) [48], or by reducing stability of anti-apoptotic and growth-inducing proteins by blocking heat shock protein 90 chaperone function (e.g. Geldanamycin) [30,31]. Therapy directed against pro-apoptotic receptors, such as FAS, has proven ineffective for thyroid cancer due to a high degree of resistance caused by the expression of labile protein inhibitors. However, inhibition of downstream anti-apoptotic pathways appears to show more promise as a clinical therapy.

Finally, gene therapy using vectors that carry cytotoxic genes ("suicide gene therapy") has been utilized to treat thyroid cancer cells in vitro, and, by direct tumor injection, in vivo. The best reported method is to induce thyroid cancer cell expression of thymidine kinase, which will uniquely sensitize the cells to treatment with the antiviral drug ganciclovir [49]. This approach has been used in xenografts as independent therapy, and also in sensitizing the cells to the effects of external irradiation. Gene therapy approaches that combine cytotoxic genes with immunomodulators have also been reported [50–52]. Tumor vaccines offer another immunotherapy model. This group of agents targeted against cell survival therefore represent an attractive option to sensitize cells to the effects of radiation and/or chemotherapy.

Other Emerging Therapies for Thyroid Cancer

Another approach for new therapies for thyroid cancer and other malignancies is to target the mechanisms by which cancer cells develop resistance to chemotherapeutic agents. For example, multiple drug resistance genes (MDR) result in resistance to a number of chemotherapy agents, such as those with documented activity for some patients with anaplastic thyroid cancer, including taxanes and doxorubicin [53–57].

Immunotherapy remains a major area of interest for thyroid cancer, and for a number of other malignancies [58,59]. The use of tumor vaccines with or without agents to enhance immune responses, or to induce thyroiditis in patients on chemotherapy using interferons, are avenues of potential treatment for thyroid cancer in the future.

Chemoprevention is another alternative for thyroid cancer that remains relatively unexplored other than the use of iodide after accidental exposure to iodine isotopes. Chemopreventive strategies could include administration of apoptotic-promoting agents after radiation exposure, to induce cell death and subsequent hypothyroidism. Or low doses of other agents that are shown to be radiation sensitizers. Finally, cyclooxygenase-2 inhibitors have been utilized as chemopreventive agents for malignancies such as colon cancer with high levels of cyclooxygenase-2 activity. Thyroid cancers also have been shown to have high levels of cyclooxygenase-2 expression and activity [60–63].

Multimodality Therapies

Based on experience with chemotherapy agents and radiation therapy, it is likely that single agent therapy may not be effective for all patients with thyroid cancers that do not respond to usual therapeutic measures. Thus, combination therapy using agents targeted against several different pathways may be needed to ultimately treat patients with these aggressive tumors. In addition, these agents may be most useful in combination with radioiodine therapy, radiation therapy, and/or traditional forms of chemotherapy, to have greatest impact on patient survival. The importance and current role of clinical trials for these patients cannot be overstated if the survival of patients with these aggressive cancers is to be enhanced.

References

1. Sherman SI, Brierley JD, Sperling M, et al. Prospective multicenter study of thyroid carcinoma treatment: initial analysis of staging and outcome. National Thyroid Cancer Treatment Cooperative Study Registry Group. Cancer 1998; 83(5):1012–1021.

2. Hundahl SA, Fleming ID, Fremgen AM, Menck HR. A National Cancer Data Base report on 53,856 cases of thyroid carcinoma treated in the US, 1985–1995. Cancer 1998; 83(12):2638–2648.

3. Hundahl SA, Cady B, Cunningham MP, et al. Initial results from a prospective cohort study of 5583 cases of thyroid carcinoma treated in the United States during 1996. US and German Thyroid Cancer Study Group. An American College of Surgeons Commission on Cancer Patient Care Evaluation study. Cancer 2000; 89(1):202–217.

4. Mazzaferri EL, Jhiang SM. Long-term impact of initial surgical and medical therapy on papillary and follicular thyroid cancer. Am J Med 1994; 97(5):418–428.

5. Braga-Basaria M, Ringel MD. Clinical review 158: Beyond radioiodine: a review of potential new therapeutic approaches for thyroid cancer. J Clin Endocrinol Metab 2003; 88(5):1947–1960.

6. Farid NR. Molecular pathogenesis of thyroid cancer: the significance of oncogenes, tumor suppressor genes, and genomic instability. Exp Clin Endocrinol Diabetes 1996; 104(Suppl 4):1–12.

7. Segev DL, Umbricht C, Zeiger MA. Molecular pathogenesis of thyroid cancer. Surg Oncol 2003; 12(2):69–90.

8. Fagin JA. Perspective: lessons learned from molecular genetic studies of thyroid cancer – insights into pathogenesis and tumor-specific therapeutic targets. Endocrinology 2002; 143(6):2025–2028.

9. Namba H, Rubin SA, Fagin JA. Point mutations of ras oncogenes are an early event in thyroid tumorigenesis. Mol Endocrinol 1990; 4(10):1474–1479.

10. Lemoine NR, Mayall ES, Wyllie FS, et al. High frequency of ras oncogene activation in all stages of human thyroid tumorigenesis. Oncogene 1989; 4(2):159–164.

11. Cohen Y, Xing M, Mambo E, et al. BRAF mutation in papillary thyroid carcinoma. J Natl Cancer Inst 2003; 95(8):625–627.

12. Fukushima T, Suzuki S, Mashiko M, et al. BRAF mutations in papillary carcinomas of the thyroid. Oncogene 2003; 22(41):6455–6457.

13. Kimura ET, Nikiforova MN, Zhu Z, et al. High prevalence of BRAF mutations in thyroid cancer: genetic evidence for constitutive activation of the RET/PTC-RAS-BRAF signaling pathway in papillary thyroid carcinoma. Cancer Res 2003; 63(7):1454–1457.

14. Nikiforova MN, Kimura ET, Gandhi M, et al. BRAF mutations in thyroid tumors are restricted to papillary carcinomas and anaplastic or poorly differentiated carcinomas arising from papillary carcinomas. J Clin Endocrinol Metab 2003; 88(11):5399–5404.

15. Trovisco V, Vieira de Castro I, Soares P, et al. BRAF mutations are associated with some histological types of papillary thyroid carcinoma. J Pathol 2004; 202(2):247–251.

16. Xing M, Vasko V, Tallini G, et al. BRAF T1796A transversion mutation in various thyroid neoplasms. J Clin Endocrinol Metab 2004; 89(3):1365–1368.

17. Xu X, Quiros RM, Gattuso P, Ain KB, Prinz RA. High prevalence of BRAF gene mutation in papillary thyroid carcinomas and thyroid tumor cell lines. Cancer Res 2003; 63(15):4561–4567.

18. Fagin JA. Tumor suppressor genes in human thyroid neoplasms: p53 mutations are associated undifferentiated thyroid cancers. J Endocrinol Invest 1995; 18(2):140–142.

19. Liaw D, Marsh DJ, Li J, et al. Germline mutations of the PTEN gene in Cowden disease, an inherited breast and thyroid cancer syndrome. Nat Genet 1997; 16(1):64–67.

20. Fagin JA, Matsuo K, Karmakar A, Chen DL, Tang SH, Koeffler HP. High prevalence of mutations of the p53 gene in poorly differentiated human thyroid carcinomas. J Clin Invest 1993; 91(1):179–184.

21. Druker BJ. STI571 (Gleevec) as a paradigm for cancer therapy. Trends Mol Med 2002; 8(4 Suppl):S14–S18.

22. Mauro MJ, O'Dwyer M, Heinrich MC, Druker BJ. STI571: a paradigm of new agents for cancer therapeutics. J Clin Oncol 2002; 20(1):325–334.

23. Sawyers CL. Cancer treatment in the STI571 era: what will change? J Clin Oncol 2001; 19(18 Suppl):13S–16S.

24. Carlomagno F, Vitagliano D, Guida T, et al. ZD6474, an orally available inhibitor of KDR tyrosine kinase activity, efficiently blocks oncogenic RET kinases. Cancer Res 2002; 62(24):7284–7290.

25. Vitagliano D, Carlomagno F, Motti ML, et al. Regulation of p27Kip1 protein levels contributes to mitogenic effects of the RET/PTC kinase in thyroid carcinoma cells. Cancer Res 2004; 64(11):3823–3829.

26. Bauer AJ, Terrell R, Doniparthi NK, et al. Vascular endothelial growth factor monoclonal antibody inhibits growth of anaplastic thyroid cancer xenografts in nude mice. Thyroid 2002; 12(11):953–961.

27. Soh EY, Eigelberger MS, Kim KJ, et al. Neutralizing vascular endothelial growth factor activity inhibits thyroid cancer growth in vivo. Surgery 2000; 128(6):1059–1065; discussion 1065–1066.

28. O'Regan RM, Khuri FR. Farnesyl transferase inhibitors: the next targeted therapies for breast cancer? Endocr Relat Cancer 2004; 11(2):191–205.

29. Mazieres J, Pradines A, Favre G. Perspectives on farnesyl transferase inhibitors in cancer therapy. Cancer Lett 2004; 206(2):159–167.

30. Workman P. Altered states: selectively drugging the Hsp90 cancer chaperone. Trends Mol Med 2004; 10(2):47–51.

31. Ringel MD, Ladenson PW. Controversies in the follow-up and management of well-differentiated thyroid cancer. Endocr Relat Cancer 2004; 11(1):97–116.

32. Dowlati A, Robertson K, Cooney M, et al. A phase I pharmacokinetic and translational study of the novel vascular targeting agent combretastatin a-4 phosphate on a single-dose intravenous schedule in patients with advanced cancer. Cancer Res 2002; 62(12):3408–3416.

33. Cooney MM, Radivoyevitch T, Dowlati A, et al. Cardiovascular safety profile of combretastatin A4 phosphate in a single-dose phase I study in patients with advanced cancer. Clin Cancer Res 2004; 10(1 Pt 1):96–100.

34. Dohan O, Baloch Z, Banrevi Z, Livolsi V, Carrasco N. Rapid communication: predominant intracellular overexpression of the Na(+)/I(−) symporter (NIS) in a large sampling of thyroid cancer cases. J Clin Endocrinol Metab 2001; 86(6):2697–2700.

35. Jhiang SM. Regulation of sodium/iodide symporter. Rev Endocr Metab Disord 2000; 1(3):205–215.

36. Ringel MD, Anderson J, Souza SL, et al. Expression of the sodium iodide symporter and thyroglobulin genes are reduced in papillary thyroid cancer. Mod Pathol 2001; 14(4):289–296.

37. Venkataraman GM, Yatin M, Marcinek R, Ain KB. Restoration of iodide uptake in dedifferentiated thyroid carcinoma: relationship to human Na+/I-symporter gene methylation status. J Clin Endocrinol Metab 1999; 84(7):2449–2457.

38. Furuya F, Shimura H, Suzuki H, et al. Histone deacetylase inhibitors restore radioiodide uptake and retention in poorly differentiated and anaplastic thyroid cancer cells by expression of the sodium/iodide symporter thyroperoxidase and thyroglobulin. Endocrinology 2004; 145(6):2865–2875.

39. Grunwald F, Pakos E, Bender H, et al. Redifferentiation therapy with retinoic acid in follicular thyroid cancer. J Nucl Med 1998; 39(9):1555–1558.

40. Schmutzler C, Winzer R, Meissner-Weigl J, Kohrle J. Retinoic acid increases sodium/iodide symporter mRNA levels in human thyroid cancer cell lines and suppresses expression of functional symporter in non-transformed FRTL-5 rat thyroid cells. Biochem Biophys Res Commun 1997; 240(3):832–838.

41. Gruning T, Tiepolt C, Zophel K, Bredow J, Kropp J, Franke WG. Retinoic acid for redifferentiation of thyroid cancer – does it hold its promise? Eur J Endocrinol 2003; 148(4):395–402.

42. Haugen BR, Larson LL, Pugazhenthi U, et al. Retinoic acid and retinoid X receptors are differentially expressed in thyroid cancer and thyroid carcinoma cell lines and predict response to treatment with retinoids. J Clin Endocrinol Metab 2004; 89(1):272–280.

43. DeGroot LJ, Zhang R. Clinical review 131: Gene therapy for thyroid cancer: where do we stand? J Clin Endocrinol Metab 2001; 86(7):2923–2928.

44. Schmutzler C, Koehrle J. Innovative strategies for the treatment of thyroid cancer. Eur J Endocrinol 2000; 143(1):15–24.

45. Ahmad M, Shi Y. TRAIL-induced apoptosis of thyroid cancer cells: potential for therapeutic intervention. Oncogene 2000; 19(30):3363–3371.

46. Mitsiades CS, Poulaki V, Mitsiades N. The role of apoptosis-inducing receptors of the tumor necrosis factor family in thyroid cancer. J Endocrinol 2003; 178(2):205–216.

47. Park JW, Wong MG, Lobo M, Hyun WC, Duh QY, Clark OH. Modulation of tumor necrosis factor-related apoptosis-inducing ligand-induced apoptosis by chemotherapy in thyroid cancer cell lines. Thyroid 2003; 13(12):1103–1110.

48. Manion MK, Hockenbery DM. Targeting BCL-2-related proteins in cancer therapy. Cancer Biol Ther 2003; 2(4 Suppl 1):S105–S114.

49. Shimura H, Suzuki H, Miyazaki A, et al. Transcriptional activation of the thyroglobulin promoter directing suicide gene expression by thyroid transcription factor-1 in thyroid cancer cells. Cancer Res 2001; 61(9):3640–3646.

50. Tanaka K, Towata S, Nakao K, et al. Thyroid cancer immuno-therapy with retroviral and adenoviral vectors expressing granulocyte macrophage colony stimulating factor and interleukin-12 in a rat model. Clin Endocrinol (Oxf) 2003; 59(6):734–742.

51. Barzon L, Bonaguro R, Castagliuolo I, et al. Gene therapy of thyroid cancer via retrovirally-driven combined expression of human interleukin-2 and herpes simplex virus thymidine kinase. Eur J Endocrinol 2003; 148(1):73–80.

52. Barzon L, Bonaguro R, Castagliuolo I, et al. Transcriptionally targeted retroviral vector for combined suicide and immunomodulating gene therapy of thyroid cancer. J Clin Endocrinol Metab 2002; 87(11):5304–5311.

53. Asakawa H, Kobayashi T, Komoike Y, et al. Establishment of anaplastic thyroid carcinoma cell lines useful for analysis of chemosensitivity and carcinogenesis. J Clin Endocrinol Metab 1996; 81(10):3547–3552.

54. Dapas B, Perissin L, Pucillo C, Quadrifoglio F, Scaggiante B. Increase in therapeutic index of doxorubicin and vinblastine by aptameric oligonucleotide in human T lymphoblastic drug-sensitive and multidrug-resistant cells. Antisense Nucleic Acid Drug Dev 2002; 12(4):247–255.

55. Massart C, Gibassier J, Raoul M, et al. Effect of S9788 on the efficiency of doxorubicin in vivo and in vitro in medullary thyroid carcinoma xenograft. Anticancer Drugs 1996; 7(3):321–330.

56. Sekiguchi M, Shiroko Y, Arai T, et al. Biological characteristics and chemosensitivity profile of four human anaplastic thyroid carcinoma cell lines. Biomed Pharmacother 2001; 55(8):466–474.

57. Sugawara I, Masunaga A, Itoyama S, Sumizawa T, Akiyama S, Yamashita T. Expression of multidrug resistance-associated protein (MRP) in thyroid cancers. Cancer Lett 1995; 95(1–2):135–138.

58. Casterline PF, Jaques DA, Blom H, Wartofsky L. Anaplastic giant and spindle-cell carcinoma of the thyroid: a different therapeutic approach. Cancer 1980; 45(7):1689–1692.

59. Schott M, Seissler J. Dendritic cell vaccination: new hope for the treatment of metastasized endocrine malignancies. Trends Endocrinol Metab 2003; 14(4):156–162.

60. Cornetta AJ, Russell JP, Cunnane M, Keane WM, Rothstein JL. Cyclooxygenase-2 expression in human thyroid carcinoma and Hashimoto's thyroiditis. Laryngoscope 2002; 112(2):238–242.

61. Ito Y, Yoshida H, Nakano K, et al. Cyclooxygenase-2 expression in thyroid neoplasms. Histopathology 2003; 42(5):492–497.

62. Quidville V, Segond N, Pidoux E, Cohen R, Jullienne A, Lausson S. Tumor growth inhibition by indomethacin in a mouse model of human medullary thyroid cancer: implication of cyclooxygenases and 15-hydroxyprostaglandin dehydrogenase. Endocrinology 2004; 145(5):2561–2571.

63. Siironen P, Ristimaki A, Nordling S, Louhimo J, Haapiainen R, Haglund C. Expression of COX-2 is increased with age in papillary thyroid cancer. Histopathology 2004; 44(5):490–497.

34

Clinical Trials for Thyroid Carcinoma: Past, Present, and Future

Steven I. Sherman

In 1999, I was asked to speak at the 72nd annual meeting of the American Thyroid Association on the selected topic of "Multicenter Clinical Trials in Thyroid Cancer." The assigned task was to summarize the state of the field and identify both the challenges to and opportunities for advancement of improved clinical care and outcomes for our patients. Surveying the medical literature of the last quarter of the 20th century in preparation for that lecture led to certain obvious yet unsatisfying conclusions about the state of affairs in 1999:

- No data existed from randomized controlled trials testing any of the primary treatments commonly used for thyroid carcinoma (surgery, radioiodine, and thyroid hormone suppression for differentiated carcinoma; surgery for medullary carcinoma; and chemotherapy and external beam radiation with or without surgery for anaplastic carcinoma).
- The few prospective clinical trials of therapies that had been performed for advanced or metastatic disease were generally unsuccessful in demonstrating treatment benefits, but these studies often were closed long before sufficient numbers of patients were enrolled to allow adequate statistical power to reject a false-negative conclusion.
- Pharmaceutical companies, with rare exception, had not developed or supported clinical trials to address new therapies for thyroid carcinoma.

- An apparent dearth of federal and other peer-reviewed funding opportunities and a common perception of bias against clinical investigators in academic career progression [1] often discouraged young physicians from pursuing a career path emphasizing clinical trials for thyroid carcinoma.

How did this quandary evolve? Five years hence, how has the landscape changed? And what scientific and organizational strategies should be pursued now and in the future to achieve the ultimate goal of eliminating morbidity and mortality from thyroid carcinoma?

From Whence We Came: 1975–1999

The formal clinical trial to test a therapy for cancer emerged in the mid 1950s when C. Gordon Zubrod, as Director of the National Cancer Institute, championed the need for prospective rather than retrospective study design [2]. He introduced application of the scientific method and statistical hypothesis testing to clinical oncology studies. Joining Zubrod in these early efforts were young oncologists such as Emil Frei III and Emil Freireich, and over a 15-year period they used these methods to identify curative regimens for childhood acute leukemias [3]. Oncologists were emboldened by these early gains, and attempted to re-create this experience with many of the common solid tumors. With recognition of the need for large numbers of patients to participate in pivotal trials, regional cooperative oncology groups were established throughout the United States, merging investigators from multiple institutions with expertise in clinical trials design, biostatistics, drug development, and patient care. During the next two decades, these groups developed and implemented multiple studies that demonstrated benefit from many of the now-standard chemotherapeutic agents for malignancies such as lymphoma, testicular carcinoma, and breast carcinoma.

From this background, cancer researchers hypothesized that some of these new cytotoxic drugs being tested in various malignancies might also benefit patients with advanced thyroid carcinomas. Beginning in the 1970s, trials were performed of single agents as well as multidrug combinations, with suggestions appearing that doxorubicin as well as bleomycin had significant activity against differentiated and medullary carcinomas. However, by reviewing the outcomes reported of 26 single agents and 17 combination therapies, it was soon realized that poor accrual was leading to disappointingly inadequate evaluations of treatment efficacy, and physicians were urged to consider increasing participation in such studies [4]. Attempts to reproduce the success of the cooperative groups with other malignancies by both the Eastern Cooperative Oncology Group (ECOG) and Southeastern Cancer Study Group (SCSG) led to multicenter trials to evaluate the combination of doxorubicin and cisplatin. Whereas the phase II SCSG study concluded that the combination had little efficacy, the larger randomized phase III ECOG study suggested that complete response could be seen in 12% after treatment with both drugs; nevertheless, the SCSG study closed having recruited only 22 of the needed 30 patients, and the ECOG protocol closed after entering only 92 of the 182 needed [5,6]. Two other NCI-sponsored phase III trials were initiated, one through Roswell Park Cancer Institute testing the combination of vincristine, doxorubicin, and methotrexate in comparison with doxorubicin alone, and one intramural study of low dose doxorubicin to augment the effectiveness of radioiodine treatment, but neither achieved full enrollment and results were not published. Unfortunately, this experience represented more the norm than the exception: of 15 clinical trials focused specifically on thyroid carcinomas that were listed through the National Cancer Institute as having been initiated between 1975 and 1999, only five led to published results [7]. This poor experience, both in terms of patient's response rates and completion of clinical trials, resulted in the widely accepted conclusion that "conventional chemotherapy has prove[n] to be ineffective for most patients with progressive metastases from thyroid cancer" [8].

Multiple factors can probably be identified that led to these unsatisfying outcomes. From a biological standpoint, most of the tested therapies were compounds that attacked dividing cells; the more rapid the cell cycle, the more cytotoxic the drug. Thyroid tumors, on the other hand, are typically slowly growing relative to many other solid tumors, and therefore thyroid cancers would not be expected to respond very significantly. However, a relatively narrow therapeutic index for anthracyclines (e.g. doxorubicin), alkylating agents (e.g. cisplatin), and antitumor antibiotics (e.g. bleomycin) led to marked side effects at doses necessary for even marginal effectiveness. Inadequate recruitment may therefore have been secondary to the emerging reality that these chemotherapies were relatively ineffective. From a trial design standpoint, many of the studies combined all of the major histologies of thyroid carcinoma in one group for analysis purposes, thus introducing considerable biological heterogeneity that may have obscured potential activity against one particular subtype of the disease. Finally, the limited participation in these trials by endocrinologists as investigators may have restricted awareness among potential referring physicians and patients, thus leading to the mistaken impression that such trials were in fact not available.

Where We Are Now: 2000–2004

By 1999, a phase I trial of a novel therapy for chronic myelogenous leukemia had been started. Imatinib mesylate (Gleevec, Novartis Oncology) was developed specifically as an inhibitor of the protein tyrosine kinase pathophysiologically linked with the leukemia, the Bcr-Abl oncoprotein [9]. The demonstration that targeting a specific abnormally expressed or activated molecular pathway could lead to successful therapy ushered in a new era in medical oncology, further enhanced by approval of other targeted tyrosine kinase inhibitors such as gefitinib (Iressa, AstraZeneca) against the epidermal growth factor receptor in non-small cell lung cancer, and bevacizumab (Avastin, Genentech) against the vascular epithelial growth factor receptor in colorectal carcinoma. Other "targeted therapies" similarly developed include drugs that promote apoptosis or inhibit cell cycle progression in malignant cells that have otherwise escaped normal regulation of such processes, and therapies to inhibit or reverse the epigenetic modifications associated with loss of differentiated phenotype in cancers.

Investigators have recognized that these same pathways of disordered intracellular signaling, promoter dysfunction, cell cycle dysregulation, and altered control of apoptosis are associated with development, maintenance, and progression of the malignant phenotype in thyroid carcinomas (for reviews, see references 8, 10–12). During the past 5 years, numerous clinical trials have been initiated by endocrinologists working in collaboration with oncologists, utilizing novel therapies targeted against these pathways to try to halt progression or induce regression of advanced thyroid carcinomas. Many of these trials have been based upon preclinical studies that have demonstrated drug activity against animal models of human thyroid cancers, although in many other malignancies such animal models have been imperfect in predicting human clinical response. Other agents have entered clinical trial based upon mechanisms of action that can be reasonably suspected to work in thyroid cancer, even in the absence of specifically demonstrated activity in preclinical models. Examples of such targeted phase II drug studies include:

- ZD6474 (AstraZeneca), an inhibitor of multiple tyrosine kinases including the ret oncoprotein, VEGF receptor, and EGF receptor, being tested in hereditary medullary carcinoma;
- decitabine, a DNA methyltransferase inhibitor, being tested in radioiodine-unresponsive differentiated carcinoma;

- imatinib being tested in anaplastic carcinoma;
- multiple single drugs, including gefitinib, bortezomib (Velcade, Millennium Pharmaceuticals), celecoxib (Celebrex, Pfizer), and sorafenib (Bayer), being tested in advanced differentiated carcinoma.

As of this writing, more than 15 phase II trials have been initiated during this 5-year period, more than tripling the rate of new study initiation of the previous time period. In contrast, however, none of these trials have been organized within the NCI-supported cooperative oncology groups. Instead, studies are being performed either as single institution protocols or as ad hoc groups. Bypassing the organized groups may provide greater flexibility to involve those institutions and investigators most likely to contribute to successful recruitment and completion of a study. However, the established expertise within the cooperative groups in trial oversight, protocol auditing, and centralized data accumulation is also lacking within such ad hoc arrangements. Similar to the earlier era, some of these current studies combine biologically dissimilar histologies without stratification in recruitment or analysis, introducing potentially significant heterogeneity that can confound results. And although most of the trials now involve or are led by endocrinologists, awareness of these studies remains limited in the absence of a complete centralized listing of open trials in thyroid cancer readily accessible to patients and the physicians who are most likely to be caring for them; even the NCI website, when searched for active clinical trials for thyroid cancer, fails to mention several of the known ongoing trials.

Where Shall We Go in the Future?

The age-adjusted incidence of thyroid cancer in the United States is increasing by 3% per year, and the disease is the most rapidly increasing malignancy diagnosed in women during the past 10 years. At our institution, more than 20% of the patients seen last year on referral for management of thyroid carcinoma had distant metastases. Yet, there remains no treatment for progressive disseminated metastatic disease proven to be more effective than the cytotoxic chemotherapies introduced decades ago, despite the promise of the ongoing clinical trials described previously.

Given this current reality, a concerted effort is necessary to enhance the approach to clinical investigation for advanced thyroid carcinomas, an effort that will require participation among clinicians, clinical researchers, translational scientists, research policy-makers, pharmaceutical companies, and thyroid cancer patient advocacy groups. Improved patient outcomes may require a combination of advances both in the knowledge of thyroid cancer biology as well as the administrative systems used to organize clinical trials. Learning from the experiences of clinical investigation in thyroid cancer for the past three decades, some of the necessary advances may include the following:

- An improved understanding of the molecular derangements contributing to thyroid cancer progression is necessary, including identification of the complex interactions among various signaling and regulatory pathways. Therapies could then be more rationally combined to provide synergistic benefit and reduce the risk of drug resistance mediated by bypassing a drug-induced blockade or inhibition. Improved pre-clinical identification of disease mechanisms and effective treatments may require development of superior animal models of disease, emphasizing the interactions between tumor cells and their microenvironment [13].

- The significance of disease mechanisms needs to be individualized, allowing the application of therapies targeted against a particular molecular pathway. Further, the illuminating example of selective sensitivity to gefitinib in lung tumors bearing activating mutations in the EGF receptor demonstrates the value of applying treatments individualized to the particular derangements active in a given patient's malignancy [14].

- Given the relatively poor predictive value of current disease description and staging systems in thyroid carcinoma [15], improved molecular profiling should allow creation of appropriately homogeneous

cohorts for prognostication as well as recruitment for clinical trials. Resources should be devoted to expanded collection of well-characterized tissue specimens to be used for genomic analysis and biomarker discovery.

- Building upon preclinical animal models, clinical trials should include molecular-genetic imaging modalities that can permit identification of appropriate patients for particular therapies, early assessment of biological response to treatment, and recognition of better correlates that predict long-term patient outcomes [16].

- Clinical trials must be optimized to enhance patient recruitment and to increase the likelihood that each study will maximally contribute to improved patient care. Although this principle should apply to all clinical research, it is particularly relevant for uncommon or rare diseases such as advanced thyroid cancer. Initiatives that may contribute to this goal include:

  - Creation of clinical trials consortia dedicated to thyroid cancer, involving endocrinologists, surgeons, oncologists, radiation specialists, imaging experts, pathologists, biostatisticians, and laboratory scientists. Particularly for trials of rarer diseases such as anaplastic carcinoma or for large phase III studies, international cooperation will be imperative.

  - Joint efforts by patient advocacy organizations such as ThyCa and professional societies such as the American Thyroid Association can contribute to patient referral for trial participation and to financial support for novel research undertakings. By broadening the sources of patient referral, participation by traditionally underrepresented minorities can be emphasized, ensuring adequate subgroup involvement so that results can be properly extrapolated to all relevant populations.

  - Phase I studies should be developed that specifically target the tumor types most likely to respond, thus creating opportunities for thyroid cancer patients to participate in the earliest human trials of new drugs. By including thyroid cancer patients in such studies, it will be more likely that phase II studies will subsequently be developed for thyroid cancer, based upon the occasional clinical response seen in the phase I trial; the current industry-sponsored phase II studies of the angiogenesis inhibitors AG-013736 and combretastatin A4 phosphate were developed on the basis of responders in the corresponding phase I studies.

– Clinical trials must be designed to maximize the likelihood of identifying effective treatments and minimize the numbers of patients exposed to ineffective ones. Smarter, more efficient phase II trial designs can be employed, utilizing randomized treatment assignment among multiple possible interventions and application of Bayesian analytical methods to continuous monitoring of multiple outcomes [17]. For a disease like papillary thyroid carcinoma, in which patients may be asymptomatic from widely metastatic disease, studies should emphasize assessment of quality of life as a key outcome measure along with tumor reduction.

– Advanced bioinformatics systems will be required, capable of standardizing and automating clinical trial data acquisition as well as integrating clinical parameters with complex data from genomic and proteomic analyses.

• New post-fellowship training programs should be developed to develop oncological endocrinologists educated in the application of oncological therapies to endocrine cancers. Clinical instruction should emphasize multidisciplinary care, and incorporation of high quality research training can lead to successful application for NIH funding to support this novel educational effort.

• Academic endocrine and oncology programs must provide greater opportunities for developing and promoting faculty members expert in clinical trials research, including more financial support for research nursing and data management, sufficient protected time particularly for junior faculty, and identification of career pathways that contribute to faculty security and innovation.

The outcomes for most patients with thyroid cancers have unfortunately not significantly improved in decades (M. Maldonado and S. I. Sherman, Clinicopathologic staging for medullary thyroid carcinoma, presented at the 72nd annual meeting of the American Thyroid Association, 1999) [18]. Nonetheless, the dramatic transformation of clinical research for these diseases during the past several years, combined with inventive approaches to applying new biological discoveries in future clinical trials, bring tremendous promise for improving care and potentially eliminating morbidity and mortality from thyroid cancer.

References

1. Mendelsohn J. Merging medicine with science: The birth of a targeted therapy in cancer. Ann Med 2004; 33(Suppl)(5):S3.
2. Frei E. In memoriam: C. Gordon Zubrod. J Clin Oncol 1999; 17(5):1331–1333.
3. Freedman MH. The cure of childhood leukemia: into the age of miracles. N Engl J Med 1996; 334(4):275.
4. Poster DS, Bruno S, Penta J, Pina K, Catane R. Current status of chemotherapy in the treatment of advanced carcinoma of the thyroid gland. Cancer Clin Trials 1981; 4(3):301–307.
5. Shimaoka K, Schoenfeld DA, DeWys WD, Creech RH, DeConti R. A randomized trial of doxorubicin versus doxorubicin plus cisplatin in patients with advanced thyroid carcinoma. Cancer 1985; 56(9):2155–2160.
6. Williams SD, Birch R, Einhorn LH. Phase II evaluation of doxorubicin plus cisplatin in advanced thyroid cancer: A Southeastern Cancer Study Group Trial. Cancer Treat Rep 1986; 70(3):405–407.
7. National Cancer Institute. Clinical trials. http://www.nci.nih.gov/clinicaltrials; last accessed 12/9/2004.
8. Braga-Basaria M, Ringel MD. Beyond radioiodine: a review of potential new therapeutic approaches for thyroid cancer. J Clin Endocrinol Metab 2003; 88(5):1947–1960.
9. Druker BJ, Lydon NB. Lessons learned from the development of an abl tyrosine kinase inhibitor for chronic myelogenous leukemia. J Clin Invest 2000; 105(1):3–7.
10. Sarlis NJ, Gourgiotis L. Molecular elements of apoptosis-regulating pathways in follicular thyroid cells: Mining for novel therapeutic targets in the treatment of thyroid carcinoma. Curr Drug Targets Immune Endocr Metab Disord 2004; 4(3):187–198.
11. Wells SA, Nevins JR. Evolving strategies for targeted cancer therapy – past, present, and future. J Natl Cancer Inst 2004; 96(13):980–981.
12. Burman KD. A new paradigm in the treatment of carcinoma: Specific molecular targeting. Endocrinology 2004; 145(3):1027–1030.

13. Baker CH, Kedar D, McCarty MF, et al. Blockade of epidermal growth factor receptor signaling on tumor cells and tumor-associated endothelial cells for therapy of human carcinomas. Am J Pathol 2002; 161(3):929–938.

14. Arteaga CL. Selecting the right patient for tumor therapy. Nat Med 2004; 10(6):577–578.

15. Sherman SI, Brierley JD, Sperling M. Prospective multicenter study of thyroid carcinoma treatment: initial analysis of staging and outcome. Cancer 1998; 83(5): 1012–1021.

16. Gelovani Tjuvajev J, Blasberg RG. In vivo imaging of molecular-genetic targets for cancer therapy. Cancer Cell 2003; 3(4):327–332.

17. Estey EH, Thall PF. New designs for phase 2 clinical trials. Blood 2003; 102(2):442–448.

18. Hay ID, Thompson GB, Grant CS, et al. Papillary thyroid carcinoma management at the Mayo Clinic during six decades (1940–1999): temporal trends in initial therapy and long term outcome in 2444 consecutively treated patients. World J Surg 2002; 26(8):879–885.

Index